SickKids Handbook of Pediatric Thrombosis and Hemostasis

3rd, revised and extended edition

SickKids Handbook of Pediatric Thrombosis and Hemostasis

3rd, revised and extended edition

Editors

Victor S. Blanchette Toronto, ON
Leonardo R. Brandão Toronto, ON
Manuel D. Carcao Toronto, ON
Riten Kumar Boston, MA
Margaret L. Rand Toronto, ON
Shoshana Revel-Vilk Jerusalem

53 figures, 35 in color, and 105 tables, 2024

Karger

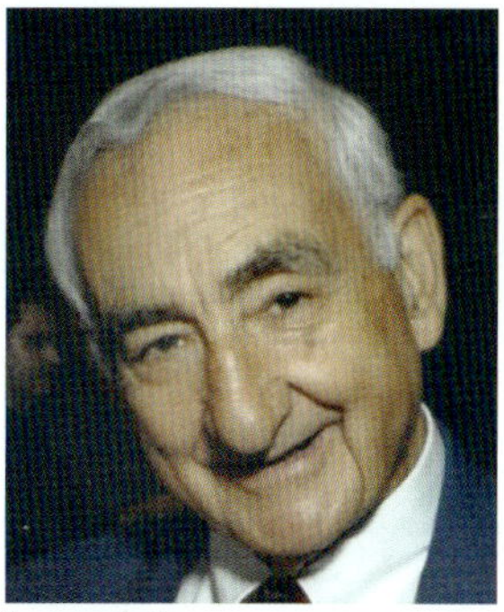

Source: private

Dr. Alvin Zipursky

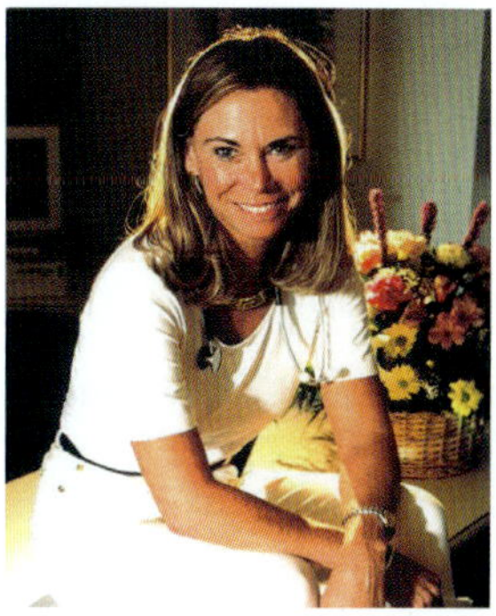

Source: private

Dr. Maureen Andrew

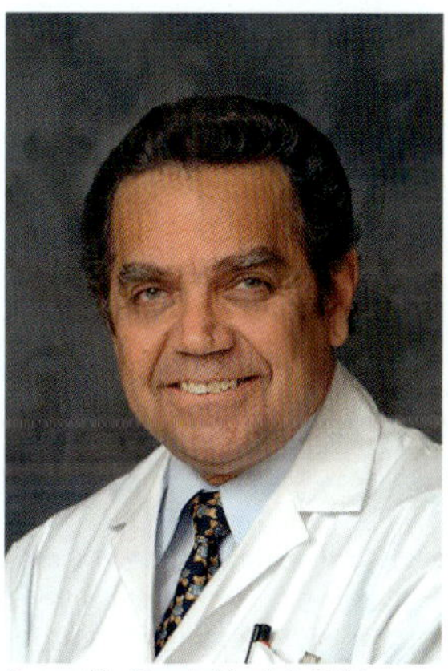

Source: The Hospital for Sick Children

Dr. Victor Blanchette

This Handbook is dedicated to the memory of Alvin Zipursky, Maureen Andrew, and Victor Blanchette, three pioneers and giants in the fields of pediatric hematology, thrombosis and hemostasis. All spent major parts of their careers at the Hospital for Sick Children (SickKids), where they nurtured the fields that we today call pediatric thrombosis and pediatric hemostasis.

Alvin had a profound influence on the development of pediatric hematology at Canadian institutions including McMaster Hospital in Hamilton, and SickKids in Toronto. In these world-renowned institutions, he mentored and recruited many hematologists/oncologists including Maureen and Victor, both of whom followed in Alvin's footsteps and further developed the fields of pediatric thrombosis (Maureen) and hemostasis (Victor). Maureen and Victor began the Pediatric Thrombosis and Hemostasis training program at SickKids, which ultimately led to the recruitment of so many trainees who have gone on to contribute in major ways to the fields of pediatric thrombosis and hemostasis all over the world; many of them are now authors of this Handbook.

The editors of this Handbook wish to acknowledge these three transforming figures and the influence that they have had on us and on all the other authors of the 3rd edition of this Handbook. For many of the Handbook authors, Alvin, Maureen, and Victor were mentors, colleagues, and friends. For those who did not know them personally, they, and all their accomplishments, remain a source of inspiration.

Victor S. Blanchette, MA, MB, BChir(Cantab), FRCP(C), FRCP (deceased)
Professor of Pediatrics
University of Toronto
McCaig Magee Family Honorary Medical Director, SickKids-Caribbean Initiative
Senior Associate Scientist Emeritus, Child Health Evaluative Sciences Program
Division of Hematology/Oncology
The Hospital for Sick Children
555 University Avenue
Toronto, ON M5G 1X8 (Canada)

Leonardo R. Brandão, MD, MSc
Professor of Pediatrics and Dalla Lana School of Public Health
University of Toronto
Thrombosis Program Director
Division of Hematology/Oncology
The Hospital for Sick Children
555 University Avenue
Toronto, ON M5G 1X8 (Canada)

Manuel D. Carcao, MD, MSc, FRCPC
Professor of Pediatrics
University of Toronto
Pediatric Hematologist/Oncologist
Director, Hemophilia Clinic
Division of Hematology/Oncology
Hak-Ming and Deborah Chiu Chair in Pediatric Translational Research
The Hospital for Sick Children
555 University Avenue
Toronto, ON M5G 1X8 (Canada)

Riten Kumar, MD, MSc
Associate Professor of Pediatrics
Harvard Medical School
Director of Thrombosis and Anticoagulation Program
Dana Farber/Boston Children's Cancer and Blood Disorders Center
300 Longwood Avenue
Boston, MA 02115 (USA)

Margaret L. Rand, PhD
Professor of Laboratory Medicine and Pathobiology, Biochemistry, and Pediatrics,
University of Toronto
Senior Associate Scientist, Translational Medicine Program
Division of Hematology/Oncology
The Hospital for Sick Children
555 University Avenue
Toronto, ON M5G 1X8 (Canada)

Shoshana Revel-Vilk, MD, PhD
Professor of Pediatrics, School of Medicine,
Hebrew University
Pediatric Hematology/Oncology Unit and Gaucher Unit
Shaare Zedek Medical Center
Shmuel Beyth St 12
Jerusalem 9103102 (Israel)

Bibliographic Indices. This publication is listed in bibliographic services, including Current Contents® and Index Medicus.

www.karger.com
Printed in Germany on acid-free and non-aging paper (ISO 9706)
ISBN 978–3–318–07272–3
e-ISBN 978–3–318–07273–0

Cover image: Colorized scanning electron micrograph of a whole blood clot showing platelets (in purple), fibrin fibres, and trapped red blood cells. Reused with permission from © Image Professionals/Anne Weston, EM STP, the Francis Crick Institute.

Contents

Appendix III

Appendix IV

Published online: December 5, 2024

Blanchette VS, Brandão LR, Carcao MD, Kumar R, Rand ML, Revel-Vilk S (eds): SickKids Handbook of Pediatric Thrombosis and Hemostasis, ed 3, rev. and ext. Basel, Karger, 2024, pp XI–XVIII (DOI: 10.1159/000538116)

Contributors

Denise M. Adams, MD
Professor of Pediatrics, University of Pennsylvania
Division of Oncology, Children's Hospital of Philadelphia
Director, Comprehensive Vascular Anomaly Program
Co-Director, CVAP Frontier Program
Alan Cohen Chair in Pediatrics
The HUB for Clinical Collaboration
Oncology, 3rd Floor, #3514
3500 Civic Center Blvd
Philadelphia, PA 19104 (USA)
adamsdm@chop.edu

Manuela Albisetti, MD
Professor of Pediatrics
University of Zurich
Director, Thrombosis and Hemophilia Care Center
Division of Hematology
University Children's Hospital
Steinwiesstrasse 75
CH–8032 Zurich (Switzerland)
manuela.albisetti@kispi.uzh.ch

Ahmad Al-Huniti, MD
Assistant Professor of Pediatrics
Mayo Clinic College of Medicine
Pediatric Hematology Oncology
Division of Pediatrics
Mayo Clinic
200 First Street SW
Rochester, MN 55905 (USA)
al-huniti.ahmad@mayo.edu

Eman Taryam AlShamsi, MD
Adjunct Clinical Professor of Paediatrics
Mohammed Bin Rashid University
Paediatric Haematologist Oncologist
Acting Head, Division of Haematology/Oncology
Al Jalila Children's Specialty Hospital
Oud Metha Road, Al Jaddaf
Dubai (United Arab Emirates)
ajch_ealshamsi@dubaihealth.ae

Azzah Alzahrani, MD
Consultant, Pediatric Hematology/Oncology & BMT
Prince Sultan Military Medical City
MPR7+4CQ, Makkah Al Mukarramah Road
Riyadh 12233 (Saudi Arabia)
azzahalzahrani@yahoo.com

Joao Guilherme Amaral, MD
Professor of Radiology
Department of Medical Imaging
University of Toronto
Pediatric Interventional Radiologist
Department of Diagnostic and Interventional Radiology
Division of Interventional Radiology/Image Guided Therapy
The Hospital for Sick Children
555 University Avenue
Toronto, ON M5G 1X8 (Canada)
joao.amaral@sickkids.ca

Ali Amid, MD, FRCPC
Assistant Professor of Pediatrics
University of British Columbia
Pediatric Hematologist, Division of Hematology/Oncology
BC Children's Hospital
4480 Oak Street
Vancouver, BC V6H 3V4 (Canada)
ali.amid@cw.bc.ca

Andrea Andrade, MD, CSCN-EEG
Associate Professor of Paediatrics and Clinical Neurological Sciences
Schulich School of Medicine and Dentistry, Western University
Director, Paediatric Epilepsy Program
Division Head, Paediatric Neurology
London Health Sciences Centre
800 Commissioners Road East
London, ON N6A 5W9 (Canada)
andrea.andrade@lhsc.on.ca

Gail Annich, MD, MS, FELSO
Professor of Pediatrics
University of Toronto
Director of CCRT & Resuscitation
Pediatric Intensivist, Critical Care Medicine
The Hospital for Sick Children
555 University Avenue
Toronto, ON M5G 1X8 (Canada)
gail.annich@sickkids.ca

Laura Avila, MD, PhD
Assistant Professor of Pediatrics and Dalla Lana School of Public Health
University of Toronto
Hematologist, Division of Hematology/Oncology
Clinician Scientist, Child Health Evaluative Sciences
The Hospital for Sick Children
555 University Avenue
Toronto, ON M5G 1X8 (Canada)
laura.avila@sickkids.ca

Riyana Babul-Hirji, MSc, CGC
Associate Professor of Molecular Genetics
University of Toronto
Genetic Counsellor, Department of Genetic Counselling
The Hospital for Sick Children
555 University Avenue
Toronto, ON M5G 1X8 (Canada)
riyana@sickkids.ca

Laura Banov, MD
Pediatric Hematologist
Hemostasis and Thrombosis Unit
Hematology and Oncology Department
Gaslini Children's Hospital
Gaslini Street 5
IT–16148 Genova (Italy)
laurabanov@gaslini.org

Chris Barnes, MBBS(Hons), FRACP, FRCPA
Pediatric Haematologist
Department of Haematology
Royal Children's Hospital
The University of Melbourne
Flemington Road
Parkville, VIC 3052 (Australia)
chris.barnes@rch.org.au

Tina Biss, BMedSci, BM BS (Hons), MD
Consultant Haematologist
Department of Haematology
The Newcastle upon Tyne Hospitals NHS Foundation Trust
Queen Victoria Road
Newcastle upon Tyne NE1 4LP (UK)
t.biss@nhs.net

Victor S. Blanchette, MA, MB, BChir(Cantab), FRCP(C), FRCP
Professor of Pediatrics
University of Toronto
McCaig Magee Family Honorary Medical Director
SickKids-Caribbean Initiative
Senior Associate Scientist Emeritus, Child Health Evaluative Sciences Program
Division of Hematology/Oncology
The Hospital for Sick Children
555 University Avenue
Toronto, ON M5G 1X8 (Canada)
victor.blanchette@sickkids.ca

Valerie Bloomfield, MD, FRCSC
Assistant Professor
McMaster University
Department of Obstetrics & Gynecology
St Joseph's Healthcare
301 James Street South, 2nd Floor Fontbonne Building
Hamilton, ON L8P 3B7 (Canada)
valerie.bloomfield@sickkids.ca

Alessandra Bosch, MD, MSc
Pediatric Hematologist/Oncologist
Division of Hematology
University Children's Hospital
Steinwiesstrasse 75
CH–8032 Zurich (Switzerland)
alessandra.bosch@kispi.uzh.ch

Vanessa Bouskill, MN, NP
Adjunct Faculty, Lawrence Bloomberg Faculty of Nursing
University of Toronto
Nurse Practitioner
Division of Hematology/Oncology
The Hospital for Sick Children
555 University Avenue
Toronto, ON M5G 1X8 (Canada)
vanessa.bouskill@sickkids.ca

Leonardo R. Brandão, MD, MSc
Professor of Pediatrics and Dalla Lana School of Public Health
University of Toronto
Thrombosis Program Director
Division of Hematology/Oncology
The Hospital for Sick Children
555 University Avenue
Toronto, ON M5G 1X8 (Canada)
leonardo.brandao@sickkids.ca

Vicky R. Breakey, MD, MEd, FRCPC
Associate Professor of Pediatrics
McMaster University
Pediatric Hematologist/Oncologist
Division of Pediatric Hematology/Oncology
McMaster Children's Hospital
HSC 3N27A – 1280 Main Street West
Hamilton, ON L8S 4K1 (Canada)
breakev@mcmaster.ca

Manuel D. Carcao, MD, MSc, FRCPC
Professor of Pediatrics
University of Toronto
Pediatric Hematologist/Oncologist
Director, Hemophilia Clinic
Division of Hematology/Oncology
Hak-Ming and Deborah Chiu Chair in Pediatric Translational Research
The Hospital for Sick Children
555 University Avenue
Toronto, ON M5G 1X8 (Canada)
manuel.carcao@sickkids.ca

Anthony K.C. Chan, MBBS, FRCPC, FCAHS, FRCPI, FRCPCH, FRCPath
Professor of Pediatrics
McMaster University
Chair, Pediatric Thrombosis and Hemostasis
Division of Pediatric Hematology/Oncology
McMaster Children's Hospital
HSC 3N27A – 1280 Main Street West
Hamilton, ON L8S 4K1 (Canada)
akchan@mcmaster.ca

Julie Curtin, MBBS (Hons I), PhD, FRACP, FRCPA
Senior Staff Specialist
Department of Haematology
The Children's Hospital at Westmead
Locked Bag 4001
Westmead, NSW 2145 (Australia)
julie.curtin@health.nsw.gov.au

Kevon Dindial, MBBS, DM
Paediatrics, Subspeciality Affiliate (Paediatric Haematology/Oncology)
Consultant Paediatric Haematologist/Oncologist
Department of Paediatrics
Eric Williams Medical Sciences Complex, JHWG+PC9
San Juan (Trinidad and Tobago)
kevon.dindial@gmail.com

Nomazulu Dlamini, MBBS, MSc, PhD
Associate Professor of Pediatrics
University of Toronto
Director, Children's Stroke Program
Division of Neurology
Senior Associate Scientist, Neuroscience and Mental Health Program
The Hospital for Sick Children
555 University Avenue, RM 6510
Toronto, ON M5G 1X8 (Canada)
nomazulu.dlamini@sickkids.ca

Samantha Gouw, MD, PhD
Pediatric Hematologist
Department of Pediatric Hematology
Emma Children's Hospital
Amsterdam University Medical Center
University of Amsterdam
Meibergdreef 9
NL–1105 AZ Amsterdam (The Netherlands)
s.c.gouw@amsterdamumc.nl

Anne-Marie Guerguerian, MD, PhD
Associate Professor of Pediatrics
University of Toronto
Staff Physician, Paediatric Intensive Care Unit
Medical Director ECLS Program
Department of Critical Care Medicine
Senior Scientist, Neuroscience and Mental Health Program
Research Institute
Peter Gilgan Centre for Research and Learning
686 Bay Street, 8th Floor South
Toronto, ON M5G 0A4 (Canada)
anne-marie.guerguerian@sickkids.ca

Rebecca Ichord, MD
Professor of Neurology
University of Pennsylvania School of Medicine
Department of Neurology, CTRB 10th Floor
Children's Hospital of Philadelphia
3501 Civic Ctr Blvd
Philadelphia, PA 19104 (USA)
ichord@emailchop.edu

Sara J. Israels, OM, MD, FRCPC
Professor of Pediatrics and Child Health
University of Manitoba
Section of Pediatric Hematology/Oncology
CancerCare Manitoba
Senior Scientist, CancerCare Manitoba Research Institute
675 McDermot Avenue
Winnipeg, MB R3E 0V9 (Canada)
sara.israels@umanitoba.ca

Melanie E. Jackson, BSc, MBBS, FRACP
Paediatric Haematologist
Kids Cancer Centre
Sydney Children's Hospital
High Street
Randwick, NSW 2066 (Australia)
melanie.jackson@health.nsw.gov.au

Paula D. James, MD, FRCPC
Professor and Deputy Head, Department of Medicine
Division of Hematology
Queen's University
94 Stuart Street
Kingston, ON K7L 3N6 (Canada)
jamesp@queensu.ca

Aamir Jeewa, MB, BCh, FAAP, FRCPC
Associate Professor of Pediatrics
University of Toronto
Section Head, Cardiomyopathy & Heart Function Program
Division of Pediatric Cardiology
The Hospital for Sick Children
175 Elizabeth Street
Toronto, ON M5G 2G3 (Canada)
aamir.jeewa@sickkids.ca

Walter H.A. Kahr, MD, PhD, FRCPC
Professor of Pediatrics and Biochemistry
University of Toronto
Hematologist, Division of Hematology/Oncology
Senior Scientist, Cell Biology Program
The Hospital for Sick Children
Peter Gilgan Centre for Research and Learning, 19.9714 686 Bay Street
Toronto, ON M5G 0A4 (Canada)
walter.kahr@sickkids.ca

Muhammad Faisal Khanani, MD, FRCPI, FRCPCH(UK)
Chief of Pediatrics, Hematology/Oncology
Tawam Hospital
Tawam Street
Al Ain (United Arab Emirates)
smilesaif@hotmail.com

Alicia Koo, PharmD, BScPhm, HonBSC
Clinical Pharmacy Specialist
Department of Pharmacy
The Hospital for Sick Children
555 University Avenue
Toronto, ON M5G 1X8 (Canada)
alicia.koo@sickkids.ca

Thomas Kühne, MD
Professor of Pediatric Oncology/Hematology
University Children's Hospital Basel
Division of Oncology/Hematology
Spitalstrasse 33
CH–4031 Basel (Switzerland)
thomas.kuehne@ukbb.ch

Riten Kumar, MD, MSc
Associate Professor of Pediatrics
Harvard Medical School
Director of Thrombosis and Anticoagulation Program
Dana Farber/Boston Children's Cancer and Blood Disorders Center
300 Longwood Avenue
Boston, MA 02115 (USA)
riten.kumar@childrens.harvard.edu

Veerle Labarque, MD, PhD
Part-time Assistant Professor
KU Leuven
Clinical Head, Department of Pediatrics
Pediatric Hemato-Oncology
University Hospitals Leuven
Herestraat 49
BE–3000 Leuven (Belgium)
veerle.labarque@uzleuven.be

Joel Livingston, MSc, MD, FRCPC
Assistant Professor of Pediatrics
University of Alberta
Pediatric Hematologist
Medical Lead, KidClot Program
Stollery Children's Hospital
3-528 ECHA 11405 87 Avenue
Edmonton, AB T6G 1C9 (Canada)
joel.livingston@ahs.ca

Lara Lobianco e Souza, MD
Advanced Clinical Fellow
Pediatric Hematology and Thrombosis Program
Hematology/Oncology Department
University of Toronto
Division of Hematology/Oncology
The Hospital for Sick Children
555 University Avenue
Toronto, ON M5G 1X8 (Canada)
lara.lobiancoesouza@sickkids.ca

Caroline Malcolmson, MD, MSc, FRCPC, FAAP
Assistant Professor of Pediatrics
University of Toronto
Pediatric Hematologist/Oncologist
Division of Hematology/Oncology
The Hospital for Sick Children
555 University Avenue
Toronto, ON M5G 1X8 (Canada)
caroline.malcolmson@sickkids.ca

Christoph Male, MD, MSc
Associate Professor of Paediatrics
Head, Pediatric Thrombosis & Haemostasis Unit
Department of Paediatrics, Medical University of Vienna
Waehringer Strasse 18-20
AT–1090 Vienna (Austria)
christoph.male@meduniwien.ac.at

Noa Mandel-Shorer, MD
Head, Pediatric Hematology Service
Department of Pediatric Hematology-Oncology
Ruth Rappaport Children's Hospital
Rambam Medical Center
Efron Street 19-27
Haifa (Israel)
n_mandel@rmc.gov.il

Natalie Mathews, MDCM, FRCPC
Assistant Clinical Professor
Department of Pediatrics
Université de Montréal
Pediatric Hematologist/Oncologist
Director of Hemophilia Centre
Division of Hematology/Oncology
Centre Hospitalier Universitaire Sainte-Justine
3175 Chem. de la Côte-Sainte-Catherine
Montréal, QC H3T 1C5 (Canada)
natalie.mathews.med@ssss.gouv.qc.ca

Brian W. McCrindle, MD, MPH
Professor of Pediatrics
University of Toronto
Section Head, Preventive Cardiology
Staff Cardiologist and Senior Scientist
Labatt Family Heart Centre
The Hospital for Sick Children
555 University Avenue
Toronto, ON M5G 1X8 (Canada)
brian.mccrindle@sickkids.ca

Roberto Mendoza-Londono, MD, MS, FRCPS, FCCMG
Associate Professor of Pediatrics and Molecular Genetics
University of Toronto
Division Head, Clinical and Metabolic Genetics
Women's Auxiliary Chair of Clinical and Metabolic Genetics
Co-Director, Translational Genomics Node
Precision Child Health
The Hospital for Sick Children
555 University Avenue
Toronto, ON M5G 1X8 (Canada)
roberto.mendoza@sickkids.ca

Paul Monagle, MBBS, MD, MSc, FRACP, FRCPA, FCCP
Professor of Paediatrics
The University of Melbourne
Paediatric Haematologist
Department of Haematology, Royal Children's Hospital
Honorary Haematologist
Kids Cancer Centre, Sydney Children's Hospital
Group Leader, Haematology Research
Murdoch Children's Research Institute
50 Flemington Road
Melbourne, VIC 3010 (Australia)
paul.monagle@rch.org.au

Rungrote Natesirinilkul, MD
Associate Professor of Pediatrics
Division of Hematology and Oncology, Faculty of Medicine
Chiang Mai University
110 Intawaroros Road
Chiang Mai 50200 (Thailand)
rungrote.n@cmu.ac.th

Constance O'Connor, MN, NP
Nurse Practitioner, Ehlers-Danlos Syndrome and
Connective Tissue Disorders Program
Department of Pediatrics
The Hospital for Sick Children
555 University Avenue
Toronto, ON M5G 1X8 (Canada)
constance.oconnor@sickkids.ca

Marie-Claude Pelland-Marcotte, MD, PhD, FRCPC
Associate Professor of Pediatrics
Université Laval
Pediatric Hematologist/Oncologist
Co-Director, Hemophilia Treatment Center
Division of Hematology/Oncology
Centre Hospitalier Universitaire de Québec
2705, Boulevard Laurier
Québec City, QC G1V 4G2 (Canada)
marie-claude.pelland-marcotte.med@ssss.gouv.qc.ca

Alyssa Power, MD, FRCPC, FACC
Assistant Professor of Pediatrics
University of Toronto
Pediatric Cardiologist, Labatt Family Heart Centre
Division of Cardiology
The Hospital for Sick Children
555 University Avenue
Toronto, ON M5G 1X8 (Canada)
alyssa.power@sickkids.ca

Victoria E. Price, MBChB, MSc, FRCPC
Professor of Pediatrics
Dalhousie University
Pediatric Hematologist/Oncologist
Head, Division of Pediatric Hematology/Oncology
IWK Health Center
5850/5980 University Avenue
P.O. Box 9700
Halifax, NS B3K 6R8 (Canada)
vicky.price@iwk.nshealth.ca

Rajiv K. Pruthi, MBBS
Professor of Medicine, Mayo Clinic College of Medicine
Consultant, Division of Hematology
Director, Mayo Comprehensive Hemophilia Center
Co-Director, Special Coagulation and
Molecular Hematopathology Laboratories
Chair, Coagulation Diseases Oriented Group (Hematology)
Mayo Clinic
200 First Street SW
Rochester, MN 55905 (USA)
pruthi.rajiv@mayo.edu

Elizabeth Pulcine, MD, MSc, FRCPC
Assistant Professor of Pediatrics
University of Toronto
Pediatric Neurologist, Division of Neurology
The Hospital for Sick Children
555 University Avenue
Toronto, ON M5G 1X8 (Canada)
liza.pulcine@sickkids.ca

Margaret L. Rand, PhD
Professor of Laboratory Medicine and
Pathobiology, Biochemistry, and Pediatrics
University of Toronto
Senior Associate Scientist, Translational Medicine Program
Division of Hematology/Oncology
The Hospital for Sick Children
555 University Avenue
Toronto, ON M5G 1X8 (Canada)
margaret.rand@sickkids.ca

Shoshana Revel-Vilk, MD, PhD
Professor of Pediatrics, School of Medicine, Hebrew University
Pediatric Hematology/Oncology Unit
Head, Gaucher Unit
Shaare Zedek Medical Center
Shmuel Beyth Street 12
Jerusalem 9103102 (Israel)
svilk@szmc.org.il

Janaina Bosso S. Ricciardi, PT, PhD
Physiotherapist, Hemophilia Treatment Center
Hemocentro UNICAMP
University of Campinas
Rua Carlos Chagas 480
Campinas, SP 13.083-878 (Brazil)
jbosso@unicamp.br

Mattia Rizzi, MD, PhD
Pediatric Hematologist/Oncologist
Pediatric Hematology/Oncology Unit
Department of Woman-Mother-Child
CHUV – Lausanne University Hospital
Rue du Bugnon 21
CH–1011 Lausanne (Switzerland)
mattia.rizzi@chuv.ch

Jeremy Robertson, MBBS, FRACP, FRCPA
Director, Haematology & Haemophilia Service
Clinical Lead, Vascular Medicine Service
Senior Staff Specialist, Paediatric Haematology
Pathologist, Department of Haematology
Queensland Children's Hospital
501 Stanley Street
South Brisbane, QLD 4101 (Australia)
jeremy.robertson@health.qld.gov.au

Nancy Robitaille, MD, FRCPC
Professor of Pediatrics
Université de Montréal
Pediatric Hematologist
Division of Hematology/Oncology
CHU Sainte-Justine
Vice-President, Transfusion Medicine
Héma-Québec
4045 Boulevard Côte-Vertu
Montréal, QC H4R 2W7 (Canada)
nancy.robitaille.md@hema-quebec.qc.ca

Christine A. Sabapathy, MD, MSc
Assistant Professor of Pediatrics
McGill University
Pediatric Hematologist-Oncologist
Division of Pediatric Hematology-Oncology
Montreal Children's Hospital
1001 Blvd Decarie
Montréal, QC H4A 3J1 (Canada)
christine.sabapathy@mcgill.ca

Markus Schmugge, MD
Associate Professor, Faculty of Medicine
University of Zurich
Head, Haematology
Department of Haematology, Oncology,
Bone Marrow Transplant, Immunology
University Children's Hospital
Steinwiesstrasse 75
CH–8032 Zurich (Switzerland)
markus.schmugge@kispi.uzh.ch

Natsaruth Songthawee, MD
Assistant Professor of Pediatrics
Prince of Songkla University
Pediatric Hematologist/Oncologist
Division of Hematology/Oncology
Department of Pediatrics
Songklanagarind Hospital
15 Karnjanavanit Road
Hat Yai, Songkhla 90110 (Thailand)
snatsaru@medicine.psu.ac.th

Michael Temple, MD
Head, Interventional Radiology
St Jude Children's Research Hospital
262 Danny Thomas Place
Memphis, TN 38105 (USA)
michael.temple@stjude.org

Mark Todd, RRT, HBSc
ECLS Coordinator and Clinical Educator
Departments of Respiratory Therapy and Critical Care
The Hospital for Sick Children
555 University Avenue
Toronto, ON M5G 1X8 (Canada)
mark.todd@sickkids.ca

Soumitra Tole, MD, MSC, FRCPC
Assistant Professor of Pediatrics
Schulich School of Medicine and Dentistry, Western University
Pediatric Hematologist/Oncologist
Division of Pediatric Hematology/Oncology
Children's Hospital, London Health Sciences Center
800 Commissioner's Road E
London, ON N6A 5W9 (Canada)
soumitra.tole@lhsc.on.ca

Christina VanderPluym, MD
Associate Professor of Pediatrics
Harvard School of Medicine
Director, Cardiac Antithrombosis Management Program
Co-Director, Stroke Center
Director, Ventricular Assist Device Program
Heart Center, Department of Cardiology
Boston Children's Hospital
300 Longwood Avenue
Boston, MA 02115 (USA)
christina.vanderpluym@cardio.chboston.org

Heleen van Ommen, MD, PhD
Associate Professor of Pediatric Hematology
Head, Department of Pediatric Hematology & Oncology
Pediatric Hematologist
Erasmus University Medical Center Sophia Children's Hospital
Wijtemaweg 80
NL–3015 CN Rotterdam (The Netherlands)
c.vanommen@erasmusmc.nl

Carolina Vargas, MD
Fellow, Pediatric Stroke Program
Division of Neurology
The Hospital for Sick Children
555 University Avenue
Toronto, ON M5G 1X8 (Canada)
carolina.vargas@sickkids.ca

Mariella Vargas-Gutierrez, MD
Assistant Professor of Pediatrics
Division of Pediatric Critical Care
Children's Hospital of Eastern Ontario
University of Ottawa
401 Smyth Road
Ottawa, ON K1H 8L1 (Canada)
mvargasgutierrez@cheo.on.ca

Jennifer Vincelli, RN(EC)
Adjunct Lecturer
University of Toronto
Pediatric Nurse Practitioner, Thrombosis
Division of Hematology/Oncology
The Hospital for Sick Children
555 University Avenue
Toronto, ON M5G 1X8 (Canada)
jennifer.vincelli@sickkids.ca

Hilary E.A. Whyte, MB, MSc, FRCPI, FRCPC
Professor of Pediatrics
University of Toronto
Neonatologist, Division of Neonatology
The Hospital for Sick Children
555 University Avenue
Toronto, ON M5G 1X8 (Canada)
hilary.whyte@sickkids.ca

Suzan Williams, MD, MSc, FRCPC
Associate Professor of Pediatrics
University of Toronto
Pediatric Hematologist
Division of Hematology/Oncology
The Hospital for Sick Children
555 University Avenue
Toronto, ON M5G 1X8 (Canada)
suzan.williams@sickkids.ca

Rochelle Winikoff, MD, FRCP, MSc
Assistant Professor of Hematology
University of Montréal
Hematology/Oncology Service
Department of Pediatrics
CHU Sainte-Justine
3175 Côte Sainte-Catherine Road
Montréal, QC H3T 1C5 (Canada)
rochelle.winikoff.med@ssss.gouv.qc.ca

Alexandra Zabeida, MD, FRCPC, MSc
Fellow, Pediatric Thrombosis and Hemostasis Program
Division of Hematology/Oncology
The Hospital for Sick Children
555 University Avenue
Toronto, ON M5G 1X8 (Canada)
alexandra.zabeida@sickkids.ca

Ester Zapotocka, MD
Senior Hematologist
Department of Pediatric Hematology and Oncology
University Hospital Motol and Second Faculty of Medicine
Charles University
V Uvalu 84
CZ–150 06 Prague (Czech Republic)
ester.zapotocka@fnmotol.cz

Published online: December 5, 2024

Blanchette VS, Brandão LR, Carcao MD, Kumar R, Rand ML, Revel-Vilk S (eds): SickKids Handbook of Pediatric Thrombosis and Hemostasis, ed 3, rev. and ext. Basel, Karger, 2024, pp XIX–XX (DOI: 10.1159/000538191)

Preface

This third edition of the Hospital for Sick Children (SickKids) Handbook of Pediatric Thrombosis and Hemostasis is dedicated to a trio of giants who collectively led to the formation of the Pediatric Thrombosis and Hemostasis Programs at SickKids: Drs. Alvin Zipursky, Maureen Andrew, and Victor Blanchette. Ultimately, it was the excellence of the programs which they collectively created and nourished that attracted and continue to attract trainees from Canada and from across the world, many of whom today are leading/working in premier pediatric thrombosis and hemostasis programs worldwide. The editors of this edition of the Handbook were all taught, mentored, inspired, and befriended by one, two, or all three of these giants.

Dr. Alvin Zipursky was recruited (from McMaster, Hamilton) to SickKids in 1981 to become head of a newly created Division of Hematology/Oncology that for the first time combined pediatric hematology together with oncology; he led the division until 1991 (see Chapter 1). Dr. Zipursky was a wonderful teacher and mentor, having the ability to draw people together and to bring out the best in them. He recognized talent and consequently, he recruited many people in both hematology and oncology including Drs. Victor Blanchette (on a full-time basis) and Maureen Andrew (on a part-time basis). Dr. Zipursky had earlier on brought Maureen to McMaster where he had been Chair of Pediatrics at McMaster University. Dr. Zipursky saw the importance of mentoring young clinicians who he knew could go on to develop the fields of pediatric thrombosis and hemostasis – the former, a field that was barely in its infancy in the 1990s. Alvin finally retired from clinical work at SickKids in 1995 – a few of us were still fortunate to have been trained by him; he went on to do much important work in global child health after "retiring" until his passing in 2021.

Maureen became a pioneer of pediatric thrombosis and she, more than anyone, put the field "on the map." It was because of her that the world began to recognize that children could indeed clot. Maureen's dynamism and dedication led to countless publications and led to trainees coming to Toronto to work and learn pediatric thrombosis from her. SickKids was the institution to which other centers turned when faced with a child with a clot; to facilitate providing recommendations to others, Maureen began the 1-800-NO-CLOTS service and developed thromboembolism and stroke protocols, which became internationally used. Despite Maureen's much too early and untimely death in 2001, the internationally recognized program that she established in pediatric thrombosis at SickKids continued to attract trainees and staff to come to the institution and work in the program that Maureen had commenced and nurtured, and to build on her legacy.

Victor was recruited to SickKids by Dr. Zipursky in 1983 to lead the Hemophilia Clinic and Pediatric Hemostasis Program. Over the next 4 decades, Victor's contributions to the field of pediatric hemostasis were innumerable. He spearheaded pivotal studies in immune thrombocytopenia, hemophilia, and other acquired/inherited bleeding disorders, and his vision led to the development of assessment tools that have become widely used in evaluating quality of life and musculoskeletal status in children with hemophilia. Yet his contributions were so much more.

He has been a leader and innovator, with the unique talent to bring people together to do collective work. In this regard he, along with Maureen, started the Canadian Pediatric Thrombosis and Hemostasis Network (CPTHN). Victor also initiated the International Prophylaxis Study Group (IPSG), was instrumental in starting the Association of Hemophilia Clinic Directors of Canada (AHCDC), and was pivotal to the formation of many other organizations and groups – in Canada and overseas in such places as Brazil, China, and many of the islands in the Caribbean including Barbados, the island of his birth. He also was a great recruiter of people, bringing many of us to SickKids as trainees or junior colleagues. In 1998, he became Chief of the Division of Pediatric Hematology/Oncology – a position he held until 2012. Victor was passionate about training the next generation and in this regard he, along with Maureen, in 2001, started a pediatric hemostasis-thrombosis training program. Victor was able to persuade an industry sponsor (Baxter Bioscience – now Takeda) to support an endowed fellowship in pediatric hemostasis thrombosis. The financial stability from this allowed for the funding of a minimum of one fellow annually; additional funding over the years came from other industry sponsors (Bayer, Pfizer, and additional funding from Takeda) along with some financial support from the Division of Hematology/Oncology. Over 50 trainees have trained at SickKids and subsequently have gone on to lead/work in pediatric hemostasis and/or thrombosis programs throughout the world.

It was Victor who conceived of inviting many of these former trainees to come together in 2010 to create a SickKids Handbook of Pediatric Thrombosis and Hemostasis.

The first edition of this handbook was published in 2013, with a second in 2017. During the past decade, the world of pediatric thrombosis and hemostasis has changed greatly with transformative changes in hemophilia care and an expansion on how to recognize and treat children at risk of, or with, thrombotic complications. As such, there was a need to update the Handbook, and hence, the impetus for this third edition to which Victor contributed greatly before his passing.

Victor's intention was to have this third edition dedicated to his mentor and friend Alvin Zipursky, but this time Victor was vetoed and instead we (Victor's former trainees and colleagues, and his dear friends) chose to dedicate this handbook collectively to him, to his dear colleague Maureen, and to their mentor – Alvin Zipursky.

We hope that you will enjoy this textbook, that you will find it useful, and that it will also inspire you to follow in the footsteps of Victor, Maureen, and Alvin in the same way they have influenced us. Please note that there is an online version of this textbook (available at http://www.karger.com/sickkids).

Manuel D. Carcao, Toronto, ON, Canada
Leonardo R. Brandão, Toronto, ON, Canada
Riten Kumar, Boston, MA, USA
Margaret L. Rand, Toronto, ON, Canada
Shoshana Revel-Vilk, Jerusalem, Israel

Chapter 1

Published online: December 5, 2024

Blanchette VS, Brandão LR, Carcao MD, Kumar R, Rand ML, Revel-Vilk S (eds): SickKids Handbook of Pediatric Thrombosis and Hemostasis, ed 3, rev. and ext. Basel, Karger, 2024, pp 1–12 (DOI: 10.1159/000538320)

Pediatric Thrombosis and Hemostasis: A Historical Perspective

Leonardo R. Brandão Victor S. Blanchette

Division of Hematology/Oncology, The Hospital for Sick Children, University of Toronto, Toronto, ON, Canada

Introduction

Throughout medical school and residency, trainees frequently hear the adage "kids are not just little adults." Nowhere in pediatrics is this truer than in the physiology of coagulation. In fact, the coagulation system evolves in utero and continues to develop over the course of childhood.

Initial studies on this subject focused on premature infants and the potential role that the differences in their coagulation system might have played in the development of intracranial hemorrhage. A second wave of studies surfaced in the 1970s, when the coagulation system in neonates started to be characterized [1–3]. In the late 1980s, Dr. Maureen Andrew and her colleagues at McMaster University studied healthy newborns and, subsequently, preterm infants to better understand postnatal development of the human coagulation system and determine age-related reference ranges [4, 5]. Additional work describing the maturation of the hemostatic system in children and adolescents was published by Andrew et al. [6] in 1992. These landmark observations were confirmed in subsequent publications that highlighted the significant and important differences in the physiology of coagulation and fibrinolysis in children, paving the way for our growing understanding of the qualitative and quantitative developmental differences that occur throughout childhood (see Chapter 2 and Appendix II).

A Pediatric Hemostasis-Thrombosis Program Is Born

In the early modern era, children in need usually received care in foundling houses. For centuries, this type of institution was the only place where children in social need could have access to medical care, and where clinical pediatrics evolved. It was only in the late modern era that the idea of having separate hospitals or outpatient facilities devoted solely to the care of sick children emerged. In London (United Kingdom), the short-lived Dispensary for the Infant Poor (1769–1781), and in Austria, the outpatient clinic called Kinder-Krankeninstitut (1787, Vienna) spearheaded the list of European inpatient/outpatient pediatric facilities, followed by the Hôpital des Enfants-Malades (1802, Paris/France) [7–9]. In North America, the Children's Hospital of Philadelphia (1855) and the Children's Hospital of Boston (1869) opened with 12 and 20 beds, respectively, influenced by the Great Ormond Street Hospital of London (1852) [10, 11]. The second pediatric hospital in the British Commonwealth and the first in Canada opened with 6 beds in Toronto in March 1875, the Victoria Hospital for Sick Children (until 1912; The Hospital for Sick Children [SickKids] thereafter), followed by two centers in Montréal, the Children's Memorial Hospital (1903; changed to Montréal Children's Hospital [1954]), and Hôpital Sainte-Justine (1907) [12].

Within the next decades, SickKids faced a dramatic growth, with the number of beds peaking at 810 in the 1970s, when the hospital became the largest pediatric facility in North America, to being strategically downsized (to 305 beds, currently) to promote an improved healthcare delivery. In its early years, blood transfusion techniques were pioneered as early as 1915, and hematology started as a laboratory-based discipline in 1932 [13]. A formal pediatric hematology service was established in 1958, becoming a combined Division of Pediatric Hematology-Oncology only in 1981, with the arrival of Dr. Alvin Zipursky (chief of the combined division from 1981 to 1991; he retired from clinical work in 1995) [14], who brought his experience of leading both pediatric hematology/oncology and the Pediatric Department at McMaster University Health Sciences Center in Hamilton, Canada. Dr. Zipursky was an accomplished clinician scientist, and his research helped to legitimize neonatal hematology as a field of its own. While his main academic interest was Rhesus (Rh) hemolytic disease of the newborn, he was also active in other areas including neonatal coagulation [15–18], and he instituted multidisciplinary sections within hematology, including the inherited bleeding disorders (focused on hemophilia) and hemoglobinopathies (focused on sickle cell disease and thalassemia), that persist to this day. During his tenure at SickKids, the then called combined Division of Pediatric Hematology/Oncology/Stem Cell Transplantation developed Canada's premier fellowship training program. During this time, Dr. Maureen Andrew was recruited in a part-time faculty position to the division. Dr. Andrew brought to the institution her legacy of working for almost one decade at the well-established evidence-based and clinical trial-driven adult thrombosis team at McMaster University Health Sciences Center, where she received mentorship from giants in the field such as Drs. Jack Hirsh and Michael Gent. Dr. Andrew initiated a pediatric thrombosis service (i.e., pediatric thrombophilia clinic) at SickKids in May 1991 (Fig. 1) and on September 28, 1995, in collaboration with Dr. Victor Blanchette, who oversaw the pediatric comprehensive care hemophilia program, the SickKids pediatric hemostasis-thrombosis service was officially announced (Fig. 2). Under Dr. Andrew's visionary leadership, the thrombosis program grew to pave the way on establishing many of the principles identified as vital by the International Society on Thrombosis and Haemostasis (ISTH) Pediatric and Neonatal Thrombosis and Haemostasis subcommittee almost two and a half decades later [19, 20]. In 1998, Dr. Blanchette was appointed as Head of the Pediatric Hematology/Oncology Division at SickKids, and one of his first initiatives was to recruit Dr. Andrew from her then part-time faculty position in the Division of Hematology/Oncology to a full-time position.

Thrombosis in Childhood

Unlike hemostatic disorders, thrombosis had long been considered a condition of adults. Unlike bleeding disorders, where inherited conditions usually present early in childhood, inherited

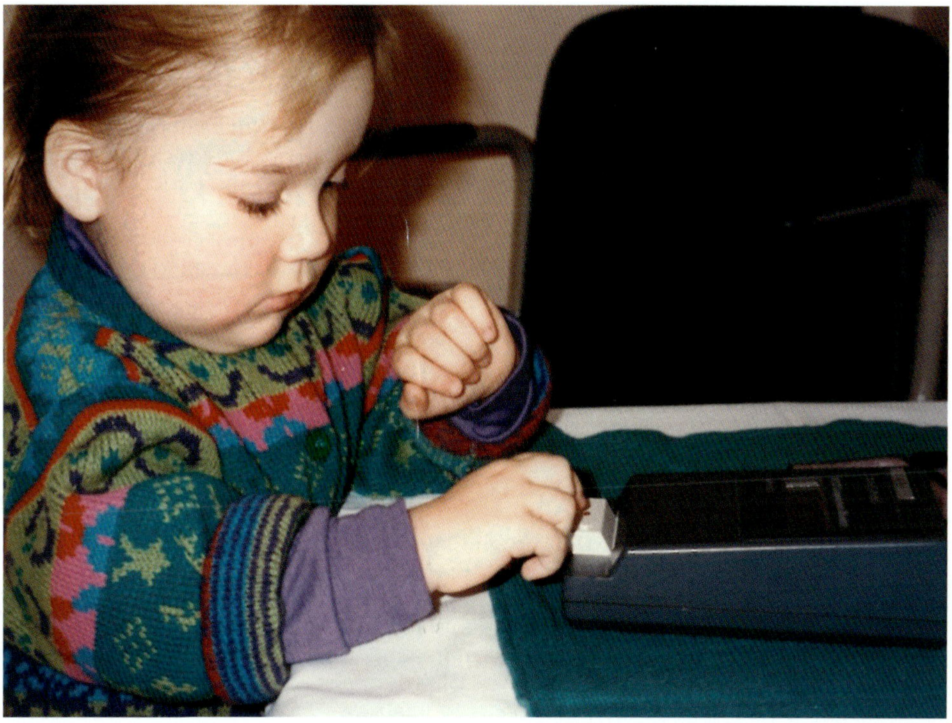

Fig. 1. Patient using a point-of-care device for anticoagulation monitoring in the thrombosis clinic (circa 1995). Whole blood prothrombin time/international normalized ratio (PT/INR) monitor, the Biotrack® 512 prototype [55, 56]. Written informed consent was obtained from the parent/legal guardian of the patient for publication of this image in research or educational materials. Copyright © SickKids Thrombosis Program.

thrombophilias most commonly first manifest during adult life, with only rare and severe deficiencies presenting spontaneously early in childhood. The first reported case of inherited thrombophilia described a Norwegian family and was published by Egeberg in 1965 [21]. Since then, variants in numerous genes have been implicated in inherited thrombophilias. In addition to the thromboembolic events (TEs) that occur solely secondary to inherited thrombophilia variants, which represent a vast minority of all pediatric cases, acquired TEs are much more prevalent during childhood [22]. This notion was not always clear to the scientific community or to patients and families, reflected in initial guidance statements recommending universal and comprehensive thrombophilia testing for children with TEs, a tendency that has significantly lessened over the years. Issues around who, and when, to test for inherited thrombophilias remain the source of much debate amongst experts in the field (see Chapter 13).

In the pediatric literature, the scarce information of TEs was in general represented by case reports or by autopsy-based manuscripts with limited value in defining the epidemiology of these events in children. From 1968 to 1971, an all-Scottish pediatric inpatient hospital database began a trend of maintaining databases of TEs in children; decades later, national and internation-

Haematology launches new program

Sick Kids has launched a new paediatric Hemostasis-Thrombosis Program. This initiative will be directed by Dr. Victor Blanchette, Haematology/Oncology, and brings together his background in bleeding disorders and transfusion medicine with expertise in clotting problems from Drs. Michael Leaker and Maureen Andrew, Haematology/Oncology. An integral component to the program is the coagulation service laboratory directed by Dr. Annette Poon, Haematology/Blood Bank.

The new HSC program will bridge state-of-the-art basic research in the field with a first-class ambulatory and in-patient consultation service utilizing innovative clinical treatment protocols. "This type of program is absolutely unique to paediatrics worldwide and is certain to advance this important field in a major way for education and training, research, and patient care," says Dr. Melvin Freedman, chief of Haematology and co-head of the Division of Haematology/Oncology.

Fig. 2. Announcement of the Pediatric Hemostasis-Thrombosis Service in the SickKids *This Week* Report. *This Week* (internal publication for staff of The Hospital for Sick Children): volume 12, number 39, September 28, 1995.

al databases started to better define the characteristics of thrombosis in children.

In the early 1990s, Dr. Andrew started the first surveillance program across Canada to determine the incidence and nature of thromboembolic diseases in childhood [22]. She and her colleagues found the incidence of deep vein thrombosis (DVT)/pulmonary embolism (PE) to be 5.3/10,000 hospital admissions or 0.07/10,000 children.

Despite the initial perceived relative rarity of thrombosis in childhood, increasing complex medical interventions, the increasing use of central venous catheters (CVCs) and cancer therapies, in particular, have led to a much higher burden of TE disease in children. Improved awareness has elevated clinical suspicion, thus increasing the diagnosis of TEs.

The "epidemic nature" of this dramatic increase in reported TEs in children was documented by a recent publication summarizing data from tertiary USA pediatric centers, confirming an overall 300% increase of pediatric venous thromboembolic events (VTE) in hospitalized patients during a 20-year period (2001–2019). We are now aware that 1 in 100 children admitted to a complex pediatric health care facility will develop a VTE [23]. Based on this increased incidence, a consensus paper on the importance of Hospital-Based Inpatient Thrombosis and Hemostasis Consultive Services was published [20].

Follow-up data on the original Canadian registry at a mean of 2.86 years gave additional insights, suggesting a heavy burden of overall mortality in this group of 16%. Death due to DVT/PE occurred in 2%, all of whom had CVC-related thrombosis. Additionally, follow-up data showed that 8% of children developed recurrent thrombosis, and 12%, post-thrombotic syndrome [24].

Building on the initial epidemiologic findings gathered by international pediatric databases, the importance of TEs in children, both subclinical and clinically overt, and their contribution to morbidity and mortality is now increasingly evident [25, 26]. More recent studies have shown that, in terms of morbidity, children with congenital cardiac defects affected by TEs spend 10 additional days in the cardiac intensive care unit, as compared with children without TEs. In regard to mortality, we are now aware that depending on the type of underlying condition predisposing the child to VTE (i.e., cardiac) and the location of the vessel occlusion (i.e., pulmonary circulation, intracardiac/cardiac shunt), the frequency of direct TE-related mortality may be as high as 7% to 9%. Finally, the initial cost estimates related to VTE alone in children in the USA, likely an underestimation, are in the order of USD 90 million per year [27].

Following the initiation of the Canadian registry, Dr. Andrew led the development of two practical clinical treatment initiatives. The first was a telephone consultation service, called "1-800-NO-CLOTS," which logged well over 4,000 international physician pediatric thrombosis consults in the first 8 years, subsequently led by Drs. Patricia Massicotte (SickKids) and Anthony K. Chan (McMaster University, Hamilton, Canada). The second initiative was the development of institutional pathways for thrombosis treatment. The latter, entitled "Thromboembolism and Stroke Protocols," had its first edition published in 1997 [28]. These initiatives were well received internationally and continue to be utilized by physicians around the world. Following the Canadian Thrombophilia registry, registries of arterial ischemic stroke and cerebral sinus venous thrombosis were set up in partnership with Dr. Gabrielle deVeber, the then head of the Paediatric Stroke Program at Sickkids, leading to the development of the International Pediatric Stroke Study [29].

Anticoagulation in Children: The Evolution of Antithrombotic Care in Children

1

While the discovery of heparin took place in the early 1900s (Jay McLean, 1916), and the initial administration of a nontoxic heparin formulation to a human was reported in Toronto in the mid-1930s (C.H. Best, May 1935), heparin gained increased clinical interest during, and after, the Second World War. By the time the first evidence-based anticoagulant guideline for the management of adults launched in 1984, in a combined effort cosponsored by the American College of Chest Physicians (ACCP) and National Heart, Lung, and Blood Institute, several randomized clinical trials involving anticoagulation (e.g., unfractionated heparin [UFH], low-molecular weight heparin [LMWH], oral vitamin K antagonists [VKAs, i.e., warfarin]) and/or antiplatelet therapy (e.g., acetylsalicylic acid) had already been conducted. Conversely, in children, sporadic case reports including anticoagulation therapy appeared in the literature only between the late 1940s and 1960s [30, 31], and only in the mid-1990s, pediatric dose-finding studies involving these agents became available, establishing age-appropriate dosing for UFH, VKA and LMWH.

Pediatric guidelines for the management of TEs were first included in the 5th edition of the ACCP Chest Guidelines for Antithrombotic and Thrombolytic Therapy, published in 1995. The 9th edition of this evidence-based guideline was published in 2012 [32]. This document became the pre-eminent resource for the management of pediatric thrombosis; however, many recommendations are still based on extrapolated adult data. Additional and similarly valuable pediatric guidelines have also been published to date, including the first American Society of Hematology (ASH) 2018 guideline for management of VTE in children, reflecting the increased degree of international awareness and clinical relevance related to this topic [33]. Despite having a more focused scope, approximately 75% of the recommendations were still graded at expert-based level (e.g., level 2C). In the near future, a second edition of the evidence-based ASH guidelines will expand the original recommendations, incorporating the recent burst of pediatric trials evaluating the role of direct oral anticoagulants (DOACs) in children with VTE (see below).

In adults, regulatory agencies such as the United States Food and Drug Administration (US FDA) and the European Medical Agency (EMA) have approved the use of DOACs (direct factor-Xa [apixaban, edoxaban, and rivaroxaban] or direct oral thrombin inhibitors [dabigatran]) for the indications of VTE treatment and prophylaxis in a number of clinical settings over the last decade. More recently, together with pharmaceutical companies, both agencies have established partnerships to evaluate DOACs in children, from phase I to IV trials, including pharmacokinetic/pharmacodynamic model studies. Furthermore, DOACs in children for specific indications (e.g., primary anticoagulant prophylaxis to prevent CVC-related thrombosis in pediatric acute lymphoblastic leukemia [PREVAPIX-ALL study], primary prophylaxis to prevent thrombi in patients with single ventricle physiology patients) have also been completed [34]. As we await the last few pediatric phase III trials to be published, to date, dabigatran and rivaroxaban have been the DOACs approved for use in children diagnosed with an acute VTE [35–38]. It is hoped that the expanding anticoagulant and antiplatelet pharmacopeia available to pediatric treaters will broaden the options of drugs available allowing them to use agents tailored to each patient, considering their underlying condition, while maximizing their efficacy and safety (see Chapter 20).

Hemostatic Disorders in Children: The Evolution of Hemophilia Care

Historically, congenital bleeding disorders like hemophilia were considered to be pediatric conditions as patients' life spans were limited due to bleeding. Over the course of the second half of the 20th century, hemophilia care saw considerable advancements, first with the discovery of cryoprecipitate in the 1960s and quickly followed thereafter with the development of easy to reconstitute and administer lyophilized factor (F)VIII and FIX plasma-derived clotting factor concentrates. Tragically, the tainted blood scandal of the 1980s resulted in the death of many young hemophilia patients who were infected with the hepatitis viruses and/or human immune deficiency virus. This devastating circumstance resulted in intense pressure to develop safe, virus-inactivated plasma-derived FVIII and FIX concentrates and subsequently to engineer synthetic, recombinant FVIII and FIX replacement products. Recombinant FVIII became available in 1992, followed by a recombinant FIX product in 1997. These synthetic products subsequently became the mainstay of hemophilia treatment in much of the developed world.

With improved accessibility to factor replacement and decreased risk of transmission of infectious diseases, the opportunities for regular replacement therapy (prophylaxis) increased. The first FVIII prophylaxis was given in the late 1950s by Inga Marie Nilsson in Sweden [39]. Early studies of prophylaxis were positive, suggesting that infusing factor regularly could dramatically improve outcomes. The Swedish group devised the Malmö protocol, which aimed to keep circulating factor levels at >1% (>0.01 IU/dL) at all times, essentially converting severe hemophiliacs to a moderate phenotype with a substantial reduction in the frequency of spontaneous bleeding. Factor was given at a dose of 25–40 IU/kg for a minimum of three times weekly for FVIII deficiency and twice weekly for FIX deficiency. Data showed that early institution of prophylaxis before bleeding was optimal for preventing joint disease. Investigators reported that anything less than full-dose prophylaxis, or prophylaxis started at an older age (>3 years), did not completely prevent significant hemophilic arthropathy in boys with severe hemophilia A [40]. Manco-Johnson et al. [41] were the first to prospectively study prophylaxis in severe hemophilia. The USA Joint Outcome Study randomized 63 boys (<30 months of age) with severe hemophilia A to one of two treatment regimens, either primary prophylaxis using the Malmö regimen, or an on-demand regimen in which they received 40 IU/kg of factor with each joint bleed, followed by 25 IU/kg the next day and after a gap of 1 day, a third infusion of 25 IU/kg. The primary outcome was preservation of normal joint structure in ankles, knees, and elbows as seen with plain-film radiography and magnetic resonance imaging at 6 years of age. Patients were enrolled in this prospective study at an average age of 18 months. The results demonstrated that prophylaxis was significantly better than on-demand therapy for preventing hemarthroses and preserving joint structure and function in boys with severe hemophilia A [41]. With prophylaxis, severe hemophilia patients have far less joint disease [42]. Consequently, their lifespan in developed countries began to approach that of the general population.

From the 1990s to the 2010s, hemophilia management primarily was focused on optimizing prophylaxis beginning in very young ages whilst dealing with complications of hemophilia management including inhibitor development. During this time, treatments available for hemophilia did not change dramatically. However, the 2010s witnessed exciting new developments in the area of hemophilia care beginning with the development of new extended half-life (EHL) FVIII and FIX coagulation factor concentrates [43]. These products, prepared using fusion technology (to IgG1 or albumin) or through coupling of FVIII/FIX to polyethylene glycol, provide an approximate 1.5-fold extension of FVIII half-life and a 3- to 5-fold extension of FIX half-life. The result is a reduction in the frequency of infusions required to maintain any given trough FVIII or FIX level or a higher trough level of FVIII/FIX if the frequency of infusions is held constant. Prospective clinical trials ensued that established the benefit of these new products with regard to long-term joint health in persons with hemophilia and to improvements in quality of life mainly due to the reduction in number of intravenous infusions (see Chapter 8).

Unfortunately, the major problems of inhibitor development and its negative impact on bleeding and long-term joint outcomes were not solved by the introduction of EHL coagulation factor concentrates. Fortunately, whilst EHL concentrates were being developed other exciting developments in the field of nonfactor therapies were occurring. These nonfactor therapies, including a FVIII mimetic emicizumab, could be used with similar effectiveness in persons with and without inhibitors to FVIII. Emicizumab was first licensed by FDA in 2017 and by EMA in 2018 for use in persons with inhibitors. Shortly thereafter, in 2018 and 2019, it was licensed by the two regulatory agencies, respectively, for use in persons without inhibitors. Very soon, other regulatory agencies including Health Canada similarly approved emicizumab under the trade name Hemlibra®. Now, as of 2023, it is estimated that there are over 20,000 persons with hemophilia A (most without inhibitors) on Hemlibra. The use of this product has greatly changed prophylaxis in young children with severe hemophilia A who are increasingly commenced on Hemlibra at even younger age than traditionally has been done with clotting factor concentrates, given that the latter must be given intravenously, whereas Hemlibra is given subcutaneously [44].

Hemlibra is just the start of many other non-factor therapies in development including not only other FVIII mimetics, but also the anti-tissue factor pathway inhibitor fitusiran, an agent that reduces the production of antithrombin, and other drugs targeting other natural anticoagulants including protein C [45]. In addition to all these new therapies being subcutaneously administered and having very long half-lives permitting very infrequent administration, in some cases, once every 2 months, they also can be used in both persons with hemophilia A or hemophilia B, unlike FVIII mimetics.

Whilst all these exciting developments have been occurring, gene therapy, which offers a one-time cure for hemophilia, has now become a reality in many adults as the first gene therapy has been approved by FDA and EMA and is now beginning to be used outside the studies. Indeed, we are now in "exciting and rapidly changing times for persons with hemophilia" [46].

Although the improvements in hemophilia management have been miraculous, they have for the most part not, as yet, been accompanied by dramatic improvements in the management of other relatively common (e.g., von Willebrand disease [VWD] and platelet disorders) and more rare bleeding disorders including severe deficiencies of rare coagulation factors.

The SickKids hemostasis group led by Dr. Blanchette has spearheaded many studies in hemophilia particularly on introduction of prophylaxis in young children. Dr. Blanchette recruited basic laboratory and clinical experts who have made significant contributions to the improved management and understanding in different areas, such as the role of the platelet function analyzer in investigating bleeding disorders, to the genetics of hemophilia, VWD, and platelet disorders, and to the increasing use of bleeding questionnaires in children. Moreover, under his guidance, SickKids led or greatly contributed to national (i.e., Association of Hemophilia Clinic Directors of Canada [AHCDC], Canadian Pediatric Thrombosis and Hemostasis Network [CPTHN]) and to global collaborative efforts (i.e., International Prophylaxis Study Group [IPSG]) on improving the management of children with inherited or acquired bleeding diatheses, including the development of a Canadian disease-specific (i.e., hemophilia) quality of life tool, and new validated physiotherapy- and radiology-based joint assessment instruments for children with hemophilia.

The Future of Pediatric Thrombosis and Hemostasis

As we move forward, two essential topics must be considered to further develop and advance the field of pediatric thrombosis and hemostasis. The first is continued research in this field, at the basic science, translational, and clinical levels. Much work is required for us to understand the physiology and pathophysiology of the hemostatic system in children, the pharmacology of antithrombotic agents, the natural history of thrombotic disorders, and the risk-benefit ratios of treatment according to type and severity of TEs. In this patient population of uncommon disorders, physicians and researchers must continue to form alliances and collaborations. We must continue to pursue representation on committees of large organizations, such as the subcommittee for pediatric and neonatal thrombosis and hemostasis of the ISTH, the American Heart Association, and other international and/or national societies representative of pediatric hematologists with expertise in pediatric hemostasis and thrombosis (e.g., American Society of Pediatric Hematology Oncology, ASH, Hemostasis Thrombosis Research Society, German Society for Thrombosis and Hemostasis, Thrombosis & Hemostasis Summit of North America, National Hemophilia Foundation) and work together with those who provide care for adults with bleeding and thrombotic disorders. In addition, research collaborations at national and international levels will increase patient enrollment numbers and promote the success of prospective clinical studies. We must find creative ways to overcome barriers beyond small numbers of patients, which include practical limitations to the number and volume of blood samples needed and financial constraints on funding for pediatric research [47].

From a hemostasis perspective, at the end of 1996, a group of European pediatric hematologists with special interests in treating children with hemophilia started a collaborative group called the Pediatric Network on Haemophilia Management (PedNet). In the following year, its first meeting gathered 21 physicians from 16 European countries. Today, the PedNet group hosts 33 participating centers from 19 countries, of which Canada is the only non-European country (SickKids and St. Justine Hospital). PedNet remains a very active and productive platform (>35 publications in high impact journals [including one *New England Journal of Medicine* manuscript] and >2,500 children with hemophilia A/B enrolled in the PedNet registry). In North America, early in the 2000s, a pilot study including eight national hemophilia treating centers in the USA evaluated the impact of their partnership to identify and solve unmet needs pertaining to children with thrombotic conditions, leveraging the infrastructure already being provided by the Centers for Disease Control. Similarly, in 2003, an international multidisciplinary meeting occurring in Montréal, QC, Canada, led to the creation of the IPSG, whose first academic output was the development of the well-accepted Hemophilia Joint Health Score tool to evaluate the musculoskeletal health of children with bleeding tendencies (see Chapter 8). To date, the IPSG continues to strive, distributing the expertise of its members within five different expert working groups (i.e., musculoskeletal health, pharmacokinetics, prophylaxis, joint imaging, and health care access) and maintaining an intense list of peer-reviewed high impact publications.

From a pediatric thrombosis perspective, a more recent effort, the International Pediatric Thrombosis Network (IPTN), is being led by Dr. Heleen van Ommen under ISTH auspices, gathering data from centers around the globe where children with thrombotic conditions are being followed [48]. Currently, over 1,250 children from 98 participating centers (29 countries) have been enrolled in the Throm-PED registry [49]. In parallel, to coordinate an effective approach to antithrombotic studies, including postmarketing trials, the Pedi-ATLAS trialists group was created [50]. By generating improved evidence, we will promote the best care for our patients.

Second, we must support trainee education and subspecialization. In pediatrics, we face an ongoing struggle to ensure that nonmalignant hematology receives sufficient attention in intensive combined pediatric hematology/oncology training curricula. If hematology is taught well by enthusiastic teachers, more trainees will opt to focus in this area. An editorial published in the *Journal of Thrombosis and Haemostasis* suggested a dramatic decline in the number of physicians interested in careers in the area of bleeding disorders, a trend that continues to date [51]. There was a call for additional fellowship programs to support the education of a new generation of specialists in this area, and it was suggested that training should not be concentrated in one area alone but should embrace both thrombosis and hemostasis, at least for young academic physicians entering the field [52]. Since that time, many additional fellowships have been started, most funded by industry sponsors and in partnership with different societies. The pursuit of grant-funded mentored fellowship training in hemostasis/thrombosis seems to deliver higher rates of academic retention within these subspecialties, as well as research productivity, in comparison to conventional hematology/oncology fellowship training [53]. Perhaps some of the advantages offered by such programs relate to the existence of a core curriculum, in addition to different degrees of research/grant writing exposure [54]. At SickKids, since its inception in 1994 and by the end of the 2026 academic year, a total of 51 individuals from 22 different countries will have been trained following this model (Americas [North: 13, South: 4]; Europe: 16; Asia: 6; Australia: 5; Middle East: 5; Africa: 2). Importantly, most of the SickKids hemostasis thrombosis fellowship alumni returned home or were hired by global academic leading institutions to become local, national, and international leaders in their field, contributing for the improvement of the lives of their patients/families and for the advancement of our field.

In summary, the history of the study and care of disorders of pediatric thrombosis and hemostasis is a tale of innovative thought, hard work, and dedication. Our predecessors were talented and driven to build the science that supports our clinical practice. The story continues to evolve, and much is left to be discovered. International research collaborations and focused efforts to mentor young academically oriented physicians will ensure that advances continue to be made in the coming years.

Acknowledgments

The authors express their appreciation for the help provided by Dr. Hugh O'Brodovich (Toronto, ON, Canada) and Velma Marzinotto (Toronto, ON, Canada), who both graciously shared valuable material pertaining to SickKids' history for this chapter. Our special thanks also go to Drs. Vicky R. Breakey and Shoshana Revel-Vilk who were authors of this chapter in the first and/or second editions of the Handbook, which provided a valuable background for this updated chapter.

Conflict of Interest Statement

Victor S. Blanchette reports receiving consultancy and speaker fees from Bayer HealthCare, Sanofi-Genzyme, Novo Nordisk, Pfizer, Roche, Takeda, and Spark Therapeutics. He is recipient of research grants from Sanofi-Genzyme, Bayer HealthCare, and Takeda, and serves as a member of Data Safety Monitoring Boards for Octapharma and Takeda. He is Chair of a nonprofit organization, the IPSG. Leonardo R. Brandão reports receiving consultancy and speaker fees from Takeda and Inari Medical. He is recipient of a research grant from Takeda and an educational grant from Inari Medical.

Author Contributions

Victor S. Blanchette drafted the chapter, critically revised the chapter, and approved the final version. Leonardo R. Brandão drafted the chapter, critically revised the chapter, and approved the final version.

Abbreviations

ACCP	American College of Chest Physicians
ASH	American Society of Hematology
CVC	Central venous catheter
DOAC	Direct oral anticoagulant
DVT	Deep vein thrombosis
EHL	Extended half-life
EMA	European Medicines Agency
FDA	Food and Drug Administration
FVIII	Factor VIII
FIX	Factor IX
IPSG	International Prophylaxis Study Group
IPTN	International Pediatric Thrombosis Network
ISTH	International Society on Thrombosis and Haemostasis
IU	International unit
LMWH	Low-molecular-weight heparin
PE	Pulmonary embolism
PedNet	Pediatric Network on Haemophilia Management
TE	Thromboembolism/thromboembolic event
VKA	Vitamin K antagonist
VTE	Venous thromboembolism/thromboembolic event
VWD	von Willebrand disease
UFH	Unfractionated heparin

References

1 Holmberg L, Henriksson P, Hans Ekelund H, Astedt B. Coagulation in the human fetus. Comparison with term newborn infants. J Pediatr. 1974;85(6):860–4.
2 Hathaway WE, Bonnar J. Perinatal Coagulation. New York: Grune and Straton, 1978.
3 Barnard DR, Simmons MA, Hathaway WE. Coagulation studies in extremely premature infants. Pediatr Res. 1979;13(12):1330–5.
4 Andrew M, Paes B, Milner R, Johnston M, Mitchell L, Tollefsen DM, et al. Development of the human coagulation system in the full-term infant. Blood. 1987;70(1):165–72.
5 Andrew M, Paes B, Milner R, Johnston M, Mitchell L, Tollefsen DM, et al. Development of the human coagulation system in the healthy premature infant. Blood. 1988;72(5):1651–7.
6 Andrew M, Vegh P, Johnston M, Bowker J, Ofosu F, Mitchell L. Maturation of the hemostatic system during childhood. Blood. 1992;80(8):1998–2005.
7 Dunn PM. George Armstrong MD (1719–1789) and his dispensary of the infant poor. Arch Dis Child Fetal Neonatol Ed. 2002;87(3):228–31.
8 Wyklicky H. Welfare service of the Emperor Joseph II for orphaned and sick children. Padiatr Padol. 1982;17(2):437–40.
9 Lereboullet O. L'Hôpital des Enfants-Malades (1802–1913). Paris Médicale. 1914;14:3.
10 Radbill SX. A history of children's hospitals. Am J Dis Child. 1955;90(4):411–16.
11 The History of The Hospital for Sick Children at Great Ormond Street (1852–1914). 2009. Historic Hospital Admission Records Project (HHARP). Available from https://www.hharp.org/library/gosh/general/history.html (Accessed February 05, 2024).
12 Adams A, Theodore D. Designing for "the little convalescents": children's hospitals in Toronto and Montréal, 1875–2006. Can Bull Med Hist. 2002;19(1):201–43.
13 O'Brodovich, H. Haematology oncology. In: O'Brodovich. Editor. Paediatricians at SickKids. The Department of Paediatrics and Its Advancements in Care at The Hospital for Sick Children 1875–2006. SickKids Archives 2019. Toronto. First edition. p. 107–18.
14 Blanchette V, Manley-Kucey M, Zipursky R, Odame I, Bhutta Z, Hitzler J, et al. Alvin Zipursky (1930–2021): an unsurpassable mentor, counselor, and child health advocate. Pediatr Res. 2022;92:902–4.
15 Luke KH, Taylor A, Hirsh J, Zipursky A. Antihemophilia globulin (AHG) response to exercise for the detection of hemophilia A carriers. Pediatr Res. 1971;5:409.
16 Barnard D, Simmons MA, Zipursky A, Hathaway WE. Physiological coagulation studies in infants 24–31 weeks gestation. Pediatr Res. 1978;12:460.
17 Schmidt BK, Muraki T, Zipursky A. Similar decrease of antithrombin III (ATIII) and albumin in birth asphyxia and presumed disseminated intravascular coagulation (DIC). Pediatr Res. 1984;18:248A.
18 Witt DR, McGillivray BC, Allanson JE, Higher HE, Hathaway WE, Zipursky A, et al. Bleeding diathesis in Noonan syndrome: a common association. Am J Med Genet. 1988;31(2):305–17.
19 Newall F, Jones S, Bauman M, Bruce A, Massicotte MP, Monagle P; Subcommittee on Perinatal and Paediatric Haemostasis. Recommendations for the development of a dedicated pediatric anticoagulation service: Communication for the SSC of the ISTH. J Thromb Haemost. 2015;13(1):155–9.
20 Woods GM, Raffini L, Brandão LR, Jaffray J, Branchford BR, Ng CJ, et al. Practical considerations and consensus opinion for children's hospital-based inpatient hemostasis and thrombosis (HAD) consultative services: communication from the ISTH SSC Subcommittee on Pediatric/Neonatal Thrombosis and Hemostasis. J Thromb Hemost. 2022;20(9):2151–8.
21 Egeberg O. Inherited antithrombin deficiency causing thrombophilia. Thromb Diath Haemorrh. 1965;13:516–30.
22 Andrew M, David M, Adams M, Ali K, Anderson R, Barnard D, et al. Venous thromboembolic complications (VTE) in children: first analyses of the Canadian Registry of VTE. Blood. 1994;83(5):1251–7.
23 O'Brien S, Stanek JR, Witmer CM, Raffini L. The continued rise of venous thromboembolism across US children's hospitals. Pediatrics. 2022;149(3):e2021054649.
24 Monagle P, Adams M, Mahoney M, Ali K, Barnard D, Bernstein M, et al. Outcome of pediatric thromboembolic disease: a report from the Canadian childhood thrombophilia registry. Pediatr Res. 2000;47(6):763–76.
25 Jones S, Butt W, Monagle P, Cain T, Newall F. The natural history of asymptomatic central venous catheter-related thrombosis in critically ill children. Blood. 2019;133(8):857–66.
26 Avila L, Amiri N, De R, Vincelli J, Pullenayegum E, Williams S, Brandao LR. Characteristics of upper- and lower-extremity deep vein thrombosis and predictors of postthrombotic syndrome in children. Blood Adv. 2021;5(19):3737–47.
27 Setty BA, O'Brien SH, Kerlin BA. Pediatric venous thromboembolism in the United States: a tertiary care complication of chronic disease. Pediatr Blood Cancer. 2011;59(2):258–64.
28 Andrew M, deVeber G. Pediatric Thromboembolism and Stroke Protocols. 1st ed. Hamilton: BC Decker; 1997.
29 Anonymous. IPSS overview. Available from: https://lab.research.sickkids.ca/ipss/about/ (Accessed February 06, 2024).
30 Keller MJ. Deep vein thrombosis in a newborn infant. J Pediatr. 1949;34(4):482–6.
31 Allen DM. Heparin therapy in purpura fulminans. Pediatrics. 1966;38(2):211–4.
32 Monagle P, Chan AK, Goldenberg NA, Ichord RN, Journeycake JM, Nowak-Gottl U, et al. Antithrombotic therapy in neonates and children: antithrombotic therapy and prevention of thrombosis, ed 9:American College of Chest Physicians Evidence-Based Clinical Practice Guidelines. Chest. 2012;141(suppl 2):e737S-801S.
33 Monagle P, Cuello CA, Augustine C, Bonduel M, Brandao LR, Capman T, et al. American Society of Hematology 2018 Guidelines for management of venous thromboembolism: treatment of pediatric venous thromboembolism. Blood Adv. 2018;2(22):3292–316.

34 O'Brien SH, Rodriguez V, Lew G, Newburger JW, Schultz CL, Orgel E, et al. Apixaban versus no anticoagulation for the prevention of venous thromboembolism in children with newly diagnosed acute lymphoblastic leukaemia or lymphoma (PREVAPIX-ALL): a phase 3, open-label, randomized, controlled trial. Lancet Haematol. 2024;11(1):e27–37.
35 Anonymous Pradaxa – dabigatran etexilate. European Medicines Agency 2018. Available from: https://www.ema.europa.eu/en/medicines/human/EPAR/pradaxa (Accessed February 06, 2024).
36 Anonymous Xarelto. European Medicines Agency 2018. Available from https://www.ema.europa.eu/en/medicines/human/EPAR/xarelto (Accessed February 06, 2024).
37 FDA approves first oral blood thinning medication for children. FDA, 2021 (cited June 21, 2021). Available from https://www.fda.gov/news-events/press-announcements/fda-approves-first-oral-blood-thinning-medication-children (Accessed February 06, 2024).
38 FDA approved drug to treat, help prevent types of blood clots in certain pediatric populations, FDA, 2021 (cited December 20, 2021). Available from https://www.fda.gov/drugs/news-events-human-drugs/fda-approves-drug-treat-help-prevent-types-blood-clots-certain-pediatric-populations (Accessed February 06, 2024).
39 Nilsson IM, Blomback M, Ahlberg A. Our experience in Sweden with prophylaxis on haemophilia. Bibl Haematol. 1970;34:111–24.
40 Nilsson IM. Experience with prophylaxis in Sweden. Semin Hematol. 1993;30 (suppl 2):16–9.
41 Manco-Johnson MJ, Abshire TC, Shapiro AD, Riske B, Hacker MR, Kilcoyne R, et al. Prophylaxis versus episodic treatment to prevent joint disease in boys with severe hemophilia. N Engl J Med. 2007;357(6):535–44.
42 Ljung R, Gretenkort Andersson N. The current status of prophylactic replacement therapy in children and adults with haemophilia. Br J Haematol. 2015;169(6):777–86.
43 Mahdi AJ, Obaji SG, Collins PW. Role of enhanced half-life factor VIII and IX in the treatment of haemophilia. Br J Haematol. 2015;169(6):768–76.
44 Mahlangu J, Iorio A, Kenet G. Emicizumab state-of-the-art update. Haemophilia. 2022;Suppl 4:103–10.
45 Gogia P, Tarantino M, Schramm M, Aledort L. New directions to develop therapies for people with hemophilia. Expert Rev Hematol. 2023;16(6):417–33.
46 Nathwani AC, Nienhuis AW, Davidoff AM. Our journey to successful gene therapy for hemophilia B. Hum Gene Ther. 2014;25(11):923–6.
47 Manco-Johnson MJ. Pediatric thrombophilia and thrombosis: an historical perspective. Hematology Am Soc Hematol Educ Program. 2008:227.
48 Van Ommen CH, Albisetti M, Bhatt M, Bonduel M, Branchford B, Chalmers E, et al. Subcommittee on Pediatric, Neonatal Thrombosis, Hemostasis. International pediatric thrombosis network to advance pediatric thrombosis research: communication from the ISTH SSC subcommittee on pediatric and neonatal thrombosis and hemostasis. J Thromb Haemost. 2021;19(4):1123–9.
49 Anonymous. International Pediatric Thrombosis Network – working together to improve care of pediatric patients with thrombosis. Available from https://pediatricthrombosis.com/ (Accessed February 05, 2024).
50 Anonymous. Pedi-ATLAS. Available from https://cpcclinicalresearch.org/pedi-atlas/ (Accessed February 06, 2024).
51 Mannucci PM, Roberts HR. Uncertain times for research on hemophilia and allied disorders. J Thromb Haemost. 2005;3(3):423.
52 Blanchette VS. Uncertain times for research on hemophilia and allied disorders. J Thromb Haemost. 2006;4:682.
53 Goldenberg NA, Kruse-Jarres R, Frick N, Pipe SW, Leissinger A, Kessler CM. Outcomes of mentored, grant-funded fellowship in haemostasis/thrombosis: findings from a nested case-control survey study. Haemophilia. 2012;18(3): 326–31.
54 Thornburg CD, Montgomery RR, Pipe SW. How we approach: training pediatric coagulationists. Pediatr Blood Cancer. 2019;66(12):e27982.
55 Jennings I, Luddington RJ, Baglin T. Evaluation of the Ciba Corning Biotrack 512 coagulation monitor for the control of oral anticoagulation. J Clin Pathol. 1991;44(11):950–3.
56 Marzinotto V, Monagle P, Chan A, Adams M, Massicotte P, Leaker M, et al. Capillary whole blood monitoring of oral anticoagulant in outpatient clinics and the home setting. Pediatr Cardiol. 2000;21(4):347–52.

Chapter 2

Published online: December 5, 2024

Blanchette VS, Brandão LR, Carcao MD, Kumar R, Rand ML, Revel-Vilk S (eds): SickKids Handbook of Pediatric Thrombosis and Hemostasis, ed 3, rev. and ext. Basel, Karger, 2024, pp 13–24 (DOI: 10.1159/000538206)

Hemostasis and Its Regulation

Margaret L. Rand[a] Shoshana Revel-Vilk[b] Sara J. Israels[c]

[a]Department of Laboratory Medicine & Pathobiology, University of Toronto, Division of Haematology/Oncology, Hospital for Sick Children, Toronto, ON, Canada; [b]Pediatric Hematology/Oncology Unit and Gaucher Unit, Shaare Zedek Medical Center, Faculty of Medicine, Hebrew University, Jerusalem, Israel; [c]Department of Pediatrics and Child Health, University of Manitoba, CancerCare Manitoba Research Institute, Winnipeg, MB, Canada

Introduction

At the site of vessel wall injury, adhesion, activation, and aggregation of platelets result in the formation of a platelet plug (primary hemostasis). Concurrent activation of the coagulation pathway results in the formation of covalently cross-linked fibrin that stabilizes the platelet plug (secondary hemostasis). Inhibitors of the coagulation cascade limit and confine the response (regulation of coagulation), and activation of the fibrinolytic pathway results in dissolution of the fibrin clot to maintain and/or restore blood vessel patency (fibrinolysis). The aim of this chapter is to summarize the complex process of hemostasis and its regulation, highlighting points that are relevant to the clinical care of the neonate, infant, and child/adolescent (<18 years of age) with reference to specific Chapters and Appendices with more detailed information or discussion.

Primary Hemostasis

Primary hemostasis is based on the formation of a platelet plug at a site of vascular injury. It has four sequential but overlapping phases: vasoconstriction, platelet adhesion, platelet activation, and platelet aggregation [1, 2].

Vasoconstriction

Immediate constriction of the vessel to temporarily decrease blood flow and pressure within the vessel occurs as a neurogenic response. Serotonin and thromboxane A_2 (TxA_2) released from activated platelets (see below) further promote and sustain vasoconstriction.

Platelet Adhesion

In the bloodstream, red blood cells (RBCs) predominate in the axial stream, with platelets marginated along the vessel wall by shear forces and collisions with RBCs. As a result, platelets are well positioned to monitor the integrity of the vessel wall. When endothelial damage occurs, platelets

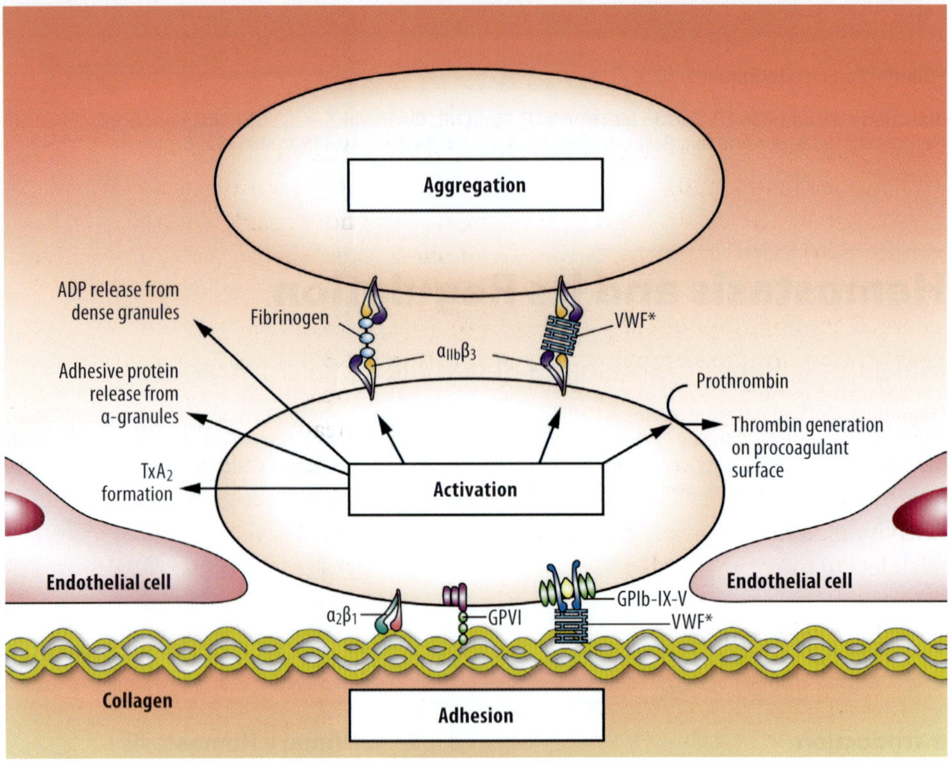

Fig. 1. A simplified diagram of platelet adhesion, activation, and aggregation in response to blood vessel wall damage and exposure of the subendothelium; the platelet plug that forms aids in the cessation of bleeding. Asterisks indicate interactions involving VWF that occur at high shear. Reproduced with permission from Israels and Rand [3]. ADP, adenosine 5′-diphosphate; GP, glycoprotein; TxA_2, thromboxane A_2; VWF, von Willebrand factor.

are captured by exposed collagen fibrils, the most thrombogenic component of the subendothelial matrix (Fig. 1). Adhesion of platelets to collagen is influenced by shear stress. At low shear, binding occurs via the integrin α2β1 (glycoprotein [GP] Ia-IIa) and GPVI receptors, while at high shear, binding occurs via the GPIb-IX-V receptor and von Willebrand factor (VWF) bound to the collagen. Platelet adhesion at the site of vessel wall damage initiates platelet activation events via intracellular signaling pathways.

Platelet Activation

Platelets adherent to the subendothelium undergo a dramatic shape change to an irregular sphere with multiple filipodia, spreading to increase their area of surface contact. During shape change, granules coalesce in the center of the platelet, fuse with the surface-connected canalicular system, and release their contents to the exterior. Secretion of adenosine 5′-diphosphate (ADP) from dense granules amplifies platelet recruitment and activation (Fig. 1). Release of VWF and fibrinogen (adhesive proteins) from α-granules enhances platelet adhesion and aggregation. Release of TxA_2, a second messenger synthesized via the cyclooxygenase (COX)-1 pathway, augments platelet activation and recruitment of additional platelets to the platelet plug (Fig. 1). Acetylsalicylic acid (ASA), the most commonly used antiplatelet drug, acts through irreversible inactivation of COX-1 (see Chapter 20).

Activated platelets undergo remodeling of the surface membrane resulting in exposure of phosphatidylserine on the cell surface. This negatively charged aminophospholipid provides a procoagulant surface for the assembly of the coagulation factors and generation of thrombin, the most potent platelet aggregating agent (Fig. 1). Thrombin triggers further secretion of storage granule contents and formation of TxA_2, both of which act to amplify platelet activation and recruit additional platelets to the primary plug.

Platelet Aggregation
Aggregation is an active process resulting from binding of the agonists ADP, TxA_2, and thrombin to their specific membrane receptors. ADP activates platelets via the P2Y1 and P2Y12 receptors; TxA_2 via the thromboxane-prostanoid (TP) receptor; and thrombin via binding to GPIb-IX-V and cleaving protease-activated receptor (PAR)1 and PAR4. The antiplatelet drugs clopidogrel, prasugrel, and ticagrelor act through blocking of the P2Y12 ADP receptor (see Chapter 20). Epinephrine stimulates aggregation via α2-adrenergic receptors, but only in the presence of other agonists. The binding of agonists to their receptors results in the activation of intracellular signaling pathways, ultimately converting integrin αIIbβ3 (GPIIb-IIIa) from a low-affinity resting state to a high-affinity activated state. Activated αIIbβ3 binds to plasma fibrinogen and VWF, the latter at high shear (Fig. 1). Divalent fibrinogen and multivalent VWF function as bridges between αIIbβ3 on adjacent activated platelets, resulting in aggregation and formation of the platelet plug. An animated summary of platelet plug formation in primary hemostasis can be viewed at the URL provided in [4]. Abnormalities of platelet adhesion, activation, and/or aggregation are associated with increased mucocutaneous bleeding [1] (see Chapter 6).

The Role of RBCs
RBCs are important contributors to platelet function; quantitative and qualitative changes in RBCs and their interactions with cellular and molecular components of the hemostatic system can impact both bleeding and thrombosis [5]. Decreased RBC mass reduces platelet margination and increases the risk of bleeding [6]; prevention and treatment of anemia in patients with bleeding disorders is of clinical benefit. RBC-related viscosity, rising nonlinearly with hematocrit, slows flow in small vessels and capillaries, and increases the risk of thrombosis. Reduced RBC deformability in acquired and inherited RBC disorders can be associated with increased risk of thrombosis.

2

Secondary Hemostasis

Secondary hemostasis results in the formation, via the coagulation pathway, of covalently cross-linked fibrin that stabilizes the platelet plug [7, 8]. The pathway is complex and involves many different proteins: zymogens (inactive precursors) of serine proteases (factor [F] II, FVII, FIX, FX, FXI, FXII), cofactors (tissue factor [TF], FVIII, FV), a transglutaminase zymogen (FXIII), and fibrinogen. A serine protease is an enzyme with the amino acid serine in its active site that hydrolyzes specific peptide bonds in proteins, and a transglutaminase is an enzyme that forms peptide bonds between the side chains of specific glutamine and lysine amino acid residues. Congenital and acquired deficiencies of FII, FV, FVII, FVIII, FIX, FX, FXI, FXIII, and fibrinogen can be associated with increased bleeding (see Chapters 8, 10, 11).

Serial activation of the serine protease zymogens and FVIII and FV, and feedback amplification loops result in the activation of FII (prothrombin) to FIIa (thrombin; Fig. 2) (note: acti-

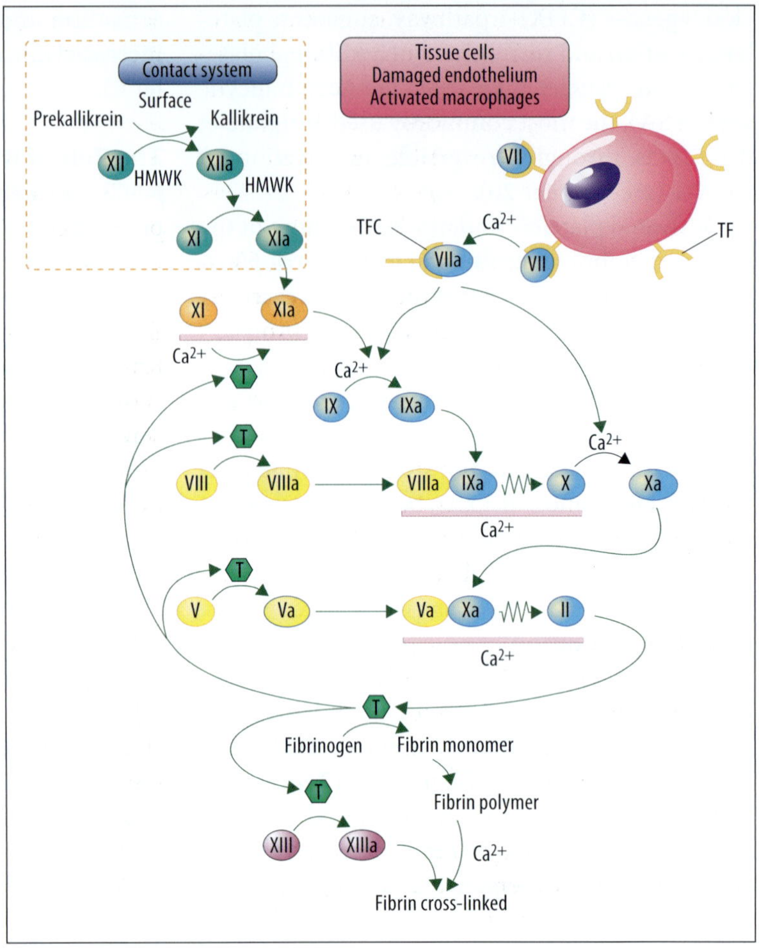

Fig. 2. Serial activation of coagulation zymogens and feedback amplification loops starting from the exposure/release of TF and ending in the generation of thrombin. The pink bars represent the negatively charged membrane surface upon which the enzyme complexes assemble. Reproduced with permission from Teitel [8]. HMWK, high-molecular-weight kininogen; T, thrombin; TF, tissue factor; TFC, tissue factor complex.

vated coagulation factors are denoted by the suffix "a"). The activation of the serine protease zymogens occurs on negatively charged phospholipid membrane surfaces of activated platelets, monocytes, and endothelial cells. Thrombin is a multifunctional enzyme that catalyzes reactions that promote coagulation, particularly the conversion of fibrinogen to fibrin monomer, and platelet activation, but also initiates pathways that limit coagulation, including activation of the natural anticoagulant protein C system.

The serine protease coagulation zymogens are synthesized in the liver. Vitamin K is an essential cofactor for γ-carboxylation of the N-terminal glutamic acid residues of the vitamin K-dependent zymogens FII, FVII, FIX, and FX; γ-carboxylation enhances the association of these factors with negatively charged phospholipid membrane surfaces. Vitamin K deficiency is associated with increased bleeding risk in newborns (see Chapter 3) and older children (see Chapter 11). Vitamin K antagonists are used for oral anticoagulation therapy (see Chapter 20). FVIII is synthesized in endothelial cells, and FV is synthesized in the liver and megakaryocytes (and stored in the α-granules of megakaryocytes and platelets). TF is an integral membrane GP that is expressed on fibroblasts and smooth muscle cells, but normally does not come into contact with flowing blood until there is endothelial cell damage.

Coagulation proceeds by the formation of three enzyme complexes on negatively charged procoagulant membrane surfaces in a Ca^{2+}-dependent fashion: the TF complex (TF/FVIIa), the tenase complex (FVIIIa/FIXa), and the prothrombinase complex (FVa/FXa). Each of these complexes involves a vitamin K-dependent protein (FVIIa, FIXa, FXa) and a cofactor (TF, FVIIIa, FVa). The coagulation pathway has three sequential overlapping phases: initiation, amplification, and propagation.

Initiation of Coagulation

At the site of vessel wall injury, blood comes into contact with cells that express TF on their surfaces, and TF-FVIIa complexes (TF/FVIIa) are formed [7, 8]. Historically referred to as the extrinsic pathway because of the extravascular location of TF, this pathway is the primary initiator of hemostasis in vivo. The TF/FVIIa complex activates small amounts of FX and FIX, forming FXa and FIXa. FXa forms a complex with FVa to convert limited amounts of FII (prothrombin) to FIIa (thrombin). Therapeutically, recombinant FVIIa can be used to promote hemostasis in patients with bleeding disorders such as hemophilia complicated by inhibitors (see Chapter 8), and Glanzmann thrombasthenia with bleeding refractory to other therapies (see Chapter 6). It also can be useful in acquired intractable or massive bleeding where standard hemostatic measures have not been adequate.

Amplification of Coagulation

Thrombin formed during initiation activates platelets, exposing the negatively charged membrane surface, releasing FV from the α-granules, and activating FXI, FVIII, and FV on the activated platelet surface.

Propagation of Coagulation

On the activated platelet surface, FIXa activated by TF/FVIIa during the initiation phase and by platelet-bound FXIa during the amplification phase binds to FVIIIa and Ca^{2+} in the tenase complex and activates FX to FXa. FXa then associates with FVa and Ca^{2+} in the prothrombinase complex, resulting in the activation of FII to form a massive amount of FIIa (thrombin burst).

The thrombin formed during the propagation phase of coagulation is of sufficient concentration to promote fibrin clot formation. Thrombin cleaves fibrinopeptides A and B from the Aα and Bβ chains, respectively, of fibrinogen to form fibrin monomer; fibrin monomers polymerize spontaneously to form an insoluble fibrin mesh. Thrombin also converts FXIII to FXIIIa, which stabilizes the fragile clot by covalently cross-linking fibrin, making the fibrin polymer resistant to lysis by fibrinolytic enzymes.

The Contact System

The contact factors (FXII, high-molecular-weight kininogen [HMWK] and prekallikrein) play a minor role in initiating coagulation in vivo (Fig. 2) [7, 8]. However, they are important in the initiation of the coagulation cascade in vitro (referred to as the "intrinsic pathway"), as measured by the activated partial thromboplastin time (aPTT).

Contact with a negatively charged surface (e.g., extracellular DNA, RNA, polyphosphate) activates FXII to FXIIa in the presence of prekallikrein and HMWK; FXIIa activates prekallikrein to kallikrein and FXI to FXIa. Kallikrein feeds back to activate additional FXII and cleaves HMWK to release bradykinin. Although in vitro activation of this pathway leads to thrombin generation, it does not play an in vivo role in the activation of FXI; deficiencies of FXII, prekallikrein, or HMWK are not associated with abnormal bleeding. However, the contact pathway is physiologically important in the activation of fibrinolysis, the complement pathway, and angiogenesis. It may also play a role in thrombosis, particularly thrombosis associated with contact activation by foreign surfaces [9].

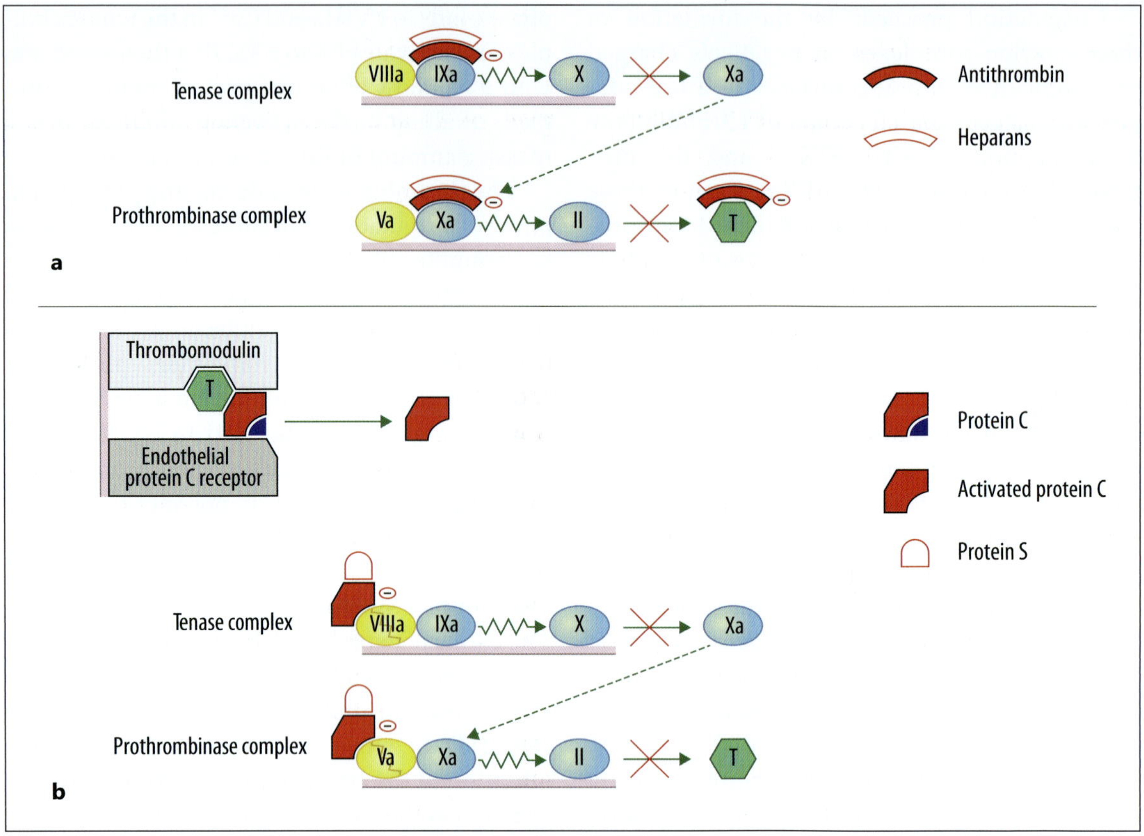

Fig. 3. Inhibitors of coagulation. **a** Antithrombin pathway. **b** Protein C pathway. The pink bars represent the negatively charged membrane surface upon which the enzyme complexes assemble. T, thrombin.

Regulators of Coagulation

Inhibitors of coagulation limit and confine the hemostatic response to sites of vascular damage by a multistep cascade [10]. There are three major endogenous anticoagulation pathways: tissue factor pathway inhibitor (TFPI), antithrombin (AT), and the protein C system (Fig. 3).

Tissue Factor Pathway Inhibitor

TFPI, the principal inhibitor of the initiation of coagulation (the TF-FVIIa pathway), inhibits FXa directly, and inhibits the activation of FIX and FX by TF/FVIIa, indirectly, through the formation of a quaternary complex FXa/TFPI/TF/FVIIa [7, 11]. TFPIα, the isoform present in plasma and released from platelets, requires protein S as a cofactor to efficiently bind and inhibit FXa. Therapeutically, inhibitors of TFPI are being evaluated in the management of bleeding in hemophilia and other inherited bleeding disorders (see Chapter 8).

Antithrombin

AT, a serine protease inhibitor (a member of the serpin superfamily), slowly reacts with, and irreversibly inhibits, the proteolytic activity of FXIa, FXa, FIXa, and FIIa (thrombin). Its inhibition of more than one factor in the coagulation cascade augments its effect [12]; it contributes the majority (approx. 75%) of antithrombin activity. Glycosaminoglycans such as heparan sulfate on the endothelial surface bind to AT and induce a conformational change that accelerates its inhibitory effect (approximately 1,000-fold in the case of thrombin inhibition) (Fig. 3a). The anticoagulant effect of therapeutic heparin is due to its enhancement of AT's inhibition of serine proteases, particularly FX and FII (see Chapter 20). Decreased plasma levels of AT are associated with an increased risk for venous thrombosis (see Chapter 13). Inhibition of AT synthesis is being pursued for therapeutic purposes in the management of bleeding in hemophilia (see Chapter 8).

Protein C System

Protein C, a vitamin K-dependent serine protease zymogen, is activated on the endothelial surface by thrombin bound to thrombomodulin. Thrombin bound to thrombomodulin gains the potential to activate protein C but loses its capacity to cleave fibrinogen. The endothelial membrane-associated protein C receptor is a cofactor that enhances the activation of protein C by thrombin/thrombomodulin (Fig. 3b). Activated protein C (APC) downregulates thrombin generation during the propagation phase of coagulation by inactivation of FVIIIa and FVa. Protein S, a vitamin K-dependent cofactor for TFPI, is also a cofactor for APC-mediated cleavage of FVIIIa and FVa and for efficient APC-dependent regulation of coagulation [13]. Decreased plasma levels of protein C or protein S are associated with increased risk for thrombosis. Recurring single nucleotide variants in FV (e.g., FV Leiden) or FVIII that result in their resistance to cleavage by APC also increase the risk of venous thrombosis (see Chapter 13).

α2-Macroglobulin

α2-Macroglobulin is a large plasma GP that inactivates a variety of proteases including thrombin and plasmin. It is synthesized in the liver and in macrophages. Plasma levels are higher in neonates and infants and remain higher than adult levels until adolescence (see Appendix II). α2-Macroglobulin compensates for lower circulating levels of AT and other protease inhibitors in the young.

Fibrinolysis

Fibrinolysis is the enzymatic pathway that cleaves fibrin, thereby localizing and limiting clot size and duration. The major enzyme of the fibrinolytic pathway is plasmin [14, 15]. It is the product of plasminogen cleavage by specific plasminogen activators, tissue plasminogen activator (tPA), and urokinase plasminogen activator (uPA) (Fig. 4). Plasmin cleaves fibrin into soluble fragments, i.e., fibrin degradation products (FDPs; the fragment most frequently measured is the D-dimer). Proteases released by neutrophils and other cells can also degrade fibrin to end products that are removed by phagocytosis, contributing to the pathophysiology of disseminated intravascular coagulation (DIC) [16] (see Chapter 11). Analogous to the coagulation system, the fibrinolytic pathway is regulated by both activators and inhibitors [17].

Plasminogen Activators

tPA, a serine protease synthesized by endothelial cells, is the primary intravascular activator of plasminogen (Fig. 4). The binding of plasminogen and tPA to fibrin forms a ternary complex, which amplifies the activity of tPA several hundred times and ensures that only fibrin-bound plasminogen is activated. When plasminogen is cleaved, the resulting plasmin remains bound to fibrin, where it is protected from inhibitors and is optimally positioned to degrade fibrin. Recombinant tPA is currently an important drug for therapeutic thrombolysis (see Chapter 20).

uPA (Fig. 4) is synthesized by monocytes/macrophages, fibroblasts, and epithelial cells, and is found in urine, plasma, and the extracellular

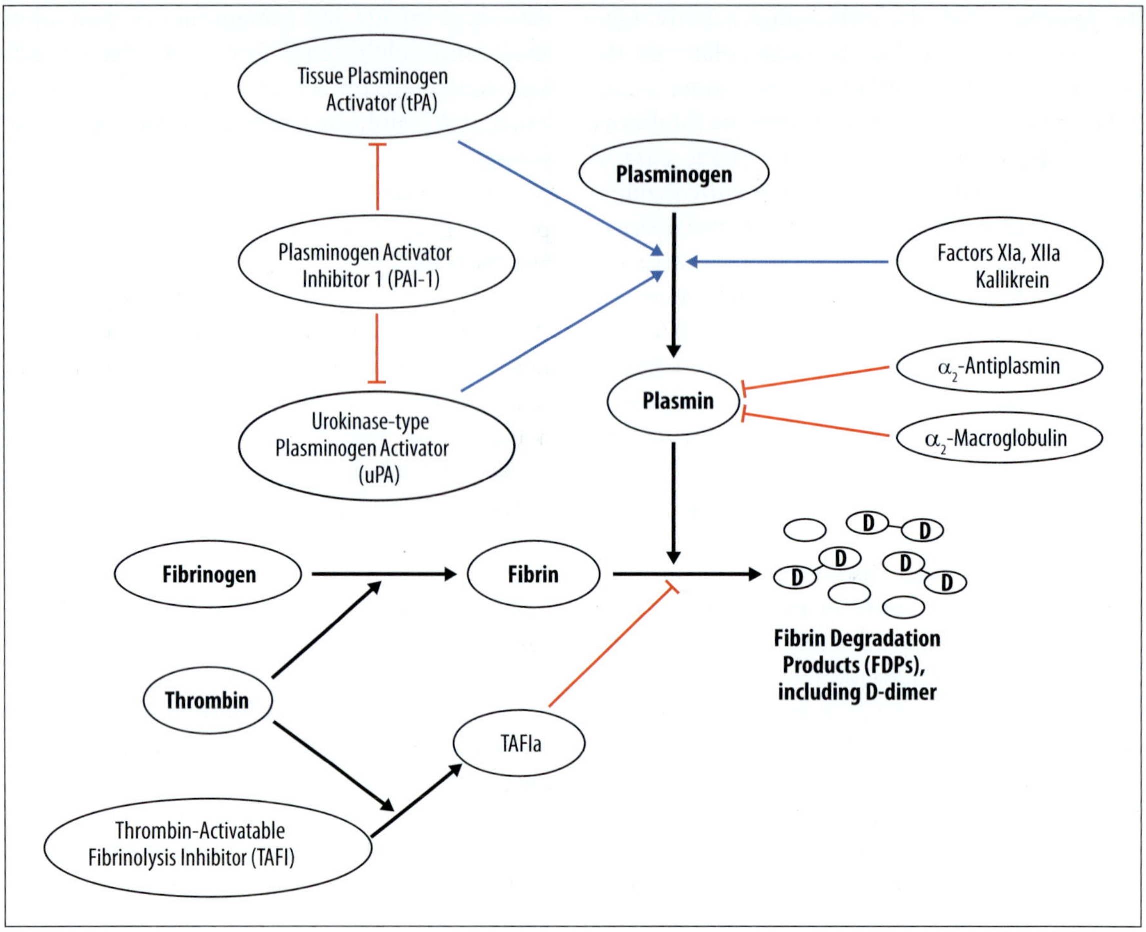

Fig. 4. The fibrinolysis pathway. FDPs, fibrin degradation products; PAI-1, plasminogen activator inhibitor type 1; TAFI, thrombin-activatable fibrinolysis inhibitor; tPA, tissue plasminogen activator; uPA, urokinase plasminogen activator.

matrix. It is secreted as an inactive single-chain molecule. At sites of vascular injury, kallikrein, FXIIIa, thrombin, or plasmin can cleave single-chain uPA into a two-chain active form. Activated uPA enhances fibrinolysis by further activation of plasminogen. The single-chain form also has enhanced activity when bound to receptors on leukocytes and platelets. In contrast to tPA, uPA can activate plasmin in the absence of fibrin. Urokinase can also be used for therapeutic thrombolysis (see Chapter 20).

Inhibitors of Plasminogen Activation

Plasminogen activator inhibitor (PAI)-1, a serpin, is the primary inhibitor of tPA and uPA (Fig. 4). It is synthesized in the liver, endothelial cells, and megakaryocytes, and is stored in endothelial cells and platelet α-granules. Fibrinolytic enzymes bound to fibrin are protected from inhibition, but PAI-1 can form stable complexes with unbound tPA and uPA that are then cleared by the liver. Deficiency of PAI-1 is associated with increased bleeding risk (see Chapter 10).

Thrombin-activatable fibrinolysis inhibitor (TAFI) inhibits fibrinolysis by interfering with formation of the fibrin-plasminogen-tPA complex. TAFI is activated by thrombin, thrombin/thrombomodulin, or plasmin (providing a link between coagulation and fibrinolysis). Reduced thrombin generation results in decreased levels of TAFIa and an increased rate of clot lysis; this mechanism may explain the premature lysis of clots in hemophilia (see Chapter 8). TAFIa is thermally unstable with a half-life of approximately 8 min and spontaneously converts to an inactive form, providing a means of autoregulation for the fibrinolytic system.

Inhibitors of Plasmin

α2-Antiplasmin (AP) (also called α2-plasmin inhibitor), a serpin, is the primary inhibitor of plasmin. It is synthesized in the liver, circulates in plasma, and is stored in platelet α-granules. α2-AP neutralizes both fibrin-bound and free (unbound) plasmin by binding to its catalytic and lysine-binding sites. The α2-AP-plasmin complexes are cleared by the liver. Deficiency of α2-AP is associated with increased bleeding risk (see Chapter 10). α2-Macroglobulin is also an important inhibitor of plasmin.

Fibrin Degradation Products

The degradation of the fibrin polymer by plasmin produces lytic fragments (FDPs), including cross-linked D-D fragments (D-dimers) (Fig. 4). Elevated plasma levels of D-dimers can be observed in the setting of thrombosis, inflammation, consumptive coagulopathy, liver disease, or malignancy (see Chapter 13) and indicate lysis of cross-linked fibrin. D-dimer measurement can be used in conjunction with additional clinical assessment to exclude the diagnosis of venous thromboembolism (see Chapter 14).

Developmental Hemostasis

Developmental hemostasis describes the evolution of the hemostatic system from fetal life to adolescence. This age-dependent development applies to all components of the hemostatic system: platelets and primary hemostatic proteins, the coagulation and fibrinolytic pathways, and their regulatory proteins [18, 19]. Although much of the evolution of hemostatic and regulatory proteins toward normal adult levels takes place within the first 6 months, some proteins do not reach adult levels until adolescence (see Appendix II).

Age-dependent differences are most significant during the neonatal period but can be considered as part of an age-appropriate balanced hemostatic system. Healthy neonates are not particularly prone to either bleeding or thrombosis. Risks of both bleeding and thrombosis are increased, however, in the setting of prematurity and illness [18, 19]. The hemostatic reserve of neonates and infants may be more easily depleted in the setting of sepsis, endothelial damage, and liver or cardiac dysfunction. Thrombocytopenia and procoagulant and anticoagulant deficiencies are common particularly in the setting of inflammatory diseases. Both hemorrhage and thrombosis can occur in these settings, sometimes both in the same patient. These scenarios are discussed more fully in Chapters 3, 14, 15, and 17.

Functionally, platelets in healthy neonates demonstrate relative in vitro hyporesponsiveness, with impaired adhesion, aggregation, and secretion. Platelet hypofunction may be compensated for by other contributors to primary hemostasis that enhance platelet/vessel wall interactions, including higher hematocrit and mean corpuscular volume (MCV), and higher levels of plasma VWF with enhanced adhesive activity due to an increased proportion of high-molecular-weight VWF multimers. Platelet hyporeactivity is more pronounced in premature infants. Platelet reactivity appears to improve during the first 2 weeks to 6 months of life [19, 20].

Hemostatic proteins do not cross the placenta; they are synthesized by the fetus and reach measurable levels at 10 weeks of gestational age. Functional levels of these proteins gradually increase during gestation and after birth, most attaining near adult values by approximately 6 months of age. Lower concentrations of coagulation proteins in healthy premature infants are compensated for by accelerated maturation, so that levels by 6 months of age are not substantially different from healthy term infants [19].

The levels of most coagulation factors increase during gestation and the postnatal period. In full term infants, levels of the vitamin K-dependent factors (FII, FVII, FIX, FX) and contact factors (FXI, FXII, prekallikrein) are approximately 50% of the levels shortly after birth, rise rapidly over the first 6 months, and then more slowly, reaching adult levels in adolescence. The activity of vitamin K-dependent factors is further reduced in preterm infants, to approximately 20–30% in 24–29 weeks' gestation infants. In contrast, levels of FVIII, FXIII, fibrinogen, and VWF in neonates are similar to levels in older children and adults (see Appendix II).

The capacity of newborn plasma to generate thrombin is decreased compared to that of adults because of decreased levels of coagulation factors, particularly prothrombin. Despite this, in vitro assays show more rapid initiation of thrombin generation, the result of decreased levels of TFPI. Decreased thrombin generation is balanced by a decreased rate of thrombin inhibition because plasma levels of AT and heparin-cofactor II are lower at birth and rise to adult levels at 3–6 months of life.

Levels of α2-macroglobulin are higher and may play a more significant role as a thrombin inhibitor in neonates and children, compensating for the low levels of AT. Levels of other endogenous anticoagulants including proteins C and S are also low at birth (see Appendix II), and mature during the first 6–12 months of life. However, protein S may be more functionally available for cofactor support of both the protein C and TFPI pathways in neonates because a higher proportion is circulating as free protein S; its plasma carrier protein, C4b-binding protein, is reduced [21].

The fibrinolytic activity of neonatal plasma is low, primarily due to plasma concentrations of plasminogen that remain low throughout the neonatal period. Levels of both fibrinolysis activators and inhibitors are not significantly different than adult levels after the first few days of life [21].

Understanding age-related differences in the hemostatic system is essential when evaluating neonates and infants with abnormal bleeding or thrombosis. The interpretation of, and response to, coagulation screening tests is a case in point. The "prolongation" of the prothrombin time (PT) and aPTT in a newborn is the result of low concentrations of many of the coagulation factors. However, this prolongation is not an accurate representation of the bleeding risk because of coexisting balanced decreases in the activity of the endogenous anticoagulants, which are not reflected in the PT and aPTT. Errors in the interpretation of these screening tests can lead to inaccurate diagnosis, unnecessary investigations, or inappropriate therapies. The use of age-specific reference intervals for hemostatic assays is key to avoiding these errors (see Appendix II).

Conclusion

Hemostasis is a complex process that relies on the equilibrium between procoagulant, anticoagulant, and fibrinolytic factors that interact to ensure appropriate hemostatic plug formation at sites of vascular injury. Disruption of this equilibrium resulting from structural abnormalities and/or aberrant concentrations of the components can lead to hemorrhage, thrombosis, or both. Understanding how the balance in the hemostatic system is maintained, and how it can be disrupted, is key to the diagnosis and management of hemostatic and thrombotic disorders in neonates, infants, and older children.

Conflict of Interest Statement

Shoshana Revel-Vilk has received research grants, speaker fees, and travel support from Pfizer, Sanofi Genzyme, and Takeda/Shire. Margaret L. Rand and Sara J. Israels have no conflicts of interest to declare.

Author Contributions

Margaret L. Rand drafted the chapter, critically revised the chapter, and approved the final version. Shoshana Revel-Vilk critically revised the chapter and approved the final version. Sara J. Israels drafted the chapter, critically revised the chapter, and approved the final version.

Abbreviations

α2-AP	α2-Antiplasmin
ADP	Adenosine 5′-diphosphate
APC	Activated protein C
aPTT	Activated partial thromboplastin time
ASA	Acetylsalicylic acid
AT	Antithrombin
COX	Cyclooxygenase
DIC	Disseminated intravascular coagulation
FDP	Fibrin degradation product
FII	Factor II (prothrombin)
FV	Factor V
FVII	Factor VII
FVIII	Factor VIII
FIX	Factor IX
FX	Factor X
FXI	Factor XI
FXII	Factor XII
FXIII	Factor XIII
GP	Glycoprotein
HMWK	High-molecular-weight kininogen
MCV	Mean corpuscular volume
PAI-1	Plasminogen activator inhibitor type 1
PT	Prothrombin time
RBC	Red blood cell
TAFI	Thrombin-activatable fibrinolysis inhibitor
TF	Tissue factor
TFPI	Tissue factor pathway inhibitor
TP	Thromboxane-prostanoid
tPA	Tissue plasminogen activator
TxA_2	Thromboxane A_2
uPA	Urokinase plasminogen activator
VWF	von Willebrand factor

2

References

1 Israels SJ, Kahr WH, Blanchette VS, Luban NL, Rivard G, Rand ML. Platelet disorders in children: a diagnostic approach. Pediatr Blood Cancer. 2011; 56(6):975–83.

2 Rand ML, Israels SJ, McNicol A. Platelet structure and function. In Israels SJ, editor: Mechanisms in Hematology, ed 4. Core Health Services; 2010. Available from: www.mechanismsinhematology.ca

3 Israels SJ, Rand ML. What we have learned from inherited platelet disorders. Pediatr Blood Cancer. 2013; 60(suppl 1):S2–7.

4 Mechanisms in Medicine: Platelet adhesion and aggregation. 2010. Available from: http://www.youtube.com/watch?v=0pnpoEy0eYE

5 Weisel JW, Litvinov RI. Red blood cells: the forgotten player in hemostasis and thrombosis. J Thromb Haemost. 2019; 17(2):271–82.

6 Thakar S, Gabarin N, Gupta A, Radford M, Warkentin TE, Arnold DM. Anemia-induced bleeding in patients with platelet disorders. Transfus Med Rev. 2021; 35(3):22–8.

7 O'Donnell JS, O'Sullivan JM, Preston RJS. Advances in understanding the molecular mechanisms that maintain normal haemostasis. Br J Haematol. 2019;186(1):24–36.

8 Teitel JM. Coagulation cascade. In Israels SJ, editor: Mechanisms in Hematology, ed 4. Core Health Services; 2010. www.mechanismsinhematology.ca

9 Hsu C, Hutt E, Bloomfield DM, Gailani D, Weitz JI. Factor XI inhibition to uncouple thrombosis from hemostasis: JACC review topic of the week. J Am Coll Cardiol. 2021;78(6):625–31.

10 Houston DS. Regulators of coagulation. In Israels SJ, editor: Mechanisms in Hematology, ed 4. Core Health Services; 2010. Available from: www.mechanismsinhematology.ca

11 Gierula M, Ahnstrom J. Anticoagulant protein S – new insights on interactions and functions. J Thromb Haemost. 2020;18(11):2801–11.

12 Rezaie AR, Giri H. Anticoagulant and signaling functions of antithrombin. J Thromb Haemost. 2020;18(12):3142–53.

13 Amiral J, Seghatchian J. Revisiting the activated protein C-protein S-thrombomodulin ternary pathway: impact of new understanding on its laboratory investigation. Transfus Apher Sci. 2019;58(4):538–44.

14 Chapin JC, Hajjar KA. Fibrinolysis and the control of blood coagulation. Blood Rev. 2015;29(1):17–24.

15 Parmar N, Albisetti M, Berry LR, Chan AK. The fibrinolytic system in newborns and children. Clin Lab. 2006;52(3–4): 115–24.

16 Popescu NI, Lupu C, Lupu F. Disseminated intravascular coagulation and its immune mechanisms. Blood. 2022; 139(13):1973–86.
17 Schaller J, Gerber SS. The plasmin-antiplasmin system: structural and functional aspects. Cell Mol Life Sci. 2011; 68(5):785–801.
18 Jaffray J, Young G. Developmental hemostasis: clinical implications from the fetus to the adolescent. Pediatr Clin North Am. 2013;60(6): 1407–17.
19 Davenport P, Sola-Visner M. Hemostatic challenges in neonates. Front Pediatr. 2021;9:627715.
20 Margraf A, Nussbaum C, Sperandio M. Ontogeny of platelet function. Blood Adv. 2019;3(4):692–703.
21 Will A. Neonatal haemostasis and the management of neonatal thrombosis. Br J Haematol. 2015;169(3):324–32.

Chapter 3

Published online: December 5, 2024

Blanchette VS, Brandão LR, Carcao MD, Kumar R, Rand ML, Revel-Vilk S (eds): SickKids Handbook of Pediatric Thrombosis and Hemostasis, ed 3, rev. and ext. Basel, Karger, 2024, pp 25–49 (DOI: 10.1159/000538217)

Bleeding in the Neonate

Natalie Mathews[a, b] Laura Avila[a, c, d] Hilary Whyte[c, e] Victor S. Blanchette[a, c]

[a]Division of Hematology/Oncology, Hospital for Sick Children, Toronto, ON, Canada; [b]Division of Hematology/Oncology, Centre Hospitalier Universitaire Sainte-Justine, Montréal, QC, Canada; [c]Department of Pediatrics, University of Toronto, Toronto, ON, Canada; [d]Child Health Evaluative Sciences, Research Institute, Hospital for Sick Children, Toronto, ON, Canada; [e]Division of Neonatology, Hospital for Sick Children, Toronto, ON, Canada

Introduction

Neonates may present at birth with a variety of bleeding manifestations, including intracranial hemorrhage (ICH), bleeding from the gastrointestinal tract, respiratory system, or skin. In the first few days of life, bleeding may also be seen at the umbilical stump or procedural site postcircumcision. Although hemostatic disorders are rare in neonates, they can be life-threatening and thus demand immediate attention once suspected. Thorough history-taking, including any family history of bleeding as well as maternal medical history and medications, can help reveal the etiology. Physical examination is also important for assessing whether the infant is unwell and for detecting the presence of bleeding sites, relevant congenital anomalies, and manifestations of systemic disease, such as hepatosplenomegaly. Laboratory values pertaining to coagulation should be interpreted in the context of the developing hemostatic system and specific neonatal reference values (see Chapter 2 and Appendix II, respectively). Among the potential causes of neonatal bleeding are neonatal thrombocytopenia, coagulation factor deficiencies, and combined disorders. These disorders may require urgent transport to a pediatric tertiary care center; transport considerations are included at the end of the chapter. Some definitions used throughout this section are listed in Table 1.

Neonatal Thrombocytopenia

Thrombocytopenia in neonates has classically been defined as an absolute platelet count below 150×10^9/L, irrespective of the gestational age (GA). However, this traditional definition remains controversial, as some studies suggest that preterm infants born before 33 weeks of gestation often have platelet count in the range of 100–150 $\times 10^9$/L [1, 2]. Irrespective of the normal reference value used, repeated platelet count lower than 100

Table 1. Definitions

Term	Definition
Neonatal period	First 28 days of extrauterine life
Low birth weight infant	Birth weight <2,500 grams
Very low birth weight infant	Birth weight <1,500 grams
Extremely low birth weight infant	Birth weight <1,000 grams
Preterm newborn	Infant born before week 37 gestational age
Term newborn	Infant born between weeks 37 and 42 gestational age
Small for gestational age infant	Infant with birth weight below the 10th percentile for gestational age
Large for gestational age infant	Infant with birth weight above the 90th percentile for gestational age

$\times 10^9$/L, confirmed in a venous blood sample and by examination of a well stained peripheral blood smear by an experienced individual, deserves further investigation.

Thrombocytopenia, as traditionally defined (i.e., platelet count <150 $\times 10^9$/L), has a relatively low incidence in the general neonatal population, occurring in 0.5–2% of unselected newborns as detected by cord blood sampling, and is severe (i.e., platelet count <50 $\times 10^9$/L) in only 30% of those cases. Conversely, thrombocytopenia is the most common abnormal hemostatic finding in the neonatal intensive care unit (NICU), affecting approximately one-third of all neonates during the course of their hospital stay. It is especially common in premature and extremely low birth weight infants, in whom thrombocytopenia may be due to one or more related etiologies. While the majority of these neonates exhibit mild (i.e., platelet count 100–150 $\times 10^9$/L) or moderate thrombocytopenia (i.e., platelet count 50–100 $\times 10^9$/L), 2% of neonates admitted to NICUs exhibit severe thrombocytopenia.

A practical approach for identifying the etiology of neonatal thrombocytopenia includes consideration of the time of onset as well as the clinical status of the neonate. Early thrombocytopenia is defined as thrombocytopenia presenting within the first 72 h of postnatal life and late thrombocytopenia as presenting thereafter. According to this approach, the most frequent causes of neonatal thrombocytopenia are summarized in Table 2.

Fetal and Early-Onset Thrombocytopenia

Chronic Fetal Hypoxia

This condition, which may develop in conjunction with maternal hypertensive disorders, maternal diabetes, or fetal growth restriction, is the most common cause of early-onset thrombocytopenia. Thrombocytopenia in the context of chronic fetal hypoxia tends to be mild to moderate. If all major hypertensive disorders of pregnancy are considered (preeclampsia, preexisting hypertension, and gestational hypertension), chronic fetal hypoxia affects approximately 10% of these newborns. Although the pathogenesis of neonatal thrombocytopenia in the context of maternal hypertension is not clear, it is thought to be associated with decreased megakaryopoiesis in the presence of normal thrombopoietin levels [3].

Not surprisingly, due to the intricate relationship between the maternal environment and fetal growth, thrombocytopenia is also seen in small for gestational age (SGA) infants. The mechanism of thrombocytopenia in SGA infants has been shown to be associated with decreased platelet production in the context of low megakaryocytic mass and inadequate thrombopoietin levels [4]. Most infants are asymptomatic, with thrombocytopenia being identified incidentally on a routine complete blood count. In general, thrombocytopenia associated with either maternal hypertension or fetal growth restriction is less severe

Table 2. Causes of neonatal thrombocytopenia by age of onset and clinical status

Onset	Disorder	Severity	Clinical findings
Fetal and early-onset thrombocytopenia (<72 h postnatal age)	Chronic fetal hypoxia (e.g., pregnancy-induced hypertension, IUGR)	Mild to moderate	Suggestive prenatal history, small for gestational age
	Alloimmune thrombocytopenia	Moderate to severe	Well-appearing
	Autoimmune thrombocytopenia	Moderate	Well-appearing
	Genetic syndromes	Moderate	Dysmorphic features, congenital anomalies
	Viral infections	Variable	Ill-appearing
	Perinatal asphyxia	Moderate	Ill-appearing
	Inherited thrombocytopenia	Variable	Well-appearing, dysmorphic features in some cases
Late-onset thrombocytopenia (>72 h of age)	Necrotizing enterocolitis	Moderate to severe	Ill-appearing
	Fungal infections/sepsis	Severe	Ill-appearing
	Drugs	Moderate to severe	Variable appearance at presentation
Variable onset	DIC	Severe	Ill-appearing
	Bacterial infections/sepsis	Variable	Ill-appearing
	KMP	Severe	Vascular tumors
	Thrombosis (e.g., portal vein, renal vein)	Moderate	Variable appearance at presentation
	Metabolic diseases	Variable	Ill-appearing
	MIS-N	Variable	Evidence of SARS-CoV-2

Modified with permission from Sola [61] and Goodnight and Hathaway [62]. DIC, disseminated intravascular coagulation; IUGR, intrauterine growth restriction; KMP, Kasabach-Merritt phenomenon; MIS-N, multisystem inflammatory disease in neonates; SARS-CoV-2, severe acute respiratory syndrome coronavirus-2.

and tends to improve spontaneously within 7–10 days after birth without requiring therapy (e.g., platelet transfusions).

Fetal and Neonatal Alloimmune Thrombocytopenia

Fetal and neonatal alloimmune thrombocytopenia (FNAIT) is the most common cause of *severe* thrombocytopenia in an otherwise *healthy* neonate, presenting in approximately 1 in 1,000–2,000 live births within the Caucasian population (the frequency is less well-known amongst other ethnicities). However, up to one-third of neonates with FNAIT have an additional condition that could account for a low platelet count. Fetuses and neonates affected by FNAIT may suffer life-threatening complications, including ICH.

FNAIT results from maternal immunization against paternally inherited fetal platelet alloantigens (shown in Fig. 1) that are not present on ma-

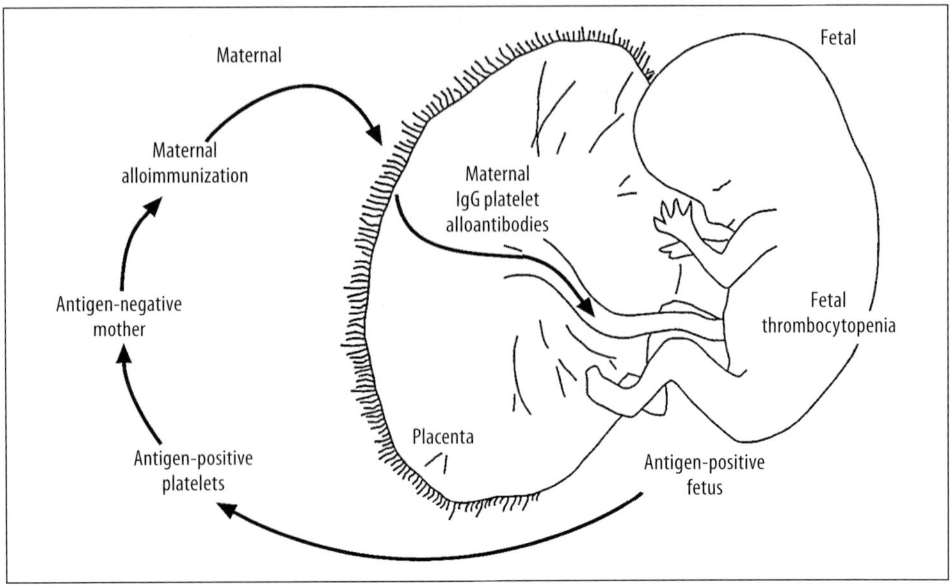

Fig. 1. Pathophysiology of fetal and neonatal alloimmune thrombocytopenia. From Dr. Victor Blanchette, with permission, personal communication. IgG, Immunoglobulin G.

ternal platelets. Fetal platelets express alloantigens early in the second trimester of gestation and cross the placenta. Exposure of a mother to fetal platelets bearing a platelet antigen of paternal origin that she does not share leads, in some cases, to maternal alloimmunization and production of alloantibodies directed against this "foreign" platelet alloantigen. Transport of maternal alloantibodies across the placenta into the fetal circulation occurs via fetal Fc receptors expressed in the placenta. The maternal alloantibodies opsonize fetal platelets leading to their accelerated removal from the circulation by phagocytic cells in the fetal reticulo-endothelial system (i.e., spleen, liver, and bone marrow). In addition, reduced platelet production due to targeting of fetal megakaryocytes by maternal alloantibodies has been described.

Human platelet antigens (HPAs), derived from glycoproteins (GPs) located in the platelet membrane, are the offending antigen in essentially all cases of FNAIT. Over thirty different HPA discordances have been implicated to date. HPA-1a is expressed on the platelets of 98% of Caucasians and is by far the most common FNAIT antigen involved in this race (80% of cases), followed by HPA-5b (10–15% of cases) [5]. FNAIT attributed to HPA-2a, HPA-3a, and HPA-15 occurs less frequently. HPA-1a antibodies are *not* typically encountered in Asian and African populations, for which HPA-5b antibodies have been commonly described [6, 7]. HPA-4b and HPA-3a antibodies are also well reported within Asian populations [7, 8], while GP IV/cluster of differentiation (CD) 36 antibodies have been implicated in individuals of both Asian and African ancestry [9]. Detailed information pertaining to FNAIT-related alloantibody discordances is unfortunately limited outside of the Caucasian population. A summary of known important alloantibodies implicated in FNAIT for various ethnic groups, and relative risks for severe bleeding, can be found in Table 3 [6, 10–14].

Table 3. Fetal and neonatal alloimmune thrombocytopenia alloantibodies reported by ethnicity and respective risks of severe bleeding [6, 10–14]

Ethnicity	Important alloantibodies to consider	Risk of severe bleeding
Caucasian	HPA-1a	High
	HPA-5b	Variable
	HPA-2a	May induce miscarriage, but no bleeding in neonates
	HPA-3a	High risk of ICH; may cause miscarriage
	HPA-15	Low
Asian	HPA-4b	Low
	HPA-5b	Variable
	HPA-3a	High risk of ICH; may cause miscarriage
	Glycoprotein IV (CD36)	Documented cases are limited; fatal ICH and severe thrombocytopenia have been reported
African	HPA-5b	Variable
	Glycoprotein IV (CD36)	Documented cases are limited; fatal ICH and severe thrombocytopenia have been reported

CD, cluster of differentiation; HPA, human platelet antigen; ICH, intracranial hemorrhage.

3

Of note, 20% of affected FNAIT cases present during the first pregnancy, which is an important distinction from the analogous alloimmune condition, hemolytic disease of the fetus/neonate, in which development of antibodies targeting fetal red blood cells during a first pregnancy is atypical. The majority of neonates with FNAIT present with cutaneous bleeding (petechiae, ecchymoses). However, 1 in 2,500 pregnancies may present with severe FNAIT (i.e., platelet count $<50 \times 10^9$/L), which is traditionally associated with HPA-1a incompatibility [10], in particular. HPA-5b mismatch has also been implicated in this severe phenotype [11]. Moreover, alloantibodies against HPA-3a and GP IV have also been associated with severe bleeding [12–14]. The most feared complication of severe FNAIT is ICH, which occurs in 10–20% of all clinically detected cases of FNAIT [15]. FNAIT is reportedly the most common cause of severe ICH in term newborns, and at least 50% of these ICH cases occur in utero. An unexplained intraparenchymal ICH in a term newborn is suggestive of FNAIT, and this diagnosis should be explored in these situations. Given the potential for developing life-threatening bleeding due to FNAIT, some experts have proposed that HPA-1a typing should be included within routine pregnancy care [16], although consensus is lacking.

Diagnosis

Diagnosing FNAIT serves two purposes: (i) to assist with the management of the index case and (ii) to help plan future pregnancies. However, es-

Table 4. Recommendations for transfusion in neonates based on clinical condition and platelet count, as published in the British guidelines [20]

Indication	Clinical condition	Threshold for platelet transfusion
Prophylaxis	High risk of bleeding (ECMO, perioperative for neurosurgery)[a]	<100 × 10^9/L
	Intermediate risk of bleeding (unstable patient, coagulopathy, invasive procedure, infants with FNAIT whose sibling has a history of ICH)[a]	<50 × 10^9/L
	Low risk (stable neonates, excluding FNAIT patients whose sibling has a history of ICH)[a]	<25 × 10^9/L
Active bleeding	Major	<100 × 10^9/L
	Nonmajor	<50 × 10^9/L

ECMO, extracorporeal membrane oxygenation; FNAIT, fetal and neonatal alloimmune thrombocytopenia; ICH, intracranial hemorrhage. [a]Thresholds for prophylactic platelet transfusion should be considered on a case-by-case basis, considering the etiology of the thrombocytopenia and local accessibility to platelets.

tablishing a laboratory diagnosis may be time-consuming and treatment of an infant for suspected FNAIT should *not* be delayed. The main component of laboratory diagnosis is based on the detection of antiplatelet alloantibodies in the maternal serum. Monoclonal antibody-specific immobilization of platelet antigens (MAIPA) is the gold standard laboratory test, but it is labor intensive. Increasingly, a solid phase enzyme-linked immunosorbent assay (ELISA) test is used. To determine the causative platelet antigen, or to further investigate a case that is highly suspicious for FNAIT despite negative antibody testing, platelet phenotyping and/or genotyping of both parents (by polymerase chain reaction [PCR], fluorescence, or ELISA-based techniques) are required and can be arranged in selected reference laboratories, such as the National Platelet Immunology Reference Laboratory through Canadian Blood Services (Winnipeg, Canada), the Versiti Blood Center (Milwaukee, USA), and Bloodworks Northwest (Seattle, USA).

Management of the Unexpected Case of FNAIT

The management plan, including the prophylactic platelet transfusion threshold, for each individual case of FNAIT, should be made in conjunction with an experienced hematologist and take into account the respective suspected or confirmed HPA discordance as well as the local accessibility of platelets, should they be required urgently. The PlaNeT-2 trial [17] established 25 × 10^9/L as a safe platelet transfusion cut-off in stable neonates. Some experts suggest that this threshold can be applied to nonbleeding neonates affected by FNAIT, although this practice is not evidence-based [18]. ICH rarely occurs in infants with FNAIT whose platelet count exceeds 30 × 10^9/L [19]. However, the British guidelines advise maintaining a platelet count above 50 × 10^9/L in neonates affected by FNAIT whose sibling has a past history of ICH [20]. Neonates with clinically significant bleeding (e.g., necessitating or prolonging admission or requiring red blood cell transfusion) should be also transfused to maintain platelet count above 50 × 10^9/L and those with diagnosed ICH should have platelet count kept above 100 × 10^9/L (see Recommendations for Platelet Transfusions section and Table 4). Since FNAIT is self-limited, and recovery of the platelet count usually occurs within 1–4 weeks, prophylactic platelet transfusion is recommended until platelet recovery. Transfusion of safe (i.e., tested for infectious diseases) HPA-typed platelets is the preferred treatment. When HPA-typed platelets are not available, irradiated and washed maternal platelets can also be used. However, these products are not available everywhere and are rarely available in the acute setting. Importantly, random donor platelets have been found to produce more modest, yet acceptable, increases in platelet count (by approximately 70×10^9/L according to a multicentered, international study for which transfusion volumes were not disclosed [21]), although the response is transient. Physicians should not hesitate to use random donor platelets when necessary. Because of the possibility of a poor response, it is generally recommended that a 30- to 60-min posttransfusion platelet count be obtained following an infusion of random donor platelets. Concomitant intravenous immunoglobulin (IVIG) at 1 g/kg daily for 1–3 days is recommended to help increase the lifespan of autologous platelets in cases that fail to respond to the initial infusion of random donor platelets, although a systematic review on postnatal treatment of FNAIT did not find clear evidence of its benefit [19]. In cases with organ or life-threatening bleeding that is refractory to random donor platelets and IVIG, every effort should be made to obtain and transfuse compatible antigen-negative platelets from the mother or a volunteer blood donor that have been tested for viral pathogens, e.g., hepatitis B, hepatitis C, and human immunodeficiency virus (HIV). Use and dosing of recombinant activated factor VII in this clinical setting remains controversial. If used, doses of 30 μg/kg every 3–4 h for up to a total of 6–7 doses, depending on clinical response, is a possible starting regimen for consideration by the clinical team caring for the affected infant.

Management of the Expected Case of FNAIT

The delivery of neonates with prenatal diagnosis of FNAIT should be planned, including, if possible, the availability of matched (antigen-negative compatible) platelets. During labor, fetal scalp monitoring should be avoided. The mode of delivery remains controversial, but elective cesarian section is often employed. In the event of vaginal delivery, the use of forceps and vacuum assistance should be avoided.

Imaging

Imaging studies, including ultrasound, magnetic resonance imaging (MRI), or computed tomography (CT), to rule out ICH in neonates with severe thrombocytopenia are recommended, as the presence of ICH guides the threshold for platelet transfusion (as above) and is the most relevant predictor of clinically relevant FNAIT for future pregnancies. Ultrasound is the most commonly used imaging technique. However, MRI and CT can also be used in this setting. CT can be performed rapidly and without sedation in the neonate, while MRI provides better resolution imaging of the brain parenchyma.

Future Pregnancies

Mothers who have delivered an infant with proven FNAIT should be referred to a specialist obstetric unit for counseling and management of future pregnancies. The risk of recurrence depends on the paternal zygosity for the pathologic platelet alloantigen. The recurrence rate of FNAIT due to HPA-1a mismatch in the Caucasian population is approximately 90% [22], and the severity of thrombocytopenia usually worsens in subsequent pregnancies. While the predictive value of high maternal HPA-1a antibody titers for severity of disease in the fetus is poor, a history of a previous child affected by ICH remains the best predictor of earlier and more severe thrombocytopenia due to FNAIT during subsequent pregnancies. Cases of FNAIT-affected fetuses whose sibling sustained ICH at 28 weeks of GA or more are considered high risk. Cases in which the sibling sustained ICH at <28 weeks are considered extremely high risk. Treatment of the mother with repeated infusions of IVIG (1–2 g/kg/week), starting at

3

12 weeks of gestation for mothers of children previously diagnosed with FNAIT *and* ICH, or at 20 weeks of gestation for mothers of children previously diagnosed with FNAIT *without* ICH in order to maintain a presumably safe fetal platelet count, is recommended in cases where the fetus is known to be antigen-positive [23]. Corticosteroid therapy (prednisone 0.5–1 mg/kg/day) should be added at 20 weeks of gestation for mothers of neonates with a previous history of ICH. It should be noted that invasive strategies, including cordocentesis to directly measure fetal platelet count and fetal platelet transfusion, are associated with significant complication rates and do not lower the risk of ICH; they are, therefore, not routinely recommended [24]. If the father is heterozygous for the offending alloantigen, PCR testing via amniocentesis for fetal platelet genotyping should be considered. Noninvasive techniques involving fetal platelet genotyping in maternal blood samples are new methods proposed in the literature. The choice of prenatal prevention strategy is based on the risk of ICH (i.e., standard, high, or extremely high risk). Further information, including detailed management algorithms, can be found in the article by Pacheco et al. [23].

Special cases of FNAIT have been reported in children born to females with platelet surface receptor disorders, such as Bernard-Soulier syndrome (BSS) and Glanzmann thrombasthenia (see below and in Chapter 6). Glanzmann thrombasthenia is a rare autosomal recessive disorder characterized by a defect in the GP IIb-IIIa receptor, which results in impaired platelet aggregation (see Chapter 6). A 2011 systematic review on the outcomes of pregnancy in women affected by Glanzmann thrombasthenia reported the presence of antibodies to GP IIb-IIIa in 73% of pregnancies [25]. Thrombocytopenia was documented in 7.5% of neonates, although most newborns were not tested. In utero deaths due to ICH occurred in 7% of the cases. In a 2010 systematic review of BSS in pregnancy, it was reported that 6 of 24 newborns in whom a platelet count was available developed FNAIT due to maternal sensitization against the GP Ib-IX-V complex [26]. Two of those cases suffered severe bleeding events (ICH and severe fetal gastrointestinal bleeding resulting in intrauterine death). Prospective registries that include imaging studies are warranted to more accurately investigate the risk of severe intrauterine bleeding in fetuses of mothers affected by these rare diseases.

Neonatal Autoimmune Thrombocytopenia

Thrombocytopenia can occur in neonates born to mothers affected by autoimmune thrombocytopenia. Maternal immune thrombocytopenia (ITP) is the most common condition, occurring at a frequency of 1/1,000–1/10,000 pregnancies, but autoimmune thrombocytopenia can also be secondary to other diseases such as systemic lupus erythematosus and autoimmune thyroid disease. Similar to FNAIT, trans-placental transport of maternal platelet antibodies (in this case, *auto*-antibodies) is implicated in the pathogenesis of neonatal autoimmune thrombocytopenia. However, in neonatal autoimmune thrombocytopenia, the decrease in platelet count tends to be mild to moderate. Approximately 10% of neonates born to mothers with ITP have been found to be thrombocytopenic at birth, with about half of those requiring treatment [27]. Whereas a clinical history of a thrombocytopenic sibling in the neonatal period is the best predictor of severe neonatal autoimmune thrombocytopenia in future pregnancies, new-onset maternal ITP, lower maternal platelet count, and history of maternal splenectomy for ITP are additional possible risk factors [27, 28].

Clinical Findings

Minor bleeding, including cutaneous bleeding and cephalohematoma, is the most common manifestation and may occur in 3% of those affected. As opposed to FNAIT, ICH is rare in neonatal autoimmune thrombocytopenia and the frequency is estimated to be at or below 1%.

Management

Neonates born to mothers with a history of ITP should have their platelet count monitored closely during the first few days of life, since the nadir of thrombocytopenia is usually reached after birth and typically during first 2–5 days of life. Resolution follows 7 days to a few weeks later. If the platelet count is below 25–30 × 10^9/L during the first week of life [17, 19], below 20 × 10^9/L after that, or if there is life-threatening bleeding, IVIG should be administered. The recommended initial dose is 1 g/kg daily, administered over 6–8 h for a total of 1–3 days. In cases with organ (e.g., ICH) or life-threatening bleeding or if IVIG is not available or fails to produce a clinically meaningful response, corticosteroid therapy (pulse intravenous [IV] methylprednisolone 30 mg/kg/dose × 1–3 days or oral prednisone 3–4 mg/kg/day divided into 3–4 doses/day × 3–4 days with no tapering) is recommended. In these emergent situations, platelet transfusion should also be administered to rapidly correct the platelet count, knowing, however, that these donor platelets will have a shortened lifespan. Head imaging studies to rule out ICH are recommended in cases of severe thrombocytopenia or if clinically indicated.

Genetic Syndromes

Thrombocytopenia has been reported in many chromosomal anomalies, including Turner syndrome, trisomy 13, trisomy 18, and triploidy. In addition to a lower platelet count, larger platelets have been reported in neonates with Down syndrome (trisomy 21). Affected infants tend to present with mild to moderately reduced platelet count and do not typically require treatment for thrombocytopenia solely attributed to a chromosomal anomaly. However, in neonates with Down syndrome, thrombocytopenia may also be associated with transient abnormal myelopoiesis (TAM), which occurs in 10% of this population (see below).

Clinical Findings

Clinical findings vary by syndrome. In any thrombocytopenic neonate with dysmorphic features and/or congenital anomalies, it is prudent to consider chromosomal syndromes that may affect platelet production and/or bone marrow function.

Management

See Recommendations for Platelet Transfusions section.

Perinatal Asphyxia

See section of Combined Disorders.

Inherited Thrombocytopenia

Inherited thrombocytopenia should be suspected in cases of persistent thrombocytopenia. The thrombocytopenia may be identified incidentally on a routine complete blood count or as part of evaluation of bleeding symptoms. Signs of cutaneous bleeding and bloody diarrhea often present in the neonatal period; bleeding from the umbilical stump or postcircumcision is also relatively common. Platelet counts at presentation may vary between mildly to severely decreased and platelet size may vary between small and large. A family history of thrombocytopenia, consanguinity, or dysmorphic features should raise the suspicion for inherited thrombocytopenia. For additional details on the different inherited thrombocytopenia syndromes, see Chapter 6.

Inherited Thrombocytopenia with Small Platelets

Syndromes Associated with the Wiskott Aldrich Syndrome Gene

Variations in the gene that encodes the Wiskott-Aldrich syndrome (WAS) protein on the short arm of the X chromosome are responsible for a wide spectrum of clinical phenotypes, characteristically encompassing classic WAS and X-linked thrombocytopenia. Approximately 4–10 in 1 million individuals will exhibit clinical manifestations relating to these disorders. Classic WAS features include thrombocytopenia in the neonatal period, susceptibility to infections due to combined immunodeficiency in early infancy, extensive eczema in infancy and childhood, and a tendency to develop malignancies (such as B cell lymphomas, leukemias) and autoimmune diseases (such as hemolytic anemia, neutropenia, arthritis, vasculitis, and inflammatory bowel disease) later in life.

Thrombocytopenia is often severe in these cases and is characterized by the presence of small platelets (3.8–5 fL, half the mean volume of normal platelets). Signs of cutaneous bleeding and bloody diarrhea often present in the neonatal period; bleeding from the umbilical stump or circumcision is also relatively common. X-linked thrombocytopenia is a milder variant, with less frequent and less severe extra-hematological manifestations, particularly eczema and infections.

Conventional supportive treatment includes IVIG and antimicrobial prophylaxis in relevant cases. With regard to thrombocytopenia, platelet transfusion is only indicated in the case of active bleeding. Platelets should be irradiated before transfusion because of the association of immunodeficiency with WAS. Additional treatment modalities beyond the neonatal period are discussed in Chapter 6.

Inherited Thrombocytopenia with Normal Size Platelets

Thrombocytopenia Absent Radius Syndrome

Thrombocytopenia absent radius (TAR) is a recessive disorder. In the majority of cases, it is caused by a compound inheritance affecting the *RBM8A* gene in chromosome 1q21.1, whereby one of the *RBM8A* copies is not functional and the expression of the other copy is reduced [29]. TAR is characterized by congenital or early thrombocytopenia and bilateral absence of the radii. The thumbs can be hypoplastic but are always present. Thrombocytopenia, due to abnormal megakaryopoiesis, is usually present at birth or develops early in infancy. Bleeding manifestations can be severe in neonates; however, platelet count can fluctuate and spontaneous improvement in the platelet count typically occurs after the first year of life. Other common manifestations include other limb, cardiac, central nervous system, and genitourinary anomalies. Interestingly, almost half of affected neonates also have associated cow's milk allergy, and thrombocytopenia can be triggered by exposure to these dairy products, including cow's milk formula. Platelet transfusions should be given in the event of bleeding episodes. Due to spontaneous improvement of platelet count over time, hematopoietic stem cell transplantation is generally not necessary.

Amegakaryocytic Thrombocytopenia with Radio-Ulnar Synostosis

Pathogenic variations within the *HOXA11* gene are responsible for this rare autosomal dominant disorder, which is characterized by early neonatal amegakaryocytic thrombocytopenia and bilateral proximal fusion of the radius and ulna. Amegakaryocytic thrombocytopenia with radio-ulnar synostosis (RUSAT1) is also associated with sensorineural hearing loss and the development of aplastic anemia in childhood.

Congenital Amegakaryocytic Thrombocytopenia

Congenital amegakaryocytic thrombocytopenia (CAMT) is an autosomal recessive disorder involving pathogenic variants in *MPL*, the thrombopoietin receptor gene, resulting in congenital severe thrombocytopenia that ultimately progresses to bone marrow failure during childhood. Newborns with CAMT can have severe bleeding episodes during the first weeks of life. Physical anomalies tend to be limited to the head region, involving the brain, eyes, or orbit [30]. Anomalies involving the skeletal, cardiac, or urogenital systems would strongly suggest a different diagnosis. During the neonatal period, management includes supportive therapy with platelet transfusion if clinical bleeding occurs; transfused platelets should be irradiated, as neonates with CAMT may require an eventual stem cell transplantation. Eventual hematopoietic stem cell transplantation remains the only curative therapy available at present.

Inherited Thrombocytopenia with Large Platelets

Myosin Heavy Chain 9-Related Disease

May-Hegglin anomaly, Sebastian platelet syndrome, Epstein syndrome, and Fechtner syndrome are a group of rare and predominantly autosomal dominant macrothrombocytopenias encompassed within myosin heavy chain 9-related disease (MYH9-RD). The finding of pathognomonic Döhle body-like neutrophil cytoplasmic inclusions in conventionally stained (i.e., May-Grünwald-Giemsa or Wright) peripheral blood smears or by immunofluorescence confirms the diagnosis of MYH9-RD. These aggregates contain myosin IIA, ribosomes, and MYH9 messenger RNA (mRNA), the latter being responsible for the appearance of the inclusions. However, mRNA is degraded with time and therefore, the inclusions may be difficult to detect in standard stains. In contrast, immunofluorescence staining is a sensitive (100%) and specific (95%) technique for detection of these inclusions. Genetic testing of the *MYH9* gene can also be performed. Apart from the presence of macrothrombocytopenia (with mean platelet volume [MPV] >12 fL) at birth, nonhematologic manifestations, including sensorineural deafness, cataracts, and nephritis, can occur and are usually detected later in life. Easy bruising can be present during the neonatal period, though bleeding is not usually a major problem; further, newborns do not seem to be at higher risk for ICH. Platelet transfusions are indicated to control bleeding complications and may be used prophylactically in the perioperative setting for at-risk neonates. Additional information pertaining to MYH9-RD can be found in Chapter 6.

Bernard-Soulier Syndrome

BSS is a rare autosomal recessive disorder secondary to quantitative or qualitative abnormalities in the platelet GPIb-IX-V complex that causes abnormal von Willebrand factor (VWF)-mediated platelet adhesion and leads to moderate to severe macrothrombocytopenia. Bleeding symptoms and signs, such as epistaxis and gingival bleeding, start early in childhood and are disproportional to the platelet count. Although it usually presents later, a few cases have been reported in the neonatal period. Diagnosis of BSS can be established by the presence of macrothrombocytopenia, reduced or absent ristocetin-induced platelet aggregation with normal aggregation in the presence of other agonists, and low or absent GPIb-IX-V complex (CD42a-d) by flow cytometry. Genetic testing for variations in *GP1BA*, *GP1BB*, and *GP9*, which encode 3 of the 4 subunits of the GPIb-IX-V complex, can also be performed. Additional information pertaining to BSS can be found in Chapter 6.

Gray Platelet Syndrome

The hallmark of this rare autosomal recessive disorder is thrombocytopenia associated with abnormally large platelets that display markedly decreased or absent alpha granules. Variants within the *NBEAL2* gene have been identified as a cause of this syndrome, which probably involves defective protein storage or packaging during biogenesis of the platelet alpha-granules. Although Gray platelet syndrome (GPS) can present soon after birth (usually with easy bruising), the mean onset is in early childhood. The severity of bleeding symptoms and the degree of thrombocytopenia vary but tend to be moderate to severe. The typical appearance of platelets on conventionally stained peripheral blood smears (i.e., pale gray and larger than normal) is highly suggestive of this syndrome. Platelet thin section electron microscopy confirms the diagnosis. Additional information pertaining to GPS can be found in Chapter 6.

Thrombocytopenia Paris-Trousseau Type and Jacobsen Syndrome
Clinical findings in these two syndromes, which are both associated to terminal 11q deletions, typically overlap. Deletion of the *FLI1* gene, in particular, is believed to be the cause of thrombocytopenia encountered in both of these syndromes [31]. Cognitive impairment, dysmorphic features, growth retardation, and cardiac abnormalities are also commonly seen in both entities. Neonates diagnosed with thrombocytopenia Paris-Trousseau type tend to present during the first month of life with severe thrombocytopenia and a mild bleeding phenotype. Dysmegakaryocytopoiesis with micromegakaryocytes is common. In Jacobsen syndrome, thrombocytopenia is also associated with dysmegakaryocytopoiesis. Clinically significant bleeding should be treated with platelet transfusions. Additional information pertaining to these disorders can be found in Chapter 6.

Platelet-Type von Willebrand Disease
Platelet-type von Willebrand disease (PT-VWD) is an autosomal dominant disorder caused by variations in the gene encoding the alpha subunit of the platelet GP Ib-IX-V complex. The abnormal GP Ib alpha receptor exhibits enhanced affinity with spontaneous binding to its ligand, VWF. As a consequence of this increased interaction, platelets and high-molecular-weight VWF multimers are cleared from circulation. Platelet-type VWD is rare, with only 55 cases reported to date. At baseline, neonates have a normal platelet count. However, under stress, they can develop macrothrombocytopenia and a mild to moderate bleeding phenotype. Importantly, platelet-type VWD is clinically indistinguishable from VWD type 2B, which similarly involves increased platelet-VWF binding, but is due to a gain-of-function variant within the *VWF* gene. Differentiating these two diagnoses is important for guiding treatment. Both disorders will reveal heightened platelet agglutination in the presence of low concentrations of ristocetin but can be distinguished through mixing platelets with normal plasma to determine if platelet aggregation returns to normal values (as in VWD type 2B), flow cytometry, and/or genetic testing. Neonates with platelet-type VWD require platelet transfusion in the case of major bleeding; adjunctive therapies (i.e., antifibrinolytic agents) can be utilized for minor bleeding events. Of note, desmopressin is *not* recommended due to risk of exacerbating thrombocytopenia. Moreover, desmopressin poses a risk of iatrogenic hyponatremia within this age group. Additional information can be found in Chapters 6 and 9.

Inherited Bone Marrow Failure Syndromes with Thrombocytopenia

CAMT, TAR syndrome, and RUSAT1 are described above.

Fanconi Anemia
Cytogenetic instability, progressive pancytopenia, and a high risk to develop malignancies, such as acute myeloblastic leukemia, characterize this autosomal recessive or, rarely, X-linked, form of inherited bone marrow failure. Several genes have been implicated, with *FANCA* variants being found in 65% of cases [32]. Phenotypic expression is highly variable: short stature, skin hyperpigmentation, abnormal thumbs and radii, microcephaly or hydrocephaly, microphthalmia, and developmental delay are commonly found congenital abnormalities. About one-third will have no additional anomalies. Hematological manifestations of Fanconi anemia usually present later in childhood. However, cases of neonatal onset have been reported and it may present as isolated thrombocytopenia. The diagnosis is typically made following abnormal chromosomal breakage analysis of lymphocytes. Management of Fanconi anemia is beyond the scope of this chapter.

Late-Onset Thrombocytopenia (>72 h)

Late-Onset Sepsis

See Combined Disorders section.

Necrotizing Enterocolitis

This disease of unclear pathophysiology almost exclusively affects very low birth weight infants, having a prevalence of 5–10%. It is characterized by the presence of an excessive inflammatory process and, therefore, systemic manifestations including hematological abnormalities are common. Moreover, necrotizing enterocolitis (NEC) is the greatest contributor to nonchronic thrombocytopenia in tertiary NICUs. Thrombocytopenia has been reported to correlate with NEC severity and mortality, and to indicate a poor prognosis. Moderate to severe thrombocytopenia (platelet count $<100 \times 10^9$/L) affects up to 95% of neonates with NEC at diagnosis [33] and usually recovers after 7–10 days. Coagulopathy is seen in up to a third of affected neonates. Peripheral platelet destruction appears to be the causative mechanism, although decreased production may contribute to thrombocytopenia. Platelet activating factors, implicated in the pathogenesis of NEC, may affect thrombopoiesis in unclear ways. The majority of infants are noted to have an incidental thrombocytopenia on a complete blood count performed as an investigation of NEC. Platelet concentrates should be administered following current neonatal transfusion guidelines (see below). In vivo survival of transfused platelets is expected to be shortened in neonates with NEC.

Drug-Induced Thrombocytopenia

Drugs administered to either the mother or the neonate can cause neonatal thrombocytopenia. Cases related to administration of vancomycin, amphotericin B, and valproic acid have been described. The frequency of thrombocytopenia in neonates receiving linezolid has been estimated to be 2% and a case of meropenem-induced pancytopenia in a preterm infant during the first week of life has been reported [34]. Indomethacin-associated thrombocytopenia has been reported in 10% of very low birth weight infants, though studies comparing surgical ligation and indomethacin in the treatment of patent ductus arteriosus did not show significant difference between groups.

Drugs administered to the mother may induce immunoglobulin G (IgG) antibodies directed against drug-epitopes that can lead to thrombocytopenia in the mother and also cross the placenta thus affecting the fetus. Cases of neonatal thrombocytopenia secondary to maternal exposure to quinine and to valproic acid have been reported.

While heparin administration can lead to heparin-induced thrombocytopenia in 0.2–5% of adults, a systematic review found no cases of heparin-induced thrombocytopenia among 325 neonates included in well-designed cohort studies [35]. Thus, other causes of thrombocytopenia are more likely and should be investigated in neonates exposed to heparin.

Variable Onset Neonatal Thrombocytopenia

Viral Infections

Neonatal TORCH (toxoplasmosis, rubella, cytomegalovirus, herpes simplex virus-2) infections can present with thrombocytopenia. Mixed mechanisms may be responsible for thrombocytopenia, including impaired platelet production due to suppression of proliferation and cytotoxic effects on megakaryocytes and their precursors, and accelerated platelet removal. Cytomegalovirus is one of the most common causes of congenital infection. The classical findings include jaundice, hepatosplenomegaly, and petechiae and occur in 10–15% of affected neonates. Platelet count less than 50×10^9/L are found in half of these cases.

Severe thrombocytopenia secondary to parvovirus B19 has been reported. Enterovirus infections have also been associated with neonatal thrombocytopenia in the context of hepatitis. HIV-associated thrombocytopenia is uncommon in affected neonates, although almost 50% of newborns exposed to HIV during pregnancy, though not necessarily infected, manifest low platelet count after birth (ranging between 50 and 150 × 10^9/L). In HIV-infected infants, thrombocytopenia should improve approximately 1 week after starting adequate antiretroviral therapy.

To date, there has not been convincing evidence that neonatal severe acute respiratory syndrome coronavirus-2 (SARS-CoV-2) infection is associated with thrombocytopenia. However, there is emerging evidence that neonates may experience systemic inflammatory responses, with associated severe thrombocytopenia, in the aftermath of an acute SARS-CoV-2 infection (see Multisystem Inflammatory Syndrome in Children/Neonate section).

Bacterial Infections
See Combined Disorders section.

Thrombosis
The main peak incidence of thrombosis in children occurs during the neonatal period, with an incidence of approximately 15.5 per 1,000 admissions to NICUs [36]. Central access devices and prematurity are major risk factors in this age group. Renal vein thrombosis, the most prevalent non-catheter-related thrombotic event in neonates, presents with a triad of thrombocytopenia, a palpable abdominal mass and hematuria, although the complete triad is present in less than a quarter of neonates. Almost 50% of neonates with renal vein thrombosis have thrombocytopenia at presentation. The large majority of cases are detected within the first 3 days of life. Platelet counts below 100 × 10^9/L have also been reported in almost 20% of neonates with portal vein thrombosis. Almost half of these neonates, however, had additional conditions (sepsis, NEC) that would account for the presence of thrombocytopenia. Diagnosis and management of neonatal venous thrombosis is reviewed in Chapters 14 and 16.

Disseminated Intravascular Coagulation
See Combined Disorders section.

Metabolic Diseases
A few inborn errors of metabolism, such as propionic acidemia, mevalonic aciduria, storage diseases, Pearson syndrome, and neonatal hemochromatosis have been reported to be associated with isolated cases of neonatal thrombocytopenia. Further description of each of these diseases is beyond the scope of this chapter.

Inherited and Acquired Thrombocytopenia Related to GATA-1 Variants
Dyserythropoietic anemia with thrombocytopenia (or X-linked macrothrombocytopenia), X-linked thrombocytopenia with beta-thalassemia, Down syndrome-associated TAM, Down syndrome-associated acute megakaryoblastic leukemia, and X-linked anemia with or without neutropenia and/or platelet abnormalities are all rare conditions caused by inherited or somatic variations within the *GATA-1* gene. Defective megakaryocyte maturation with severe thrombocytopenia and bleeding since birth has been reported in cases of dyserythropoietic anemia with thrombocytopenia. Moderate thrombocytopenia due to dysmegakaryocytopoiesis, platelet dysfunction, reticulocytosis, and globin synthesis imbalance resembling beta-thalassemia have been described among neonates with X-linked thrombocytopenia with beta-thalassemia.

Down syndrome-associated TAM occurs in 10–30% of newborns with constitutional or mosaic trisomy 21 [37]. The median age at diagnosis is 3 days of life [38] and the median platelet count ranges between 96 and 125 × 10^9/L in reported series [38–40]; 41% of cases present with platelet count below 100 × 10^9/L [38]. Common findings are hepatosplenomegaly, pleural or pericardial effusions, ascites, and liver fibrosis secondary to megakaryocytic infiltration, jaundice, vesiculopapular skin lesions, anemia, leukocytosis, and thrombocytopenia. The hematological abnormalities associated with TAM often resolve spontaneously within two to three months. However, early mortality occurs in 10–20%, and 20% of affected neonates develop acute myeloid leukemia within the first 4 years of life [38–40]. Low-dose cytarabine should be considered for neonates with risk factors for early death including hyperleukocytosis (white blood cell count >100 × 10^9/L), hydrops, liver failure, ascites, pericardial or pleural effusion not secondary to cardiac failure, renal dysfunction, bleeding diathesis, and preterm delivery [40].

Kasabach-Merritt Phenomenon

See Combined Disorders section.

Multisystem Inflammatory Syndrome in Children/Neonate

Multisystem inflammatory disease in children (MIS-C) is a new diagnosis in the wake of the SARS-CoV-2 pandemic and is characterized by the presence of fever, multiorgan inflammation, and SARS-CoV-2 infection. A systematic review of multisystem inflammatory disease in neonate (MIS-N) divided this diagnosis into early and late MIS-N, depending on whether the diagnostic criteria were met within or after the first 72 h of life [41]. Cardiovascular, respiratory, and/or gastrointestinal involvement presented most commonly. Thrombocytopenia was reported in just over one-quarter of neonates, and need for platelet transfusion has been rarely reported [42, 43]. Management has included anti-inflammatory and antimicrobial medications as well as supportive care. Mortality is markedly higher in neonates than in older children at 9.2–11% versus 1.9%, respectively [41, 44].

Recommendations for Platelet Transfusions

Transfusion of platelet concentrates is the only therapy available for management of many causes of neonatal thrombocytopenia. However, careful consideration should be given prior to administration of platelets, as associated risks include transfusion reactions and transmission of viral or bacterial infections. Furthermore, platelet nadirs have not been shown to be predictors of clinically significant bleeding in the premature neonatal population [45].

In the past, guidelines for prophylactic platelet transfusions (i.e., the neonate is not bleeding) were based almost entirely on expert opinion. In 2019, the results of the multicenter randomized clinical trial, the PlaNeT-2 study, were published [17]. PlaNeT-2 compared two different platelet transfusion thresholds (50 × 10^9/L and 25 × 10^9/L) in premature neonates (<34 weeks GA), demonstrating a higher rate of mortality or major bleeding episodes over the subsequent 28 days in those who were transfused to maintain a platelet count of 50 × 10^9/L. This liberal transfusion group was also found to have a higher incidence of bronchopulmonary dysplasia. These findings suggest that a prophylactic platelet transfusion of 50 × 10^9/L is an inappropriately high threshold in nonbleeding neonates. However, both the clinical condition of the neonate and the availability of platelets for transfusion need to be taken into consideration when recommending thresholds for platelet transfusions (see Table 4). Importantly, the strategy described in Table 4 does not consider abnormalities in platelet function.

Platelets for neonatal transfusions should be, if possible, single donor, Rhesus (Rh) compatible, and ABO blood type-specific. ABO compatibility of the plasma present in the platelet product is an important consideration when ABO blood type-specific products are not available. Group O platelets administered to group A or B neonates can cause hemolysis because of the passive transfer of anti-A or anti-B present in the plasma and, thus, platelets

3

should be volume reduced in this situation. Platelets should be irradiated if administered to neonates with congenital immunodeficiency, malignancy, or conditions associated with bone marrow failure as well as in cases of transfusions from family members, particularly when maternal platelets are transfused to newborns with FNAIT. Some centers irradiate all platelet transfusions administered to neonates in order to prevent transfusion-associated graft-versus-host disease in potentially not-yet-diagnosed cases of cellular immunodeficiency or bone marrow failure. Cytomegalovirus-seronegative or leukoreduced (to obtain a white cell count $<5 \times 10^6$/unit) products, which are standard of care in many countries, are recommended, especially for low birth weight infants. Pathogen-reduced platelet systems, which are aimed to decrease the incidence of transfusion-associated infections, have been associated with similar adverse reaction rates to those seen with conventional platelets [46]. The recommended volume of transfusion ranges between 10 and 20 mL/kg [18], with 10 mL/kg being standard dosing for neonates in North America (see Appendix III). While dosing can vary, depending on the product available in the local blood bank, the question of whether a lower volume (5 mL/kg) is safer and more efficacious for neonates than a standard volume (15 mL/kg) will be explored in the upcoming PlaNcT-3 study [47]. While evidence on transfusion duration in neonates is lacking, some experts recommend transfusing platelets over 2–3 h in neonates to reflect a maximum rate of 5 mL/kg/h to mitigate intraventricular hemorrhage risk due to circulatory overload [48].

Inherited Coagulation Factor Deficiencies

von Willebrand Disease

VWD Type 1, the most common type of VWD, is not usually recognized in the neonatal period due to increased VWF levels at this age. Type 3, the most severe form, in which VWF is <5%, is an autosomal recessive or compound heterozygous disorder that may manifest in newborns, but has rarely been reported (see Chapter 9). Type 2B VWD, which is of interest in the newborn period due to its association with thrombocytopenia, is reviewed in Chapter 9.

Hemophilia A and B

These two X-linked disorders are increasingly diagnosed at earlier ages, either secondary to prenatal diagnosis (known carriers or a positive family history) or due to early bleeding events. Hemophilia is the most common inherited bleeding disorder manifesting in neonates.

Delivery of the Infant with Possible/Confirmed Hemophilia

The delivery of any infant with possible hemophilia should occur in a hospital setting. Once delivery is imminent, it is critical to notify the blood bank, neonatology team, and hemophilia treatment team. The optimal mode of delivery is a matter of debate. The risk of ICH in neonates with hemophilia at delivery has been reported at 0.8–2.3% versus <0.2% in the general population [49]. A study of 926 neonates with moderate or severe hemophilia reported ICH rates of 2.4% and 1.7% in those delivered by spontaneous vaginal delivery and cesarian section, respectively, and major bleeding in 4.2% and 5.8%, respectively; however, neither of these differences were statistically significant [50]. For infants with hemophilia who are born via spontaneous delivery, the use of instrumentation has been shown to increase ICH risk by 10.6-fold [51]. Instrumentation, as well as invasive monitoring and scalp blood sampling, should be avoided in this population. The British Guidelines [52] recommend a case-by-case approach for delivery of infants in which a diagnosis of moderate or severe hemophilia is suspected, taking into account obstetric indications, fetal hemophilia status, and sex to decide the mode of delivery (spontaneous vaginal delivery or planned cesarian section).

Table 5. Guide to surgical prophylaxis during neonatal circumcision for severe hemophilia A and B

Severe hemophilia A	On the day of the procedure, have the neonate arrive to the hospital early in the morning to receive FVIII.		
	Verify that FVIII (__________= brand name) is available.		
	Administer bolus dose of FVIII 250 IU IV prior to the procedure.		
	Commence oral tranexamic acid 1 h prior to the procedure 50 mg* three times daily for 10 doses.		
	Avoid topical sealants (to minimize exposure to plasma products).		
	In most cases, the neonate can be discharged the same day if there are no bleeding concerns.		
	If necessary, administer a second bolus of FVIII 250 IU the following day.		
Severe hemophilia B	On the day of the procedure, have the neonate arrive to the hospital early in the morning to receive FIX.		
	Verify that FIX (__________= brand name) is available.		
	Select one of the following:	FIX *not* conjugated to polyethylene glycol	Administer bolus dose of 80–100 IU/kg IV prior to the procedure.
		FIX conjugated to polyethylene glycol	Administer bolus dose of 40 IU/kg (typically 250 IU) IV prior to the procedure.
	Commence oral tranexamic acid 1 h prior to the procedure 50 mg* three times daily for 10 doses.		
	Avoid topical sealants (to minimize exposure to plasma products).		
	In most cases, the neonate can be discharged the same day if there are no bleeding concerns.		
	If necessary, administer a second bolus of FIX the following day.		

Adapted and modified with permission from current clinical practice at The Israel National Hemophilia Center, Sheba Medical Center, Tel Hashomer, Israel. FVIII, factor VIII; FIX, factor IX; IU, international units; IV, intravenous. *In the absence of syrup, the liquid from the vial can be used. In older children, weight-adjusted dose of antifibrinolytic agent should be used (see Appendix III).

Management of Infants Born to Known Carriers

A cord blood sample should be obtained to measure activated partial thromboplastin time (aPTT) and factors VIII (FVIII) or IX (FIX) levels (see Appendix II for age-specific reference values). Since FVIII levels are not low at birth, diagnosis is relatively simple in suspected cases of hemophilia A. Levels of FIX in newborns, on the other hand, are 35–70% that of adults, rendering the diagnosis of milder forms of hemophilia B more difficult. Admission to the NICU is recommended for any infant who is considered to have a significant risk of bleeding or a history of prematurity, traumatic delivery, or facial bruising [53]. Although vitamin K is typically administered by the intramuscular (IM) route in otherwise healthy neonates, there are three options for the route of administration in neonates suspected for hemophilia: IM or subcutaneously, each using a 27-gauge needle and followed by compression for 5–10 min, or orally for a total of 3 doses (see below) [53]. Bleeding events occurring during the neonatal period should be managed with immediate administration of recombinant or plasma-derived virus-inactivated FVIII or FIX products. Where these treatment options are available, the use of cryoprecipitate (for hemophilia A cases) and fresh frozen plasma (FFP) (for hemophilia B cases) is not recommended since these blood products carry a risk, albeit small, of transmitting viral infections such as HIV and hepatitis C. The half-life of the factor is expected to be shorter in newborn infants for several reasons, including larger plasma volume, volume of distribution, and liver-to-body ratio with increased weight-adjusted clearance. Therefore, close monitoring of factor levels is warranted. Short-term primary prophylaxis may be indicated in cases of traumatic or instrumental delivery. If circumcision is planned, the procedure should be performed electively under the care of an experienced surgeon and hematologist working out of a hemophilia treatment center, with appropriate accommodations to minimize bleeding risks (Table 5). Performing a head ultrasound is recommended prior to discharge, or preferably on the first day of life, for neonates with moderate or severe hemophilia.

Index Cases Presenting with Bleeding Events

The diagnosis of hemophilia during the neonatal period is based on the presence of hemorrhagic manifestations in one-third of the cases. Among such manifestations, bleeding following circumcision, ICH, and heel stick bleeding are the most commonly reported initial sites of bleeding. Hemophilia should be suspected on the basis of an aPTT that is prolonged beyond age-appropriate normal ranges, and confirmation of the diagnosis with factor level determination should follow.

Further details, including differential diagnosis and management of bleeding in neonates and children with hemophilia, are reviewed in detail in Chapter 8.

Deficiencies of Other Coagulation Factors

Other rare inherited coagulation factor deficiencies that may present in the neonatal period are reviewed in Chapter 10.

Acquired Coagulation Factor Deficiencies

Vitamin K Deficiency Bleeding

Vitamin K serves as a co-factor for the gamma-carboxylation of procoagulant proteins (factor II [FII], factor VII [FVII], FIX, and factor X [FX]) and of natural anticoagulants (proteins C, S, and Z). This posttranslational modification allows calcium-mediated binding of these proteins to negatively charged phospholipids, which is key to their hemostatic activity. Formerly known as "hemorrhagic disease of the newborn," vitamin K deficiency bleeding (VKDB) encompasses three syndromes classified according to the time of onset: early, classic, and late VKDB. These syndromes have in common a reduction of vitamin K-dependent factor activity levels, which is correctable after vitamin K administration.

Clinical Findings

Early VKDB occurs in the first day of life and is seen in neonates born to mothers receiving medication that interferes with vitamin K activity, such as anti-tuberculosis drugs, some antibiotics, and vitamin K antagonists. Anticonvulsants have also been traditionally implicated; however, evidence is limited. Early VKDB is often severe and associated with cephalohematoma, ICH, and intra-abdominal bleeding, including adrenal hemorrhage, which can have catastrophic consequences if not recognized early. Classic VKDB presents between the second and seventh day of life and is secondary to inadequate or delayed feeding. Clinical manifestations are milder; mucocutaneous and gastrointestinal bleeding are more common, but ICH can occur. It can be prevented with administration of vitamin K prophylaxis (see below). Late VKDB is defined as presenting between the 1st and the 12th week of life, but it usually manifests between the 2nd and 8th week. The incidence of late VKDB has been estimated at 4.4–7.2 per 100,000 births [54]. It is more common in males and conveys a substantial risk of ICH (approximately 50%) and high mortality, estimated at 20%.

Late VKDB is seen in exclusively breastfed infants, in children with underlying disorders associated with abnormal vitamin K absorption, and in children who did not receive vitamin K prophylaxis following delivery. Breastfed infants are at greater risk of VKDB due to inadequate intake, since breast milk has a lower concentration of vitamin K compared to commercial formula, and due to lower vitamin K production by their intestinal flora. It is imperative to properly explore any reasons for hesitancy of prophylactic vitamin K administration and ensure that parents and/or guardians are able to make informed decisions.

Diagnosis
Diagnosis of VKDB is based on the presence of prolonged prothrombin time (PT)/international normalized ratio (INR) with a normal platelet count and fibrinogen level. The aPTT is also prolonged in severe cases. Rapid normalization of the abnormal laboratory findings (within hours) following vitamin K administration confirms the diagnosis. Alternatively, protein induced by vitamin K absence (PIVKA) testing can be performed via high-performance liquid chromatography (HPLC), ELISA, or immunoelectrophoresis. The abnormal presence of PIVKA resolves within 5 days of vitamin K treatment [55].

Prevention
Early VKDB can be prevented by daily oral administration of 10 mg of vitamin K to pregnant women at risk during the 2 weeks prior to delivery. Classic and late VKDB can be effectively prevented with IM administration of 0.5–1 mg of vitamin K at birth. Oral or subcutaneous administration can be used in some cases, such as neonates with hemophilia. However, to ensure protection with oral vitamin K, 2 mg should be administered at birth, and again at 2–4 weeks and at 6–8 weeks [55]. The recommended dose for premature infants weighing less than 1,000 g is a one-time administration of 0.3 mg/kg IM (preferred route) or 0.2 mg IV [56].

Management
Treatment of symptomatic VKDB consists of IV or subcutaneous vitamin K at 0.25–0.3 mg/kg, with a single dose of 1–2 mg considered to be sufficient for an infant of 6 months of age or younger [57]; the IM route should be avoided due to the risk of bleeding. Plasma concentrates containing the vitamin K-dependent coagulation factors may be indicated in severe or life-threatening bleeding (see Appendix III).

Combined Disorders

Microbial Infections and Sepsis

Sepsis is a systemic inflammatory response syndrome that occurs in the presence of, or as a result of, a suspected or proven infection. Thrombocytopenia can be found in the course of sepsis, with or without the presence of disseminated intravascular coagulation (DIC). Bacterial sepsis has been associated with low platelet count in approximately 20–60% of cases. The risk and severity of thrombocytopenia is reportedly higher with Gram-negative and fungal infections compared to Gram-positive infections. Candidiasis is responsible for 5–10% of sepsis occurring after 72 h of life among very low birth weight infants, and harbors a high risk of death. Less common fungi, *Pantoea agglomerans* and *Malassezia furfur* have been reported in neonates with thrombocytopenia and other associated conditions. Thrombocytopenia in neonatal sepsis is also associated with increased risk of death [58]. The duration of thrombocytopenia is variable, but is generally short (<5 days); increased MPV is a common finding due to the release of new platelets. Thrombocytopenia is thought to be multifactorial, and causes include enhanced peripheral clearance (secondary to endothelial damage with platelet activation, direct effect of toxins, and DIC) and decreased platelet production. In the case of DIC, coagulation factors and fibrinogen are also consumed, predisposing the neonate to both bleeding and microvascular clotting (see below).

Asphyxia

Perinatal asphyxia is associated with moderate neonatal thrombocytopenia. Thrombocytopenia has been reported to occur in up to one-third of preterms with perinatal asphyxia as compared to 5% of matched controls, and has been described to reach its nadir on the third day of life, recovering by the 3rd week of life. Different injury patterns have been described in the literature pertaining to fetal asphyxia, based on fetal heart rate and/or timing of the neurological insult. Injury can occur (1) before hospital admission (preadmission), (2) during delivery, accompanied by a relatively prolonged change in fetal heart rate (intrapartum), or (3) acutely intrapartum, associated with a catastrophic event (acute asphyxia). Studies have shown that platelet count is lower in newborns sustaining preadmission or intrapartum injury of some duration in comparison to newborns suffering acute asphyxia, thus suggesting that low platelet count may be a marker to date the insulting event. The potential role of fibrinolytic system activation in cases of injury of some duration has been raised. In fact, asphyxiated newborns have reportedly lower fibrinogen levels and higher D-dimers in cord blood. Animal studies suggest decreased platelet survival in hypoxemic conditions, which could be related to activation of fibrinolysis or to antibody-mediated removal. In some cases, asphyxia can lead to DIC, thus accentuating coagulation abnormalities. Endothelial damage is another possible mechanism of hemostatic derangement.

Induced hypothermia (whole-body or head) is a therapeutic approach that aims to improve the neurological outcome of neonates with hypoxic-ischemic events. It has been suggested that induced hypothermia increases the incidence of thrombocytopenia, but does not increase the risk of coagulopathy in newborns with perinatal asphyxia.

Disseminated Intravascular Coagulation

DIC is an acquired disorder characterized by massive inflammatory response with microvascular endothelial damage and systemic activation of coagulation that can lead to organ dysfunction. In neonates, it can be secondary to several underlying conditions, such as sepsis, respiratory distress, severe asphyxia, NEC, liver dysfunction, and vascular tumors. Laboratory findings include thrombocytopenia resulting from platelet consumption, microangiopathic hemolytic anemia, prolonged PT/INR and aPTT, elevated D-dimers, and a low fibrinogen level. The interpretation of all coagulation-related laboratory results requires comparison with age-appropriate reference values (see Appendix II). The treatment of DIC primarily involves treatment of the underlying condition and supportive care, including replacement of blood products for neonates with bleeding diatheses (see Chapter 11). Some experts have suggested exchange transfusion for neonates experiencing DIC with hemorrhaging, typically associated with cardiovascular collapse following an ischemic event, to avoid fluid overload [59].

Neonatal Liver Failure

Coagulopathy due to hepatic dysfunction is one of the essential components of the diagnosis of this rare disorder. The presence of hemostatic abnormalities is largely explained by the crucial role of the liver in the synthesis and posttranslational modification of the majority of the proteins that belong to secondary and tertiary hemostasis (i.e., coagulation factors, natural anticoagulants, and proteins of fibrinolysis). Hemochromatosis and viral infections are the most common causes of liver failure among newborns. Further details, including management of liver-related coagulopathy, are reviewed in Chapter 11.

Kasabach-Merritt Phenomenon

Kasabach-Merritt phenomenon (KMP) is characterized by the presence of microangiopathic hemolytic anemia, consumptive coagulopathy, and

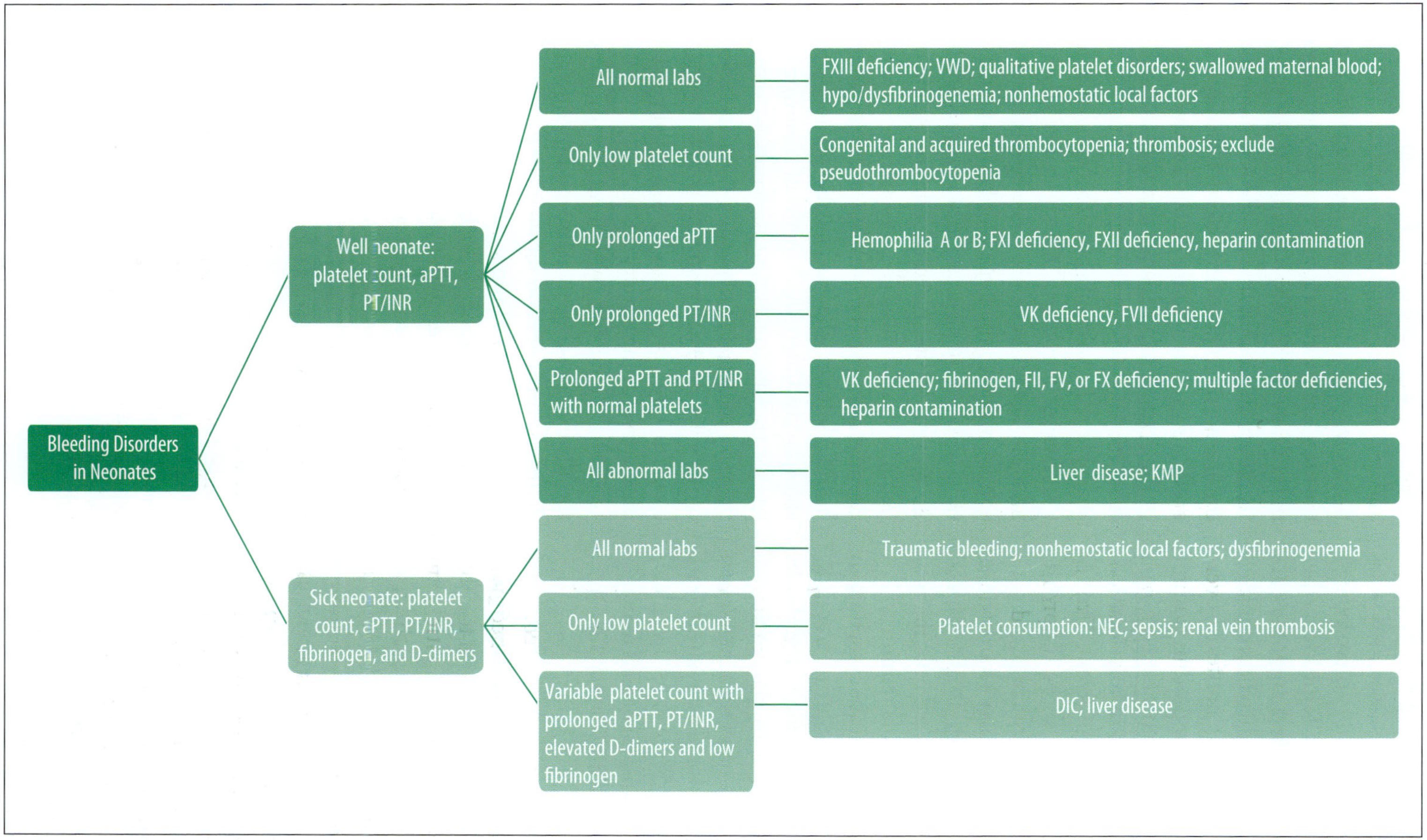

Fig. 2. Diagnosis of bleeding disorders in neonates. Used with permission of Natalie Mathews, from Disorders of Hemostasis and Thrombosis: A Clinical Guide, Goodnight and Hathaway [62]; permission conveyed through Copyright Clearance Center, Inc. The blood volumes required to perform laboratory tests should be taken into account, particularly in relation to premature infants. Although the amount of blood needed for these assays varies from laboratory to laboratory, most laboratories require 0.5 mL to perform a complete blood count and 1 mL to run standard coagulation tests (including PT/INR, aPTT, fibrinogen, and D-dimers). The anticoagulant recommended for the standard coagulation tests is 3.2% tri-sodium citrate. In these containers, a 9:1 ratio of blood to anticoagulant is critical for valid coagulation test results. aPTT, activated partial thromboplastin time; DIC, disseminated intravascular coagulation; FII, factor II; FV, factor V; FVII, factor VII; FX, factor X; FXI, factor XI; FXII, factor XII; FXIII, factor XIII; INR, international normalized ratio; KMP, Kasabach-Merritt phenomenon; NEC, necrotizing enterocolitis; PT, prothrombin time; VK, vitamin K; VWD, von Willebrand disease.

3

severe thrombocytopenia in the presence of an enlarging vascular tumor. KMP-associated mortality may be as high as 30% and is often related to bleeding complications [60]. Kaposiform hemangioendotheliomas and tufted angiomas are the vascular tumors underlying this disorder [60]. These two rare vascular tumors are most commonly present at birth and show predilection for the upper body (trunk and extremities), although vascular lesions can be present in any location, including internal sites (e.g., the liver). The lesions are usually unifocal and can be differentiated from their benign equivalent (e.g., hemangiomas) based on clinical findings (hard, violaceous red tumors, present at birth). MRI with and without gadolinium is the preferred imaging modality for evaluation of the vascular tumor.

The pathophysiology of thrombocytopenia in KMP is primarily a result of platelet trapping, probably due to enhanced adhesion to the abnormal endothelium, which leads to platelet activation and subsequent activation of the coagulation and fibrinolytic system. Increased shear rate within the tumor may contribute to further platelet activation. Further details, including management of KMP, are reviewed in Chapter 12.

Diagnostic Algorithm: Approach to Bleeding in the Neonate

To summarize some of the concepts discussed, we present in Figure 2 a general approach to the diagnosis of bleeding disorders, which combines standard and broadly available laboratory tests and the most common disorders found in neonates.

Transport Considerations

There are no published guidelines for managing neonates with bleeding disorders during the interhospital transport process. However, transfer of a neonate to a tertiary center for diagnostic workup and treatment is frequently required. The usual principles of stabilization, focusing on airway, breathing, and circulation, still apply, regardless of the etiology of the baby's bleeding tendency. Correction of the underlying problem will depend on the diagnostic ability of the referring facility and the availability of the required blood products locally. In the event of hypovolemia due to blood loss, uncross matched Group O-negative blood is usually available at the hospital's blood bank for emergency transfusion. However, "blood on board" critical care air ambulances are becoming increasingly common due to the large number of nursing stations with little or no access to blood or its products. To prevent further bleeding, administration of vitamin K should always be considered. In addition, administration of FFP is usually possible within the hospital setting, whereas platelets are rarely available quickly. Often, the benefits of acquiring platelets for transfusion during transport far outweigh the risks of delaying departure from the referring center by 1 or 2 h. Treatment with crossmatched blood or other blood products is usually deferred until arrival at the tertiary NICU.

While the neonate may have already suffered significant bleeding in utero and/or during the delivery, consideration must still be given to minimize the risks of trauma to the infant during interfacility transport. Such accommodations should be discussed with the neonatology team at the receiving tertiary care center.

Acknowledgments

We thank Dr. Sara Israels (Winnipeg, Canada), Dr. Veerle Labarque (Leuven, Belgium), Dr. Margaret Rand (Toronto, Canada), Dr. Nancy Robitaille (Montréal, Canada), Dr. Claudio Solana (Buenos Aires, Argentina), and Dr. Alexandra Zabeida (Toronto, Canada) for providing insightful comments on the third version of this chapter.

Conflict of Interest Statement

Natalie Mathews has received financial support from the Garron Family Cancer Center Clinical Advisor Council for research unrelated to this manuscript. Laura Avila holds official copyrights for CAPTSure©. Hilary Whyte reports no relevant conflicts of interest. Victor Blanchette reports receiving consultancy and speaker fees from Bayer Healthcare, Sanofi-Genzyme, Novo Nordisk, Pfizer, Roche, Takeda and Spark Therapeutics. He is a recipient of research grants from Sanofi-Genzyme, Bayer HealthCare, and Takeda, and he serves as a member of Data Safety Monitoring Boards for Octapharma and Takeda. He is chair of a nonprofit organization, the International Prophylaxis Study Group.

Author Contributions

Natalie Mathews drafted the chapter, critically revised the chapter, and approved the final version. Laura Avila planned the original layout of this chapter and drafted earlier editions of this chapter. For the 3rd edition, she critically revised the chapter and approved the final version. Hilary Whyte drafted the Transport Considerations section of the chapter, critically revised the chapter, and approved the final version. Victor Blanchette planned the original layout of this chapter. For the 3rd edition, he critically revised the chapter and approved the final version.

Abbreviations

aPTT	Activated partial thromboplastin time
BSS	Bernard-Soulier syndrome
CAMT	Congenital amegakaryocytic thrombocytopenia
CD	Cluster of differentiation
CT	Computed tomography
DIC	Disseminated intravascular coagulation
ELISA	Enzyme-linked immunosorbent assay
FII	Factor II (prothrombin)
FV	Factor V
FVII	Factor VII
FVIII	Factor VIII
FIX	Factor IX
FX	Factor X
FXI	Factor XI
FXII	Factor XII
FXIII	Factor XIII
FNAIT	Fetal and neonatal alloimmune thrombocytopenia
FFP	Fresh frozen plasma
GA	Gestational age
GP	Glycoprotein
GPS	Gray platelet syndrome
HIV	Human immunodeficiency virus
HPA	Human platelet antigen
HPLC	High-performance liquid chromatography
ICH	Intracranial hemorrhage
IgG	Immunoglobulin G
IM	Intramuscular
ITP	Immune thrombocytopenia
IV	Intravenous
IVIG	Intravenous immunoglobulin
KMP	Kasabach-Merritt phenomenon
MAIPA	Monoclonal antibody-specific immobilization of platelet antigens
MIS-C	Multisystem inflammatory disease in children
MIS-N	Multisystem inflammatory disease in neonates
MPV	Mean platelet volume
MRI	Magnetic resonance imaging
mRNA	Messenger RNA
MYH9-RD	Myosin heavy chain 9-related disease
NEC	Necrotizing enterocolitis
NICU	Neonatal intensive care unit
PCR	Polymerase chain reaction
PIVKA	Protein induced by vitamin K absence
PT/INR	Prothrombin time/international normalized ratio
PT-VWD	Platelet-type von Willebrand disease
RUSAT1	Amegakaryocytic thrombocytopenia with radio-ulnar synostosis
SARS-CoV-2	Severe acute respiratory syndrome coronavirus-2
SGA	Small for gestational age
TAM	Transient abnormal myelopoiesis
TAR	Thrombocytopenia absent radius
TORCH	Toxoplasmosis, rubella, cytomegalovirus, herpes simplex virus-2
VKDB	Vitamin K deficiency bleeding
VWD	von Willebrand disease
VWF	von Willebrand factor
WAS	Wiskott-Aldrich syndrome

References

1 Christensen RD. Platelet transfusion in the neonatal intensive care unit: benefits, risks, alternatives. Neonatology. 2011;100(3):311–8.
2 Chakravorty S, Roberts I. How I manage neonatal thrombocytopenia. Br J Haematol. 2012;156(2):155–62.
3 Sola-Visner M, Sallmon H, Brown R. New insights into the mechanisms of nonimmune thrombocytopenia in neonates. Semin Perinatol. 2009;33(1):43–51.
4 Takeshita S, Kakita H, Asai S, Asai T, Mori M, Ueda H, et al. Thrombocytopenia and insufficient thrombopoietin production in human small-for-gestational-age infants. Pediatr Res. 2023;93(3):619–24.
5 Regan F, Lees CC, Jones B, Nicolaides KH, Wimalasundera RC, Mijovic A, et al. Prenatal management of pregnancies at risk of fetal neonatal alloimmune thrombocytopenia (FNAIT): scientific Impact Paper No. 61. BJOG. 2019;126(10):e173–85.
6 Ohto H, Miura S, Ariga H, Ishii T, Fujimori K, Morita S, et al. The natural history of maternal immunization against foetal platelet alloantigens. Transfus Med. 2004;14(6):399–408.
7 Peterson JA, McFarland JG, Curtis BR, Aster RH. Neonatal alloimmune thrombocytopenia: pathogenesis, diagnosis and management. Br J Haematol. 2013;161(1):3–14.
8 Ohto H. Neonatal alloimmune thrombocytopenia. Nihon Rinsho. 1997;55(9):2310–4.
9 Petermann R, Bakchoul T, Curtis BR, Mullier F, Miyata S, Arnold DM, et al. Investigations for fetal and neonatal alloimmune thrombocytopenia: communication from the SSC of the ISTH. J Thromb Haemost. 2018;16(12):2526–29.
10 de Vos TW, Winkelhorst D, de Haas M, Lopriore E, Oepkes D. Epidemiology and management of fetal and neonatal alloimmune thrombocytopenia. Transfus Apher Sci. 2020;59(1):102704.
11 de Vos TW, Porcelijn L, Hofstede-van Egmond S, Pajkrt E, Oepkes D, Lopriore E, et al. Clinical characteristics of human platelet antigen (HPA)-1a and HPA-5b alloimmunised pregnancies and the association between platelet HPA-5b antibodies and symptomatic fetal neonatal alloimmune thrombocytopenia. Br J Haematol. 2021;195(4):595–603.
12 Curtis BR, Ali S, Glazier AM, Ebert DD, Aitman TJ, Aster RH. Isoimmunization against CD36 (glycoprotein IV): description of four cases of neonatal isoimmune thrombocytopenia and brief review of the literature. Transfusion. 2002;42(9):1173–9.
13 Zdravic D, Yougbare I, Vadasz B, Li C, Marshall AH, Chen P, et al. Fetal and neonatal alloimmune thrombocytopenia. Semin Fetal Neonatal Med. 2016;21(1):19–27.
14 Bertrand G, Renac V, Lefaix M-C, Nivet C, Trudel E, Richard L. Neonatal intracranial hemorrhage with a dramatic outcome due to maternal anti CD36 antibodies. Reports. 2019;2(1):7.
15 Kato S, Sugiura T, Ueda H, Ito K, Kakita H, Kato I, et al. Massive intracranial hemorrhage caused by neonatal alloimmune thrombocytopenia associated with anti-group A antibody. J Perinatol. 2013;33(1):79–82.
16 Bussel JB, Vander Haar EL, Berkowitz RL. New developments in fetal and neonatal alloimmune thrombocytopenia. Am J Obstet Gynecol. 2021;225(2):120–27.
17 Curley A, Stanworth SJ, Willoughby K, Fustolo-Gunnink SF, Venkatesh V, Hudson C, et al. Randomized trial of platelet-transfusion thresholds in neonates. N Engl J Med. 2019;380(3):242–51.
18 New HV, Stanworth SJ, Gottstein R, Cantwell C, Berryman J, Chalmers EA, et al. British Society for Haematology Guidelines on transfusion for fetuses, neonates and older children (Br J Haematol. 2016;175:784–828). Addendum August 2020. Br J Haematol. 2020;191(5):725–7.
19 Baker JM, Shehata N, Bussel J, Murphy MF, Greinacher A, Bakchoul T, et al. Postnatal intervention for the treatment of FNAIT: a systematic review. J Perinatol. 2019;39(10):1329–39.
20 New HV, Berryman J, Bolton-Maggs PH, Cantwell C, Chalmers EA, Davies T, et al. Guidelines on transfusion for fetuses, neonates and older children. Br J Haematol. 2016;175(5):784–828.
21 Bakchoul T, Bassler D, Heckmann M, Thiele T, Kiefel V, Gross I, et al. Management of infants born with severe neonatal alloimmune thrombocytopenia: the role of platelet transfusions and intravenous immunoglobulin. Transfusion. 2014;54(3):640–5.
22 Bussel JB, Primiani A. Fetal and neonatal alloimmune thrombocytopenia: progress and ongoing debates. Blood Rev. 2008;22(1):33–52.
23 Pacheco LD, Berkowitz RL, Moise KJ Jr, Bussel JB, McFarland JG, Saade GR. Fetal and neonatal alloimmune thrombocytopenia: a management algorithm based on risk stratification. Obstet Gynecol. 2011;118(5):1157–63.
24 Winkelhorst D, Murphy MF, Greinacher A, Shehata N, Bakchoul T, Massey E, et al. Antenatal management in fetal and neonatal alloimmune thrombocytopenia: a systematic review. Blood. 2017;129(11):1538–47.
25 Siddiq S, Clark A, Mumford A. A systematic review of the management and outcomes of pregnancy in Glanzmann thrombasthenia. Haemophilia. 2011;17(5):e858–69.
26 Peitsidis P, Datta T, Pafilis I, Otomewo O, Tuddenham EG, Kadir RA. Bernard Soulier syndrome in pregnancy: a systematic review. Haemophilia. 2010;16(4):584–91.
27 Rottenstreich A, Israeli N, Roth B, Elchalal U, Amsalem H, Da'as N, et al. Risk factors associated with neonatal thrombocytopenia in pregnant women with immune thrombocytopenic purpura. J Matern Fetal Neonatal Med. 2020;33(9):1572–78.
28 Point F, Terriou L, Rakza T, Drumez E, Alluin G, Garabedian C, et al. Risk factors for severe neonatal thrombocytopenia in cases of maternal immune thrombocytopenia. Acta Paediatr. 2022;111(5):985–91.
29 Albers CA, Paul DS, Schulze H, Freson K, Stephens JC, Smethurst PA, et al. Compound inheritance of a low-frequency regulatory SNP and a rare null mutation in exon-junction complex subunit RBM8A causes TAR syndrome. Nat Genet. 2012;44(4):435–9, S1–2.
30 Germeshausen M, Ballmaier M. CAMT-MPL: congenital amegakaryocytic thrombocytopenia caused by MPL mutations – heterogeneity of a monogenic disorder – a comprehensive analysis of 56 patients. Haematologica. 2021;106(9):2439–48.
31 Vo KK, Jarocha DJ, Lyde RB, Hayes V, Thom CS, Sullivan SK, et al. FLI1 level during megakaryopoiesis affects thrombopoiesis and platelet biology. Blood. 2017;129(26):3486–94.

32 Dokal I, Tummala H, Vulliamy TJ. Inherited bone marrow failure in the pediatric patient. Blood. 2022;140(6):556–70.

33 Maheshwari A. Immunologic and hematological abnormalities in necrotizing enterocolitis. Clin Perinatol. 2015; 42(3):567–85.

34 Hussain K, Salat MS, Mohammad N, Mughal A, Idrees S, Iqbal J, et al. Meropenem-induced pancytopenia in a preterm neonate: a case report. J Med Case Rep. 2021;15(1):25.

35 Avila ML, Shah V, Brandao LR. Systematic review on heparin-induced thrombocytopenia in children: a call to action. J Thromb Haemost. 2013;11(4):660–9.

36 Bhat R, Kwon S, Zaniletti I, Murthy K, Liem RI. Risk factors associated with venous and arterial neonatal thrombosis in the intensive care unit: a multicentre case-control study. Lancet Haematol. 2022;9(3):e200–7.

37 Roberts I, Alford K, Hall G, Juban G, Richmond H, Norton A, et al. GATA1-mutant clones are frequent and often unsuspected in babies with Down syndrome: identification of a population at risk of leukemia. Blood. 2013;122(24): 3908–17.

38 Klusmann JH, Creutzig U, Zimmermann M, Dworzak M, Jorch N, Langebrake C, et al. Treatment and prognostic impact of transient leukemia in neonates with Down syndrome. Blood. 2008;111(6): 2991–8.

39 Massey GV, Zipursky A, Chang MN, Doyle JJ, Nasim S, Taub JW, et al. A prospective study of the natural history of transient leukemia (TL) in neonates with Down syndrome (DS): Children's Oncology Group (COG) study POG-9481. Blood. 2006;107(12):4606–13.

40 Gamis AS, Alonzo TA, Gerbing RB, Hilden JM, Sorrell AD, Sharma M, et al. Natural history of transient myeloproliferative disorder clinically diagnosed in Down syndrome neonates: a report from the Children's Oncology Group Study A2971. Blood. 2011;118(26): 6752–9; quiz 996.

41 Shaiba LA, More K, Hadid A, Almaghrabi R, Al Marri M, Alnamnakani M, et al. Multisystemic inflammatory syndrome in neonates: a systematic review. Neonatology. 2022;119(4):405–17.

42 Zhu H, Wang L, Fang C, Peng S, Zhang L, Chang G, et al. Clinical analysis of 10 neonates born to mothers with 2019-nCoV pneumonia. Transl Pediatr. 2020; 9(1):51–60.

43 Lakshminrusimha S, Hudak ML, Dimitriades VR, Higgins RD. Multisystem inflammatory syndrome in neonates following maternal SARS-CoV-2 COVID-19 infection. Am J Perinatol. 2022; 39(11):1166–1171.

44 De Rose DU, Pugnaloni F, Calì M, Ronci S, Caoci S, Maddaloni C, et al. Multisystem inflammatory syndrome in neonates born to mothers with SARS-CoV-2 infection (MIS-N) and in neonates and infants younger than 6 months with acquired COVID-19 (MIS-C): a systematic review. Viruses. 2022; 14(4):750.

45 Sola-Visner M, Bercovitz RS. Neonatal platelet transfusions and future areas of research. Transfus Med Rev. 2016;30(4): 183–8.

46 Lasky B, Nolasco J, Graff J, Ward DC, Ziman A, McGonigle AM. Pathogen-reduced platelets in pediatric and neonatal patients: demographics, transfusion rates, and transfusion reactions. Transfusion. 2021;61(10):2869–76.

47 Moore CM, Curley AE. Neonatal platelet transfusions: starting again. Transfus Med Rev. 2021;35(3):29–35.

48 Ferrer-Marín F, Sola-Visner M. Neonatal platelet physiology and implications for transfusion. Platelets. 2022;33(1):14–22.

49 Leebeek FWG, Duvekot J, Kruip MJHA. How I manage pregnancy in carriers of hemophilia and patients with von Willebrand disease. Blood. 2020;136(19): 2143–50.

50 Andersson NG, Chalmers EA, Kenet G, Ljung R, Mäkipernaa A, Chambost H, et al. Mode of delivery in hemophilia: vaginal delivery and Cesarean section carry similar risks for intracranial hemorrhages and other major bleeds. Haematologica. 2019;104(10):2100–6.

51 Chalmers EA, Alamelu J, Collins PW, Mathias M, Payne J, Richards M, et al. Intracranial haemorrhage in children with inherited bleeding disorders in the UK 2003–2015:a national cohort study. Haemophilia. 2018;24(4):641–7.

52 Chalmers E, Williams M, Brennand J, Liesner R, Collins P, Richards M, et al. Guideline on the management of haemophilia in the fetus and neonate. Br J Haematol. 2011;154(2):208–15.

53 Moorehead PC, Chan AKC, Lemyre B, Winikoff R, Scott H, Hawes SA, et al. A practical guide to the management of the fetus and newborn with hemophilia. Clin Appl Thromb Hemost. 2018;24(9_suppl):29S-41S.

54 Van Winckel M, De Bruyne R, Van De Velde S, Van Biervliet S. Vitamin K, an update for the paediatrician. Eur J Pediatr. 2009;168(2):127–34.

55 Ng E, Loewy AD. Position statement: guidelines for vitamin K prophylaxis in newborns—a joint statement of the Canadian Paediatric Society and the College of Family Physicians of Canada. Can Fam Physician. 2018;64(10):736–9.

56 Hand I, Noble L, Abrams SA. Vitamin K and the newborn infant. Pediatrics. 2022;149(3):e2021056036.

57 Araki S, Shirahata A. Vitamin K deficiency bleeding in infancy. Nutrients. 2020;12(3):780.

58 Ree IMC, Fustolo-Gunnink SF, Bekker V, Fijnvandraat KJ, Steggerda SJ, Lopriore E. Thrombocytopenia in neonatal sepsis: incidence, severity and risk factors. PLoS One. 2017;12(10): e0185581.

59 Zipursky A, deSa D, Hsu E, Johnston M, Milner R. Clinical and laboratory diagnosis of hemostatic disorders in newborn infants. Am J Pediatr Hematol Oncol. 1979;1(3):217–26.

60 Ryan C, Price V, John P, Mahant S, Baruchel S, Brandao L, et al. Kasabach-Merritt phenomenon: a single centre experience. Eur J Haematol. 2010; 84(2):97–104.

61 Sola MC. Evaluation and treatment of severe and prolonged thrombocytopenia in neonates. Clin Perinatol. 2004;31(1): 1–14.

62 Goodnight SH, Hathaway WE. Disorders of Hemostasis and Thrombosis: A Clinical Guide. 2nd ed. McGraw-Hill; 2001.

Chapter 4

Published online: December 5, 2024

Blanchette VS, Brandão LR, Carcao MD, Kumar R, Rand ML, Revel-Vilk S (eds): SickKids Handbook of Pediatric Thrombosis and Hemostasis, ed 3, rev. and ext. Basel, Karger, 2024, pp 50–59 (DOI: 10.1159/000538214)

An Approach to the Bleeding Child

Caroline Malcolmson[a] Melanie Jackson[a] Sara J. Israels[b] Margaret L. Rand[a]
Shoshana Revel-Vilk[c, d]

[a]Division of Hematology/Oncology, The Hospital for Sick Children, University of Toronto, Toronto, ON, Canada; [b]Department of Pediatrics and Child Health, University of Manitoba, Winnipeg, MB, Canada; [c]Pediatric Hematology/Oncology Unit and Gaucher Unit, Shaare Zedek Medical Center, Jerusalem, Israel; [d]Faculty of Medicine, Hebrew University, Jerusalem, Israel

Introduction

Bleeding in a child can be a diagnostic challenge because of the wide range of possible causes, but making a specific diagnosis is clinically important in order to provide appropriate therapy and counseling. An excessive bleeding response to commonly encountered challenges suggests the possibility of an underlying bleeding disorder. Symptoms such as bruising, gingival bleeding, and epistaxis frequently occur in children without underlying bleeding disorders, so determining which child requires further investigation can be difficult. Even when initial symptoms appear unimpressive, children with underlying bleeding disorders may be at increased risk for significant bleeding associated with surgical procedures, trauma, menses, or future obstetric procedures.

Bleeding disorders can be inherited or acquired and include quantitative and qualitative defects in the components of primary and secondary hemostasis (see Chapter 2). Inherited disorders can be recessive or dominant, autosomal or X-linked, and often occur sporadically due to de novo genetic variants. von Willebrand disease (VWD) and mild platelet defects are the most common inherited bleeding disorders seen in clinical practice in children (see Chapters 6 and 9). The coexistence of two inherited and/or acquired bleeding disorders should also be considered in specific situations. The evaluation of a child presenting with abnormal bleeding should include a comprehensive medical and bleeding history, a complete family history, a detailed physical examination, and selected laboratory tests as outlined in Figure 1.

History

Medical History

Clinical evaluation of a bleeding patient begins with a detailed history, emphasizing the child's age, sex, past medical history, clinical presentation, bleeding symptomatology, and family history.

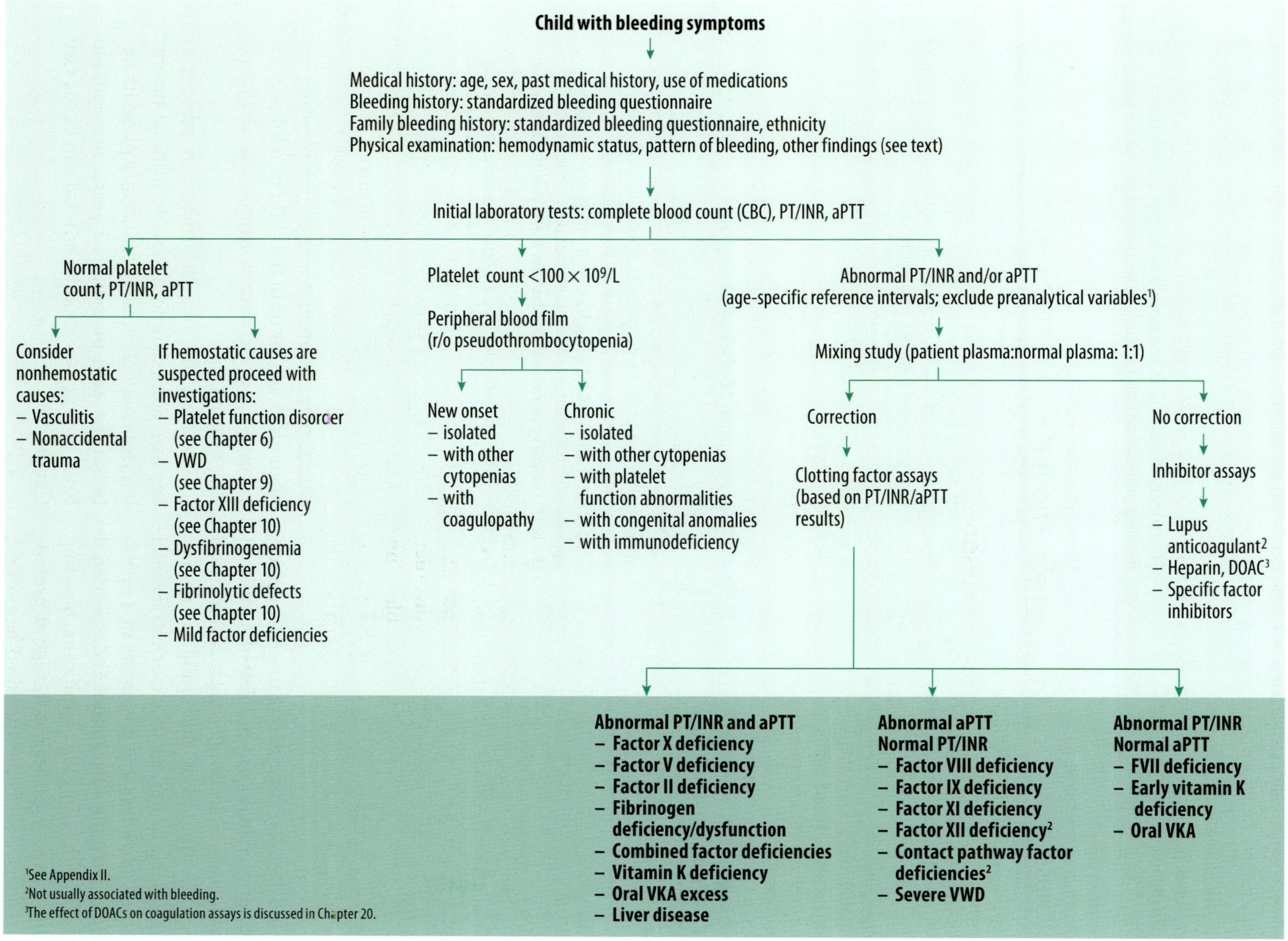

Fig. 1. Evaluation of a child presenting with bleeding symptoms. aPTT, activated partial thromboplastin time; DOAC, direct oral anticoagulant; PT/INR, prothrombin time/international normalized ratio; VKA, vitamin K antagonists; VWD, von Willebrand disease.

4

Table 1. Clinical abnormalities associated with inherited bleeding disorders with a single hemostatic defect

	Nonbleeding manifestations
Coagulation defects	
Factor XIII deficiency	Poor/delayed healing of the umbilical stump, poor wound healing, abnormal scar formation, recurrent pregnancy loss
Platelet function defects	
Hermansky-Pudlak syndrome	Oculocutaneous albinism
Chediak-Higashi syndrome	Oculocutaneous albinism, increased risk of infections, neutrophil peroxidase-positive inclusions
Arthrogryposis-renal dysfunction-cholestasis (ARC) syndrome	Arthrogryposis, renal dysfunction, cholestasis
Myosin heavy chain 9 (MYH9)-related disease	Cataracts, sensorineural hearing defect, nephritis
Leukocyte adhesion deficiency type III	Recurrent severe infections, delayed separation of the umbilical cord, delayed wound healing, neutrophilia
Thrombocytopenia	
Wiskott-Aldrich syndrome (WAS)	Eczema, immunodeficiency
Thrombocytopenia absent radius	Skeletal defects
Amegakaryocytic thrombocytopenia with radioulnar synostosis	
X-linked thrombocytopenia and dyserythropoiesis with or without anemia/X-linked thrombocytopenia-thalassemia	Microcytosis of red blood cells, unbalanced hemoglobin chain synthesis resembling β-thalassemia minor
Trisomy 21	Cognitive impairment, hearing loss, hypothyroidism, cardiac abnormalities, gastroenteric defects, hypotonia, cataracts, leukopenia/neutropenia, increased risk of leukemia
Trisomy 18	Cleft lip and palate, polydactyly, rocker-bottom feet, cutis aplasia, omphalocele, cardiac abnormalities, neural tube defects, severe growth restriction/low birth weight, cognitive impairment
Trisomy 13	Dolichocephaly, micrognathia, cleft lip and palate, overriding fingers, cardiac abnormalities, horse-shoe kidney, psychomotor retardation

Age

Most cases of severe inherited hemostatic defects will be diagnosed in infancy because of significant mucocutaneous bleeding, post-circumcision bleeding, bleeding from the umbilical stump, bleeding/oozing from heel sticks, or intracranial hemorrhage. However, the possibility of a severe inherited hemostatic defect should be considered in a child with clinically significant bleeding symptoms/signs, regardless of the age at presentation. Moderate and mild inherited hemostatic defects may not present with clinical bleeding until an older age, or until the child or adolescent is exposed to a significant hemostatic challenge, e.g., surgery.

Acquired bleeding disorders can present at any age. For example, although immune thrombocytopenia (ITP) most commonly presents between the ages of 2 and 10 years, presentation from the age of 3 months onward can occur (see Chapter 7).

Sex

Some of the inherited bleeding disorders are X-linked-recessive and thus are generally only seen in males. These include hemophilia A (factor VIII [FVIII] deficiency), hemophilia B (factor IX [FIX] deficiency), Wiskott-Aldrich syndrome (WAS)/X-linked thrombocytopenia, and X-linked thrombocytopenia with dyserythropoiesis. In rare instances, these disorders can affect females due to other genetic anomalies, including skewed X-inactivation, or absence of the second X chromosome (e.g., Turner syndrome). A family history of bleeding limited to males suggests an X-linked disorder. All other inherited and acquired hemostatic defects occur in both sexes, although there is an elevated rate of diagnosis of VWD, platelet defects, and factor XI (FXI) deficiency in women because of heavy menstrual bleeding (HMB) and bleeding related to childbirth [1].

General Medical History

Presentation of signs and symptoms other than bleeding can provide a clue to the diagnosis of inherited hemostatic disorders and genetic disorders associated with hemostatic disorders (Table 1) [2]. A detailed medical history is essential for the diagnosis of acquired hemostatic disorders. A history of weakness, fever, weight loss, etc. can suggest malignancy. Liver disease affects the synthesis of multiple coagulation factors. Cholestasis, fat malabsorption, or antibiotic use can cause vitamin K deficiency. Sepsis is associated with consumptive coagulopathy and thrombocytopenia. Uremia can be associated with acquired platelet dysfunction. Splenomegaly can cause thrombocytopenia due to hypersplenism. The use of medications can be associated with drug-induced thrombocytopenia or platelet dysfunction.

Bleeding History

The type and pattern of bleeding are important indicators of possible diagnoses. Mucocutaneous bleeding such as petechiae, bruising, epistaxis, gingival bleeding, gastrointestinal bleeding, and/or HMB suggests disorders of platelets, von Willebrand factor (VWF), or connective tissue/vascular disorders such as hereditary hemorrhagic telangiectasia or Ehlers-Danlos syndrome (see Appendix IV). Additionally, in these disorders, there may be prolonged bleeding following surgery and/or dental extractions. In contrast, spontaneous or excessive bleeding into soft tissues, muscles, and joints or delayed surgical bleeding suggests disorders of coagulation factors. It should be noted that coagulation factor disorders may also cause mucocutaneous bleeding, epistaxis, or gastrointestinal bleeding. Neonatal intracranial hemorrhage, or post-circumcision or severe mucosal bleeding in early infancy requires immediate investigation for a severe bleeding disorder, specifically a coagulation factor deficiency. Excessive bleeding from the umbilical cord stump within the first days of life is strongly suggestive of factor XIII (FXIII) deficiency, factor X (FX) deficiency, congenital afibrinogenemia, or antiplasmin deficiency.

The onset and acuity of bleeding may also indicate a specific diagnosis. Acquired disorders may have an acute onset (e.g., ITP) compared with inherited disorders where symptoms are present for months or years. Challenges to the hemostatic system are often required to make a bleeding disorder clinically evident so that mild/moderate bleeding disorders may not be appreciated until events such as trauma, surgery, or menarche occur.

The recognition of significant clinical bleeding is the first step in the diagnosis of bleeding disorders. In children with severe bleeding disorders, the bleeding history is usually clear. However, children presenting with mild/moderate bleeding symptoms may have bleeding symptoms such as recurrent epistaxis or bruises that are also common among healthy children. In these instances, the diagnosis may be challenging, and the distinction between normal children and those with bleeding disorders can be difficult to make.

Table 2. Clinical abnormalities associated with inherited bleeding disorders with multiple hemostatic defects

Disorder	Hemostatic abnormalities[a]	Non-bleeding manifestations
Noonan syndrome	Thrombocytopenia Low factor XI, factor XII, factor XIII Abnormal platelet function Acquired von Willebrand syndrome[b]	Short stature ± growth hormone deficiency Abnormal facies and eye anomalies Cardiac abnormalities Learning disability and developmental delay Hearing impairment Lymphedema and lymphangiectasia
Turner syndrome	Thrombocytopenia Low factor VIII/factor IX (in hemophilia carriers) Acquired von Willebrand syndrome[b]	Short stature Dysmorphic facies and webbed neck Cardiac abnormalities Delayed puberty Gonadal dysfunction Lymphedema
Di George (22q11.2 deletion syndrome; velocardiofacial syndrome)	Thrombocytopenia Abnormal platelet function Acquired von Willebrand syndrome[b]	Palatal abnormalities (cleft palate, bifid uvula) Immune dysfunction Cardiac abnormalities Abnormal facial features Learning difficulties Hearing loss Hypocalcemia
Jacobsen (11q23 deletion) syndrome	Thrombocytopenia Acquired von Willebrand syndrome[b]	Growth retardation Developmental delay Abnormal facial features Cardiac abnormalities

[a]These abnormalities have been observed in some but not all individuals with the diagnosis. [b]Acquired von Willebrand syndrome in these syndromes is associated with the presence of cardiac abnormalities that cause high shear stress resulting in qualitative abnormalities of von Willebrand factor.

The use of standardized scores to quantitate bleeding symptoms is recommended. A validated pediatric bleeding assessment tool, the Pediatric Bleeding Questionnaire, that addresses pediatric-specific symptoms [3–5], has been incorporated into the International Society of Thrombosis and Haemostasis (ISTH) Bleeding Assessment Tool (ISTH-BAT) for both children and adults (see Appendix I) [6, 7]. Symptom-specific bleeding scores for HMB (the Pictorial Blood Loss Assessment Chart) and epistaxis are useful for describing the severity of the specific bleeding symptom (see Appendix I).

Family History

In addition to the child's bleeding history, the family history may provide important clues about the potential inheritance of an underlying bleeding disorder. For example, an autosomal-dominant inheritance pattern would be in keeping with type 1 VWD and some platelet function disorders, and an X-linked pattern with FVIII or FIX deficiency. Consanguinity in a family increases the risk of autosomal-recessive disorders. Evaluation of the bleeding history in family members by a validated bleeding questionnaire could be useful for appreciating the significance of the family's bleeding history.

Generally, there is little racial or ethnic predisposition to bleeding disorders. However, a few rare bleeding disorders are more prevalent in certain populations, e.g., FXI deficiency among Jews of Ashkenazi (European) origin, the Basque population of south-western France and north-eastern Spain. Autosomal-recessive bleeding disorders can be more common in small, geographically or ethnically isolated communities sharing common genetic variants.

Physical Examination

A careful physical examination for the evaluation of clinical bleeding and associated abnormalities is an essential part in the diagnosis of hemostatic disorders. Mucocutaneous bleeding suggests a disorder of primary hemostasis, i.e., VWD or platelet dysfunction/deficiency, or connective tissue/vascular disorders such as hereditary hemorrhagic telangiectasia or Ehlers-Danlos syndrome (see Appendix IV). In males, deep hematomas, hemarthroses, or evidence of chronic joint abnormalities suggests FVIII or FIX deficiency. Acquired bleeding disorders may present in the context of coexisting illnesses such as autoimmune conditions or post-viral infections. Lymphadenopathy and/or organomegaly suggest an infiltrative process such as malignancy or a storage disease. Signs of liver failure suggest acquired coagulation factor deficiencies. Additional congenital anomalies and dysmorphic features may suggest the presence of a syndromic bleeding disorder (Table 2).

A pattern of bruising that is not consistent with accidental injury should raise concerns about nonaccidental trauma.

Laboratory Investigations

Laboratory screening tests for suspected bleeding disorders provide additional diagnostic indicators that direct more specific investigations. Figure 1 provides an approach to the evaluation of a child with bleeding symptoms. Preanalytical variables that may affect coagulation testing in children are discussed in Appendix II.

Screening Tests

Initial tests to screen for bleeding disorders should include a complete blood count (CBC), blood smear, prothrombin time/international normalized ratio (PT/INR), and activated partial thromboplastin time (aPTT).

A *CBC (blood collected into ethylenediaminetetraacetic acid [EDTA])* is performed to exclude thrombocytopenia. It should be noted, however, that automated cell counters (counters based on impedance rather than optical technology) may underestimate platelet count and under- or overestimate mean platelet volume when platelet size is outside of the established reference range. The CBC also provides information about additional cytopenias, and other white blood cell (WBC) and red blood cell (RBC) abnormalities.

Peripheral blood smear (blood collected into EDTA) provides additional information regarding platelet number, size, clumping and granularity (the platelet count can be estimated by the number of platelets per ×100 field multiplied by 20×10^9/L). Pseudothrombocytopenia resulting from clumping of platelets collected in EDTA anticoagulant can be identified by examination of the blood smear and confirmed by recollecting a specimen in citrate anticoagulant in which clumping will not occur. Examination of the peripheral blood smear is essential in the evaluation of a child with a suspected platelet disorder. If true thrombocytopenia is diagnosed, the next step is to differentiate between new-onset acquired thrombocytopenia, chronic acquired thrombocytopenia, and congenital thrombocytopenia (Fig. 1).

Evaluation of WBC morphology allows identification of malignant blasts, granulocyte inclusions, such as Döhle-like bodies, or other WBC abnormalities. Evaluation of RBC morphology is important to exclude a microangiopathic process

4

as evidenced by the presence of fragmented RBCs, microcytosis, macrocytosis, and other RBC abnormalities.

PT/INR (blood collected into citrate) measures the extrinsic and common pathways in the coagulation cascade (tissue factor, factor VII [FVII], FX, factor V [FV], factor II [FII], fibrinogen). Results should be compared with age-specific laboratory reference ranges (Appendix II) and are reported in seconds and/or as a percentage of a normal control sample. The INR is a standardized version of the PT, calculated by the ratio of a patient's PT to a normal control sample, raised to the power of the international sensitivity index (ISI) of the thromboplastin value for the analytical system used. The INR was developed for standardizing and guiding management in patients treated with oral vitamin K antagonists (VKAs) and was not meant to be used for evaluation of bleeding. However, as some laboratories now report only the INR and not the PT, it has been included in Figure 1. An isolated prolonged PT/high INR (with normal aPTT) suggests FVII deficiency, vitamin K deficiency (nutritional or caused by VKAs such as warfarin) or liver disease.

aPTT (blood collected into citrate) measures the intrinsic and common pathways of coagulation (factor XII [FXII], FXI, FIX, FVIII, FX, FV, FII, and fibrinogen). Results are reported in seconds and should be compared with age-specific laboratory reference ranges (see Appendix II). The aPTT is less sensitive than the PT to deficiencies of the common pathway factors. An isolated abnormally prolonged aPTT (with a normal PT/INR) suggests FVIII or FIX deficiency (see Chapter 8), FXI deficiency (see Chapter 10), or contact pathway deficiency [8]. Importantly, an aPTT within the reference range does not exclude mild FVIII, FIX, or FXI deficiency. Therefore, factor assays should be performed if specific deficiencies are suspected.

Deficiency of factors in the contact pathway, i.e., FXII, plasma prekallikrein, and high-molecular-weight kininogen, commonly prolong the aPTT, but do not cause clinically significant bleeding. A prolonged aPTT can occur in severe VWD, as a result of the associated FVIII deficiency (see Chapter 9).

The aPTT is also prolonged in the presence of inhibitors, including heparin, direct oral anticoagulants (DOACs), and lupus anticoagulant (LAC) (Fig. 1). Heparin contamination occurs most often in specimens drawn from arterial or central venous catheters. To avoid heparin contamination, an adequate volume of blood should be removed from the catheter prior to sampling. Where that is not possible, heparin neutralization can be performed in the laboratory, usually by adding heparinase to the sample plasma. The use of DOACs interferes with the correction of mixing studies [9]. Selecting alternatives to clot-based hemostasis assays in patients taking DOACs and sample collection when the patient is off or at the expected drug trough are optional ways to avoid DOAC interference [9]. To avoid an incidental prolonged aPTT secondary to LAC, reagents with low LAC sensitivity can be used when screening for coagulation factor deficiencies [10].

Combined prolongation of PT/INR and aPTT can result from inherited deficiencies of individual factors in the common pathway: FX, FV, FII, and fibrinogen, or from the rare inherited deficiency of the vitamin-K-dependent coagulation factors (see Chapter 10). More commonly, combined abnormalities of aPTT and PT/INR are the result of acquired deficiencies of multiple coagulation factors such as that caused by severe vitamin K deficiency, liver disease, or disseminated intravascular coagulation (see Chapter 11).

A *mixing study (patient plasma 1:1 normal plasma) (blood collected into citrate)* is performed when an abnormal PT and/or aPTT is identified. The patient's plasma is mixed with normal plasma in a 1:1 ratio, and the screening tests are repeated. This test helps to differentiate between factor deficiency (mixing corrects the PT or aPTT) and the presence of an inhibitor (mixing does not correct the PT or aPTT). The most common inhibitor that results in noncorrection of the aPTT with mixing is presence of an LAC. This is often an incidental finding in children post viral infections and is not associated with clinical bleeding and/or risk of thrombosis. It should be appreciated that a low-titer antiphospholipid antibody may prolong the aPTT but may still show correction in a mixing study. If clinically indicated, specialized assays will confirm its presence (see Chapter 13). Specific factor inhibitors also interfere with correction of screening tests by mixing with normal plasma. Confirmation requires specific inhibitor assays.

The laboratory reagents used for PT and aPTT testing vary in their sensitivity to coagulation factors, and insensitive reagents may result in false-negative (i.e., normal) results for mild deficiencies. If there is a strong suspicion of a coagulation factor deficiency, specific factor assays should be performed.

The decision to proceed to further testing should depend on clinical suspicion of a bleeding disorder. Repeating screening tests because of mild abnormalities is not warranted in a child without a significant bleeding history and no family history of a bleeding disorder. For children/adolescents with clinical indicators of a bleeding disorder and a positive ISTH-BAT score (see Appendix I), more specific diagnostic tests may be more cost-effective.

Thrombin time (TT) (blood collected into citrate) measures the thrombin-induced conversion of fibrinogen to fibrin. A prolonged TT suggests a quantitative or qualitative abnormality of fibrinogen or the presence of heparin or a thrombin inhibitor such as dabigatran in the sample.

Fibrinogen measurement (blood collected into citrate) is most commonly performed as a functional fibrinogen test, generally available in coagulation laboratories. A fibrinogen antigen level for quantitative measurement of fibrinogen is generally available only in a reference coagulation laboratory (see Chapter 10).

The PT, aPTT, and TT do not screen for FXIII deficiency. Specific tests for FXIII are discussed in Chapter 10.

Testing for Defects in Primary Hemostasis

Bleeding time (using a device appropriate for the age of a neonate/child/adolescent) is measured using a lancet device to make a standardized cut on the volar surface of the forearm, and the time it takes for bleeding to stop is measured. The bleeding time test was widely used as a screening test for primary hemostasis disorders but is much less often used now because of difficulties in standardization. The bleeding time is operator dependent and is affected by other factors such as the amount of fatty tissue in the area of puncture, the temperature of the skin, etc. In current times, it is more likely to be utilized in resource-limited locations.

Platelet function analyzer, PFA-100®/200® (blood collected into citrate), is an instrument in which primary, platelet-related hemostasis is simulated. A small sample of anticoagulated whole blood (0.8 mL) is aspirated via a narrow-diameter capillary through a microscopic aperture cut into a membrane coated with the platelet agonists collagen and epinephrine or collagen and adenosine 5′-diphosphate (ADP). The high shear rate generated under the standardized flow conditions and presence of the chemical stimuli result in platelet adhesion, activation, and aggregation at the aperture, building a stable platelet plug. The time required to obtain full occlusion of the aperture is reported as the closure time. The closure time is prolonged by low levels or activity of VWF, thrombocytopenia, decreased hematocrit, and by some platelet function abnormalities (e.g., severe disorders such as Bernard-Soulier syndrome and Glanzmann thrombasthenia). Due to issues of both sensitivity and specificity, the use of the PFA-100®/200® as a routine screening test is still debated; in particular, PFA-100®/200® closure times lack sensitivity/specificity for mild platelet disorders [11]. However, the small blood volume needed for this test compared with the much larger volume required for platelet function testing by aggregometry (10 mL or more) is an advantage, especially for screening very young

4

children for severe VWD or platelet function disorders such as Glanzmann thrombasthenia or Bernard-Soulier syndrome.

VWF antigen and activity (blood collected into citrate): These tests measure the level and the activity of VWF for the diagnosis of VWD. The von Willebrand factor ristocetin cofactor (VWF:RCo) level was previously the most commonly used measure to assess VWF activity. Currently, newer, more specific VWF assays are increasingly used (see Chapter 9). Specialized laboratory evaluations of VWF, such as a FVIII binding assay and VWF multimer analysis, to determine the VWD subtype are discussed in Chapter 9. ABO blood group influences plasma levels of VWF, which are approximately 25% lower in healthy blood group O compared with healthy blood group non-O individuals. Current diagnostic guidelines do not require ABO blood group determination to establish a diagnosis of VWD (see Chapter 9). However, identifying the ABO blood group can aid the interpretation of test results for VWF antigen and activity testing with an understanding of the influence of blood group status on VWF antigen and activity levels.

Light transmission aggregometry (blood collected into citrate) is the most common method of assessing platelet function, in which the increase in light transmission through a rapidly stirred sample of citrated platelet-rich plasma is recorded as platelets aggregate. As a fresh blood sample is needed for aggregation testing, the patient may have to be referred to a center with a specialized laboratory [12] (see Chapter 6).

Specialized testing of platelet function including measurement of granule secretion (e.g., lumi-aggregrometry), flow cytometric assessment of surface receptors and activation markers, and evaluation of platelet ultrastructure by transmission electron microscopy and immunofluorescence are discussed in Chapter 6.

Fibrinolysis Inhibitors

Rare abnormalities of fibrinolysis inhibitors (blood collected into citrate), such as α2-antiplasmin and plasminogen activator inhibitor type 1 (PAI-1) deficiencies and the Québec platelet disorder, can cause bleeding disorders because of increased fibrinolysis and decreased clot stability (see Chapter 10).

Genetic Testing

The genetic variants associated with inherited hemostatic disorders are increasingly being revealed, and genetic testing is becoming more readily available in many centers. If available, genetic analysis aids in accurate diagnosis and improves genetic counseling and prenatal diagnosis (see Chapter 21). Next-generation sequencing panels that are now available offer an efficient approach to the molecular diagnosis of selected coagulation and platelet disorders. Recommendations for genetic testing for specific disorders are provided in the relevant chapters in this handbook. Advances in genotyping and sequencing technologies are aiding in the discovery of new genes that play a role in hemostasis and thrombosis. The ISTH Subcommittee on Genomics in Thrombosis and Hemostasis has developed a tool to capture the genomic variants detected in patients with bleeding, thrombotic, and platelet disorders identified by the ISTH community [13] (https://www.isth.org/page/GinTh_GeneLists).

Conflict of Interest Statement

Caroline Malcolmson, Melanie Jackson, Sara J. Israels, and Margaret L. Rand report no conflict of interest. Shoshana Revel-Vilk received grant/research support, honoraria, and advisory fee from Takeda, Pfizer, and Sanofi/Genzyme.

Author Contributions

Shoshana Revel-Vilk wrote the first draft of the chapter. Caroline Malcolmson critically revised the chapter and approved the final version. Melanie Jackson critically revised the chapter and approved the final version. Sara J. Israels critically revised the chapter and approved the final version. Margaret L. Rand critically revised the chapter and approved the final version.

Abbreviations

ADP	Adenosine 5′-diphosphate
aPTT	Activated partial thromboplastin time
BAT	Bleeding assessment tool
CBC	Complete blood count
DOAC	Direct oral anticoagulant
EDTA	Ethylenediaminetetraacetic acid
FII	Factor II (prothrombin)
FV	Factor V
FVII	Factor VII
FVIII	Factor VIII
FIX	Factor IX
FX	Factor X
FXI	Factor XI
FXII	Factor XII
FXIII	Factor XIII
HMB	Heavy menstrual bleeding
INR	International normalized ratio
ISI	International Sensitivity Index
ISTH	International Society on Thrombosis and Haemostasis
ITP	Immune thrombocytopenia
LAC	Lupus anticoagulant
PAI-1	Plasminogen activator inhibitor type 1
PFA	Platelet function analyzer
PT	Prothrombin time
RBC	Red blood cell
TT	Thrombin time
VKA	Vitamin K antagonist
VWD	von Willebrand disease
VWF	von Willebrand factor
WAS	Wiskott-Aldrich syndrome
WBC	White blood cell

4

References

1 Atiq F, Saes JL, Punt MC, van Galen KPM, Schutgens REG, Meijer K, et al. Major differences in clinical presentation, diagnosis and management of men and women with autosomal inherited bleeding disorders. EClinicalMedicine. 2021;32:100726.

2 Sarangi SN, Acharya SS. Bleeding disorders in congenital syndromes. Pediatrics. 2017;139(2):e20154360.

3 Biss TT, Blanchette VS, Clark DS, Bowman M, Wakefield CD, Silva M, et al. Quantitation of bleeding symptoms in children with von Willebrand disease: use of a standardized pediatric bleeding questionnaire. J Thromb Haemost. 2010;8(5):950–6.

4 Biss TT, Blanchette VS, Clark DS, Wakefield CD, James PD, Rand ML. Use of a quantitative pediatric bleeding questionnaire to assess mucocutaneous bleeding symptoms in children with a platelet function disorder. J Thromb Haemost. 2010;8(6):1416–9.

5 Levy E, Kuperman A, Sela E, Kashkoush A, Miari AD, Hana RY, et al. Utility of the pediatric bleeding questionnaire in predicting posttonsillectomy bleeding. Otolaryngol Head Neck Surg. 2022; 167(3):576–82.

6 Bidlingmaier C, Grote V, Budde U, Olivieri M, Kurnik K. Prospective evaluation of a pediatric bleeding questionnaire and the ISTH bleeding assessment tool in children and parents in routine clinical practice. J Thromb Haemost. 2012; 10(7):1335–41.

7 Rodeghiero F, Tosetto A, Abshire T, Arnold DM, Coller B, James P, et al. ISTH/SSC bleeding assessment tool: a standardized questionnaire and a proposal for a new bleeding score for inherited bleeding disorders. J Thromb Haemost. 2010;8(9):2063–5.

8 Barbosa ACN, Montalvao SAL, Barbosa KGN, Colella MP, Annichino-Bizzacchi JM, Ozelo MC, et al. Prolonged APTT of unknown etiology: a systematic evaluation of causes and laboratory resource use in an outpatient hemostasis academic unit. Res Pract Thromb Haemost. 2019;3(4):749–57.

9 Moser KA, Smock KJ. Direct oral anticoagulant (DOAC) interference in hemostasis assays. Hematology. 2021;2021(1): 129–33.

10 Fritsma GA, Dembitzer FR, Randhawa A, Marques MB, Van Cott EM, Adcock-Funk D, et al. Recommendations for appropriate activated partial thromboplastin time reagent selection and utilization. Am J Clin Pathol. 2012;137(6): 904–8.

11 Hayward CP, Harrison P, Cattaneo M, Ortel TL, Rao AK. Platelet function analyzer (PFA)-100 closure time in the evaluation of platelet disorders and platelet function. J Thromb Haemost. 2006;4(2): 312–9.

12 Hvas AM, Grove EL. Platelet function tests: preanalytical variables, clinical utility, advantages, and disadvantages. Methods Mol Biol. 2017;1646:305–20.

13 Megy K, Downes K, Morel-Kopp M-C, Bastida JM, Brooks S, Bury L, et al. GoldVariants, a resource for sharing rare genetic variants detected in bleeding, thrombotic, and platelet disorders: communication from the ISTH SSC Subcommittee on Genomics in Thrombosis and Hemostasis. J Thromb Haemost. 2021;19(10):2612–7.

Chapter 5

Published online: December 5, 2024

Blanchette VS, Brandão LR, Carcao MD, Kumar R, Rand ML, Revel-Vilk S (eds): SickKids Handbook of Pediatric Thrombosis and Hemostasis, ed 3, rev. and ext. Basel, Karger, 2024, pp 60–69 (DOI: 10.1159/000538199)

Heavy Menstrual Bleeding in Adolescents

Caroline Malcolmson[a] Vanessa Bouskill[a] Eman Taryam AlShamsi[b]
Valerie Bloomfield[c] Rochelle Winikoff[d] Shoshana Revel-Vilk[e, f]

[a]Division of Hematology/Oncology, The Hospital for Sick Children, University of Toronto, Toronto, ON, Canada; [b]Department of Pediatric Hematology/Oncology, Al Jalila Children's Specialty Hospital, Dubai, United Arab Emirates; [c]Division of Gynecology, The Hospital for Sick Children, University of Toronto, Toronto, ON, Canada; [d]Department of Pediatrics, CHU Sainte-Justine, Université de Montréal, Montréal, QC, Canada; [e]Pediatric Hematology/Oncology Unit and Gaucher Unit, Shaare Zedek Medical Center, Jerusalem, Israel; [f]Faculty of Medicine, Hebrew University, Jerusalem, Israel

Introduction

Women with bleeding disorders can manifest a multitude of bleeding symptoms, including but not limited to gingival bleeding, epistaxis, easy bruising, minor wound bleeding, hemarthrosis, perioperative/postoperative, and dental bleeding; however, unique to women is the manifestation of gynecological bleeding, such as heavy menstrual bleeding (HMB). Approximately 15–30% of women with HMB will be diagnosed with a bleeding disorder, wherein, in many cases, HMB is the first and most common bleeding manifestation [1, 2]. Still, the true prevalence of bleeding disorders in women is unknown and is estimated to be grossly underdiagnosed [2, 3]. Many women with bleeding disorders experience years of delay from the time of presentation to the time of diagnosis [2, 4].

Pre-adolescent females with diagnosed bleeding disorders and their families should be educated about the risk of HMB ahead of menarche. It is important to counsel them about the signs and symptoms of HMB and when medical care should be sought. They should know that various medications can manage HMB and that these options are similar to those of adolescents without bleeding disorders, with few exceptions. In select cases of severe bleeding disorders, menstrual suppression at menarche may be considered.

This chapter reviews the evaluation and management of HMB in adolescents, emphasizing the importance of the specialized, multidisciplinary care required to meet diverse women's needs.

In this chapter, we will use the term women to address medical concerns related to persons assigned sex female and persons with a uterus. We wish to acknowledge, however, that not all persons assigned sex female identify as such.

Evaluation of Heavy Menstrual Bleeding

Normal Menstruation

Menstruation represents a bleeding challenge that occurs cyclically in women. Menarche, the first menstrual period, usually occurs 2–3 years after the initial onset of pubertal changes and typically occurs between the ages of 10 and 16, with the average age of onset being 12.5 years [5, 6]. The normal menstrual cycle length ranges from 24 to 38 days, with an average of 32 days [6, 7]. Within the first 3 years of menarche, it is common for adolescents to describe menstrual irregularity secondary to anovulatory cycles due to an immature hypothalamic pituitary-ovarian axis. With time, the hormonal signaling pathways mature and ovulatory cycles establish regularity [6]. Most menstruation lasts for less than 8 days [7]. Typically, no more than three to six regular pads or tampons are needed per day, and normal blood loss should be <80 mL per cycle [6]. Blood volume loss may vary from cycle to cycle.

Heavy Menstrual Bleeding

Abnormal uterine bleeding (AUB) is a term used to describe aberration in the volume, duration, or timing of menstruation [6]. HMB is defined objectively as >80 mL of blood loss per cycle. The clinical correlates of HMB include needing to change products such as a pad or tampon frequently (every 1–2 h), flooding, duration >7 days, passing of clots larger than 2.5 cm (1 inch) in diameter, or blood loss that interferes with subjective physical, social, and emotional wellbeing and/or resulting in iron deficiency. HMB may be associated with other symptoms such as dysmenorrhea, premenstrual symptoms, and/or premenstrual dysphoric disorder [7]. Overall, an estimated 30–40% of women will have HMB at some point.

It is important to note that by far the most common cause of AUB or HMB in adolescents is the result of anovulatory menstrual cycles or other gynecologic pathology such as polycystic ovarian syndrome (PCOS). In a typical ovulatory menstrual cycle, estrogen allows the growth of the endometrial lining while progesterone stabilizes the endometrium. There is cyclic estrogen and progesterone secretion, and when progesterone levels fall, menses occur. In anovulatory menstrual cycles, the midcycle surge of luteinizing hormone is absent, resulting in sustained production of estrogen and lack of progesterone. The endometrium then proliferates, and irregular heavy bleeding occurs when the endometrium becomes unstable. Approximately 85% of cycles are anovulatory in the first year after menarche; however, cycles may remain irregular for up to 3 years after the onset of menarche [6]. Anovulatory cycles, while one possible explanation for HMB, do not exclude the possibility of a concurrent bleeding disorder [1].

Multidisciplinary Care

Management of adolescents with HMB is best undertaken in a multidisciplinary care clinic involving specialties such as hematology, adolescent medicine, gynecology, social work, and nursing [8]. Multidisciplinary clinics should have access to laboratories specializing in coagulation testing for diagnosing bleeding disorders. When relevant, transitioning between pediatric and adult multidisciplinary clinics is essential to ensure proper care.

Psychosocial Impact

HMB can have a significant psychosocial impact [9]. Women with HMB have been found to have a significantly lower health-related quality of life and increased incidence of depression, anxiety, and absence from school and work. Thus, it is important to have a high index of suspicion for adverse psychosocial outcomes in women with HMB and consider the incorporation of validated patient self-reported screening questionnaires such as the menstrual bleeding questionnaire (MBQ), the adolescent menstrual bleeding questionnaire (aMBQ) [10], and the pediatric quality of life inventory (PedsQL).

5

Table 1. Menstrual history

- Age at menarche
- Cycle length and regularity
- Number of days of menstrual blood flow
- Number of sanitary protections (pads, diva cup, and/or tampons) changed per day
- Passage of clots, flooding/leaking
- Associated symptoms/dysmenorrhea (pelvic/lower abdominal pain, back pain)
- Signs and symptoms of iron deficiency (with or without anemia)
- Signs and symptoms of possible associated disorders (premenstrual dysphoric disorder, thyroid disease, liver disease, polycystic ovary syndrome [PCOS], tendency to extragenital bleeding)

Iron Deficiency

Iron deficiency with and without anemia is a major sequela for women with HMB that is often overlooked [11]. While definitions of iron deficiency can vary, more recent studies suggest a ferritin cutoff of <30 μg/L for women of reproductive age [12]. Signs and symptoms of iron deficiency with or without anemia can include fatigue/generalized weakness, decreased exercise tolerance, dyspnea, pallor, headache, irritability/depression, restless leg syndrome, vertigo, tachycardia, cardiac murmur, pica, and pagophagia [13]. Some adolescents may be asymptomatic. Thus, iron stores should be routinely monitored and repleted in adolescents with HMB.

Clinical History

The menstrual cycle should be considered a "fifth vital sign," along with blood pressure, body temperature, heart rate, and respiratory rate in all adolescents [14]. A detailed menstrual history should be part of the routine practice (Table 1).

Teaching women to track their menstrual cycles and accompanying symptoms, as well as number of products used, can be a powerful way for women to convey to their healthcare providers the extent of bleeding symptoms without relying on mental recall. This can be done with a traditional paper diary, bleeding questionnaires, or menstrual bleeding applications on an electronic device.

Validated bleeding questionnaires play an important role in determining the severity of bleeding as they help standardize subjective bleeding experiences. Subjective HMB may be normalized within a family of women who all experience HMB similarly. The Pictorial Blood Loss Assessment Chart (PBAC) is a validated semi-objective visual scoring system that depicts a graded series of soiled tampons and/or towels (see Appendix I). A PBAC score of >100 has been previously validated as both sensitive and specific for detecting HMB [15]. This score has been updated for the inclusion of modern menstrual products [16].

A careful bleeding history should include detailed timing and specifics of any other bleeding events (see Chapter 4 and Appendix I). Special care must be taken to inquire about hemarthroses and/or muscular hematomas, which may be overlooked in women (see Chapter 8).

A detailed family history should be obtained identifying: consanguinity and family history of abnormal bleeding or known bleeding disorders; requirements for transfusion; HMB; postpartum hemorrhage; history of hysterectomy or other invasive procedures for HMB; and a history of anemia requiring iron replacement therapy.

Laboratory Investigations

The initial laboratory tests for adolescents with HMB include a complete blood count (CBC), reticulocyte count, ferritin, transferrin, soluble transferrin receptor, and basic coagulation stud-

Table 2. Laboratory tests for diagnosis of a bleeding disorder

Tier	Tests	Comments
1	CBC aPTT, PT/INR VWF:Ag, VWF:Act, FVIII:C Blood type	- Abnormal CBC, aPTT and/or PT/INR may lead to further testing (see Chapter 4, Fig. 1) - Normal aPTT may miss mild coagulation deficiencies, testing is recommended in relevant cases (see Chapter 10) - Testing for von Willebrand disease is discussed in Chapter 9 - Blood type is useful to interpret VWF:Ag, VWF:Act and FVIII:C (see Chapter 9)
2	Platelet aggregation Platelet function analyzer-100®/200®	- Testing for platelet dysfunction is discussed in Chapter 6 - The use of NSAIDs and the presence of iron deficiency anemia may impact platelet function testing
3	Fibrinogen Factor XIII Fibrinolysis testing Bleeding disorder genetic testing	- Testing for inherited rare coagulation disorders is discussed in Chapter 10 - If there is a high index of clinical suspicion or family history of a bleeding disorder, proceed to genetic testing (see Chapter 21)

aPTT, activated partial thromboplastin time; CBC, complete blood count; FVIII:C, factor VIII activity; NSAIDs, nonsteroidal anti-inflammatory drugs; PT/INR, prothrombin time/international normalized ratio; VWF:Ag, von Willebrand factor antigen; VWF:Act, von Willebrand factor activity.

Table 3. Pre-analytic variables that can increase VWF and FVIII:C levels

- Pregnancy
- Oral contraceptive (estrogen dose >35 μg)[a]
- Physical and emotional stress
- Active bleeding
- Infection, inflammatory diseases (e.g., inflammatory bowel disease, lupus)

FVIII:C, factor VIII activity; VWF, von Willebrand factor. [a]Most commonly prescribed oral contraceptives have 30 μg of ethinyl estradiol.

ies (Table 2, Tier 1). Pregnancy testing, prolactin, and thyroid-stimulating hormone should be considered. Pre-analytic variables can impact von Willebrand factor (VWF) and factor VIII (FVIII) levels (Table 3). It may, therefore, be necessary to repeat these tests once these pre-analytic variables have been resolved [17].

Additional testing (Table 2, Tiers 2–3) is recommended in patients with a personal or family history of bleeding, significant HMB (e.g., causing anemia or iron deficiency, requiring hospitalization), or for persons >3 years from menarche with chronic HMB [17].

Management of Heavy Menstrual Bleeding

Medical Management of Acute Heavy Menstrual Bleeding

Optimal management of acute HMB includes rapid intervention and access to multidisciplinary care involving Pediatric Hematology and Gynecology or Adolescent Gynecology services. The development of in-house hospital protocols for the management of acute HMB is encouraged [18].

General Care Principles

Most acute HMB can be stopped with a combination of hormonal therapy and an intravenous/oral antifibrinolytic agent.

Hormonal therapy such as intravenous conjugated equine estrogen, 25 μg every 4–6 h, or monophasic combined oral contraceptives (COCs), 30 to 50 μg of an ethinyl estradiol formulation every 6–8 h, may be used until the bleeding has halted. A tapering regimen should begin after bleeding has stopped, usually within 24 to 48 h. Nausea and vomiting are common with high-dose estrogen therapy and can be exacerbated by oral iron therapy. Nausea can be managed by advising taking the medication immediately before sleep or with a short course of anti-emetics until developing tolerance. If these measures fail or an adolescent has a contraindication or intolerance to estrogen, they can be treated with progesterone-only therapy of oral medroxyprogesterone, 10 to 20 mg every 6–12 h, or norethindrone, 5–10 mg, every 6 h [19].

Ultrasonography can guide procedural management in adolescents who do not respond to medical therapy. For life-threatening HMB, endometrial balloon tamponade or additional surgical interventions may be considered in consultation with gynecology.

Transfusion of blood products should be reserved for life-threatening bleeds. Red blood cell (RBC) transfusion should be given if the patient is hemodynamically unstable. Avoiding RBC transfusion in children and adolescents with iron deficiency anemia is recommended when there is no evidence of hemodynamic instability or active bleeding [20]. Exposure to frozen plasma/fresh frozen plasma or cryoprecipitate should be limited to specific cases of severe factor deficiencies with life-threatening uncontrolled bleeding in the absence of factor concentrate.

Platelet transfusions may be used for platelet function disorders if the above measures do not control life-threatening bleeding and should be used cautiously in Bernard-Soulier syndrome and Glanzmann thrombasthenia (see Chapter 6). Human leukocyte antigens-matched platelets are preferred to avoid alloimmunization (and possible subsequent fetal neonatal alloimmune thrombocytopenia in pregnancy); however, this testing is time-consuming and not readily available. Platelet matching should not delay platelet transfusion in life-threatening bleeding. Women who are Rhesus D (RhD) negative should receive Rh immunoglobulin to reduce the risk of RhD sensitization if exposed to RhD-positive blood products (see Appendix III). Women who may become exposed to blood products should receive routine immunizations for hepatitis B.

Diagnosis-Specific Therapy Options

HMB in adolescents with factor deficiencies may be treated with factor concentrates specific to their deficiency, as outlined in the relevant chapters (see Chapters 8–10). Adolescents with severe platelet function disorders, such as Glanzmann thrombasthenia, may be treated with recombinant factor VIIa [21] (see Chapter 6).

Medical Management of Chronic Heavy Menstrual Bleeding

Once acute HMB is controlled and hormonal therapy has been tapered (usually over 1 to 2 weeks), maintenance therapy options should be based on the underlying diagnosis. A shared decision-making model incorporating adolescent and family preferences is suggested. Collaboration with gynecology, pediatric gynecology, and adolescent medicine, where available, can aid in counseling and help tailor therapy to target symptoms of bleeding and other menstrual-related concerns such as dysmenorrhea and/or the need for contraception.

Cultural Considerations of Menstrual Suppression

There are a multitude of personal, social, and cultural practices and beliefs surrounding menstruation and fertility. Providers must be open to adolescent and family preferences and support them in their decision-making. Information should be evidence-based, culturally safe, and tailored to the adolescent's needs. There are additional issues in women of childbearing age who wish to conceive but experience HMB. Pregnancy is not contraindicated in women with bleeding disorders but requires an appropriate choice of treatment for HMB and a multidisciplinary approach. A pre-pregnancy discussion with a multidisciplinary medical care team is ideal. The values, beliefs, and individual needs of each case should be sought, and decisions about the care and treatment options chosen should be respected.

Hormonal Therapy Options

Combined Oral Contraceptives

COCs are the first-line therapy for the management of HMB. They are effective and safe unless specifically contraindicated (e.g., thrombotic risk, history of cancer, migraine with aura). In addition to the effects on the uterine lining, these agents also increase FVIII and VWF plasma levels (Table 3). Reported side effects include mood changes, headaches, nausea, fluid retention, and breast tenderness. COCs (monophasic) may be used for a fixed period followed by a hormone-free interval (e.g., 42 days on, followed by a 3-day hormone-free interval) or continuously to extend the intervals between menstruation. A common side effect of continuous use is irregular spotting or breakthrough bleeding. Breakthrough bleeding can be ignored if mild, but if troublesome, a gynecology consult is advised.

Transdermal Contraceptive Patch

Transdermal patches contain combined estrogen-progesterone medication and are applied once weekly via a cutaneous patch that is highly adherent. Similar to COCs, the patch can be used to extend the cycle interval (e.g., one patch weekly for 6 weeks, followed by 1 week off). The side effect profile is similar to COCs.

Oral Progestins

For adolescents unable to tolerate estrogen-containing therapy or have a contraindication, oral progesterone-only pills, such as norethindrone, 5 to 15 mg/day, can be used for menstrual suppression. Unlike COCs, these medications are taken daily with no hormone-free interval. Common side effects include headache, nausea/vomiting, mood changes, and spotting.

Depot Medroxyprogesterone Acetate

Depot medroxyprogesterone acetate (DMPA) is an injectable progestin that offers high rates of reversible amenorrhea. DMPA can be administered intramuscularly (150 mg) or subcutaneously (104 mg) every 10 to 12 weeks. In women with bleeding disorders not on prophylaxis therapy, the subcutaneous route is preferred, and pressure should be applied to the injection site for 15 min or more. If given intramuscularly, a 27-gauge needle should be used. Around a third of women experience unscheduled bleeding while on therapy, which generally improves with continued use. Other common side effects include weight gain, headache, and mood changes; these symptoms may persist for several months. DMPA induces a hypoestrogenic state, and studies have demonstrated a reversible reduction in bone mineral density, which is thought to recover once this medication is discontinued. Adolescents should be counseled to optimize bone health with vitamin D supplementation and ensure sufficient dietary calcium.

Levonorgestrel-Releasing Intrauterine System

Levonorgestrel-releasing intrauterine system (LNG-IUS) is a small device placed within the endometrial cavity. It releases a low dose of levonorgestrel daily to induce endometrial atrophy. It is inserted into the uterus transvaginally. This insertion can occur in the office or hospital setting with or without sedation, patient dependent. For women with severe bleeding disorders, the use of antifibrinolytic agents around LNG-IUS insertion may be considered. The LNG-IUS may remain in place for years (duration specific to the product monograph). It can significantly reduce menstrual bleeding, clotting, and dysmenorrhea. LNG-IUS may be a good option for adolescents with poor compliance with oral hormonal therapies or who have a contraindication for COCs. Given the local effects of the LNG-IUS, systemic side effects (such as headache or mood changes) are uncommon. In the months following insertion, adolescents may experience irregular spotting and cramping. This improves with continued use.

Implant

The progesterone-only implant is a small rod inserted in the upper arm which releases progesterone continuously. Like other progestin methods, this serves to induce endometrial atrophy and may suppress ovulation. The implant may stay in place for years (depending on the specific drug monograph). Reported side effects may include but are not limited to mood alterations, headaches, vaginal dryness, breast tenderness, nausea, abdominal pain, and back pain.

Gonadotropin-Releasing Hormone Analogs

Gonadotropin-releasing hormone analogs (GnRHa) interrupt follicular development and ovulation, resulting in hypoestrogenism and, ultimately, secondary amenorrhea. These medications have significant side effects, including bone loss and menopausal symptoms such as hot flashes and vaginal dryness, and are typically reserved for adolescents who have failed other hormonal therapies.

Nonhormonal Therapy Options

Antifibrinolytic Agents

Nonhormonal therapies include antifibrinolytic agents, which substantially reduce fibrinolysis, decreasing menstrual blood loss [22]. They are effective in adolescents with and without underlying bleeding disorders and can be used in acute and chronic settings. Placebo-controlled studies have demonstrated up to a 40–60% reduction in menstrual losses. Antifibrinolytic agents can be used as monotherapy or in conjunction with other hormonal therapies (see Appendix III for doses). Although there is a theoretical concern about thrombotic events with concurrent use of COCs and antifibrinolytic agents, the available literature does not demonstrate increased risk. Common side effects include abdominal/pelvic pain, headaches, and nausea.

Desmopressin (DDAVP)

DDAVP (1-deamino-8-D-arginine vasopressin) is a synthetic analog of vasopressin that releases VWF and FVIII from storage in the endothelial Weibel-Palade bodies. It is given via the intranasal, intravenous, or subcutaneous route. It is reserved as a treatment strategy for persons with Type 1, 2A, or 2M von Willebrand disease or mild FVIII deficiency, including carriers of hemophilia A (see Chapters 8 and 9). It may also be considered for patients with mild platelet dysfunction and rare coagulation factor deficiencies (see Chapters 6 and 10).

DDAVP should be administered at the onset of bleeding and can be repeated at 24 h to a maximum of three doses to minimize the risk of tachyphylaxis, fluid retention, and hyponatremia. Doses of DDAVP are detailed in Appendix III. The side effects of DDAVP include facial flushing, headaches, nausea, menstrual-like cramps, and minor changes in pulse and blood pressure. Women receiving DDAVP must be monitored for fluid overload and should be fluid restricted.

Factor Therapies

Factor replacement prophylaxis should be considered for patients with relevant coagulation defects with low factor levels and in whom antifibrinolytic agents, DDAVP, and hormonal therapy failed to control the bleeding (see Chapters 8–10).

Nonsteroidal Anti-inflammatory Drugs

Nonsteroidal anti-inflammatory drugs (NSAIDs) inhibit cyclooxygenase, reduce endometrial prostaglandin levels, and interfere with platelet aggregation. NSAIDs can be modestly effective in reducing HMB and have a beneficial effect on painful menstrual periods [23]. NSAIDs should be used with caution in treating dysmenorrhea in women with bleeding disorders because of the additive effects on hemostasis.

Iron Therapy
Iron deficiency is common in women with chronic HMB, and regular monitoring of iron stores is important. Dietary advice should be reviewed, and oral or intravenous iron therapy should be administered as needed.

Hormonal Therapy and Thrombosis Risk

Women receiving COCs have a 4-fold increased risk of venous thromboembolism (VTE) compared to nonusers [24]. The estrogen dose and subtype of progesterone play a major role in thrombotic risk with COCs. Low-dose progestin-only pills are not associated with an increased risk of VTE. However, the risk of VTE is increased by about 2-fold with DMPA. LNG-IUS does not seem to increase the risk of VTE.

Providers who prescribe hormonal therapies should be familiar with indications and contraindications, such that a thorough discussion of benefits and risks can be undertaken. In addition to a comprehensive medical and surgical history, adolescents should be asked about a personal and family history of thrombotic events, personal history of migraine with aura, and smoking. All adolescents prescribed an estrogen-containing therapy should be counseled about the signs and symptoms of VTE, including but not limited to calf pain or swelling, chest pain, and shortness of breath. There is no indication for routine thrombophilia testing before COC initiation in adolescents without a family history of thrombotic events and/or thrombophilia traits (see Chapter 13).

Anticoagulant-Associated Heavy Menstrual Bleeding

Adolescents should be advised of the potential effect of anticoagulant therapy on menstrual bleeding at the time of treatment initiation. The exact rate in adolescents is unknown; however, among adult women taking oral anticoagulants, the rate of HMB was reported to be up to 70% [25]. The rate differs between types of studies. Vitamin K antagonists were reported to be associated with HMB as high as 67% in some studies and less than 10% in studies using more strict definitions. Data from large registry studies have demonstrated an increased risk of HMB in women taking oral factor Xa inhibitors as compared to warfarin, rivaroxaban (odds ratio [OR] 2.1), edoxaban (OR 1.26), and apixaban (OR 1.18) [25]. The reported risk was lower for women taking an oral direct thrombin inhibitor, such as dabigatran (OR 0.59).

Evaluation
The first assessment for HMB should be conducted at the time of initiation of anticoagulation using similar questions as described above (see Clinical History, Table 1). Assessment should include current and past menstrual-related symptoms, use of hormonal therapy, bleeding tendency, and symptoms/signs of anemia [26]. As described above, laboratory evaluation for bleeding disorder should be conducted if clinically suspected.

HMB assessment must be reviewed at each clinic visit to ensure no new symptoms develop during anticoagulant therapy. Iron deficiency with or without anemia needs to be monitored periodically.

Management
Adolescent women with HMB receiving anticoagulation therapy should be managed with a multidisciplinary approach, including hematology (preferably experts in pediatric hemostasis), adolescent medicine, and gynecology. The need for

ongoing anticoagulation and the intensity of anticoagulation should be assessed [26].

Hormonal therapies are the first-line option for managing HMB and should not be stopped in therapeutically anticoagulated women. Consideration should be given to either continuing the current hormone therapy regimen or rapidly transitioning to an alternative therapy, such as a progestin-based option. COCs should be discontinued before anticoagulation withdrawal, preferably in the setting of a transition to an alternative agent, such as the LNG-IUS or estrogen-free contraception.

Current evidence does not support the hypothesis that antifibrinolytic agents are associated with an unacceptable risk of VTE in women who received anticoagulants [25]. Antifibrinolytic agents can be given during only the heaviest days of the cycle.

Modification of Anticoagulation

Temporary or early discontinuation of anticoagulation has been shown to increase the risk of recurrent VTE, especially during the active treatment period. Therapeutic anticoagulation duration and switching of prophylaxis dose or discontinuation should be evaluated on a case-to-case basis taking into consideration the thrombotic and bleeding risks [25, 26]. Differences may exist in bleeding profiles with different formulations of anticoagulants [27–29] (see Chapter 20).

Conflict of Interest Statement

Caroline Malcolmson and Vanessa Bouskill report receiving consultancy and speaker fees from Takeda, NovoNordisk, Roche, Bayer Healthcare, Pfizer, and Sanofi/Genzyme. They are the recipients of research grants from Takeda, NovoNordisk, Roche, Bayer Healthcare, Pfizer, and Sanofi/Genzyme. Eman Taryam Al-Shamsi, Valeri Bloomfield, and Rochelle Winikoff declare no conflict of interest. Shoshana Revel-Vilk reports receiving consultancy and speaker fees from Takeda, Pfizer, and Sanofi/Genzyme. Shoshana Revel-Vilk reports receiving research grants from Takeda, Pfizer, and Sanofi/Genzyme.

Author Contributions

Caroline Malcolmson, Vanessa Bouskill, and Eman Taryam AlShamsi drafted the chapter, critically revised the chapter, and approved the final version. Shoshana Revel-Vilk critically revised the chapter, and approved the final version. Valerie Bloomfield critically revised the chapter, and approved the final version. Rochelle Winikoff critically revised the chapter, and approved the final version.

Abbreviations

aMBQ	Adolescent menstrual bleeding questionnaire
AUB	Abnormal uterine bleeding
CBC	Complete blood count
COCs	Combined oral contraceptives
DMPA	Depot medroxyprogesterone acetate
DDAVP	1-Deamino-8-D-arginine vasopressin (desmopressin)
FVIII	Factor VIII
GnRHa	Gonadotropin-releasing hormone analogs
HMB	Heavy menstrual bleeding
LNG-IUS	Levonorgestrel-releasing intrauterine system
MBQ	Menstrual bleeding questionnaire
NSAIDs	Nonsteroidal anti-inflammatory drugs
OR	Odds ratio
PBAC	Pictorial Blood Loss Assessment Chart
PCOS	Polycystic ovarian syndrome
PedsQL	Pediatric quality of life inventory
RBC	Red blood cell
RhD	Rhesus D
VTE	Venous thromboembolism/thromboembolic event
VWF	von Willebrand factor

References

1 Zia A, Jain S, Kouides P, Zhang S, Gao A, Salas N, et al. Bleeding disorders in adolescents with heavy menstrual bleeding in a multicenter prospective US cohort. Haematologica. 2020;105(7):1969–76.
2 James PD. Women and bleeding disorders: diagnostic challenges. Hematology Am Soc Hematol Educ Program. 2020; 2020(1):547–52.
3 Sidonio RF Jr, Zia A, Fallaize D. Potential undiagnosed VWD or other mucocutaneous bleeding disorder cases estimated from private medical insurance claims. J Blood Med. 2020;11:1–11.
4 Atiq F, Saes JL, Punt MC, van Galen KPM, Schutgens REG, Meijer K, et al. Major differences in clinical presentation, diagnosis and management of men and women with autosomal inherited bleeding disorders. EClinicalMedicine. 2021;32:100726.
5 Martinez GM. Trends and patterns in menarche in the United States: 1995 through 2013–2017. Natl Health Stat Report. 2020;146:1–12.
6 Borzutzky C, Jaffray J. Diagnosis and management of heavy menstrual bleeding and bleeding disorders in adolescents. JAMA Pediatr. 2020;174(2):186–94.
7 Munro MG, Critchley HOD, Fraser IS, Committee FMD. The two FIGO systems for normal and abnormal uterine bleeding symptoms and classification of causes of abnormal uterine bleeding in the reproductive years: 2018 revisions. Int J Gynaecol Obstet. 2018;143(3):393–408.
8 Zia A, Lau M, Journeycake J, Sarode R, Marshall J, De Simone N, et al. Developing a multidisciplinary Young Women's Blood Disorders Program: a single-centre approach with guidance for other centres. Haemophilia. 2016;22(2):199–207.
9 Rae C, Furlong W, Horsman J, Pullenayegum E, Demers C, St-Louis J, et al. Bleeding disorders, menorrhagia and iron deficiency: impacts on health-related quality of life. Haemophilia. 2013; 19(3):385–91.
10 Pike M, Chopek A, Young NL, Usuba K, Belletrutti MJ, McLaughlin R, et al. Quality of life in adolescents with heavy menstrual bleeding: validation of the Adolescent Menstrual Bleeding Questionnaire (aMBQ). Res Pract Thromb Haemost. 2021;5(7):e12615.
11 Zia A, Stanek J, Christian-Rancy M, Savelli S, O'Brien SH. Iron deficiency and fatigue among adolescents with bleeding disorders. Am J Hematol. 2022; 97(1):60–7.
12 MacLean B, Sholzberg M, Weyand AC, Lim J, Tang G, Richards T. Identification of women and girls with iron deficiency in the reproductive years. Int J Gynaecol Obstet. 2023;162(S2):58–67.
13 Houston BL, Hurrie D, Graham J, Perija B, Rimmer E, Rabbani R, et al. Efficacy of iron supplementation on fatigue and physical capacity in non-anaemic iron-deficient adults: a systematic review of randomised controlled trials. BMJ Open. 2018;8(4):e019240.
14 ACOG Committee Opinion No. 651:Menstruation in girls and adolescents: using the menstrual cycle as a vital sign. Obstet Gynecol 2015;126(6): e143–6.
15 Higham JM, O'Brien PM, Shaw RW. Assessment of menstrual blood loss using a pictorial chart. Br J Obstet Gynaecol. 1990;97:734–9.
16 Spence M, de Repentigny K, Bowman M, Hopman W, Thibeault L, James P. Validation of the pictorial blood loss assessment chart using modern sanitary products. Haemophilia. 2021;27(5):e632–5.
17 Zia A, Kouides P, Khodyakov D, Dao E, Lavin M, Kadir RA, et al. Standardizing care to manage bleeding disorders in adolescents with heavy menses – a joint project from the ISTH pediatric/neonatal and women's health SSCs. J Thromb Haemost. 2020;18(10):2759–74.
18 ACOG Committee Opinion No. 557: Management of acute abnormal uterine bleeding in nonpregnant reproductive-aged women. Obstet Gynecol. 2013; 121(4):891–6.
19 Costlow L. Heavy menstrual bleeding in adolescents: ACOG management recommendations. Am Fam Physician. 2020; 101(10):633–5.
20 O'Brien SH, Badawy SM, Rotz SJ, Shah MD, Makarski J, Bercovitz RS, et al. The ASH-ASPHO Choosing Wisely Campaign: 5 hematologic tests and treatments to question. Blood Adv. 2022; 6(2):679–85.
21 Tarawah A, Owaidah T, Al-Mulla N, Khanani M, Elhazmi J, Albagshi M, et al. Management of Glanzmanns thrombasthenia; guidelines based on an expert panel consensus from gulf cooperation council countries. J Appl Hematology. 2019;10(1):1–9.
22 Lethaby A, Farquhar C, Cooke I. Antifibrinolytics for heavy menstrual bleeding. Cochrane Database Syst Rev. 2000;(4):CD000249.
23 Bofill Rodriguez M, Lethaby A, Farquhar C. Non-steroidal anti-inflammatory drugs for heavy menstrual bleeding. Cochrane Database Syst Rev. 2019;9: CD000400.
24 Keenan L, Kerr T, Duane M, Van Gundy K. Systematic review of hormonal contraception and risk of venous thrombosis. Linacre Q. 2018;85(4):470–7.
25 Samuelson Bannow B. Management of heavy menstrual bleeding on anticoagulation. Hematology Am Soc Hematol Educ Program. 2020;2020(1):533–7.
26 Boonyawat K, O'Brien SH, Bates SM. How I treat heavy menstrual bleeding associated with anticoagulants. Blood. 2017;130:2603–9.
27 Huisman MV, Ferreira M, Feuring M, Fraessdorf M, Klok FA. Less abnormal uterine bleeding with dabigatran than warfarin in women treated for acute venous thromboembolism. J Thromb Haemost. 2018;16(9):1775–8.
28 Jacobson-Kelly AE, Samuelson Bannow BT. Abnormal uterine bleeding in users of rivaroxaban and apixaban. Hematology Am Soc Hematol Educ Program. 2020;2020(1):538–41.
29 Weaver J, Shoaibi A, Truong HQ, Larbi L, Wu S, Wildgoose P, et al. Comparative risk assessment of severe uterine bleeding following exposure to direct oral anticoagulants: a network study across four observational databases in the USA. Drug Saf. 2021;44(4):479–97.

Chapter 6

Published online: December 5, 2024

Blanchette VS, Brandão LR, Carcao MD, Kumar R, Rand ML, Revel-Vilk S (eds): SickKids Handbook of Pediatric Thrombosis and Hemostasis, ed 3, rev. and ext. Basel, Karger, 2024, pp 70–96 (DOI: 10.1159/000538188)

Inherited Platelet Disorders

Veerle Labarque[a] Ahmad Al-Huniti[b] Azzah Al-Zahrani[c] Walter H.A. Kahr[d]

[a]Department of Pediatric Hematology-Oncology, University Hospitals Leuven, Leuven, Belgium; [b]Department of Pediatric Hematology-Oncology, Mayo Clinic, Rochester, MN, USA; [c]Department of Pediatric Hematology-Oncology, Prince Sultan Military Medical City, Riyadh, Saudi Arabia; [d]Departments of Pediatrics and Biochemistry, University of Toronto, The Hospital for Sick Children, University of Toronto, Toronto, ON, Canada

Introduction

Platelets, the second most abundant cells in the blood, are essential in stopping bleeding and initiating hemostasis after being rapidly recruited to areas of vessel injury, where they contribute to the formation of the primary hemostatic plug (see Chapter 2). This process involves a sequence of platelet functional responses that include platelet adhesion (platelet-vessel wall interactions), platelet spreading, secretion of granular contents, platelet aggregation (platelet-platelet interactions), procoagulant surface exposure facilitating local thrombin generation, clot formation, and clot retraction. To support effective hemostasis, sufficient numbers of functional platelets must be present [1].

Platelet disorders may be inherited, but they are more frequently acquired. Given the impact on surveillance, therapeutic choices, and counseling, it is crucial to distinguish the cause of a disorder. Inherited platelet disorders (IPDs) are rare and include quantitative, qualitative, and combined platelet disorders. IPDs may lead to increased bleeding (depending on the defect) and can be accompanied by other congenital manifestations. They can also be associated with serious pathologies such as a high risk of malignancy. It is estimated that between $1:10^4$ and $1:10^6$ individuals suffer from an IPD. Mild and moderate platelet function disorders (PFDs) are more common and may go unnoticed, whereas severe disorders such as Glanzmann thrombasthenia (GT) and Bernard-Soulier syndrome (BSS) would more likely come to medical attention. High-throughput sequencing (HTS) has greatly facilitated the genetic diagnosis of IPDs, where variants in genes associated with platelet disorders are estimated to occur in 0.33% of the general population [2]. In this chapter, we give an overview of the most frequently occurring IPDs, including inherited thrombocytopenias (ITs), and PFDs. We summarize their pertinent features and discuss diagnostic techniques and therapeutic options. Acquired platelet disorders will be discussed in Chapter 7.

Inherited Thrombocytopenias

ITs mostly result from a deficit in platelet production, but some cases may be linked to reduced platelet lifespan. Understanding of the genetic basis of IT has greatly improved with the introduction of HTS. However, in daily practice it may not always be straightforward to recognize the hereditary character of thrombocytopenia, where acquired forms (e.g., immune thrombocytopenia) are much more common (see Chapter 7). Features that should raise the consideration of IT include a lifelong bleeding history, bleeding not in keeping with platelet counts, associated congenital abnormalities suggestive of a syndromic form, an informative family history, and abnormal platelet morphology (e.g., small/large or pale/gray platelets).

Classification of IT can readily be done on the basis of platelet size. Alternatively, IT can be classified as: (i) characterized by a platelet deficit only; (ii) associated with congenital abnormalities (syndromic form); or (iii) associated with an increased risk of complications such as malignancies. Note that several disorders affect both the number and function of platelets. An overview of the most common reported forms of IT and their main characteristics is presented in Table 1. A regularly updated list of genes related to bleeding disorders can be found online (https://www.isth.org/page/GinTh_GeneLists).

ITs with Normal Platelet Size

Congenital Amegakaryocytic Thrombocytopenia

Congenital amegakaryocytic thrombocytopenia (CAMT) is an autosomal recessive disorder that presents with severe thrombocytopenia and bleeding manifestations prenatally or at birth, with progression to bone marrow failure and pancytopenia during childhood [3]. Cardiac defects (atrial and ventricular septal defects), abnormalities of the central nervous system (cerebral and cerebellar hypoplasia), and retardation of psychomotor development have been reported in a minority of cases. CAMT is caused by a pathogenic variant in the *MPL* gene, resulting in the expression of a dysfunctional thrombopoietin (TPO) receptor. Levels of TPO in plasma are characteristically elevated. There is a genotype-phenotype correlation, which has led to the clinical description of two types of CAMT: *type I* presents with severe bleeding episodes prenatally or during the first weeks of life, platelet counts usually below 20×10^9/L, and early severe pancytopenia; *type II* is characterized by milder manifestations, with transient increases in platelet counts during the first year of life and severe thrombocytopenia and/or pancytopenia occurring later in childhood. Patients with frameshift or nonsense variants have a rapid progression to bone marrow failure, while the phenotype of patients with missense variants may be milder [3]. Allogeneic hematopoietic stem cell transplantation (HSCT) is the only curative treatment option for patients diagnosed with CAMT due to *MPL* variants.

TPO-Related Thrombocytopenia

TPO-related thrombocytopenia (TPO-RT) is associated with autosomal dominant or recessive variants in the *THPO* gene encoding TPO [4]. Monoallelic variants present with mild thrombocytopenia, whereas biallelic variants resemble CAMT; making the correct diagnosis is crucial for treatment, as patients with TPO-RT with complete loss of *THPO* can be treated with TPO receptor agonists including romiplostim (Nplate) and eltrombopag (Revolade).

ITs with Predisposition to Hematological Neoplasms

This group of diseases contains three autosomal dominant inherited disorders: familial platelet disorder with a propensity to acute myelogenous leukemia (FPD-AML); ankyrin repeat domain 26-related thrombocytopenia (ANKRD26-RT); and ETV6-related thrombocytopenia (ETV6-RT) [5]. Bleeding is generally mild in patients with ANKRD26-RT or ETV6-RT, while heterogenous

6

Table 1. Inherited thrombocytopenias classified by platelet size

Disease	Inheritance – gene (locus) and pathophysiology	Clinical characteristics	Laboratory characteristics	Treatment
Normal platelet size				
Congenital amegakaryocytic thrombocytopenia (CAMT) [3]	Autosomal recessive *MPL* (1p34.2) Dysfunctional thrombopoietin (THPO) receptor	Severe bleeding from birth Evolution into bone marrow failure in infancy or early childhood	Severe thrombocytopenia Reduced/absent bone marrow megakaryocytes	Supportive care Antifibrinolytics Platelet transfusion HSCT
TPO-related thrombocytopenia (TPO-RT) [4]	Autosomal dominant or recessive *THPO* (3q27) Defective TPO production	Severe bleeding from birth (mild bleeding if monoallelic) Evolution into bone marrow failure in infancy or early childhood	Mild to severe thrombocytopenia Reduced/absent bone marrow megakaryocytes	Supportive care Antifibrinolytics Platelet transfusion TPO receptor agonists might be an option
IT with predisposition to hematological neoplasms (subtypes below) [5]				
Familial platelet disorder with propensity to acute myelogenous leukemia (FPD-AML)	Autosomal dominant *RUNX1* (21q22) Defective RUNX1 protein resulting in granule deficiency and abnormal RUNX1 target signaling	Abnormal bruising or bleeding present in 90% of patients Bleeding disproportionate to platelet count High predisposition to malignancy or MDS (25–50% with average age of 33 years)	Mild to moderate thrombocytopenia ($50–150 \times 10^9$/L) but some patients have normal platelet counts Platelet aggregation: impaired response to collagen and arachidonic acid and absent/decreased second wave to ADP and epinephrine Decreased/absent α- and/or dense granules Atypical megakaryocytes in the bone marrow	Supportive care Antifibrinolytics DDAVP Platelet transfusion
Ankyrin repeat domain 26-related thrombocytopenia (ANKRD26-RT)	Autosomal dominant *ANKRD26* (10p12) Defective ANKRD26 binding to RUNX1 and FLI1 causing overexpression of ANKRD26 protein and defective pro-platelet formation as well as increased signaling through the TPO/MPL and MAPK/ERK pathways	Mild bleeding Predisposition to myeloid malignancy (8% with average age of 45 years)	Mild to moderate thrombocytopenia ($50–150 \times 10^9$/L); some patients have lower ($<10 \times 10^9$/L) and some have transient normal platelet counts Erythrocytosis and/or leukocytosis is possible	Supportive care Antifibrinolytics DDAVP Platelet transfusion
ETV6-related thrombocytopenia (ETV6-RT)	Autosomal dominant *ETV6* (12p13) Defective ETV6 function	Mild bleeding Predisposition to hematological malignancy (30%) esp. childhood B-cell ALL	Mild to moderate thrombocytopenia ($>75 \times 10^9$/L) Occasionally high MCV	Supportive care Antifibrinolytics DDAVP Platelet transfusion
Thrombocytopenia absent radius (TAR) [6,7]	Autosomal recessive *RBM8A* (1q21) Unknown pathophysiology	Severe bleeding Bilateral radial aplasia with presence of both thumbs Cow's milk allergy is common 15–20% with cardiac anomalies	Platelet count ($<50 \times 10^9$/L) that rises overtime (most patients have normal platelet count by school age)	Supportive care Antifibrinolytics Platelet transfusion

Table 1 (continued)

Disease	Inheritance – gene (locus) and pathophysiology	Clinical characteristics	Laboratory characteristics	Treatment
MECOM-related thrombocytopenia (MECOM-RT) [4]	Autosomal dominant *MECOM* (3q26) Impaired maintenance of hematopoietic stem cells due to abnormal zinc finger transcription factor	Severe bleeding from birth Possible evolution into bone marrow failure in infancy or early childhood Radius and ulna synostosis with/without other skeletal malformations	Severe neonatal thrombocytopenia Reduced/absent bone marrow megakaryocytes with/without hyporegenerative anemia	Supportive care Antifibrinolytics Platelet transfusion HSCT
Amegakaryocytic thrombocytopenia with radio-ulnar synostosis (RUSAT1) [4]	Autosomal dominant *HOXA11* (7p15) Defect in megakaryocytic differentiation	Severe bleeding from birth Radius and ulna synostosis with/without other skeletal malformations Possible evolution into bone marrow failure in infancy or early childhood	Severe neonatal thrombocytopenia Reduced/absent bone marrow megakaryocytes	Supportive care Antifibrinolytics Platelet transfusion HSCT
IKZF5-related thrombocytopenia (IKZF5-RT) [4]	Autosomal dominant *IKZF5* (10q26) Defective IKAROS Family Zinc Finger 5 (pegasos) transcription factor	Absent bleeding	Mild to moderate thrombocytopenia Decreased α- and dense granules	None
CYCS-related thrombocytopenia (CYCS-RT) [4]	Autosomal dominant *CYCS* (7p15) Pathophysiology incompletely understood	Absent bleeding	Mild to moderate thrombocytopenia	None
KDSR-related thrombocytopenia (KDSR-RT) [4]	Autosomal recessive *KDSR* (18q21.33) Defective sphingolipid synthesis	Moderate to severe bleeding Variable hyperkeratosis	Early severe thrombocytopenia Defective platelet function	Supportive care Antifibrinolytics Platelet transfusion
Quebec platelet disorder [22]	Please see Table 2			
Small platelets				
Wiskott-Aldrich syndrome (WAS)-related disorders (including X linked thrombocytopenia) [8]	X-linked *WAS* gene (Xp11.22) Absent/defective WAS protein (WASp) causing defective actin remodeling through actin-related protein 2/3 (Arp2/3) complex	Severe bleeding Eczema, recurrent infections, autoimmune disorders, lymphoma/malignancy Genotype-phenotype correlation: some variants present with only thrombocytopenia and less severe bleeding (X-linked thrombocytopenia)	Moderate to severe thrombocytopenia (usually <70 × 10^9/L) Reduced WASp expression Abnormal lymphocytes	Supportive care Antifibrinolytics Platelet transfusion TPO receptor agonists HSCT Splenectomy (not recommended)
ARPC1B deficiency [9]	Autosomal recessive *ARPC1B* (7q22.1) Absent/reduced ARPC1B in hematopoietic cell Arp2/3 complex required for actin filament branching	Moderate bleeding Inflammatory disease, recurrent infections, small vessel vasculitis	Moderate to severe thrombocytopenia (normal platelet counts in some patients) Decreased dense granules Absent/decreased ARPC1B on cell lysate immunoblot	Supportive care Antifibrinolytics Platelet transfusion HSCT
FYB-related thrombocytopenia (FYB-RT) [4]	Autosomal recessive *FYB* (5p13.1) Defective adhesion and degranulation-promoting adaptor protein (ADAP)	Mild to moderate bleeding	Moderate to severe thrombocytopenia Impaired activation of αIIbβ3	Supportive care Antifibrinolytics Platelet transfusion

Table 1 (continued)

Disease	Inheritance – gene (locus) and pathophysiology	Clinical characteristics	Laboratory characteristics	Treatment
PTPRJ-related thrombocytopenia (PTPRJ-RT) [4]	Autosomal recessive *PTPRJ* (11p11) Loss of PTPRJ expression leading to deficient SRC-type kinase activation	Mild to moderate bleeding	Moderate to severe thrombocytopenia Platelet aggregation: impaired response to collagen and convulxin	Supportive care Antifibrinolytics Platelet transfusion
Large platelets				
MYH9-RD [10]	Autosomal dominant *MYH9* (22q12-13) Malfunctioning nonmuscle myosin IIA motor protein (NMMIIA)	Absent to mild bleeding Variable degree of renal disease, sensorineural hearing loss, presenile cataract with genotype-phenotype correlation	Thrombocytopenia (platelet count underestimated by automated cell counters) Döhle-like inclusions can be seen in neutrophils on blood smears via immunofluorescence microscopy after staining for MYH9; not always present	Supportive care Antifibrinolytics Platelet transfusion TPO receptor agonists DDAVP (limited data)
Bernard-Soulier syndrome (BSS) [11]	Autosomal recessive *GP1BA* (17p13) *GP1BB* (22q11) *GP9* (3q21) Autosomal dominant *GP1BA* (17p13) *GP1BB* (22q11) Defective GPIb-IX-V receptor, impaired adhesion to VWF	Severe bleeding Bleeding disproportionate to degree of thrombocytopenia *GP9* variants might cause a milder phenotype	Moderate to severe thrombocytopenia Platelet aggregation: absent ristocetin-induced response Flow cytometry: reduced or absent CD42a (GPIX)/CD42b (GP1bα)	Supportive care Antifibrinolytics DDAVP (limited data) Platelet transfusion (risk of alloantibodies) rFVIIa (off-label use)
Thrombocytopenia Paris-Trousseau Type/Jacobsen syndrome [12]	Autosomal dominant Deletion of chromosome 11q23-24 Hemizygous deletion of *FLI1* (11q24.1-q24.3) Unknown pathophysiology	Mild to severe bleeding Cognitive, cardiac, facial, gastrointestinal, genitourinary, and central nervous system abnormalities	Thrombocytopenia might improve over time but platelet dysfunction persists Large fused α-granules on transmission electron microscopy	Supportive care Antifibrinolytics Platelet transfusion
ACTN1-related thrombocytopenia (ACTN1-RT) [13]	Autosomal dominant *ACTN1* (14q24) Disorganization of actin filaments in the cytoskeleton, defective proplatelet formation	Absent or mild bleeding	Mild to moderate thrombocytopenia Platelet anisocytosis Normal platelet function	Supportive care Antifibrinolytics
ITGA2B/ITGB3-related thrombocytopenia (ITGA2B/ITGB3-RT) [14]	Autosomal dominant *ITGA2B* (17q21) *ITGAB3* (17q21) Defective proplatelet formation	Mild to moderate bleeding	Variable degree of thrombocytopenia that may worsen at times of increased thrombopoietic demand Platelet anisocytosis Flow cytometry: low expression of CD41/CD61 (GPIIb-IIIa; αIIbβ3) Defective platelet function	Supportive care Antifibrinolytics Platelet transfusion
GFI1b-related thrombocytopenia (GFI1b-RT) [4]	Autosomal dominant or recessive *GFI1b* (9q34.13) Deficient growth factor independent 1B (GFI1B) transcription factor	Absent to severe bleeding	Mild to severe thrombocytopenia Anisopoikilocytosis and dysplastic megakaryocytes Variable α- and dense granule deficiency Abnormal expression of CD34	Supportive care Antifibrinolytics Platelet transfusion

Table 1 (continued)

Disease	Inheritance – gene (locus) and pathophysiology	Clinical characteristics	Laboratory characteristics	Treatment
GATA1-related disorders [4]	X-linked *GATA1* (Xp11.23) Deficient GATA1 transcription factor	Mild to severe bleeding	Mild to severe thrombocytopenia Dyserythropoiesis with or without anemia Dysplastic megakaryocytes Defective platelet function, α-granule deficiency	Supportive care Antifibrinolytics Platelet transfusion
TUBB1-related thrombocytopenia (TUBB1-RT) [4]	Autosomal dominant *TUBB1* (20q13) Defective β-1 tubulin	Absent to mild bleeding	Mild to moderate thrombocytopenia (normal platelet counts in some patients)	Supportive care Antifibrinolytics
PRKACG-related thrombocytopenia (PRKACG-RT) [4]	Autosomal recessive *PRKACG* (9q21.11) Defect in proplatelet formation	Severe bleeding	Severe thrombocytopenia	Supportive care Antifibrinolytics Platelet transfusion
TRPM7-related thrombocytopenia (TRPM7-RT) [4]	Autosomal dominant *TRPM7* (15q21.2) Defect of a constitutively active cation channel (transient receptor potential melastatin-like 7 [TRPM7])	Absent to mild bleeding	Moderate thrombocytopenia	Supportive care Antifibrinolytics
TPM4-related thrombocytopenia (TPM4-RT) [4]	Autosomal dominant *TPM4* (19q13.33) Dysregulated cytoskeleton function and proplatelet formation	Absent to mild bleeding	Mild thrombocytopenia	Supportive care Antifibrinolytics
SLFN14-related thrombocytopenia (SLFN14-RT) [42]	Autosomal dominant *SLFN14* (17q12) Defect in proplatelet formation and mitochondrial organization due to increased rRNA degradation	Moderate to severe bleeding	Mild to moderate thrombocytopenia Deficiency of dense granules	Supportive care Antifibrinolytics Platelet transfusion
SRC-related thrombocytopenia (SRC-RT) [4]	Autosomal dominant *SRC* (20q11.23) Overactive SRC causes reduction in proplatelet formation	Mild to severe bleeding Myelofibrosis, early edentulism, facial dysmorphia	Mild to severe thrombocytopenia Megakaryocytes with hypolobulated nuclei Deficiency of α-granules	Supportive care Antifibrinolytics Platelet transfusion
FLI-related thrombocytopenia (FLI-RT) [4]	Autosomal dominant or recessive *FLI1* (11q24.3) Maturation defect, reduced proplatelet formation, and defect in dense granule biosynthesis	Absent to moderate bleeding	Mild to moderate thrombocytopenia Giant α-granules in some platelets and deficiency of dense granule	Supportive care Antifibrinolytics Platelet transfusion
FLNA-related thrombocytopenia (FLNA-RT) [4]	X-linked *FLNA* (Xq28) Altered platelet production and modified platelet–vessel wall interaction due to impaired binding of GPIbα and integrin αIIbβ3 to the cytoskeleton	Mild bleeding Nodular periventricular heterotopia, cognitive impairment, skeletal malformations, heart valve dystrophy, intestinal obstruction, bone dysplasia	Moderate thrombocytopenia	Supportive care Antifibrinolytics

Table 1 (continued)

Disease	Inheritance – gene (locus) and pathophysiology	Clinical characteristics	Laboratory characteristics	Treatment
ACTB-related thrombocytopenia (ACTB-RT) [4]	Autosomal dominant *ACTB* (7p22.1) Inhibition of final steps in platelet maturation by compromising microtubule organization	Absent bleeding Facial anomalies, developmental delay, cognitive impairment, microcephaly (Baraitser-Winter syndrome 1)	Mild to moderate thrombocytopenia Eosinophilia or leukopenia	None
GALE-related thrombocytopenia (GALE-RT) [43]	Autosomal recessive *GALE* (1p36.11) Abnormal glycosylation of GPIbα and β1 integrin leading to decreased proplatelet formation	Severe bleeding	Severe thrombocytopenia Anemia, neutropenia Galactosemia	Supportive care Antifibrinolytics Platelet transfusion
SLC35A-related thrombocytopenia (SLC35A1-RT) [4]	Autosomal recessive *SLC35A1* (6p15) Reduced sialic acid biosynthesis, which causes altered platelet formation and increased clearance of platelets	Mild bleeding Developmental delay, epilepsy, ataxia and microcephaly	Moderate thrombocytopenia	Supportive care Antifibrinolytics
GNE-related thrombocytopenia (GNE-RT) [4]	Autosomal recessive *GNE* (9p13.3) Reduced sialic acid biosynthesis, which causes altered platelet formation and increased clearance of platelets	Mild to severe bleeding Myopathy in early adulthood	Severe thrombocytopenia	Supportive care Antifibrinolytics Platelet transfusion
MPIG6B-related thrombocytopenia (MPIG6B-RT) [4]	Autosomal recessive *MPIG6B* (6p21.33) Deficient megakaryocyte and platelet inhibitory receptor G6b	Mild to moderate bleeding	Mild to severe thrombocytopenia Atypical megakaryocytes, microcytic anemia, leukocytosis, myelofibrosis	Supportive care Antifibrinolytics Platelet transfusion
ABCG5/ABCG8-related thrombocytopenia (ABCG5/ABCG8-RT) [4]	Autosomal recessive *ABCG5* or *ABCG8* (2p21) Disorder of lipid metabolism	Mild bleeding Xanthelasmas and tendinous or tuberous xanthomas	Mild to moderate thrombocytopenia Increased plasma levels of plant sterols Blood film: stomatocytes	Supportive care Antifibrinolytics
Takenouchi-Kosaki syndrome [4]	Autosomal dominant *CDC42* (1p36) Impaired regulation of cell cycle and actin cytoskeleton	Absent bleeding May include abnormalities of brain, face, muscle, and skeletal tissues May be associated with immunodeficiency, eczema, hearing/visual impairment, lymphedema, cardiac, or genitourinary malformations	Moderate thrombocytopenia	None
DiGeorge/velocardiofacial syndrome [4]	Autosomal dominant 22q11.2 deletion (including *TBX1* and *GP1BB*) Defective GPIb-IX-V receptor	Mild to severe bleeding Cardiac abnormalities, parathyroid and thymus insufficiency, developmental delay, cleft palate, dysmorphic facial features	Moderate thrombocytopenia	Supportive care Antifibrinolytics Platelet transfusion

Table 1 (continued)

Disease	Inheritance – gene (locus) and pathophysiology	Clinical characteristics	Laboratory characteristics	Treatment
DIAPH1-related thrombocytopenia (DIAPH1-RT) [4]	Autosomal dominant *DIAPH1* (5q31) Defective actin filament nucleation and elongation	Absent or mild bleeding Hearing loss in early childhood	Mild thrombocytopenia (normal platelet counts in some patients) Variable neutropenia	Supportive care Antifibrinolytics
Gray platelet syndrome [19, 20]	Please see Table 2			
Arthrogryposis, renal dysfunction, cholestasis (ARC) syndrome [21]	Please see Table 2			

ACTN1, α-actinin 1; ADAP, adhesion and degranulation-promoting adaptor protein; ADP, adenosine 5′-diphosphate; ALL, acute lymphoblastic leukemia; ANKRD26, ankyrin repeat domain 26; ARC, arthrogryposis-renal dysfunction-cholestasis; Arp 2/3, actin-related protein 2/3; BSS, Bernard-Soulier syndrome; CAMT, congenital amegakaryocytic thrombocytopenia; CD, cluster-of-differentiation; CDC42, cell division cycle 42; CYCS, cytochrome c, somatic; DDAVP, 1-deamino-8-D-arginine vasopressin; ETV6, ETS variant transcription factor 6; FDP-AML, familial platelet disorder with propensity to acute myelogenous leukemia; FLI1, Friend leukemia virus integration 1; FLNA, filamin A; GALE, uridine diphosphate-galactose-4-epimerase; GFI1b, growth factor-independent 1b; GNE, glucosamine-2-epimerase/*N*-acetylmannosamine kinase; GP, glycoprotein; HSCT, hematopoietic stem cell transplantation; IKZF5, IKAROS Family Zinc Finger 5; IT, inherited thrombocytopenia; KDSR, 3-keto-dihydrosphingosine reductase; MCV, mean corpuscular volume; MDS, myelodysplastic syndrome; MECOM, MDS1 and EVI1 complex locus; MPIG6B, megakaryocyte and platelet inhibitory receptor G6b; MYH9-RD, myosin heavy chain 9-related disease; NMMIIA, nonmuscle myosin IIA motor protein; PRKACG, protein kinase, cyclic adenosine monophosphate-dependent, catalytic, gamma; PTPRJ, protein-tyrosine phosphatase, receptor-type, J; rFVIIa, recombinant activated factor VII; RT, related thrombocytopenia; RUSAT1, amegakaryocytic thrombocytopenia with radio-ulnar synostosis; SLC35A, solute carrier family 35 member A1; SLFN14, Schlafen 14; TAR, thrombocytopenia absent radius; TBX1, T-box transcription factor 1; TPO, thrombopoietin; TPM4, tropomyosin 4; TRPM7, transient receptor potential melastatin-like 7; TUBB1, tubulin, β1; VWF, von Willebrand factor; WAS, Wiskott-Aldrich syndrome; WASp, WAS protein.

platelet function in FPD-AML (caused by a *RUNX1* variant) leads to bleeding of varying severity. Note that some patients with a germline *RUNX1* variant have normal platelet counts. FPD-AML has the highest risk of acquired hematological malignancies (25–50% lifetime risk) and predisposes primarily to myeloid malignancies, which can present at all ages – most frequently in the third decade of life. On the other hand, ETV6-RT predominantly predisposes to lymphoid malignancies, which may occur during childhood or adulthood. It is estimated that 30% of ETV6-RT develop a hematologic malignancy. ANKRD26-RT has the lowest risk, and the prevalence of acute myelogenous leukemia (AML) or myelodysplastic syndromes (MDSs) among individuals with ANKRD26-RT is about 8% with a median age of 45 for AML progression. No consistent genotype-phenotype correlations are known for RUNX1-RT, ETV6-RT, and ANKRD26-RT. There are currently no data on an evidence-based approach for surveillance, but a clinical examination and complete blood count with differential is advised every 6 to 12 months. A bone marrow examination could be considered annually, but the frequency must be weighed against the burden of a screening protocol, particularly in young children, and should be determined on a case-by-case basis.

Thrombocytopenia Absent Radius

Thrombocytopenia absent radius (TAR) is an autosomal recessive disorder characterized by thrombocytopenia and bilateral absence of the radii with the presence of both thumbs. In most individuals, platelet counts remain low during the first 2 years of life, then increase to near-normal levels. There can also be abnormalities of the lower limbs, ribs, vertebrae, heart, and kidney, and agenesis of the uterus, cervix, and upper part of the vagina [6, 7]. The bleeding phenotype can be severe. TAR is most commonly caused by compound heterozygosity with a microdeletion involving the *RBM8A* gene (null allele) on one

6

chromosome and a single nucleotide polymorphism affecting expression of *RBM8A* (hypomorphic allele) on the other [6].

Amegakaryocytic Thrombocytopenia with Radio-Ulnar Synostosis
Amegakaryocytic thrombocytopenia with radio-ulnar synostosis (RUSAT1) is an autosomal dominant disorder associated with variants in the *HOXA11* gene causing severe neonatal thrombocytopenia that progresses to pancytopenia [4]. Bleeding tendency is severe. Radius and ulnar synostosis or proximal fusion of the radius and ulna may be accompanied by other skeletal malformations.

ITs with Small Platelets
Wiskott-Aldrich Syndrome
Wiskott-Aldrich syndrome (WAS) is an X-linked disease caused by a molecular defect in the *WAS* gene (Xp11.22) [8], encoding a protein, WASp (Wiskott-Aldrich syndrome protein), that serves as a nucleation promoting factor for actin cytoskeletal filament formation. WAS is characterized by moderate to severe thrombocytopenia in the neonatal period, susceptibility to infections due to combined immunodeficiency in early infancy, extensive eczema in infancy and childhood, and increased tendency to develop malignancies and autoimmune diseases later in life. A correlation between the genotype and phenotype has been described [8]: variants having the greatest effect on WASp expression or functionality are associated with a more severe phenotype, while variants resulting in a reduced level of protein activity lead to a less severe disease with only isolated thrombocytopenia, also called X-linked thrombocytopenia (XLT). In contrast, gain-of-function variants in *WAS* do not cause bleeding symptoms but are associated with X-linked neutropenia, which is characterized by hyperactive neutrophils, reduced myelopoiesis, and low blood neutrophil counts.

ARPC1B-Related Thrombocytopenia
ARPC1B-related thrombocytopenia (ARPC1B-RT) is an autosomal recessive disease causing moderate to severe thrombocytopenia in some patients. The defect is due to depletion of ARPC1B, a component of the Arp2/3 complex required for actin filament branching; its loss causes immune-mediated inflammatory disease, splenomegaly, lymphadenopathy, and impaired growth [9]. As in WAS, there is eosinophilia, and platelets are small and are deficient in dense granules.

ITs with Large Platelets
Myosin Heavy Chain 9-Related Disease
This autosomal dominant macrothrombocytopenia encompasses what were previously known as May-Hegglin anomaly, Fechtner syndrome, Sebastian platelet syndrome, and Epstein syndrome, which all involve variants of the *MYH9* gene [10]. Myosin heavy chain 9-related disease (MYH9-RD) is the most frequent cause of IT worldwide. Cytochemical or immunofluorescence microscopy detection of pathognomonic neutrophilic Döhle-like inclusion bodies on a blood smear (as shown in Fig. 1g, h) confirms the diagnosis, although this is not always detected. Macrothrombocytopenia of varying degree is present from birth, and the platelet count may be underestimated by automated cell counters. Apart from bleeding manifestations that are usually not a major problem in these patients, sensorineural deafness, cataracts, nephritis, and transaminitis can occur, which are mostly detected later in life. The onset of hearing loss occurs any time between the first and sixth decade. Nephropathy also presents at variable age, with a mean age at onset of 27 years. The mean age of cataracts is 37 years. However, congenital cataracts have also been reported. Interestingly, the risk and age of onset of extra-hematological symptoms varies with the location of pathogenic variants in *MYH9,* with N-terminus variants causing more severe and systemic disease owing to effects on the function of the myosin motor head. Recommended sur-

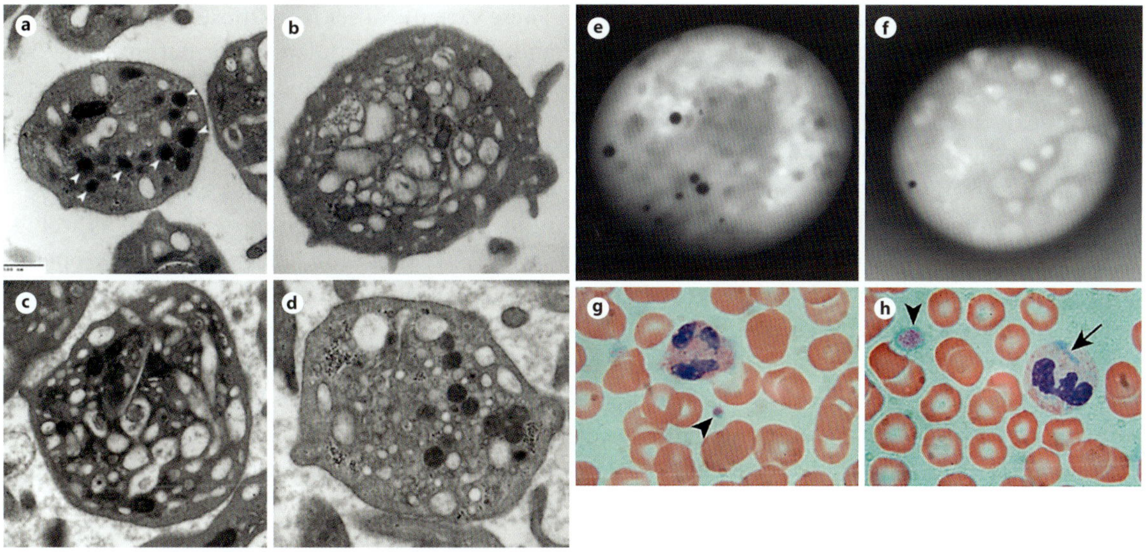

Fig. 1. Examples of diagnostic electron microscopy images of platelets. **a–d** Transmission electron microscopy images (40,000×) of platelets from a normal donor showing abundant alpha (α) granules (arrows, **a**), platelets from a patient with GPS, showing lack of α-granules and extensive vacuoles (**b**), which are also observed in platelets from a patient with ARC with a pathogenic *VIPAS39* (VPS16B) variant (**c**) and a pathogenic *VPS33B* variant (**d**) (scale bar = 500 nm); reproduced without modifications from Chen et al. [41]. **e, f** Whole-mount electron microscopy images of platelets for dense granule evaluation showing a normal platelet with dense granules appearing as electron-dense black spots (**e**) and an abnormal platelet with dense granule deficiency showing a single black spot (**f**). **g, h** Blood smear of a normal subject (**g**) revealing normal-sized platelets (arrowhead) and neutrophil and of a patient with MYH9-related disease (**h**) revealing a large platelet (arrowhead) and neutrophil containing a Döhle-like inclusion body (arrow). ARC, arthrogryposis-renal dysfunction-cholestasis; GPS, gray platelet syndrome.

veillance includes annual screening (or every 6 months in patients with high-risk *MYH9* genotypes [10]) for nephropathy, and screening every 3 years for hearing loss and cataracts. Older individuals may have elevated liver enzymes.

Bernard-Soulier Syndrome

BSS is a mostly autosomal recessive disorder secondary to the absence or nonfunctionality of the platelet glycoprotein (GP)Ib-IX-V complex, leading to abnormal von Willebrand factor (VWF)-mediated adhesion to the exposed vascular endothelium [11]. BSS is primarily caused by loss-of-function *GP1BA*, *GP1BB*, or *GP9* variants, although autosomal dominant inheritance of monoallelic *GP1BA* or *GP1BB* variants has also been described. Platelet agglutination with ristocetin is absent and not restored with the addition of normal plasma, while the response to other agonists is normal. Quantitative flow cytometry measuring GPIb-IX-V on the platelet surface can confirm the diagnosis, and molecular analysis of the respective genes can be performed. Affected patients usually have moderate to severe macrothrombocytopenia. Bleeding symptoms start early in childhood and are severe and disproportionate to the degree of thrombocytopenia. However, patients with a *GP9* variant may have a milder phenotype. Also, the monoallelic forms have been reported to result in less severe or absent bleeding symptoms.

Paris-Trousseau Thrombocytopenia/Jacobsen Syndrome
Paris-Trousseau syndrome, also called Jacobsen syndrome, is an autosomal dominant IT caused by chromosome 11q23 terminal deletions of variable length affecting many genes, including the gene encoding the Friend leukemia virus integration 1 transcription factor (FLI1) [12]. Homozygous missense variants in *FLI1* have also been reported. Most patients affected are diagnosed during the first year of life and present with severe thrombocytopenia. The bleeding tendency is mild to severe. Other clinical findings include cognitive impairment, dysmorphism of the face and digits, cardiac abnormalities, and malformations of the gastrointestinal tract, central nervous system, kidney, urinary tract, and/or skeleton, as well as growth delay. Thrombocytopenia is associated with defective platelet function due to large fused α-granules. Cardiac abnormalities associated with high-shear blood flow can also lead to acquired von Willebrand syndrome (see Chapter 11). Thrombocytopenia improves and may even resolve over time in these patients, but platelet dysfunction usually persists.

α-Actinin 1-Related Thrombocytopenia
α-Actinin 1-related thrombocytopenia (ACTN1-RT) is an autosomal dominant cause of mild to moderate macrothrombocytopenia, which is accompanied by anisocytosis [13]. Variants in the *ACTN1* gene, encoding for α-actinin 1, lead to disorganized actin filaments in the cytoskeleton and defective proplatelet formation. Bleeding symptoms in affected patients are absent or mild and no apparent in vitro defects in platelet function are present. Genetic testing should be performed to diagnose patients with ACTN1-RT.

ITGA2B/ITGB3-Related Thrombocytopenia
Heterozygous *ITGA2B* or *ITGB3* variants cause autosomal dominant ITGA2B/ITGB3-related thrombocytopenia (ITGA2B/ITGB3-RT) or Glanzmann thrombasthenia-like syndrome [14]. These variants differ from those causative for GT, and they affect proplatelet formation. They are invariably hypomorphic, which implies either a product leading to reduced αIIbβ3 activity, or decreased protein expression resulting in reduced αIIbβ3 on the platelet surface. Patients have a mild to moderate bleeding tendency, as well as variable degree of macrothrombocytopenia, platelet anisocytosis, and impaired platelet function measured by platelet function analyzer-100®/200® (PFA-100®/200®), light transmission aggregometry (LTA), and adenosine 5′-triphosphate (ATP) release. Note that the degree of thrombocytopenia can worsen at times of increased thrombopoietic demand (e.g., infections, surgery, pregnancy).

DiGeorge/Velocardiofacial Syndrome
DiGeorge/velocardiofacial syndrome, also known as 22q11.2 deletion syndrome, is caused by a microdeletion on the long arm of chromosome 22. Deletions include *TBX1* and *GP1BB* genes. It is associated with moderate thrombocytopenia, cardiac abnormalities, parathyroid and thymus insufficiency, developmental delay, cleft palate, and dysmorphic facial features [4]. It is an autosomal dominant condition, where the majority of cases are a result of de novo deletions and only 10% are inherited. Bleeding can be mild to severe.

Inherited Platelet Function Disorders

Inherited PFDs, especially secretion defects and nonspecific aggregation abnormalities, are very common and may collectively be as prevalent as mild type 1 von Willebrand disease (VWD) (see Chapter 9). Nevertheless, prevalence in the general population has not been established. Due to the challenges of diagnostic evaluation and the requirement for specialized laboratory testing, many patients are undiagnosed. Table 2 provides a list of the most frequent PFDs categorized according to the underlying pathophysiology.

Table 2. Platelet function disorders classified based on underlying pathophysiology

Disease	Inheritance – gene (locus) and pathophysiology	Clinical characteristics	Laboratory characteristics	Bleeding treatment
Glycoprotein defects				
Defects in platelet adhesion				
Bernard-Soulier syndrome (BSS) [11]	Please see Table 1			
Platelet-type von Willebrand disease (PT-VWD) [15]	Autosomal dominant *GP1BA* (17p13) Hyperresponsive GPIb-IX-V gain-of-function interaction between VWF and GP1bα	Mild to moderate bleeding	Normal platelet count in many patients but may decrease under stress conditions Platelet clumping Low VWF activity compared to VWF antigen and reduced high-molecular-weight VWF multimers Platelet aggregation: increased low-dose ristocetin-induced platelet agglutination (also after mixing platelets with normal plasma)	Supportive care Antifibrinolytics Platelet transfusion +/− VWF (if activity is low) rFVIIa (off-label use)
Collagen receptor defects [4]	Autosomal recessive *GP6* (19q13.4) Defective GPVI receptor, impaired response to collagen	Mild to moderate bleeding	Platelet aggregation: abnormal response to collagen and collagen related peptide	Supportive care Antifibrinolytics DDAVP Platelet transfusion
Ephrin type-B receptor 2 defect [4]	Autosomal recessive *EPHB2* (1p36.12) Impaired GPVI and αIIbβ3 signaling	Moderate to severe bleeding	Normal platelet count and morphology Platelet aggregation and secretion: decreased response to multiple agonists	Supportive care Antifibrinolytics DDAVP Platelet transfusion
Defects in platelet aggregation				
Glanzmann thrombasthenia (GT) [17]	Autosomal recessive *ITGA2B* (17q21.32) *ITGB3* (17q21.32) Defective integrin αIIbβ3 (GPIIb-IIIa, CD41/CD61) causing impaired fibrinogen/VWF-mediated platelet aggregation	Severe bleeding Most patients diagnosed before 5 years of age	Normal platelet count and morphology Abnormal PFA-100®/200® Platelet responses: absent to all agonists except ristocetin Flow cytometry: absent or reduced CD41 and CD61	Supportive care Antifibrinolytics rFVIIa (considered first line to avoid exposure to platelets) Platelet transfusion (risk of formation of platelet alloantibodies) – may need higher dose of platelets than usual (see text)
Defects in agonist receptors				
Adenosine 5′-diphosphate (ADP) receptor defects [4]	Autosomal recessive (or dominant) *P2RY12* (3q23–25) Defective ADP receptor	Mild bleeding	Normal platelet count Platelet aggregation: abnormal response to ADP Flow cytometry: reduced P2Y12 receptor	Supportive care Antifibrinolytics DDAVP Platelet transfusion
Thromboxane-prostanoid (TP) receptor defects [4]	Autosomal recessive or dominant *TBXA2R* (19p13.3) Defective TP receptor	Mild bleeding	Normal platelet count Platelet aggregation: abnormal response to arachidonic acid and U46619; normal or reduced second wave to other agonists	Supportive care Antifibrinolytics DDAVP Platelet transfusion

Table 2 (continued)

Disease	Inheritance – gene (locus) and pathophysiology	Clinical characteristics	Laboratory characteristics	Bleeding treatment
Defects in platelet signaling pathways				
G-protein defects [4]	Complex inheritance pattern *GNAS* (20q13.32) *GNAQ* (9q21.2) *GNAZ* (22q11.22-q11.23) *GNAI1* (7q21.11) Defects in G-protein signaling	Moderate bleeding, mostly linked to hemostatic challenges Association with neurological and other abnormalities	Normal platelet count Platelet aggregation: reduced to multiple agonists	Supportive care Antifibrinolytics DDAVP Platelet transfusion
CalDAG-GEFI defect [4]	Autosomal recessive *RASGRP2* (11q13.1) Defective Rap1 (small GTPase) and integrin activation	Moderate to severe bleeding	Normal platelet count Platelet aggregation: decreased response to ADP, epinephrine, low-dose collagen Impaired αIIbβ3 activation	Supportive care Antifibrinolytics DDAVP rFVIIa (off-label use) Platelet transfusion not efficacious
Leukocyte adhesion deficiency syndrome type 3 (LADIII) [18]	Autosomal recessive *FERMT3* (11q13.1) Impaired adhesion of leukocytes and platelets	Severe bleeding Infections, abnormal healing, osteopetrosis	Normal platelet count Platelet response: nonresponsive to all agonist except ristocetin Flow cytometry: normal levels of CD41/CD61 (GPIIb-IIIa; αIIbβ3)	Supportive care Antifibrinolytics Platelet transfusion rFVIIa (off-label use) HSCT
Platelet granule defects				
Defects in α-granules				
Gray platelet syndrome [19, 20]	Autosomal recessive *NBEAL2* (3p21) Defective development of α-granules, loss of α-granule cargo proteins into bone marrow and spleen	Mild to moderate bleeding Splenomegaly due to extramedullary hematopoiesis Immune dysregulation/autoimmunity	Mild to moderate macrothrombocytopenia; often worsening with age Progressive myelofibrosis Absent to severely reduced α-granules on TEM	Supportive care Antifibrinolytics DDVAP Platelet transfusion Splenectomy (in rare cases)
Arthrogryposis, renal dysfunction, cholestasis (ARC) syndrome [21]	Autosomal recessive *VPS33B* (15q26) *VIPAS39* (14q24) Abnormal membrane fusion and intracellular vesicle trafficking	Renal tubular dysfunction, cholestasis, joint contractures, failure to thrive, ichthyosis, central nervous system, cardiac abnormalities, and bleeding Lethal early in life (certain variants are associated with attenuated phenotype)	Thrombocytopenia Large platelets on blood film Absent α-granules on TEM Variable results of platelet aggregation	Supportive care Antifibrinolytics Platelet transfusion
Quebec platelet disorder (QPD) [22]	Autosomal dominant Tandem duplication of *PLAU* (10q22.2) Hyperfibrinolysis caused by abnormal secretion of urokinase from platelets upon clot formation	Delayed-onset bleeding not responding to platelet transfusion Joint bleed and hematuria common Delayed wound healing in about 25% of patients	Mild thrombocytopenia to normal platelet count Abnormal levels of urokinase in platelets detected with immunoblot or ELISA Platelet aggregation: abnormal response to epinephrine	Supportive care Antifibrinolytics
Defects in dense granules or secretion defects				
Nonsyndromic secretion defects of dense granule deficiency ("storage pool disease")	Variable inheritance pattern Responsible genes largely unknown	Mild mucocutaneous bleeding but more significant bleeding following surgery or trauma	Normal platelet count Platelet aggregation: variable abnormalities Decreased numbers of dense granules (dense granule deficiency) Lumiaggregometry: impaired release of ATP (secretion defects)	Supportive care Antifibrinolytics DDAVP Platelet transfusion

Table 2 (continued)

Disease	Inheritance – gene (locus) and pathophysiology	Clinical characteristics	Laboratory characteristics	Bleeding treatment
Hermansky-Pudlak syndrome (HPS) [24]	Autosomal recessive HPS1–11 (*HPS1, AP3B1, HPS3, HPS4, HPS5, HPS6, DTNBP1, BLOC1S3, BLOC1S6, AP3D1*, and *BLOC1S5*) Defective biogenesis of lysosome and lysosome-related organelle and intracellular protein trafficking including δ-granules and melanosomes	Mild to moderate bleeding Oculocutaneous albinism Pulmonary fibrosis, interstitial lung disease, granulomatous colitis, neutropenia, and/or immune defects associated with certain HPS variants	Normal platelet count Decreased to absent dense granules on whole-mount EM Lumiaggregometry: decreased/absent ATP release	Supportive care Antifibrinolytics DDAVP Platelet transfusion
Chediak-Higashi syndrome (CHS) [25]	Autosomal recessive *LYST* (1q42–1q42.2) Defective vesicular protein and membrane trafficking resulting in giant granules	Mild bleeding Oculocutaneous albinism Immunodeficiency Risk of developing HLH Neurological manifestation	Normal platelet count Giant eosinophilic inclusions in neutrophils Decreased to absent δ-granules Lumiaggregometry: decreased/absent ATP release	Supportive care Antifibrinolytics DDAVP Platelet transfusion
Defects in procoagulant activity				
Scott syndrome [26]	Autosomal recessive *ANO6* (12q12) Defective expression of TMEM16F protein; impaired calcium-mediated procoagulant phosphatidylserine exposure on platelets and other blood cells	Mild bleeding disorder Postoperative, heavy menstrual bleeding, and postpartum hemorrhage are most common manifestations	Normal platelet count Absent phosphatidylserine expression on activated platelets' surface by flow cytometry	Supportive care

ADP, adenosine 5′-diphosphate; ARC, arthrogryposis-renal dysfunction-cholestasis; ATP, adenosine 5′ triphosphate; BSS, Bernard-Soulier syndrome; CalDAG-GEFI, calcium and diacylglycerol-regulated guanine exchange factor I; CD, cluster-of-differentiation; CHS, Chediak-Higashi syndrome; DDAVP, 1-deamino-8-D-arginine vasopressin; ELISA, enzyme-linked immunosorbent assay; EM, electron microscopy; EPHB2, ephrin type-B receptor 2; GP, glycoprotein; GT, Glanzmann thrombasthenia; HLH, hemophagocytic lymphohistiocytosis; HPS, Hermansky-Pudlak syndrome; HSCT, hematopoietic stem cell transplantation; LADIII, leukocyte adhesion deficiency syndrome type 3; PFA-100®/200®, platelet function analyzer-100®/200®; PT-VWD, platelet-type von Willebrand disease; QPD, Quebec platelet disorder; RASGRP2, RAS guanyl releasing protein 2; rFVIIa, recombinant activated factor VII; TEM, transmission electron microscopy; TP, thromboxane-prostanoid; VWF, von Willebrand factor.

Glycoprotein Defects

These defects can be categorized as defects in platelet adhesion, defects of aggregation, defects of agonist receptor, and defects of signaling pathways. For this group of disorders, LTA is a useful tool to identify specific functional defects (shown in Fig. 2). Flow cytometry can be used to quantify receptors on the platelet surface.

Defects in Platelet Adhesion

Bernard-Soulier Syndrome

As described above, BSS is a bleeding disorder secondary to the absence or nonfunction of GPIb-IX-V complex that combines thrombocytopenia with platelet dysfunction (see above).

Platelet-Type von Willebrand Disease

Platelet-type von Willebrand disease (PT-VWD) is a rare autosomal dominant disorder characterized by a gain-of-function GPIb-IX-V platelet receptor, which binds spontaneously to VWF. It is caused by variants affecting the VWF-binding domains of *GP1BA* [15]. PT-VWD should be distinguished from VWD type 2B, which is caused by gain-of-function variants in exon 28 of the *VWF* gene. Patients affected with PT-VWD have a mild to moderate bleeding phenotype that is usually less severe than that of VWD type 2B. The platelet count is normal in many patients, but may decrease in stressful situations. Blood smears from patients often show platelet clumps, and laboratory investigations typically reveal low VWF activity relative to VWF antigen, reduced high-molecular-weight VWF multimers, and enhanced platelet agglutination in response to low-dose ristocetin. In contrast to what is seen in VWD type 2B, mixing platelets from PT-VWD patients with normal plasma does not resolve platelet clumping. Note that DDAVP (1-deamino-8-D-arginine vasopressin; desmopressin) treatment may exacerbate thrombocytopenia and thus it is generally not recommended for these patients.

Collagen Receptor Defects

Integrin α2β1and GPVI are platelet collagen receptors. Variants causing defects in either receptor are inherited in an autosomal recessive manner, and result in mild to moderate bleeding symptoms mostly associated with dental interventions or surgery. In aggregation studies, platelets show an isolated abnormal response to collagen and collagen-related peptide [4].

Defects in Platelet Aggregation

Glanzmann Thrombasthenia

GT is a rare autosomal recessive disorder with an estimated prevalence of about 1:1,000,000 in the general population. However, in populations with an increased incidence of consanguinity or founder effects, the prevalence can be 1:200,000 or higher, as in Iraqi Jews, Jordanian Arabs, and the Gypsy population [16]. GT is caused by defects of the integrin αIIbβ3 (GPIIb-IIIa) receptor resulting in reduced/absent platelet aggregation [16]. The defect can be quantitative (<5% of normal GPIIb-IIIa in type I, and 5–20% of normal GPIIb-IIIa in type II) and/or qualitative (type III). Platelet count and morphology in patients with GT are normal. In healthy individuals, the activated receptor binds to fibrinogen or VWF, which cross-links platelets to form aggregates. Integrin αIIbβ3 also provides a link between fibrin and the intracellular cytoskeletal proteins that mediate clot retraction, a process that fails to occur in patients with severe GT. Patients with GT commonly present with severe mucocutaneous bleeding. Most GT patients present in the neonatal period with purpura or petechiae, or in early childhood with excessive bruising, epistaxis, gingival bleeds, heavy menstrual bleeding (HMB) or bleeding after trauma or surgery. Dental extractions and exfoliation of deciduous teeth may be associated with excessive bleeding. Iron deficiency anemia is common in children with GT, due to blood loss. Fortunately, major bleeding complications during the neonatal period, such as intracranial hemorrhage (ICH), are rare. Heterozygotes are usually asymp-

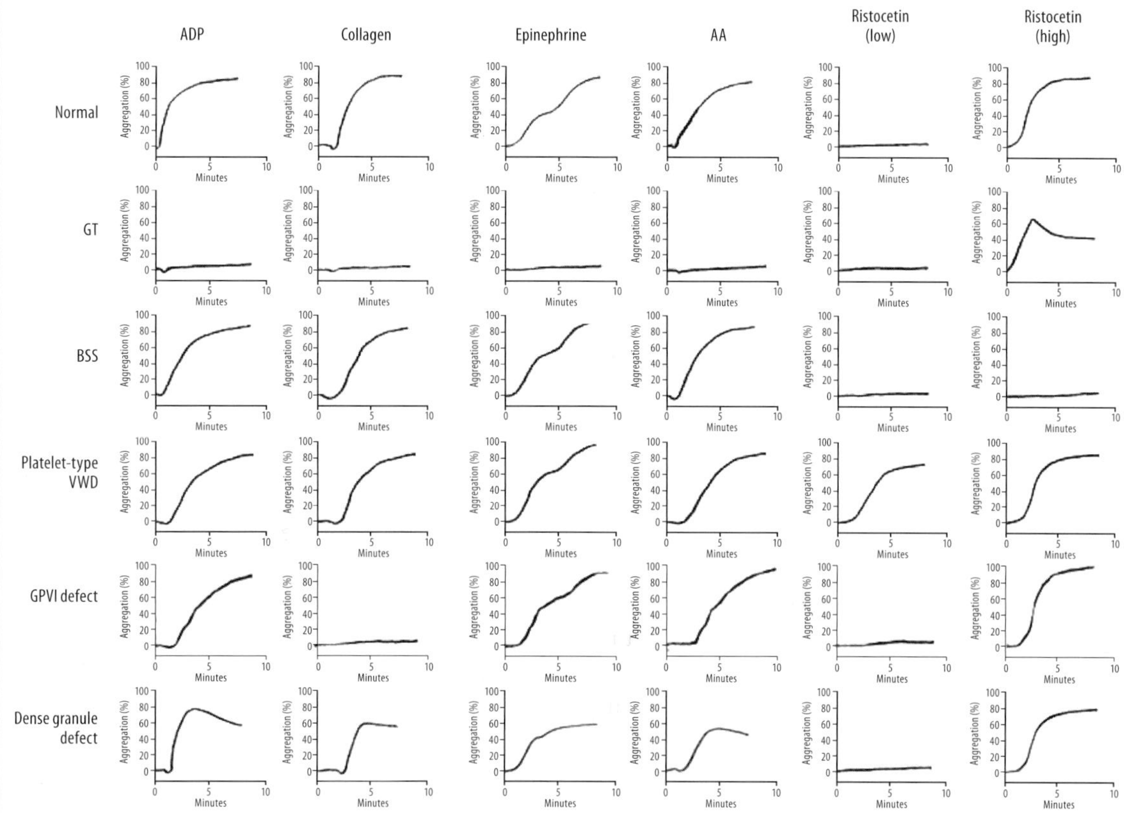

Fig. 2. Aggregation tracings for PFDs. Adapted with permission from Harrison et al. [30]. AA, arachidonic acid; ADP, adenosine 5′-diphosphate; BSS, Bernard-Soulier syndrome; GPVI, glycoprotein VI; GT, Glanzmann thrombasthenia; PFDs, platelet function disorders; VWD, von Willebrand disease.

tomatic. PFA-100®/200® closure times are significantly prolonged, typically >300 s (i.e., nonclosure) with both the collagen/epinephrine and collagen/adenosine 5′-diphosphate (ADP) cartridges. Platelet aggregation studies reveal absent aggregation with all agonists, although ristocetin-induced agglutination (GPIb-IX-V-mediated) is unaffected. αIIbβ3 deficiency can also be assessed by platelet flow cytometry or Western blotting of lysates, which typically indicate absence of platelet αIIbβ3. Genetic analysis confirms identification of *ITGA2B* or *ITGB3* gene variants.

Defects in Agonist Receptors

ADP Receptor Defects

Human platelets possess two ADP receptors: P2Y1 and P2Y12. While variants in *P2Y1* have not yet been linked to disease, *P2RY12* variants have been linked to both quantitative and qualitative abnormalities in P2Y12 [4]. These variants are usually inherited in an autosomal recessive manner, but autosomal dominant inheritance has been reported. Patients have mild bleeding symptoms after trauma or surgery. In response to ADP, platelet aggregation is slight and rapidly reversible. Reduced expression of the P2Y12 receptor can be confirmed by flow cytometry. Clopidogrel (Plavix) and ticagrelor (Brilinta) are P2Y12 receptor antagonists used to inhibit platelets in patients with cardiovascular disease.

Thromboxane A_2 Receptor Defects

Variants in the thromboxane A_2 (TxA_2) receptor gene (*TBXA2R*) are associated with a mild, predominantly postsurgical bleeding phenotype, due to a quantitative or qualitative defect in the receptor [4]. The mode of inheritance can be autosomal recessive or dominant. Affected platelets show an abnormal aggregation in response to arachidonic acid and U46619, and a normal response or reduced second wave to other agonists.

Defects in Platelet Signaling Pathways

CalDAG-GEFI Defect

CalDAG-GEFI is an autosomal recessive disorder caused by pathogenic variants of *RASGRP2. RASGRP2* encodes the calcium and diacylglycerol-regulated guanine exchange factor I (CalDAG-GEFI). Platelet counts and morphology are normal. There is decreased platelet aggregation with ADP, epinephrine, and low-dose collagen, and impaired integrin αIIbβ3 activation. Bleeding starts early in life and is moderate to severe [4]. Lack of efficacy of platelet transfusion has been reported in a large kindred.

Leukocyte Adhesion Deficiency Syndrome Type 3 (LADIII)

Leukocyte adhesion deficiency syndrome type 3 (LADIII) is an autosomal recessive disorder caused by pathogenic variants in *FERMT3,* which encodes intracellular kindlin-3 that interacts with β-integrins in hematopoietic cells. In LADIII, the adhesive functions of integrins on leukocytes and platelets are disrupted. Patients have infections, healing abnormalities, and osteopetrosis [18]. There is a severe bleeding tendency. Platelets are nonresponsive to all agonists except ristocetin, thus recapitulating GT. Here, flow cytometry would detect normal levels of CD41/CD61 (integrin αIIbβ3).

Platelet Granule Defects

Platelets contain two main types of storage/secretory granules. *α-Granules* contain proteins synthesized by megakaryocytes or acquired via endocytosis, including coagulation factors (fibrinogen, VWF), growth factors, angiogenic factors, immune modulators, and cytokines. *Dense (δ) granules* contain calcium and other ions, as well as small molecules including ADP/ATP, polyphosphate, and serotonin. During platelet activation, granules are centralized and fuse with the open canalicular system and plasma membrane, and release their contents. α-Granules can be visualized by light microscopy of blood smears owing to their dark blue appearance within platelets; accurate assessments can be made by thin-section transmission electron microscopy (TEM), flow cytometry, and immunofluorescence microscopy. Dense granule quantification can be performed by whole-mount electron microscopy (shown in Fig. 1e, f), flow cytometry, or immunofluorescence microscopy. Reduced ATP release from dense granules in patients with secretion defects can be measured by lumiaggregometry.

Defects in α-Granules

Gray Platelet Syndrome

Gray platelet syndrome (GPS) is an autosomal recessive disorder characterized by progressive macrothrombocytopenia, and bone marrow fibrosis and extramedullary hematopoiesis leading to splenomegaly, usually later in life [19, 20]. Dysregulation of the immune system with autoimmune disorders may also be present. The clinical course in GPS patients is variable, but bleeding symptoms tend to be mild to moderate. A blood smear reveals abnormally large and pale platelets; deficiency of α-granules can be demonstrated by TEM (shown in Fig. 1a, b) and immunofluorescence microscopy. The underlying defects in GPS are associated with loss-of-function variants in the *NBEAL2* gene [20].

Arthrogryposis, Renal Dysfunction, and Cholestasis Syndrome

Arthrogryposis, renal dysfunction, and cholestasis (ARC) syndrome is a severe, autosomal recessive multisystem disorder that is usually fatal early in life [21]. The molecular basis is loss-of-function variants affecting *VPS33B* or *VIPAS39* (VPS16B). ARC syndrome is characterized by a classical triad of arthrogryposis, renal tubular abnormalities in the form of Fanconi syndrome, and neonatal cholestatic jaundice. Associated features include failure to thrive, cerebral malformations, hypotonia, ichthyosis, secondary infections, dysmorphic features, congenital heart disease, and a bleeding diathesis. As in GPS, a blood smear reveals abnormally pale platelets, and absence of α-granules can be demonstrated by TEM (Fig. 1c, d). Dense granules are present in normal to increased numbers.

Quebec Platelet Disorder

Quebec platelet disorder (QPD) is an autosomal dominant disorder caused by tandem duplication of the *PLAU* gene, resulting in abnormal expression of urokinase in megakaryocytes and its secretion by activated platelets [22]. This results in activation of plasminogen to plasmin within clots, leading to hyperfibrinolysis. Bleeding in patients with QPD is delayed (1–3 days) after surgery or trauma, and is not responsive to platelet transfusion. Antifibrinolytic agents are very effective, and hence are the treatment of choice. Joint bleeds and hematuria are common, and about 25% of patients have delayed wound healing. Patients have a variable degree of thrombocytopenia and may have normal platelet counts. Platelet aggregation in response to epinephrine is abnormal, and abnormally high levels of urokinase in platelet lysates can be confirmed by enzyme-linked immunosorbent assay (ELISA) or Western blots.

Defects in Dense Granules or Secretion Defects

Nonsyndromic Secretion Defects and/or Deficiencies of Dense Granules

Defects of secretion and/or deficiencies of dense granules are the most common inherited PFDs, and are more common than defects in dense granules as part of the Hermansky-Pudlak or Chediak-Higashi syndrome. They were in the past often labelled "storage pool disorders" and are characterized by mild mucocutaneous bleeding and possibly HMB, while more significant bleeding may occur following surgery or trauma. Platelet function testing typically shows variable aggregation abnormalities by LTA, and dense granule deficiency/malfunction is specifically indicated by impaired release of ATP detected by lumiaggregometry. If lumiaggregometry indicates decreased/absent ATP release, whole-mount platelet electron microscopy can confirm either a dense granule deficiency or a secretion defect. A robust marker of platelet dense granules is RAB27B (Ras associated binding protein 27B), whereby immunofluorescence microscopy can be used to quantify dense granules in platelets [23]. The inheritance pattern of nonsyndromic dense granule and/or secretion defects is variable, and for many the specific gene variants involved are unknown.

Hermansky-Pudlak Syndrome

Hermansky-Pudlak syndrome (HPS) is a rare autosomal recessive multisystem disorder characterized by platelet-dependent bleeding, oculocutaneous albinism, and variable hypopigmentation of the skin and hair. The bleeding phenotype may be mild to moderate, and heterozygous carriers may show minor bleeding symptoms such as gingival bleeding and easy bruising. Eye abnormalities include reduced iris and retina pigmentation, foveal hypoplasia with significant reduction in visual acuity, and nystagmus. The proteins that form pigments in these tissues are the same as those forming megakaryocyte and platelet dense granules, thus defects can cause intracellu-

6

lar protein trafficking abnormalities in both platelet dense granules and melanosomes [24]. Currently, 11 HPS-associated genes have been identified (*AP3B1, AP3D1, BLOC1S3, BLOC1S5, BLOC1S6, DTNBP1, HPS1, HPS3, HPS4, HPS5, HPS6*). An up-to-date summary of the HPS pathogenic variants and clinical findings is provided in Gene Reviews® (https://www.ncbi.nlm.nih.gov/books/NBK1287/). Platelet abnormalities can be identified by determining reduced/absent dense granules via whole-mount electron microscopy (Fig. 1c, d), reduced/absent ATP release with lumiaggregometry, and reduced aggregation and/or absence of a second wave with weak/low dose agonists (Fig. 2). Depending on the genetic defect individuals may also have ceroid-lipofuscin storage in the reticuloendothelial system of multiple organs (e.g., kidney and bone marrow), pulmonary fibrosis, interstitial lung disease, granulomatous colitis, neutropenia, and/or immune defects. This makes early molecular diagnosis particularly important.

Chediak-Higashi Syndrome

Chediak-Higashi syndrome (CHS) is an autosomal recessive disorder. In addition to a defect in platelet dense granules, this disorder is characterized by recurrent bacterial infections, progressive neurological abnormalities, oculocutaneous albinism, and a high risk for developing (often fatal) hemophagocytic lymphohistiocytosis [25]. CHS arises from variants affecting *LYST*. The presence of giant eosinophilic granules inside neutrophils is the pathognomonic hallmark for this disease; platelet dense granules are reduced to absent.

Defects in Procoagulant Activity

Scott syndrome is a very rare autosomal recessive platelet-dependent bleeding disorder [26]. Gene variants of *ANO6*, encoding a multipass transmembrane protein (TMEM16F), result in abrogated protein expression leading to absent phosphatidylserine exposure by activated platelets, which is required for binding of coagulation factors (factors VIIIa/IXa and factors Va/Xa) to facilitate the conversion of prothrombin to thrombin. Thus, thrombin generation is impaired in the presence of normal coagulation factors. Platelet counts/morphology/aggregation, and prothrombin time (PT) and activated partial thromboplastin time (aPTT) are all normal. Spontaneous mucocutaneous bleeding is rare in these patients, whereas HMB and postpartum hemorrhage are marked; bleeding after surgery or trauma is the predominant clinical finding. Suspicion of this extremely rare condition can be confirmed by the assessment of activated platelet phosphatidylserine exposure via annexin A5 binding detected by flow cytometry [26]. Other diagnostic aspects including platelet count, morphology, adhesion, secretion, and aggregation are largely unaffected.

Diagnosis of Inherited Platelet Disorders

As described above, IPDs are a heterogeneous group of inherited diseases characterized by mucocutaneous and (early) postsurgical bleeding of variable severity. However, common bleeding symptoms such as epistaxis and bruising can also occur in a high proportion of healthy children, making differentiation from pathological bleeding challenging (see Chapter 4). A sequential approach beginning with a thorough patient and family history, including a bleeding score (see Appendix I) and a detailed medication history, and continuing with a multistep laboratory workup, will guide physicians to a diagnosis of IPD (see Chapter 4) [27]. Platelet aggregometry is the first step in evaluating platelet function.

Platelet Count and Morphology

An accurate assessment of platelet size, number, and morphology is an important initial step in the laboratory evaluation of a child with a suspected IPD. Automated cell counters can underestimate platelet counts when the platelet size is outside the normal reference range, leading to large platelets being incorrectly counted as white blood cells. Similarly, the mean platelet volume may be inaccurate if abnormally large and/or small platelets are excluded from the analysis. Importantly, a peripheral blood smear stained with Wright's or May-Grünwald-Giemsa and examined using a light microscope provides reasonable estimates of platelet count and size, identifies clumps and pseudothrombocytopenia, and may reveal additional important information regarding other blood cells. For example, Döhle-like inclusions in neutrophils indicate MYH9-RD (Fig. 1g, h; Table 1), large pale platelets are characteristic of GPS (Table 2), and small platelets are compatible with WAS, ARPC1B-RT, FYB-RT, and PTPRJ-RT (Table 1). If pseudo-thrombocytopenia is suspected from the blood smear examination (i.e., platelet clumping or rosettes around white blood cells), this can be confirmed by analyzing the platelet count or blood smear from a blood sample collected in 3.2% sodium citrate, heparin, or direct application on a slide. On the other hand, platelet clumps could be suggestive of either PT-VWD or type 2B VWD.

TEM of thin sections is used to examine the platelet ultrastructure, whereas whole-mount electron microscopy of platelets is the gold standard test to quantify dense granules [28]. Immunofluorescence staining of a blood smear can also be helpful in diagnosing IPDs. Briefly, fixed blood cells are stained with monoclonal antibodies specific for platelet proteins of interest, including membrane receptors, dense and/or α-granule membrane proteins, lysosome membrane components, cytoskeletal markers, or the stem cell antigen CD34 [29].

PFA-100®/200® Closure Times

Some laboratories use closure times determined with the PFA-100®/200® as a screen for platelet function and as an alternative to bleeding time. The advantage of the PFA-100®/200® test is its requirement for only a small volume of blood (0.8 mL per cartridge). The disadvantage is its lack of sensitivity for mild IPDs such as dense granule deficiency and secretion defects (where PFA-100®/200® closure times can be normal, abnormal, or even variable over time), and false prolongation in patients with thrombocytopenia (platelets <50 × 10^9/L) or anemia (hematocrit < 25%). However, the PFA-100®/200® test can be a useful screening test to rule out VWD or a severe platelet dysfunction such as GT or BSS (see Chapter 4).

Platelet Aggregation

Platelet aggregation and secretion are assessed in vitro using platelet aggregometry. To minimize preanalytical variables such as platelet activation or hemolysis, blood should be collected in 3.2% sodium citrate using a standardized atraumatic protocol, kept at room temperature (20–25 °C), and ideally analyzed between 30 min and 2 h of collection (not more than 4 h) [30]. Antiplatelet drugs (nonsteroidal anti-inflammatory drugs [NSAIDs] including aspirin [acetylsalicylic acid (ASA)]; clopidogrel, prasugrel, cangrelor, ticagrelor), anticoagulants (heparinoids, vitamin K antagonists, direct thrombin inhibitors), as well as other drugs such as caffeine and nicotine should be avoided (for a complete list refer to Table 1 in Harrison et al. [30]).

Light Transmission Aggregometry

LTA is considered the gold standard to assess platelet function in vitro. It measures the change in light transmission through rapidly stirred platelet-rich plasma (PRP) after addition of various platelet agonists. The aggregation tracing is observed for 5–10 min to monitor the lag phase, shape change (negative deflection), primary and secondary waves of aggregation, and any other platelet responses (e.g., reversible or spontaneous aggregation). International consensus recommendations for standardizing LTA, including a basic agonist panel, have been published [31]. LTA requires a relatively large volume of blood (10–15 mL) to allow for sufficient PRP; hence feasibility for thrombocytopenic patients depends on the degree of thrombocytopenia,

6

Table 3. Nomenclature of major platelet surface glycoproteins and their main agonists

Glycoprotein	CD	Integrin	Main activating ligand(s)
GPIb-IX-V	CD42a-d		VWF, thrombin
GPIIb-IIIa	CD41/61	$\alpha_{IIb}\beta_3$	Fibrinogen, VWF
GPIa-IIa		$\alpha_2\beta_1$	Collagen
GPVI	CD36		Collagen

CD, cluster-of-differentiation; GP, glycoprotein; VWF, von Willebrand factor.

ability to adjust the platelet count in PRP, and the agonist responses of interest: results should be treated with caution if the platelet count in PRP is below 100 × 10^9/L. In addition, as pre-analytical and analytical variables can significantly affect the results obtained from LTA, abnormal responses should be confirmed at least once. Characteristic aggregation tracings can be indicative of specific platelet disorders (shown in Fig. 2).

Whole-Blood Aggregometry
Whole-blood aggregometry (WBA) might be a valid alternative to LTA. It measures aggregation in saline-diluted anticoagulated whole blood (50:50) as the change in electrical impedance between electrodes. The Multiplate® analyzer is a 5-channel impedance aggregometer that uses standardized reagents. By omitting the centrifugation step, this technique requires smaller volumes of blood (0.3 mL or even 0.175 mL using a special mini-test cell) and may thus be very useful for pediatric applications [32].

Lumiaggregometry
Lumiaggregometry is a useful test in the identification of platelet dense granule secretion defects. The lumiaggregometer measures platelet aggregation (using whole blood or PRP) and secretion of ATP by the dense granules simultaneously. Released ATP oxidizes a luciferin-luciferase reagent to generate proportional chemiluminescence, which can be quantified relative to an ATP standard. If secretion is abnormal, quantification of platelet dense granules by whole-mount electron microscopy (see above) is required to distinguish a dense granule secretion defect from absent or decreased dense granules.

Flow Cytometry
This method is a long-established tool to assess expression of platelet surface antigens and activation markers that are detected via fluorochrome-conjugated antibodies. The platelet surface antigens that can be assessed include receptors such as the GPIb-IX-V complex (VWF receptor; CD42a-d; low to absent in BSS) and integrin $\alpha IIb\beta 3$ (also known as GPIIb-IIIa and CD41/CD61, receptor for fibrinogen and VWF; low to absent in GT), and activation markers such as CD62P (P-selectin) and the activated form of GPIIb-IIIa (absent in GT). Nomenclature of the most important GPs and their agonists is summarized in Table 3. After incubation with antibodies, cell suspensions are injected into the flow cytometer instrument that rapidly analyzes single cells as they flow past single or multiple lasers, thus quantifying the tagged platelet surface proteins or activation markers. Testing can be carried out in whole blood, PRP, or washed platelets, and requires very small sample volumes (0.5 mL), making it useful in children and neonates. Flow cytometry is a useful option for testing platelet activation, especially in thrombocytopenic or young patients [33].

Genetic Evaluation

Sanger sequencing has long been available for IPDs with well-defined genetic causes, and recent advances in the molecular characterization of IPDs and the identification of disease-associated gene variants by HTS have improved the molecular diagnosis of both previously recognized and newly identified disorders. Molecular diagnosis also contributes to improved genetic counseling and prenatal diagnosis (see Chapter 21). Whole-exome, whole-genome, and targeted HTS panels are currently available (e.g., https://www.preventiongenetics.com/customPanels and https://blueprintgenetics.com/tests/panels/hematology/) and are increasingly used in clinical practice, although ethical issues and counseling should be considered prior to genetic testing, particularly in (young) children (see Chapter 21). Also, the large amount of data generated by whole-genome sequencing, including variants of unknown significance, require sophisticated analyses. HTS has largely replaced Sanger sequencing and is now routinely requested early in the assessment of subjects with IT; however, it is not frequently utilized in investigating patients with PFD, those who do not have severe functional defects, or those who do not have accompanying clinical findings.

Management

Supportive Care

Patients with IPDs should be managed by multidisciplinary teams with expertise in bleeding disorders and registered with a bleeding disorders clinic, if possible. Patients and parents should be educated and provided with written information. A medical alert bracelet (for severely affected patients) and/or card (for severely affected patients and those with a milder phenotype) are recommended. Antiplatelet medications should be avoided. Maintaining good dental hygiene and regular dental visits are essential in preventing the need for invasive dental procedures. Patients with severe IPDs (GT, BSS, severe forms of WAS) should avoid high-risk contact sports or activities that would place the patient at risk for trauma or head injuries. On the other hand, participating in common activities (e.g., soccer, basketball) with their peers at school or friends at home is permitted for patients with mild IPDs, provided they wear appropriate protective equipment (e.g., a helmet when bike riding) and avoid situations such as repeated heading of a soccer ball.

It is also important to regularly monitor and treat iron deficiency in patients with chronic or repetitive mucosal bleeding symptoms. Moreover, as patients with severe IPDs such as GT are likely to be repeatedly exposed to blood products, they should at least receive hepatitis B immunizations. As transfusion-borne hepatitis A infection has also been reported, hepatitis A vaccination should be considered for patients with severe IPDs who may require repeated transfusions over time.

Management of Bleeding Episodes

Guidelines or expert recommendations for the management of children and adolescents with IPDs, especially those with severe disorders, are important but rare [34]. The treatment options to be considered depend on the degree of bleeding as well as on the specific diagnosis. If bleeding is mild to moderate, local measures such as suturing, compression, nasal packing, or use of gelatin sponge, gauze soaked in topical antifibrinolytic agents or topical recombinant human thrombin, applied to superficial wounds or nasal mucosa may suffice. Mouthwash with tranexamic acid may help to stop gum bleeding. For more details on these topical products, refer to Appendix III. Antifibrinolytic agents (tranexamic acid [Cyklokapron, Exacyl] or ε-aminocaproic acid [Amicar]) are the first-line systemic drugs for controlling mild to moderate bleeding at mucosal sites in all patients. When systemic antifibrinolytic agents alone are ineffective, DDAVP may be the next

6

agent of choice in some patients with a PFD; it is contraindicated in PT-VWD. Studies suggest that DDAVP markedly enhances platelets to form procoagulant surfaces with increased platelet-dependent thrombin generation, contributing to establishing hemostasis [35].

If the above approaches fail, and in case of severe, life-threatening bleeding in patients with an IPD, a platelet transfusion is required even if the platelet count is normal. For most IPD, an infusion of 10–15 mL/kg suffices, but in the case of GT, it is suggested to transfuse 30 mL/kg; i.e., 30 $\times 10^9$ platelets/kg [36]. The rationale is that while GT platelets are able to adhere at wound sites, they are unable to aggregate as they lack integrin αIIbβ3, thus patients require higher numbers of transfused normal platelets to outcompete the GT platelets and facilitate hemostasis. Importantly, the risk/benefit should always be considered when transfusing platelets, including the risk of the development of alloantibodies to absent platelet surface GPs in BSS and GT. The only exception to platelet transfusion in life-threatening bleeding is in QPD, where the treatment of choice is antifibrinolytic agents (as for minor bleeds), given the fibrinolytic basis of this IPD. Refer to Appendix III for details on the available products and dosages.

Note that recombinant activated factor VII (rFVIIa) (90 μg/kg every 2–6 h until hemostasis is achieved) is also licensed in Europe and North America for use in GT patients who have become refractory to platelet transfusions. However, it is not licensed for treatment of other platelet disorders, although there are some published data on its use in BSS. Assessing platelet refractoriness has only been established in the context of thrombocytopenia. Therefore, establishing resistance to platelet transfusions in patients with PFD is more challenging and should be based on the clinical recognition of an inadequate response to platelet transfusion (i.e., when it does not result in cessation of bleeding). The decision to use rFVIIa off-license must be weighed against the potential for antiplatelet antibody formation associated with repeated platelet transfusions [37]. Recent data suggest that rFVIIa with/without antifibrinolytic agents may be considered as first-line treatment for bleeds in patients with GT/BSS regardless of whether they have platelet alloantibodies [38]. Nevertheless, because the correlation between the presence of platelet alloantibodies and the clinical response to platelet transfusions is not strong in multi-transfused cases with GT/BSS, platelets should not be withheld in cases with positive antiplatelet antibodies who present with organ- or life-threatening bleeding.

Epistaxis/Gingival Bleeds/Tonsillar Bleed

Young children with epistaxis may lose much more blood than is clinically apparent. Therefore, treatment with local measures and systemic antifibrinolytic agents should be started promptly. When these measures fail to achieve hemostasis within 1–2 h, DDAVP can be tried in patients with PFD. Further treatment options include a platelet transfusion, rFVIIa, or a combination of these. Otolaryngology services (if available) should be involved in management of such bleeding.

Heavy Menstrual Bleeding

Young women with HMB should be managed jointly with (pediatric) gynecology services to assess acute bleeding quickly, and to provide maintenance therapy once bleeding is controlled. Treatment options are described in Chapter 5. Note that cultural and social issues may influence treatment decisions. Furthermore, in patients with underlying severe IPD, platelet transfusion may be required when antifibrinolytic and hormonal agents do not promptly control bleeding. Additional approaches may also include the use of DDAVP and rFVIIa.

Dental Procedures

Good oral hygiene is essential for patients with bleeding disorders. Dental procedures should be planned in advance and in consultation with a (pediatric) hematologist, whenever possible. Mandibular nerve blocks should be avoided. Local hemostatic measures are important therapeutic adjuncts. In addition, an oral antifibrinolytic agent should be started prior to the procedure and should be continued in the postprocedure period. For patients with a less severe PFD (e.g., platelet secretion defect), DDAVP may be an additional option. rFVIIa may be used for prophylactic treatment in patients with GT and BSS. If bleeding is not controlled with several doses of rFVIIa or DDAVP, the patient likely requires platelet transfusion. Patients should be kept under close clinical observation following the procedure.

Minor Surgery

Minor surgical interventions, such as wound closure, abscess drainage, removal of skin lesions, removal of ingrown toe nails, placement of ear tubes, hernia repairs, skin biopsies, etc., can be managed with antifibrinolytic agents pre/post-procedure in most patients. Patients with mild PFDs may also benefit from DDAVP. Patients with GT or BSS or those who are refractory to platelet transfusion may benefit from treatment with rFVIIa, with repeat dosing as required until bleeding is controlled.

Major Surgery

Major surgery includes neurosurgery; thoracic, abdominal, and pelvic surgery; vascular surgery; adenoidectomy; tonsillectomy; spinal/epidural anesthesia; and solid organ biopsy. Most patients will benefit from preoperatively initiated systemic antifibrinolytic agents, continued for 7–14 days after surgery. Patients with a mild bleeding tendency may also be given one or possibly two doses of DDAVP, depending on previously known responses. Due to uncertainties concerning the efficacy of rFVIIa for treatment of severe PFDs, it is recommended that platelet transfusion be used for major surgery. A transfusion should be given immediately prior to the procedure and further platelet transfusions given based on clinical need. rFVIIa may be given in cases with clinically significant bleeding not controlled by platelet transfusions.

Disorder-Specific Therapies

As described above, the management of IPDs is usually directed at the clinical bleeding symptoms rather than the underlying diagnosis, as there are few disorder-specific therapies [37]. For ITs with progression to severe pancytopenia, such as CAMT, MECOM-associated syndrome, and RUSAT1, or associated with immunodeficiency and severe infections (e.g., classic WAS), allogeneic HSCT should be considered. Gene therapy could potentially become an alternative to HSCT in patients with severe ITs and is already under investigation for some cases of WAS. Splenectomy has been used in patients with GPS who develop massive splenomegaly associated with severe thrombocytopenia and increased bleeding. Finally, the use of TPO receptor agonists (at doses comparable to those in patients with immune thrombocytopenia) has been explored in some patients with IT (MYH9-RD, ANKRD26-RT, XLT/WAS, monoallelic BSS, and ITGB3-RT) and frequent and/or serious episodes of spontaneous bleeding, and in patients in preparation for elective surgery [39, 40]. Eltrombopag (Revolade) leads to an increase in platelet counts in most patients and decreased bleeding without significant side effects, and its administration in the perioperative setting appeared to be sufficient to avoid the use of prophylactic platelet transfusions, providing an option in patients with refractoriness to platelet transfusions [39]. In addition, romiplostim (Nplate) was shown to induce a trilineage hematological response and remission of bleeding symptoms and infections in patients with a CAMT variant due to *THPO* variants and generalized bone marrow aplasia [40]. Nevertheless, more clinical experience is needed, particularly regarding the use of TPO receptor agonists in ITs predisposing to hematological malignancies, and their efficacy in disorders combining quantitative and qualitative platelet defects.

Conclusion

IPDs include thrombocytopenia, abnormalities of platelet function, or a combination of both. They present with the common signs and symptoms of mucocutaneous and perioperative bleeding. IT can be classified according to platelet size and may be one aspect of a broader syndrome. Diagnosis of PFDs requires a systematic approach, and algorithms aimed at guiding the process are available [27]. In some congenital PFDs (GT and BSS), bleeding may be severe and require repeated intervention. More common are patients with mild/moderate PFDs that require management during episodes of hemostatic stress, such as surgery. Several hemostatic drugs are available that can reduce the requirement for blood products in the management of these disorders.

Acknowledgments

Our special thanks go to Viola van Eimeren, Sara J. Israels, and Victor S. Blanchette who were authors of this chapter in the first and/or second editions of this Handbook, which provided a valuable background for this updated chapter. We also thank Sara J. Israels, Margaret L. Rand, and Yigal Dror for helpful insights during the reviewing process of this edition's chapter.

Conflict of Interest Statement

Veerle Labarque reports receiving speaker and/or consultancy fees from Bayer, Novartis, NovoNordisk, Octapharma, Roche, Sobi, and Takeda, and has received financial support for travel, accommodations, and expenses from Jazz Pharmaceuticals, Roche, and Sobi. She is recipient of a research grant from CSL Behring. Ahmad Al-Huniti, Azzah Al-Zahrani, and Walter H.A. Kahr have no conflicts of interest to declare.

Author Contributions

Veerle Labarque designed, drafted, revised, and approved the final version of chapter. Ahmad Al-Huniti designed and drafted the tables, revised the chapter, and approved the final version. Azzah Al-Zahrani revised and approved the final version. Walter H.A. Kahr contributed substantially to the conception/design of the chapter, revised the chapter, and approved the final version.

Abbreviations

ACTN1-RT	α-Actinin 1-related thrombocytopenia
ADP	Adenosine 5′-diphosphate
AML	Acute myelogenous leukemia
ANKRD26-RT	Ankyrin repeat domain 26-related thrombocytopenia
aPTT	Activated partial thromboplastin time
ARC	Arthrogryposis-renal dysfunction-cholestasis
ASA	Acetylsalicylic acid
ATP	Adenosine 5′-triphosphate
BSS	Bernard-Soulier syndrome
CalDAG-GEFI	Calcium and diacylglycerol-regulated guanine exchange factor I
CAMT	Congenital amegakaryocytic thrombocytopenia
CHS	Chediak-Higashi syndrome
DDAVP	1-Deamino-8-D-arginine vasopressin (desmopressin)
ELISA	Enzyme-linked immunosorbent assay
ETV6-RT	ETV6-related thrombocytopenia
FLI1	Friend leukemia virus integration 1
FPD-AML	Familial platelet disorder with propensity to acute myelogenous leukemia
GP	Glycoprotein
GPS	Gray platelet syndrome
GT	Glanzmann thrombasthenia
HMB	Heavy menstrual bleeding
HPS	Hermansky-Pudlak syndrome
HSCT	Hematopoietic stem cell transplantation
HTS	High-throughput sequencing
ICH	Intracranial hemorrhage
IPD	Inherited platelet disorder
IT	Inherited thrombocytopenia
ITGA2B/ITGB3-RT	ITGA2B/ITGB3-related thrombocytopenia
LADIII	Leukocyte adhesion deficiency syndrome type 3
LTA	Light-transmission aggregometry
MDS	Myelodysplastic syndrome
MECOM	MDS1 and EVI1 complex locus
MYH9-RD	Myosin heavy chain 9-related disease
NSAIDs	Nonsteroidal anti-inflammatory drugs
PFA-100®/200®	Platelet function analyzer-100®/200®

PFD	Platelet function disorder	TEM	Transmission electron microscopy
PT-VWD	Platelet-type von Willebrand disease	TPO	Thrombopoietin
PRP	Platelet-rich plasma	TPO-RT	TPO-related thrombocytopenia
PT	Prothrombin time	TxA_2	Thromboxane A_2
QPD	Quebec platelet disorder	VWD	von Willebrand disease
RAB27B	Ras associated binding protein 27B	VWF	von Willebrand factor
rFVIIa	Recombinant activated factor VII	WAS	Wiskott-Aldrich syndrome
RUSAT1	Amegakaryocytic thrombocytopenia with radio-ulnar synostosis	WASp	Wiskott-Aldrich syndrome protein
TAR	Thrombocytopenia absent radius	WBA	Whole-blood aggregometry
TBX1	T-box transcription factor 1	XLT	X-linked thrombocytopenia

References

1 Jackson SP. The growing complexity of platelet aggregation. Blood. 2007; 109(12):5087–95.
2 Oved JH, Lambert MP, Kowalska MA, Poncz M, Karczewski KJ. Population based frequency of naturally occurring loss-of-function variants in genes associated with platelet disorders. J Thromb Haemost. 2021;19(1):248–54.
3 Ballmaier M, Germeshausen M. Congenital amegakaryocytic thrombocytopenia: clinical presentation, diagnosis, and treatment. Semin Thromb Hemost. 2011;37(6):673–81.
4 Palma-Barqueros V, Revilla N, Sánchez A, Zamora Cánovas A, Rodriguez-Alén A, Marín-Quílez A, et al. Inherited platelet disorders: an updated overview. Int J Mol Sci. 2021;22(9):4521.
5 Galera P, Dulau-Florea A, Calvo KR. Inherited thrombocytopenia and platelet disorders with germline predisposition to myeloid neoplasia. Int J Lab Hematol. 2019;41 Suppl 1:131–41.
6 Albers CA, Paul DS, Schulze H, Freson K, Stephens JC, Smethurst PA, et al. Compound inheritance of a low-frequency regulatory SNP and a rare null mutation in exon-junction complex subunit RBM8A causes TAR syndrome. Nat Genet. 2012;44(4):435–9, S1–2.
7 Toriello HV. Thrombocytopenia-absent radius syndrome. Semin Thromb Hemost. 2011;37(6):707–12.
8 Massaad MJ, Ramesh N, Geha RS. Wiskott-Aldrich syndrome: a comprehensive review. Ann N Y Acad Sci. 2013; 1285:26–43.
9 Kahr WH, Pluthero FG, Elkadri A, Warner N, Drobac M, Chen CH, et al. Loss of the Arp2/3 complex component ARPC1B causes platelet abnormalities and predisposes to inflammatory disease. Nat Commun. 2017;8:14816.
10 Balduini CL, Pecci A, Savoia A. Recent advances in the understanding and management of MYH9-related inherited thrombocytopenias. Br J Haematol. 2011;154(2):161–74.
11 Pham A, Wang J. Bernard-Soulier syndrome: an inherited platelet disorder. Arch Pathol Lab Med. 2007;131(12): 1834–6.
12 Mattina T, Perrotta CS, Grossfeld P. Jacobsen syndrome. Orphanet J Rare Dis. 2009;4:9.
13 Kunishima S, Okuno Y, Yoshida K, Shiraishi Y, Sanada M, Muramatsu H, et al. ACTN1 mutations cause congenital macrothrombocytopenia. Am J Hum Genet. 2013;92(3):431–8.
14 Morais S, Oliveira J, Lau C, Pereira M, Gonçalves M, Monteiro C, et al. αIIbβ3 variants in ten families with autosomal dominant macrothrombocytopenia: expanding the mutational and clinical spectrum. PLoS One. 2020;15(12): e0235136.
15 Othman M, Gresele P. Guidance on the diagnosis and management of platelet-type von Willebrand disease: a communication from the Platelet Physiology Subcommittee of the ISTH. J Thromb Haemost. 2020;18(8):1855–8.
16 Fiore M, Pillois X, Nurden P, Nurden AT, Austerlitz F. Founder effect and estimation of the age of the French Gypsy mutation associated with Glanzmann thrombasthenia in Manouche families. Eur J Hum Genet. 2011;19(9):981–7.
17 Franchini M, Favaloro EJ, Lippi G. Glanzmann thrombasthenia: an update. Clin Chim Acta. 2010;411(1–2):1–6.
18 Yahya AM, AlMulla AA, AlRufaye HJ, Al Dhaheri A, Elomami AS, Al-Hammadi S, et al. Case report: a case of leukocyte adhesion deficiency, Type III presenting with impaired platelet function, lymphocytosis and granulocytosis. Front Pediatr. 2021;9713921.
19 Nurden AT, Nurden P. The gray platelet syndrome: clinical spectrum of the disease. Blood Rev. 2007;21(1):21–36.
20 Pluthero FG, di Paola J, Carcao MD, Kahr WHA. NBEAL2 mutations and bleeding in patients with gray platelet syndrome. Platelets. 2018;29(6):632–5.
21 Penon-Portmann M, Westbury SK, Li L, Pluthero FG, Liu RJY, Yao HHY, et al. Platelet VPS16B is dependent on VPS33B expression, as determined in two siblings with arthrogryposis, renal dysfunction, and cholestasis syndrome. J Thromb Haemost. 2022;20(7):1712–9.
22 Kahr WH, Zheng S, Sheth PM, Pai M, Cowie A, Bouchard M, et al. Platelets from patients with the Quebec platelet disorder contain and secrete abnormal amounts of urokinase-type plasminogen activator. Blood. 2001;98(2):257–65.
23 Pluthero FG, Kahr WHA. Evaluation of human platelet granules by structured illumination laser fluorescence microscopy. Platelets. 2023;34(1):2157808.
24 Li W, Hao C-J, Hao Z-H, Ma J, Wang QC, Yuan YF, et al. New insights into the pathogenesis of Hermansky-Pudlak syndrome. Pigment Cell Melanoma Res. 2022;35(3):290–302.
25 Kaplan J, de Domenico I, Ward DM. Chediak-Higashi syndrome. Curr Opin Hematol. 2008;15(1):22–9.

26 Zwaal RFA, Comfurius P, Bevers EM. Scott syndrome, a bleeding disorder caused by defective scrambling of membrane phospholipids. Biochim Biophys Acta. 2004;1636(2–3):119–28.

27 Israels SJ, Kahr WHA, Blanchette VS, Luban NLC, Rivard GE, Rand ML. Platelet disorders in children: A diagnostic approach. Pediatr Blood Cancer. 2011; 56(6):975–83.

28 Chen D, Uhl CB, Bryant SC, Krumwiede M, Barness RL, Olson MC, et al. Diagnostic laboratory standardization and validation of platelet transmission electron microscopy. Platelets. 2018;29(6): 574–82.

29 Greinacher A, Pecci A, Kunishima S, Althaus K, Nurden P, Balduini CL, et al. Diagnosis of inherited platelet disorders on a blood smear: a tool to facilitate worldwide diagnosis of platelet disorders. J Thromb Haemost. 2017;15(7): 1511–21.

30 Harrison P, Mackie I, Mumford A, Briggs C, Liesner R, Winter M, et al. Guidelines for the laboratory investigation of heritable disorders of platelet function. Br J Haematol. 2011;155(1):30–44.

31 Cattaneo M, Cerletti C, Harrison P, Hayward CP, Kenny D, Nugent D, et al. Recommendations for the standardization of light transmission aggregometry: a consensus of the Working Party from the Platelet Physiology Subcommittee of SSC/ISTH. J Thromb Haemost. 2013;11: 1183–9.

32 Halimeh S, Angelis G de, Sander A, Edelbusch C, Rott H, Thedieck S, et al. Multiplate whole blood impedance point of care aggregometry: preliminary reference values in healthy infants, children and adolescents. Klin Padiatr. 2010; 222(3):158–63.

33 Sharma P, Sachdeva MUS, Kumar N, Bose S, Bose P, Uppal V, et al. A comparative study between light transmission aggregometry and flow cytometric platelet aggregation test for the identification of platelet function defects in patients with bleeding. Blood Res. 2021; 56(2):109–18.

34 Tarawah A, Owaidah T, Al-Mulla N, Khanani MF, Elhazmi J, Albagshi M, et al. Management of Glanzmann's thrombasthenia – guidelines based on an expert panel consensus from gulf cooperation council countries. J Appl Hematol. 2019;10(1):1–9.

35 Colucci G, Stutz M, Rochat S, Conte T, Pavicic M, Reusser M, et al. The effect of desmopressin on platelet function: a selective enhancement of procoagulant COAT platelets in patients with primary platelet function defects. Blood. 2014; 123(12):1905–16.

36 Al-Battat S, Rand ML, Bouskill V, Lau W, Blanchette VS, Kahr WHA, et al. Glanzmann thrombasthenia platelets compete with transfused platelets, reducing the haemostatic impact of platelet transfusions. Br J Haematol. 2018; 181(3):410–3.

37 Almeida AM, Khair K, Hann I, Liesner R. The use of recombinant factor VIIa in children with inherited platelet function disorders. Br J Haematol. 2003;121(3): 477–81.

38 di Minno G. Eptacog alfa activated: a recombinant product to treat rare congenital bleeding disorders. Blood Rev. 2015;29 Suppl 1:S26–33.

39 Pecci A, Balduini CL. Inherited thrombocytopenias: an updated guide for clinicians. Blood Rev. 2021;48:100784.

40 Zaninetti C, Gresele P, Bertomoro A, Klersy C, De Candia E, Veneri D, et al. Eltrombopag for the treatment of inherited thrombocytopenias: a phase II clinical trial. Haematologica. 2020;105(3): 820–8.

41 Chen CH, Lo RW, Urban D, Pluthero FG, Kahr WHA. α-Granule biogenesis: from disease to discovery. Platelets. 2017;28(2):147–54.

42 ver Donck F, Ramaekers K, Thys C, Van Laer C, Peerlinck K, Van Geet C, et al. Ribosome dysfunction underlies SLFN14-related thrombocytopenia. Blood. 2023;141(18):2261–74.

43 Marín-Quílez A, di Buduo CA, Díaz-Ajenjo L, Sierra-Aisa C, Male C, Fernández-Mosteirin N, et al. Novel variants in GALE cause syndromic macrothrombocytopenia by disrupting glycosylation and thrombopoiesis. Blood. 2023; 141(4):406–21.

Chapter 7

Published online: December 5, 2024

Blanchette VS, Brandão LR, Carcao MD, Kumar R, Rand ML, Revel-Vilk S (eds): SickKids Handbook of Pediatric Thrombosis and Hemostasis, ed 3, rev. and ext. Basel, Karger, 2024, pp 97–116 (DOI: 10.1159/000538202)

Acquired Platelet Disorders

Vicky R. Breakey[a] Thomas Kühne[b] Natsaruth Songthawee[c] Julie Curtin[d] Victor S. Blanchette[e]

[a]Division of Pediatric Hematology/Oncology, McMaster University, McMaster Children's Hospital, Hamilton, ON, Canada; [b]Division of Oncology/Hematology, University Children's Hospital Basel, Basel, Switzerland; [c]Division of Hematology/Oncology, Department of Pediatrics, Prince of Songkla University, Songkhla, Thailand; [d]Department of Haematology, The Children's Hospital at Westmead, Sydney Children's Hospitals Network, Sydney, NSW, Australia; [e]Department of Pediatrics, University of Toronto and Division of Pediatric/Hematology/Oncology, The Hospital for Sick Children, Toronto, ON, Canada

Introduction

Acquired platelet disorders occur in childhood. The clinical approach to a child with a suspected acquired platelet disorder includes a careful history, a detailed physical examination, and focused laboratory investigations. Immune thrombocytopenia (ITP) is the most common acquired platelet disorder and it varies from benign and self-resolving to refractory. Treatment of ITP has evolved, and current recommendations focus on the treatment of symptomatic children only. Other acquired platelet disorders are less common, including acquired thrombocytopenia and impaired platelet function that result from a variety of causes, such as medications, dietary supplements, procedures, and systemic diseases. Non-immune acquired thrombocytopenias are discussed in Chapter 11. Heparin-induced thrombocytopenia (HIT) is very rare in childhood but should be considered in children with new-onset thrombocytopenia in the setting of heparin exposure.

Immune Thrombocytopenia

ITP, previously referred to as "idiopathic thrombocytopenic purpura," occurs with an incidence of 5–10 per 100,000 children. ITP can be an isolated primary condition, or it may be secondary to other conditions. In 70–80% of children, ITP is self-limited, with resolution generally occurring within six months. Chronic ITP is more common in older children and adolescents, with a minority having treatment-refractory disease. While ITP is one of the most common conditions encountered by pediatric hematologists, clinicians face ongoing challenges with respect to the diagnosis and treatment of ITP.

Of note, neonates may also have antibody-mediated thrombocytopenia. Fetal and neonatal alloimmune thrombocytopenia (FNAIT) and neonatal autoimmune thrombocytopenia are reviewed in detail in Chapter 3.

Pathophysiology

ITP is an acquired autoimmune process in which autoantibodies target platelets in the blood circulation and megakaryocytes in the bone marrow resulting in thrombocytopenia. There are many pathological mechanisms, often reflecting a dysregulated immune system. The following review gives a detailed overview of the possible known mechanisms of ITP [1].

Clinical Presentation

The clinical spectrum of children with ITP can vary enormously and ranges from asymptomatic to life-threatening bleeding. Bleeding is a key feature of ITP and includes several bleeding phenotypes. Skin manifestations are most common, including petechiae (spontaneous tiny skin or mucous membrane bleedings), purpura, and bruising. Petechiae are rather specific to platelet disorders. They are usually not palpable and do not blanch. If palpable lesions are present, the clinician should consider the possibility of a vasculitic disorder. Mucous membrane bleeding includes nosebleeds, gum bleeding, gastrointestinal loss, hematuria, and heavy menstrual bleeding (HMB). While bruising is benign, mucosal bleeding, particularly hematuria, is associated with a higher spontaneous bleeding risk and is, therefore, a reason to consider intervention. It has been shown that children with hematuria and post head trauma are at increased risk for intracranial hemorrhage (ICH) [2]. Hematomas and joint bleeding (hemarthrosis) are atypical in acquired thrombocytopenia and more in keeping with an underlying coagulation disorder. In pediatric ITP, there are two commonly used bleeding scores: the Buchanan and the Bolton-Maggs scores [3, 4].

Fatigue occurs in some children with ITP and may manifest as changes in behavior in younger children [5]. Diminished Health-related Quality of Life (HRQoL) is multifactorial and due to uncertainty around the risk of bleeding, limits on physical activities, and the burden of medical interventions. The Kids ITP Tool is a validated disease-specific tool that can be used clinically or in the setting of research to assess the impact of ITP on HRQoL [6].

ITP Definitions

The Vicenza conference attempted to harmonize the language used in ITP and published definitions [7]. See Table 1 for the definitions proposed.

If thrombocytopenia (platelet count $<100 \times 10^9/L$) recurs after remission of ITP, "relapsing ITP" is diagnosed. The definition of "refractory ITP" remains debated. The Vicenza conference defined it as failure of, or relapse after, splenectomy and the presence of severe thrombocytopenia or risk of bleeding that in the opinion of the attending physician requires therapy. However, since splenectomy is restrictively used in children, this definition is suboptimal for pediatric refractory ITP.

Diagnosis

The diagnosis of primary ITP is a diagnosis of exclusion. There is no single laboratory test or a combination of tests that establishes a diagnosis of ITP. The clinician must consider the children's personal and family history, physical examination findings, and the complete blood count (CBC) including interpretation of a blood smear.

The physical examination should be normal, with the exception of possible manifestations of bleeding and/or bruising. If there are other signs and symptoms, a diagnosis other than ITP has to be considered. The differential diagnosis of pediatric primary ITP is extensive (Table 2).

Besides a detailed history and a physical examination, a CBC and a blood smear examination must be performed. In individuals with ITP, platelets are frequently larger, exhibiting an increased mean platelet volume (MPV), and macrothrombocytes on the blood smear. It is important to note that the blood smear of subjects with congenital macrothrombocytopenias, e.g., myosin heavy chain 9 (MYH9) disease, Bernard-Sou-

Table 1. Definitions of ITP

Primary ITP	Primary ITP is an autoimmune disorder characterized by isolated thrombocytopenia (peripheral blood platelet count $<100 \times 10^9$/L) in the absence of other causes or disorders that may be associated with thrombocytopenia
Secondary ITP	All forms of immune-mediated thrombocytopenia except primary ITP[a]
Phases of the disease	**Newly diagnosed ITP:** within 3 months from diagnosis **Persistent ITP:** between 3 to 12 months from diagnosis. Includes patients not reaching spontaneous remission or not maintaining complete response off therapy **Chronic ITP:** lasting for more than 12 months **Severe ITP:** Presence of bleeding symptoms at presentation sufficient to mandate treatment, or occurrence of new bleeding symptoms requiring additional therapeutic intervention with a different platelet-enhancing agent or an increased dose

ITP, immune thrombocytopenia. [a]The acronym ITP should be followed by the name of the associated disease (for thrombocytopenia after exposure to drugs, the terms "drug-induced" should be used) in parentheses: for example, "secondary ITP (lupus-associated)," "secondary ITP (HIV-associated)," and "secondary ITP (drug-induced)." For manuscript titles, abstracts, and so on, definitions such as lupus-associated ITP or HIV-associated ITP can also be used.

Table 2. Differential diagnosis for thrombocytopenia in children

Increased destruction of platelets	Primary ITP Secondary ITP: SLE, RA, APLA, drug-induced ITP, ALPS, CVID Microangiopathy: DIC, TTP, HUS Mechanical: cardiac valvular dysfunction, endocarditis, Kasabach-Merritt phenomenon or LIC in the setting of vascular malformations
Decreased production of platelets	Congenital thrombocytopenias Bone marrow failure: congenital, acquired Marrow infiltration: leukemias, lymphomas, neuroblastoma, MDS, storage disease Infections: viral (HIV, HCV, EBV, CMV), bacterial sepsis, tuberculosis, malaria, babesiosis Nutritional: vitamin B12, folate, copper deficiencies Drugs: chemotherapy, vancomycin, sulfa drugs, quinine, valproic acid, others
Splenic sequestration of platelets	Cirrhosis with portal hypertension Other causes of splenomegaly (e.g., Gaucher disease)

ALPS, autoimmune lymphoproliferative syndrome; APLA, antiphospholipid antibodies; CMV, cytomegalovirus; CVID, common variable immunodeficiency; DIC, disseminated intravascular coagulation; EBV, Epstein-Barr virus; HCV, hepatitis C virus; HIV, human immunodeficiency virus; HUS, hemolytic uremic syndrome; ITP, immune thrombocytopenia; LIC, localized intravascular coagulation; MDS, myelodysplastic syndrome; RA, rheumatoid arthritis; SLE, systemic lupus erythematosus; TTP, thrombotic thrombocytopenic purpura.

lier syndrome, shows platelets that are uniformly large on a blood smear, whereas in ITP there is typically a heterogeneity in platelet size. The immature platelet fraction (IPF), if reported, is often elevated, suggesting increased platelet turnover. One key differentiating point between ITP and congenital thrombocytopenias is that in the former, there is often a history of normal platelet

Table 3. Differentiating ITP vs. congenital thrombocytopenia

Clues on history for type of thrombocytopenia	ITP	Congenital thrombocytopenia
Family history of thrombocytopenia/excessive bleeding?	No	Sometimes
Consanguinity in parents?	No	Sometimes
History of a normal platelet count?	Yes	No
Congenital anomalies (associated with thrombocytopenia/bone marrow dysfunction)?	No	Sometimes
Acute onset of symptoms?	Yes	No
Large fluctuations in platelet count?	Yes	No
Response to frontline ITP therapy (corticosteroids, IVIG)?	Yes	No
Response to platelet transfusion?	No/minimal/brief	Yes

ITP, immune thrombocytopenia; IVIG, intravenous immunoglobulin.

counts. Additionally, in ITP, the platelet count shows a higher degree of fluctuation. See Table 3 for a summary of differences between congenital and acquired thrombocytopenias. If there are other unexplained cytopenias or changes to the red cell indices, such as macrocytosis, a diagnosis other than ITP needs to be considered.

According to many practice guidelines, no other laboratory tests are needed for the diagnosis of "primary ITP." Consideration of a direct antiglobulin test (Coombs test) to rule out Evans syndrome (a combination of ITP and autoimmune hemolytic anemia) and quantitative immunoglobulin levels, particularly before treatment with intravenous immunoglobulin (IVIG), to rule out underlying immunodeficiency are justified. Based on the child's history, a search for viral infections, such as human immunodeficiency virus (HIV), hepatitis C, and others, can be considered. Testing for causes of secondary ITP should be individualized and based on symptoms (see section below on secondary ITP).

A bone marrow aspirate/biopsy is not indicated for primary ITP, even if corticosteroids are used as initial therapy. However, if any doubt is raised through the clinical history, physical examination, or available laboratory tests, bone marrow testing in individuals with ITP will typically demonstrate increased platelet production and rule out underlying production issues.

There is currently no internationally accepted algorithm for diagnostic steps in children with persistent and chronic ITP. A recent review suggests key features to help to differentiate primary ITP from inherited platelet disorders and primary immunodeficiencies [8].

Predicting the Natural History of ITP

Risk factors for chronic ITP include older age (more than 10 years), higher platelet count at initial presentation, and absence of preceding infection or vaccination. Potential risk factors with weaker validity for chronicity include insidious onset of bleeding and/or thrombocytopenia (>2 weeks) and female sex. Spontaneous remission may occur at any time, even many years from diagnosis.

There are no clear factors that predict bleeding. Risk factors for bleeding include extrinsic factors (e.g., trauma, infections, and drugs that affect the number and function of platelets) and intrinsic factors (e.g., age, anemia, genetic factors, and anatomical abnormalities, such as arterio-venous malformations).

Management of ITP

General Considerations

While the majority of ITP is self-limiting and can be managed with little or no therapy, clinicians must provide education and support to families as they adjust to the diagnosis. Low platelet counts may lead to significant anxiety in parents and affected children. Regular monitoring of blood counts may be helpful initially, but stable cases should have blood work less often or only in the setting of symptoms.

While there are limited data on the safety of various physical activities, children and adolescents with ITP should be counseled to avoid high-risk contact sports, particularly those with increased risk of head trauma or injury. At a minimum, if the child insists on engaging in these activities, then they should be cautioned to wear appropriate protective equipment for the activity. Other activities should be encouraged to promote general health and socialization. Children should not be withdrawn from kindergarten or school, but staff should be notified to have a low threshold to call parents if an injury occurs.

Medications that affect platelet function, such as acetylsalicylic acid (ASA) and nonsteroidal anti-inflammatory drugs (NSAIDs), should be avoided during periods of thrombocytopenia. Complementary and alternative medicines should be reviewed to ensure there are no ingredients that may contribute to antiplatelet activity.

Vaccinations should not be withheld. Intramuscular injections are allowed; however, many inactivated vaccines may be given subcutaneously. A small gauge needle should be used and local pressure should be applied to the injection site for a minimum of 5 min. It has been suggested that children who have received one measles, mumps, rubella (MMR) vaccine and show evidence of immunity may be excused from booster doses [9].

Oral hygiene is important to prevent inflammation, periodontal disease, and subsequent gingival bleeding. While dental cleaning and minor interventions, such as the filling of caries, are generally safe with platelet counts $>10 \times 10^9$/L, dental extractions should be avoided while the platelet count is $<50 \times 10^9$/L. Mandibular blocks are contraindicated unless the platelet count is above 100×10^9/L.

In addition to the frontline therapies outlined below, other hemostatic agents, including oral antifibrinolytic agents such as tranexamic acid and epsilon aminocaproic acid, can be prescribed on an as-needed basis for gum bleeding or HMB. For details regarding dosing see Appendix III.

First-Line Therapies for ITP

Current guidelines suggest that children with newly diagnosed ITP and minimal bleeding symptoms (i.e., skin manifestations) do not need hospitalization and can be managed with observation alone, regardless of platelet count [10]. If the diagnosis is uncertain, or if there are challenging social circumstances, hospitalization may be necessary initially to ensure that appropriate education and follow-up plans can be made. The child and family HRQoL should also be considered.

If there is significant bleeding, there are several options for first-line therapies. Corticosteroids are generally favored over IVIG and rhesus immune globulin (RhIG), but all three are effective and may be useful in different clinical scenarios [10]. A review of common therapies can be found in Table 4. Mechanisms of action for ITP therapies are outlined in Figure 1.

Corticosteroids

Oral corticosteroids are effective in increasing platelet counts in ITP and are easy to administer in the home setting. Shorter course, higher dose steroids have been shown to be effective and well tolerated in children, increasing platelet counts in 70–80%. One study used oral prednisone 4 mg/kg/day for 4 days in children with a platelet count of $<20 \times 10^9$/L and showed that within 24 and 48 h from starting treatment, 38% and 83%, respectively, of children already showed a platelet count

Table 4. Common therapies used in pediatric immune thrombocytopenia (ITP)

Therapy	Typical dosing regimen	Available dosage forms	Comments
a Corticosteroids			
Prednisone	2–4 mg/kg/day, PO (max 120 mg daily), divide BID, for 4–7 days	1 mg, 2.5 mg, 5 mg, 10 mg, 20 mg, 50 mg tablets, 5 mg/mL suspension	Suspension or crushed tablets have bitter taste compared to prednisolone
Prednisolone	2–4 mg/kg/day, PO (max 120 mg daily), divide BID, for 4–7 days	1 mg/mL liquid	Used preferentially in children with taste aversion to prednisone
Methylprednisolone	30 mg/kg/dose, once daily, IV over 1 h (max 1 g/dose) for 1–3 days	Injectable vials	Used in the setting of organ/life-threatening bleeding in children with ITP to rapidly increase the circulating platelet count
Dexamethasone	0.6 mg/kg/day, PO (max 40 mg daily), for 4 days	0.5 mg/5mL, 1 mg, 2 mg/mL suspension 0.5 mg, 0.75 mg, 2 mg, 4 mg tablets	Generally, less well studied in children and less well tolerated with significant side effects. ASH guideline panel suggests prednisone over dexamethasone [10]
b Thrombopoietin receptor agonists (TPO-RA)			
Eltrombopag	25–75 mg, once daily, PO	12.5 mg and 25 mg packets 12.5 mg, 25 mg, 50 mg, 75 mg tablets	Starting dose: 25 mg/day (age 1–6 years), 50 mg/day (>6 years); max 75 mg/day 50% decrease in starting dose in East-/Southeast-Asian ancestry Adjust dose based on platelet count (goal 50–200 × 10^9/L) Administer on an empty stomach; at least 2 h before or 4 h after antacids, foods, or supplements containing polyvalent cations; do not administer more than one dose within 24 h May need dose adjustment depending on hepatic impairment and/or drug interaction May lower iron absorption
Romiplostim	1–10 μg/kg/dose, once weekly, SC	125 μg, 250 μg, 500 μg vial	Starting dose: 3 μg/kg/dose with fairly rapid escalation up to 10 μg/kg/dose based on follow-up platelet counts at weekly time points Adjust dose based on platelet count (goal 50–200 × 10^9/L)
c Immunotherapies			
IVIG	0.8 1 g/kg/dose, IV	Round up to nearest vial (1 g, 2.5 g, 5 g, 10 g, 20 g, 30 g vials)	Infusion reactions (fever, headache, malaise, etc.), allergic reactions, rarely aseptic meningitis Can also result in hemolysis/autoimmune hemolytic anemia and/or neutropenia
Rituximab	375 mg/m²/dose, once weekly, IV (max 1 g/dose) for 4 weeks Lower doses may also be effective (see text)	100 mg, 500 mg vial	Short-term side effects include infusion reactions, allergic reactions Longer term: possibility of B cell aplasia

ASH, American Society of Hematology; BID, twice a day; IV, intravenous; IVIG, intravenous immunoglobulin; max, maximum; PO, per oral; SC, subcutaneous.

of ≥20 × 10^9/L. Overall 88% of children responded well, achieving platelet counts >20 × 10^9/L within 1 week of starting therapy [11]. The American Society of Hematology (ASH) guidelines favor corticosteroids over both IVIG and RhIG. Prednisone (2–4 mg/kg/day; maximum dose 120 mg daily, for 4–7 days, with no tapering) is favored over pulse high-dose dexamethasone, which is generally less well studied in children and less well tolerated with significant side effects. Prednisolone liquid is equivalent to prednisone, and the taste is generally preferred by toddlers

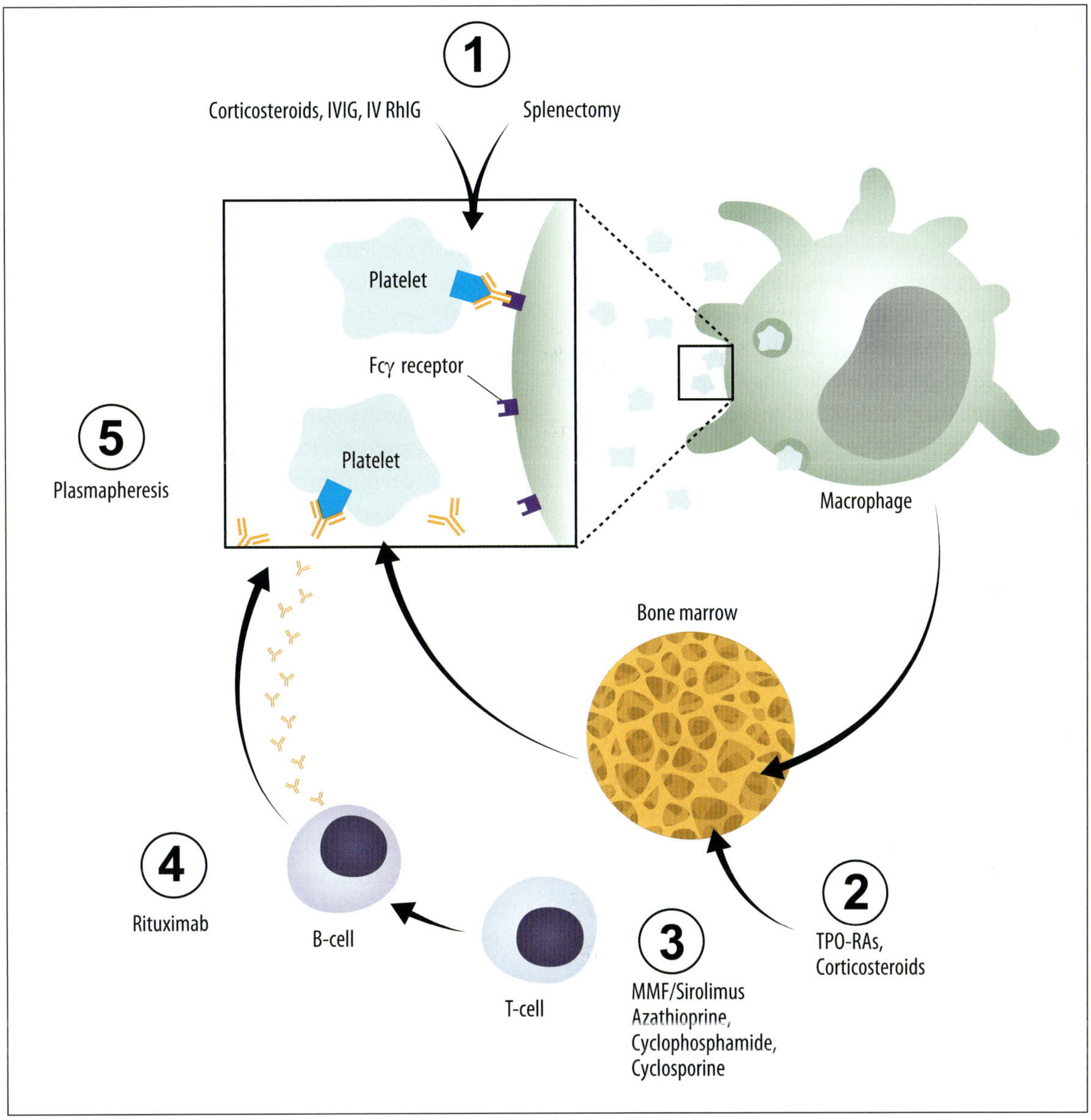

Fig. 1. Mechanisms of action of various therapies for immune thrombocytopenia. 1. Decreased clearance of autoantibody-sensitized platelets by phagocytic cells in the spleen (splenectomy) or by blockade of phagocytic cells in the reticuloendothelial system (corticosteroids, IVIG, IV RhIG). 2. Stimulation of platelet production from megakaryocytes (TPO-RAs, corticosteroids). 3, 4. Decreased production of pathologic platelet autoantibodies (rituximab, MMF, sirolimus, azathioprine, cyclophosphamide, cyclosporine). 5. Removal of pathologic platelet autoantibodies. IV, intravenous; IVIG, intravenous immunoglobulin; MMF, mycophenolate mofetil; RhIG, Rh immune globulin; TPO-RAs, thrombopoietin receptor agonists.

and young children. Few side effects are noted and settle shortly after completing the short course. Antacid blockers are generally not needed in this approach but can be added if there are gastrointestinal complaints suggestive of gastritis. Corticosteroids are much less costly than other alternative first-line therapies.

Intravenous Immunoglobulin

IVIG is also an effective frontline therapy to increase platelet counts in children with acute ITP, but it requires intravenous administration, is more expensive, and has significant short-term side effects, including headaches, malaise, and nausea/vomiting [12]. While corticosteroids are generally preferable for the above reasons, IVIG is thought to have a quicker onset of action and is sometimes used in inpatient settings. A single dose of 0.8–1 g/kg IVIG is standard and leads to an increase in platelet counts >20 × 10^9/L in 90% of children with acute ITP within 48–72 h [13]. IVIG carries a risk of infusion reactions and rarely anaphylaxis. Occasionally significant intravascular hemolysis may occur when IVIG is given to a non-O blood type individual and can result in clinically significant anemia. Clues to this complication include the development of dark-colored urine (hemoglobinuria) and a positive direct antiglobulin test with an accompanying reticulocytosis. Risk of hemolysis increases if the treatment is given more than once in a short period of time. Autoimmune neutropenia can also be seen post-IVIG. New cytopenias may worry clinicians if they are not aware of these side effects. IVIG-related aseptic meningitis is a rare but significant complication of IVIG therapy that leads to severe headache (usually onset is about 12–24 h postadministration), which can result in the child being seen in the Emergency Department or even being hospitalized. Due to the increased risk of ICH in children with ITP, children who present with headaches from IVIG often get unnecessary head computed tomography (CT) scans to rule out bleeding.

Rh Immunoglobulin

RhIG (50–75 μg/kg/dose) is also effective in increasing platelet counts in children with ITP who are Rh-positive with an intact spleen. RhIG should be avoided in children whose baseline hemoglobin is <100 g/L or in those with a positive direct antiglobulin test as it can cause intravascular hemolysis. This rare but potentially lethal side effect has resulted in a black box warning issued in 2010, which suggests children who receive RhIG should be monitored for hemolysis in hospital for at least 8 h after infusion. Although RhIG is effective in children with ITP who meet the above parameters, the risk of severe hemolysis and need for monitoring has resulted in significantly decreased usage of this intervention in the last decade.

Persistent, Chronic, and Refractory ITP

ITP that fails to respond to first-line therapies and causes persistent symptoms is a significant challenge for the pediatric hematologist. The definition of "refractory ITP" has not been standardized, but clinicians generally agree that children with ITP who have ongoing bleeding and/or diminished HRQoL in spite of treatment require special consideration and thoughtful management.

Options for treatment of symptomatic refractory/persistent/chronic ITP include thrombopoietin receptor agonists (TPO-RA), rituximab, immunosuppressive therapies, and splenectomy. Many children will require more than one modality of treatment. The order in which treatments are tried is influenced by side effect profile, medication accessibility, cost, child and family preference, and provider experience. In general, older therapies have been replaced by newer treatments in recent years [10]. The clinician must balance the risks and logistics of each therapy and discuss with the child and family to decide how best to manage refractory ITP on a case-to-case basis.

Thrombopoietin Receptor Agonists

When considering second-line therapies for symptomatic refractory ITP, the ASH guidelines suggest a preference for TPO-RA when compared to rituximab [10]. A recent systematic review comparing TPO-RA to rituximab in pediatric ITP found similar platelet response rates, but TPO-RAs were superior in the rate of partial response and obviating the need for rescue therapy [14]. Evidence also suggests that TPO-RA may reduce bleeding in ITP more than rituximab. In addition, the ASH guidelines support both TPO-RAs and rituximab over splenectomy in children. However, limitations around funding for these expensive drugs influence decision making in many countries.

TPO-RAs are among the newest ITP therapies and the most effective. TPO-RAs activate the thrombopoietic pathway and stimulate hematopoietic stem cells and megakaryocytes resulting in a massive increase in platelet production overwhelming the antiplatelet antibodies.

Currently, two TPO-RAs are licensed for use in children with chronic ITP: eltrombopag and romiplostim. Both drugs have been studied and shown to be safe and effective for long-term use [10]. Avatrombopag is a more potent oral TPO-RA with no dairy restrictions that is approved for use in adults with chronic ITP and is currently being studied for use in children. Unfortunately, the largest barrier to prescribing TPO-RA is the high cost and need for ongoing treatment, making the medications inaccessible to many individuals.

Eltrombopag is given orally, starting at a dose of 50 mg/day for children aged 6 years or older and 25 mg/day for children aged 1 to 6 years of age. Doses should be titrated every 2 weeks to achieve a platelet count of 50–200 × 10^9/L. Therapy in children of East Asian descent should be initiated at 50% of the usual dose due to differences in metabolism. Children may prefer oral eltrombopag over romiplostim, which requires a weekly injection. Younger children may not be able to take eltrombopag as it is only available in tablet form, and it must not be taken with dairy products. It should be administered 2 h prior to or 4 h after meals.

Romiplostim is a TPO-RA that is given by subcutaneous injection once per week. Initial clinical trials started romiplostim at 1 μg/kg/dose with dose adjustment to achieve a platelet count of 50–200 × 10^9/L, but subsequently, a starting dose of 2–3 μg/kg/dose has been found to be safe with the option to titrate as needed.

The adverse-effect profiles for the TPO-RAs are significantly better than those for alternative treatments. Eltrombopag can cause transaminitis that is reversible with dose reduction or drug cessation. Routine monitoring of liver function tests at baseline, with dose escalation, and every 3 months during therapy is recommended. The medication should be held if alanine aminotransferase levels reach three times the upper limit of normal and are progressive, persistent (≥4 weeks), and/or associated with direct hyperbilirubinemia. Eltrombopag has also been associated with iron deficiency anemia. There is evidence to show that adults treated with TPO-RA have an elevated risk of thrombotic complications compared to those not treated with TPO-RA [15], but this has not been shown in pediatric trials.

Rituximab

Rituximab is a monoclonal anti-CD20 antibody that targets B lymphocytes and causes Fc-mediated cell lysis. It was initially developed for the treatment of B-cell non-Hodgkin lymphoma. Administered at a standard dose of 375 mg/m^2 weekly for 4 weeks, approximately 50–60% of children with ITP will respond to this therapy [16]. Of those who respond, approximately 25% will have a durable long-term response. Rituximab may be repeated if there is a response followed by relapse. Emerging evidence suggests lower doses are also effective in ITP (100 mg or 100 mg/m^2 weekly × 4) [17]. Infusion reactions and allergies can occur but more severe side effects, such as serum sickness and B-cell aplasia, are rare. While rituximab is reported to cause periventricular leukomalacia very rarely, this has not been reported in any children with ITP to our knowledge. Rituximab is used in other autoimmune conditions, and there is evidence to support its use in children with ITP secondary to rheumatological conditions and ITP in children with autoimmune lymphoproliferative syndrome (ALPS).

Splenectomy

A registry study showed a 93% partial/complete response to splenectomy in children with chronic ITP [18]. Despite high efficacy, pediatric hematologists generally avoid splenectomy in children with primary ITP until all other available medical therapies have failed due to the associated infectious and thrombotic risks. The risk of serious bacterial infections is highest in the first 5 years of life following splenectomy, with a lifetime risk of approximately 5%. ASH guidelines suggest a minimum of 1 year from diagnosis prior to considering elective splenectomy. Before splenectomy, all vaccines for encapsulated bacteria should be administered a minimum of 2 weeks prior to surgery [19]. As immunizations do not fully protect, antibiotic prophylaxis is recommended with penicillin or amoxicillin. Duration of prophylaxis is controversial but should be continued for all children less than 5 years of age and for a minimum of 1–2 years postsplenectomy when the risk of overwhelming sepsis is highest [19]. In addition, postsplenectomy ITP patients are at increased risk for thromboembolism.

Immunosuppressive Agents

Immunosuppressive agents can be effective in treating refractory/chronic symptomatic ITP. Therapies with documented effects on improving platelet count in ITP include azathioprine, cyclophosphamide, cyclosporin A, danazol, dapsone, mycophenolate mofetil (MMF), and vinca alkaloids. These immunosuppressive agents have variable efficacy and side effect profiles. While no specific recommendations were made in the ASH guidelines due to a lack of comparable evidence, a systematic review of each agent is provided in a supplement to the primary document [10]. Given the stronger evidence for other therapies, these medications are sometimes considered "third-line treatments." They are often used in combination with other modalities and reserved for the most difficult cases. More recently, sirolimus (rapamycin) has been shown to be particularly effective when ITP occurs along with other immune cytopenias (e.g., autoimmune hemolytic anemia, Evans syndrome, and/or neutropenias) [20]. There is also evidence that sirolimus can be effective in ITP secondary to several primary immune deficiencies, such as ALPS [20, 21].

Emergency Management of Severe Bleeding

Although bleeding in children with ITP is rare, occasionally severe life-threatening bleeding may occur. Currently, there is no consensus on the best approach to managing severe bleeding in ITP.

If a child with ITP is having significant organ/life-threatening bleeding, a multimodal treatment approach including high-dose corticosteroids (intravenous methylprednisolone 30 mg/kg to a maximum dose of 1 g over 30–60 min), followed by platelet transfusion (double/triple dose) and then IVIG 1 g/kg, is a reasonable initial approach [22]. Continuous platelet transfusion, antifibrinolytic agents, and recombinant activated FVII (rFVIIa) can also be considered. See Appendix III for platelet transfusion and antifibrinolytic agents dosing. Empiric dosing for rFVIIa can be derived from the hemophilia literature: 15–30 μg/kg every 2 h × 3 doses or 270 μg/kg once by IV push in extreme circumstances [23]. TPO-RAs can be used but the response is delayed by at least a few days. Emergency splenectomy may also be considered in selected cases or if medical measures are unsuccessful.

While ICH is rare in children with ITP (0.2–1%), it can result in poor neurological outcomes or death. If a head injury occurs in a child known to have severe/refractory ITP, platelet transfusion and other emergency treatments (high-dose methylprednisolone and IVIG) and emergency imaging with a CT scan should be prioritized, even prior to obtaining a platelet count.

Secondary ITP

The distinction between primary and secondary ITP is important because the treatment of secondary ITP is often targeted to the underlying disorder (Table 2). It is important to recognize that immune-mediated thrombocytopenia may precede other manifestations of the underlying disorder by months or even years. Periodic re-evaluation of a child thought to have primary ITP is required to identify possible secondary causes of ITP. Secondary ITP can be broadly categorized by the different causes. There is, however, overlap between these categories, for example, HIV, an infectious disease, results in acquired immune dysregulation.

Etiologies of Secondary ITP

Infections

Acute infections with viruses such as Epstein-Barr virus, cytomegalovirus, varicella zoster, rubella, COVID-19, and chronic infections with viruses such as hepatitis C and HIV have been well documented in association with ITP [24]. In addition to viral infections, other infections have also been reported in association with ITP including brucellosis, tuberculosis, and *H. pylori* infection.

Chronic infection with *H. pylori*, a globally endemic bacterium associated with upper gastrointestinal disease, has been associated with a number of extragastric manifestations, including ITP. The role of *H. pylori* infection in childhood chronic ITP has been studied with conflicting results, which mirrors the data in adults with ITP. The 2019 ASH guidelines did not address the issue of *Helicobacter* infection in children contributing to chronic ITP; however, the 2011 guideline recommended against routine testing for *H. pylori* infection in children with chronic ITP. The 2016 joint European Society for Paediatric Gastroenterology, Hepatology and Nutrition and North American Society for Pediatric Gastroenterology, Hepatology and Nutrition [25] and the Japanese guidelines for *H. pylori* infection in childhood ITP recommend testing for *H. pylori* active infection by noninvasive methods when investigating causes of chronic ITP. The Japanese guidelines recommend eradication therapy for *H. pylori*-infected children with chronic ITP as the first-line therapy [26].

Connective Tissues Diseases

Systemic lupus erythematosus (SLE) is a systemic autoimmune disorder with variable multisystem involvement that is frequently associated with thrombocytopenia due to peripheral destruction of platelets mediated by autoantibodies. The onset of immune-mediated thrombocytopenia may be the first manifestation of SLE in up to 16% of cases, and it may precede the diagnosis of SLE by months or many years. This is important to appreciate when an initial diagnosis of primary ITP is being made and long-term follow-up planned.

Drug-Induced

Numerous drugs have been associated with the development of immune-mediated thrombocytopenia in both children and adults. A list of medications associated with ITP has been published by the World Health Organization [27]. The diagnosis of drug-associated ITP remains challenging because of patient comorbidities, multiple potential agents, and the challenges of stopping essential medications. The prognosis of drug-associated ITP is generally favorable when the suspected drug is withdrawn. HIT is described below.

Immune Dysregulation

Autoimmune cytopenias, including ITP, are common presentations of immune disorders in the pediatric age group. The number of inborn errors of immunity continues to expand each year as advances in discovering the genetic causes of human disease continue and the International Union of Immunological Societies Expert Committee produces regular updates of the classification of inborn errors of immunity, including those that cause immune dysregulation [28]. The autoimmune cytopenias in these disorders often have a more severe, chronic and relapsing course and frequently are refractory to treatment. ITP may be the first manifestation of the underlying inborn error of immunity. The coexistence of multiple cytopenias (e.g., Evan's syndrome) is a warning sign for the presence of an underlying immune disorder with pathogenic variants in multiple genes, including *TNFRSF6*, *CTLA4*, *STAT3*, *PIK3CD*, *CBL*, *ADAR1*, *LRBA*, *RAG1*, and *KRAS*. Humoral and cell-mediated immune defects such as reduced serum immunoglobulin levels or low T cell counts may be an indication of an underlying immune disorder.

Increasingly it is being recognized that immune dysregulation may result from an acquired disorder such as HIV infection. It has been recognized that an acquired disorder of immune regulation can also result from somatic variants (e.g., in the *FAS* gene) in cells of the immune system resulting in ALPS-like disease with lymphoproliferation and autoimmunity (see below).

Lymphoproliferative Disorders

ALPS is a disorder of immune dysregulation due to a defect in lymphocyte apoptosis, which results in a lymphoproliferative disease that is characterized by lymphadenopathy, splenomegaly, hepatomegaly, and autoimmune diseases (typically involving hematopoietic cell lines). It is characterized by elevations of CD3 positive T-cell receptor $\alpha\beta^+$ double negative T cells. Classical ALPS is due to a germline or somatic variant in the first apoptosis signal (*FAS*) receptor signaling pathway. Germline variants in *FASL* and *CASP10* also give rise to the typical ALPS phenotype because of the disruption of this apoptotic pathway. In addition to classical ALPS, there are other ALPS-like syndromes involving variants in genes involved in immune checkpoints (e.g., *CTLA4* and *LRBA*) that can be clinically similar to ALPS but are genetically and biologically different [29]. Management of cases with ALPS or ALPS like-syndromes is often challenging and is best achieved by multidisciplinary teams that include health care professionals with expertise and experience dealing with these challenging cases, e.g., hematologists, immunologists. Use of medications such as MMF and sirolimus need to be considered early in the management of these cases and splenectomy should be avoided because of the enhanced risk of overwhelming postsplenectomy sepsis.

Malignancy

Autoimmune cytopenias have been reported as a paraneoplastic phenomenon in malignant lymphomas, such as Hodgkin lymphoma. The ITP may occur prior to, concurrent with, at the time of recurrence, or in complete remission after treatment. ITP in a child with Hodgkin lymphoma generally responds to anti-lymphoma treatment. Posttreatment ITP in children who are in remission following Hodgkin lymphoma therapy generally respond easily and durably to steroids.

Acquired Platelet Function Disorders

Acquired platelet function disorders include acquired thrombocytopenia and/or impaired platelet function that result from medications, dietary supplements, procedures, and systemic diseases.

Diagnosis

The detailed medical history and current medications/dietary supplements should be carefully reviewed. A basic laboratory investigation includes a CBC, blood smear, prothrombin time/international normalized ratio (PT/INR), activated partial thromboplastin time (aPTT), and renal and liver function tests. A screening test using the closure times of the platelet function analyzer (PFA-100®/200®) may be performed [30]. It was shown that in ITP, PFA-100®/200® closure times remain normal, provided the platelet count was >50 × 10^9/L. However, this test is not specific for platelet function disorders caused by platelet granule deficiencies and/or secretion defects. For such conditions, light transmission platelet aggregation testing, lumiaggregometry and quantitation of platelet granule content are considered the gold standard. The limitation of these specialized platelet tests is that they require fresh blood samples and results are influenced by the presence of thrombocytopenia. Platelet function tests assessed by whole blood flow cytometry was found to be associated with bleeding severity in ITP, independent of platelet count [31].

Some children with ITP who have relatively higher platelet counts (>50 × 10^9/L) may report much more bleeding than expected. In such cases, the PFA-100®/200® might be useful as very abnormal closure times in such a setting may be the clue to a condition referred to as acquired Glanzmann thrombasthenia, which alternatively has also been referred to as ITP with platelet dysfunction. The disorder arises due to autoantibodies binding to and blocking integrin αIIbβ3. This is a notoriously difficult diagnosis to make and to manage, as improving the platelet count does not lessen the bleeding symptomatology [32]. Platelet aggregation testing is useful in such a setting but may be problematic in the setting of thrombocytopenia. Flow cytometric assessment of surface receptors and activation markers may be useful [31].

Etiologies

Drugs, Foods, and Dietary Supplements

Many drugs, foods, and dietary supplements have been reported to impair platelet function, some of which are given with therapeutic intent. Others have platelet inhibition as a side effect (Table 5) [33].

ASA is one of the most widely used antiplatelet agents; it inhibits formation of the platelet aggregating agent thromboxane A_2 by irreversibly inhibiting cyclooxygenase-1 (COX-1) conversion of arachidonic acid to prostaglandin G_2/prostaglandin H_2. Other NSAIDs, such as ibuprofen and naproxen, inhibit COX-1 reversibly, while COX-2 inhibitors have minimal antiplatelet activity.

Bleeding is minimal in children on a single antiplatelet agent, but significant bleeding can occur in children treated with antiplatelet agents who have underlying inherited/acquired bleeding disorders, including those who have not been diagnosed previously. As such, it is important to assess whether there are any underlying bleeding disorders that might be the real cause of the bleeding.

Management: Whenever possible, discontinue drugs that cause bleeding secondary to platelet dysfunction. Platelet transfusion is usually preserved for significant bleeding (see Appendix III). However, interruption of antiplatelet therapy and platelet transfusion should be made on an individual basis after carefully balancing the benefits and risks of both options with regard to their potential prothrombotic risks.

Chronic Renal Failure

The mechanism of bleeding in children with chronic renal failure is still unclear, but uremia-related platelet dysfunction is a major contributing factor. There appear to be several platelet defects in adhesion and secretion, mediated by increased platelet cyclic adenosine monophosphate. As a result of elevated prostacyclin (prostaglandin I_2) and nitric oxide levels, acquired dense granule disorder may result in decreased adenosine 5′-diphosphate (ADP) and serotonin levels, and reduced thromboxane A_2 levels in platelets. In addition, anemia reduces platelet-endothelial interactions and impairs platelet adhesion [34].

Management: see Chapter 11.

Table 5. Drugs, foods, and dietary supplements that can impair platelet function

Antiplatelet agents	COX-1 inhibitors: aspirin, ibuprofen, naproxen, indomethacin, diclofenac $P2Y_{12}$ receptor inhibitors: thienopyridines (clopidogrel, prasugrel), non-thienopyridines (ticagrelor, cangrelor) Integrin αIIbβ3 inhibitors: abciximab, tirofiban, eptifibatide PDE inhibitors: dipyridamole, cilostazol
Other drugs	Beta-lactam antibiotics, SSRIs, dextran, calcium channel blockers, beta blockers, milrinone, tricyclic antidepressants, inhaled nitric oxide, nitrates
Foods and dietary supplements	Alcohol, ginkgo, garlic, blueberry, ginger, dong quai, feverfew, ginseng, cumin, turmeric, meadowsweet, willow, black tree fungus, omega-3 fatty acids, onion

COX, cyclooxygenase; PDE, phosphodiesterase; SSRIs, selective serotonin reuptake inhibitors.

Liver Disease

Bleeding in children with liver disease is multifactorial. In addition to coagulopathy, thrombocytopenia and platelet dysfunction also contribute to bleeding. Thrombocytopenia is common in children with liver disease, and many studies have shown a correlation with liver dysfunction and fibrosis, and splenic sequestration (see Chapter 11). In some children with severe liver disease, platelet dysfunction has also been observed. Mechanisms include impaired thromboxane A_2 synthesis, platelet granule and secretion defects and glycoprotein Ib abnormalities [34]. Additionally, hyperfibrinolysis in children with advanced liver disease results in an accumulation of fibrin degradation products, which can impair platelet function.

Management: see Chapter 11.

Congenital Heart Disease and Mechanical Circulatory Support

Children with certain types of congenital heart disease, including valve stenosis/regurgitation, restrictive septal defects, and narrowed shunt or conduits, can have multiple acquired hemostatic abnormalities as a result of turbulent flow and high shear conditions. The abnormalities include thrombocytopenia, platelet dysfunction, acquired von Willebrand syndrome (see Chapter 11), local intravascular coagulation, and primary hyperfibrinolysis. Similarly, these abnormalities can occur in children who are on mechanical circulatory support, such as cardiopulmonary bypass, extracorporeal membrane oxygenation (ECMO) and ventricular assist devices (see Chapter 19). More than 75% of children on ECMO have evidence of platelet dysfunction. The mechanisms involved in platelet dysfunction during ECMO include exposure of blood to artificial surfaces and oxidative stress leading to platelet activation and dysfunction [35]. Additionally, the absence of in vivo platelet agonists also contributes to platelet dysfunction.

Management: see Chapter 19.

Gaucher Disease

Bleeding is common in children with Gaucher disease, which is usually attributed to thrombocytopenia, but some children experience bleeding symptoms despite having relatively high platelet counts and normal coagulation tests, suggesting platelet dysfunction [36].

Management: Following enzyme replacement therapy, it has been demonstrated that platelet counts and function improved, and there was cessation of bleeding [36]. Some children may experience bleeding tendencies while on enzyme replacement therapy. Antifibrinolytic agents and platelet transfusion may be required for the management of significant bleeding.

Myelodysplastic Syndrome

Thrombocytopenia is typically the cause of bleeding in individuals with myelodysplastic syndrome (MDS). However, MDS can cause abnormal thrombopoiesis, which results in platelet dysfunction, including reduced alpha granules and abnormalities of the dense tubular system [37]. Although reported pediatric cases with platelet dysfunction are limited, approximately 75% of adults with MDS have evidence of platelet dysfunction. If the severity of the bleeding is more than would be expected, given the degree of thrombocytopenia, platelet dysfunction should be suspected.

Management: Specific treatment for MDS can correct thrombocytopenia and platelet dysfunction but platelet transfusion may be required in children with significant bleeding.

Myeloproliferative Neoplasms

Variable degree of platelet dysfunction has been described in myeloproliferative neoplasms (MPN). Platelet dysfunction in subjects with MPN may occur in certain situations, particularly those who have thrombocytosis such as essential thrombocythemia [38]. High platelet counts can result in spontaneous binding between platelets and high-molecular-weight von Willebrand factor (HMW VWF) multimers, which leads to the increased clearance of the HMW VWF multimers and results in acquired von Willebrand syndrome (see Chapter 11). In addition, spontaneous platelet activation and the release of the contents of platelet granules lead to acquired platelet dysfunction. Nonspecific abnormalities of platelet aggregometry, including loss of the secondary wave of aggregation with epinephrine and ADP, have been reported in subjects with MPN but there is no correlation between PFA-100®/200® closure times and bleeding symptoms.

Management: Specific treatment for MPN such as cytoreductive therapy to reduce platelet count to $<1,000 \times 10^9/L$ can reduce the risk of bleeding, but platelet transfusions may be required in subjects with significant bleeding.

Eosinophilia

Acquired platelet dysfunction with eosinophilia is a well-described acquired bleeding disorder among children aged 3–7 years, most commonly diagnosed in Southeast Asia [39]. Spontaneous ecchymosis is the presenting symptom in most children, although some also experience mucosal bleeding. Most children have a parasitic infestation, which leads to the production of eosinophilia, elevated serum IgE levels, and the formation of antibodies and immune complexes. Immune complexes bind to platelets, causing platelet activation and degranulation, which results in acquired platelet dysfunction as well as increased platelet clearance in the reticuloendothelial system.

The diagnosis can be made using a history of acquired bleeding, eosinophilia, hypogranular and bizarre-shaped platelets on peripheral blood smears, and impaired platelet function tests. The impaired platelet aggregation induced by collagen is the most sensitive test, although impaired platelet aggregation induced by ADP and epinephrine and impaired adenosine 5′-triphosphate secretion are also observed. Some children have decreased or absence of dense granules as determined by platelet electron microscopy. Additionally, stool examination is recommended to evaluate parasitic infestation.

Management: Bleeding symptoms are generally mild and transient and usually require no treatment, but platelet transfusion may be needed in children with significant bleeding. Therapy with antiparasitic agents is recommended in children who are at risk or have evidence of parasitic infestation. The majority of children have spontaneous remission within 3–6 months, which is correlated with a decline in the absolute eosinophil count, and recurrence is uncommon [39].

Heparin-Induced Thrombocytopenia

HIT is an immune-mediated complication of heparin therapy resulting in a prothrombotic state that may cause life- and limb-threatening complications. In adults, clinical complications of HIT are seen in ~0.2–3% of those exposed to heparin [40]. The incidence of HIT in the pediatric population appears to be significantly lower. Nevertheless, it has been well-documented to occur in children of all ages (including neonates) and needs to be considered in the appropriate clinical setting.

HIT can occur after any exposure to heparin, including heparin flushes and heparin-coated catheters, but the risk is highest with exposure to unfractionated heparin (UFH) and is significantly less with low-molecular-weight heparin (LMWH). The formation of complexes between platelet factor 4 (PF4), an α-granule protein, and heparin results in the formation of an immunogenic neoantigen. In some children, the formation of immunoglobulin G (IgG) antibodies against the PF4/heparin complex leads to the creation of an immune complex that can activate platelets and monocytes resulting in both thrombosis and thrombocytopenia [41, 42].

The pathognomonic clinical feature of HIT is the development of thrombocytopenia and/or thrombosis in temporal association with heparin therapy. The diagnosis is rarely straightforward because there are often other causes of thrombocytopenia (infection, medications, surgery, etc.) that need to be considered. The risk of children developing HIT is related to the extent of heparin exposure. In the pediatric population, there is a bimodal frequency of HIT occurrence in neonates and adolescents, which are the two pediatric populations most at risk of thrombosis and likely to be receiving heparin.

The typical onset, as seen in two-thirds of children with HIT, is a decline in platelet count (an absolute drop in platelet count ($<150 \times 10^9$/L) or a relative decline of 30–50% from baseline counts) beginning 5 to 10 days after heparin initiation. Previously sensitized children may have a more rapid onset of thrombocytopenia. The platelet nadir is usually in the moderate range ($50–70 \times 10^9$/L) and is typically not associated with bleeding complications. Severe thrombocytopenia ($<20 \times 10^9$/L) is rare but can occur as a manifestation of fulminant thrombotic disease [43].

Thrombosis is the most severe complication of HIT and can be venous, arterial, and/or microcirculation thrombosis. Thrombosis is characteristically severe and can occur at unusual sites. In children, venous thromboses are more commonly observed and include thrombi in the subclavian and femoral veins (sites of vascular injury from catheters) [41]. The thrombotic complications typically occur concurrently with the onset of thrombocytopenia.

Diagnosis

Laboratory testing for suspected HIT involves both immune (with poor specificity) and functional assays (which are technically complex and, therefore, not routinely available in many centers). Scoring systems (e.g., the 4T system) have been developed and validated in adults to aid in decision making around the likelihood of HIT and cessation of heparin [43] (Table 6). Such scoring systems may be helpful in children.

Laboratory Tests

Immunoassays detect the presence of PF4/heparin antibodies using a variety of antibody capture platforms (e.g., ELISA). These assays are generally available in most clinical laboratories and are highly sensitive but have a low specificity (30–70%) for the diagnosis of HIT. The test has a negative predictive value of more than 97–99% and, therefore, is useful to rule out the diagnosis of HIT. Functional assays test the ability of the heparin-IgG-PF4 complex to activate platelets via FcγRII receptors. The serotonin release assay is considered the gold standard test though more

Table 6. The 4Ts score for heparin-induced thrombocytopenia (HIT)

Category	2 points	1 point	0 points
Thrombocytopenia	Platelet count decrease of >50% and platelet nadir ≥20 × 10^9/L	Platelet count decrease of 30–50% OR platelet nadir 10–19 × 10^9/L	Platelet count decrease of <30% or platelet nadir <10 × 10^9/L
Timing of decrease in platelet count	Clear onset between days 5–10 OR platelet decrease of ≤1 day with heparin exposure within 30 prior days	Decrease in platelet count consistent with onset between days 5 to 10, but timing is not clear owing to missing platelet counts OR decrease in platelet count after day 10 of heparin exposure OR decrease in platelet counts ≤1 day with prior heparin exposure between 30 and 100 days ago	Platelet count decrease of <4 days without recent heparin exposure
Thrombosis	New thrombosis, skin necrosis or acute systemic reaction after heparin exposure	Progressive/recurrent thrombosis or unconfirmed but clinically suspected thrombosis	No thrombosis or thrombosis preceding heparin exposure
Other causes for thrombocytopenia	None apparent	Possible other causes present	Probably other causes present

The 4Ts score is a sum of the points for each of the four categories. Scores of 1–3 are low, 4–5 intermediate, and 8 is high. Modified with permission from Cuker et al. [43].

recently flow-based platelet activation assays are being increasingly used. The functional assays offer high specificity (>95%) but lower sensitivity than the immunoassays [44].

Management

The management of HIT in children is extrapolated from adult data. If HIT is highly suspected, all forms of heparin exposure should be eliminated, and an alternative anticoagulant should be initiated at a therapeutic dose (even in the absence of clinical thrombosis because of the high rate of thrombosis on cessation of heparin in this patient population). Selection of alternative parenteral anticoagulation agents is largely based on drug availability and patient comorbidities and includes direct thrombin inhibitors such as argatroban or bivalirudin, indirect factor Xa inhibitors such as danaparoid or fondaparinux, or a direct oral anticoagulant (DOAC) [45]. Vitamin K antagonists should be avoided until the HIT has abated because they increase the risk of venous limb gangrene and limb loss. Prophylactic platelet transfusions should be avoided in children with HIT because the risk of bleeding is very low, and platelet transfusions can increase the risk of thrombosis. For children with thrombosis, anticoagulation is recommended for a duration appropriate for the thrombotic event (see Chapter 20). In children with acute isolated HIT and no asymptomatic DVT identified by screening compression ultrasonography, the ASH guideline panel suggests that anticoagulation be continued, at a minimum, until platelet count recovery (usually a platelet count of ≥150 × 10^9/L). The ASH guideline panel suggests against continuing treatment of ≥3 months unless the patient has persisting HIT without platelet count recovery (conditional recommendations, very low certainty in the evidence) [45].

Conclusion

Acquired platelet disorders occur in children. ITP is the most common cause of acquired thrombocytopenia in pediatric hematology. Recent developments of new therapies have provided more options for treatment of ITP, but the general approach has been to treat only children with bleeding symptoms. Treatment of secondary causes of ITP should address the underlying process. Acquired nonimmune thrombocytopenia and platelet dysfunction occur especially in hospitalized children/adolescents and may contribute to significant bleeding. HIT is a very rare entity in children, but should be considered in those exposed to heparin.

Acknowledgment

The authors would like to express their appreciation to Dr. Cindy Neunert, New York, USA, for her thoughtful review of this chapter.

Conflict of Interest Statement

Vicky R. Breakey declares no conflict of interest. Thomas Kühne received research funds from Amgen and Novartis and served on advisory boards for UCB Biosciences and SOBI. Natsaruth Songthawee declares no conflict of interest. Julie Curtin received research funds from Sanofi, Roche, and CSL Behring and served on advisory boards for CSL Behring, Novo Nordisk, and Sanofi. Victor S. Blanchette reports receiving consultancy and speaker fees from Bayer HealthCare, Sanofi, Novo Nordisk, Pfizer, Roche, Takeda, and Spark Therapeutics. He is recipient of research grants from Sanofi, Bayer HealthCare, and Takeda, and serves as a member of Data Safety Monitoring Boards for Octapharma and Takeda. He is Chair of a nonprofit organization, the International Prophylaxis Study Group (IPSG).

Author Contributions

Vicky R. Breakey coordinated writing and revision of the manuscript, co-wrote the section on ITP, and finalized the manuscript for submission. Thomas Kühne co-wrote the section on ITP, revised the completed draft, and provided feedback for revisions. Natsaruth Songthawee wrote the section on acquired disorders of platelet function and reviewed the completed draft with feedback provided for revisions. Julie Curtin wrote the sections on secondary ITP and HIT, reviewed the completed draft and provided feedback for revisions. Victor S. Blanchette revised the completed draft and provided feedback for revisions.

Abbreviations

ADP	Adenosine 5′-diphosphate
ALPS	Autoimmune lymphoproliferative disorder
aPTT	Activated partial thromboplastin time
ASA	Acetylsalicylic acid
ASH	American Society of Hematology
CBC	Complete blood count
COX	Cyclooxygenase-1
CT	Computed tomography
DOAC	Direct oral anticoagulant
ECMO	Extracorporeal membrane oxygenation
FNAIT	Fetal and neonatal alloimmune thrombocytopenia
HIT	Heparin-induced thrombocytopenia
HMB	Heavy menstrual bleeding
HMW	High-molecular-weight
HIV	Human immunodeficiency virus
HRQoL	Health-related quality of life
ICH	Intracranial hemorrhage
IgG	Immunoglobulin G
INR	International normalized ratio
IPF	Immature platelet fraction
ITP	Immune thrombocytopenia
IVIG	Intravenous immunoglobulin
LMWH	Low-molecular-weight heparin
NSAIDs	Nonsteroidal anti-inflammatory drugs
MDS	Myelodysplastic syndrome
MMF	Mycophenolate mofetil
MMR	Measles, mumps, rubella
MPN	Myeloproliferative neoplasm
MPV	Mean platelet volume
MYH9	Myosin heavy chain 9
PF4	Platelet factor 4
PFA	Platelet function analyzer
PT	Prothrombin time
rFVIIa	Recombinant activated FVII
RhIG	Rhesus (Rh) immune globulin
TPO-RA	Thrombopoietin receptor agonist
SLE	Systemic lupus erythematosus
UFH	Unfractionated heparin
VWF	von Willebrand factor

References

1 Provan D, Semple JW. Recent advances in the mechanisms and treatment of immune thrombocytopenia. eBioMedicine. 2022;76:103820.

2 Neunert CE, Buchanan GR, Imbach P, Bolton-Maggs PH, Bennett CM, Neufeld EJ, et al. Severe hemorrhage in children with newly diagnosed immune thrombocytopenic purpura. Blood. 2008;112:4003–8.

3 Buchanan GR, Adix L. Grading of hemorrhage in children with idiopathic thrombocytopenic purpura. J Pediatr. 2002;141:683–8.

4 Bolton-Maggs, P. Severe bleeding in idiopathic thrombocytopenic purpura. J Pediatr Hematol Oncol. 2003;25:S47–51.

5 Grace RF, Klaassen RJ, Shimano KA, Lambert MP, Grimes A, Bussel JB, et al. Fatigue in children and adolescents with immune thrombocytopenia. Br J Haematol. 2020;191:98–106.

6 Klaassen JR, Blanchette V, Burke TA, Wakefield C, Grainger JD, Gaedicke G, et al. Quality of life in childhood immune thrombocytopenia: international validation of the kids' ITP tools. Pediatr Blood Cancer. 2013;60:95–100.

7 Rodeghiero F, Stasi R, Gernsheimer T, Michel M, Provan D, Arnold DM, et al. Standardization of terminology, definitions and outcome criteria in immune thrombocytopenic purpura of adults and children: report from an international working group. Blood 2009;113:2386–93.

8 Grace RF, Lambert MP. An update on pediatric ITP: differentiating primary ITP, IPD, and PID. Blood 2022;140:542–55.

9 Neunert C, Lim W, Crowther M, Cohen A, Solberg L Jr, Crowther MA. The American Society of Hematology 2011 evidence-based practice guideline for immune thrombocytopenia. Blood. 2011;117:4190–207.

10 Neunert C, Terrell DR, Arnold DM, Buchanan G, Cines DB, Cooper N, et al. American Society of Hematology 2019 guidelines for immune thrombocytopenia. Blood Adv. 2019;3:3829–66.

11 Carcao M, Zipursky A, Butchart S, Leaker M, Blanchette V. Short-course oral prednisone therapy in children presenting with acute immune thrombocytopenic purpura (ITP). Acta Pædiatr Suppl. 1998;87:71–4.

12 Blanchette VS, Luke B, Andrew M, Sommerville-Nielsen S, Barnard D, de Veber B, et al. A prospective, randomized trial of high-dose intravenous immune globulin G therapy, oral prednisone therapy, and no therapy in childhood acute immune thrombocytopenic purpura. J Pediatr. 1993;123:989–95.

13 Blanchette V, Imbach P, Andrew M, Adams M, McMillan J, Wang E, et al. Randomised trial of intravenous immunoglobulin G, intravenous anti-D, and oral prednisone in childhood acute immune thrombocytopenic purpura. Lancet. 1994:344:703–7.

14 Ayad N, Grace RF, Al-Samkari H. Thrombopoietin receptor agonists and rituximab for treatment of pediatric immune thrombocytopenia: a systematic review and meta-analysis of prospective clinical trials. Pediatr Blood Cancer. 2022;69:e29447.

15 Tjepkema M, Amini S, Schipperus M. Risk of thrombosis with thrombopoietin receptor agonists for ITP patients: a systematic review and meta-analysis. Crit Rev Oncol Hematol. 2022;171:103581.

16 Harris EM, Hillier K, Al-Samkari H, Berbert L, Grace RF. Response to rituximab in children and adults with immune thrombocytopenia (ITP). Res Pract Thromb Haemost. 2021;5:e12587.

17 Li Y, Shi Y, He Z, Chen Q, Liu Z, Yu L, et al. The efficacy and safety of low-dose rituximab in immune thrombocytopenia: a systematic review and meta-analysis. Platelets. 2019;30:690–7.

18 Avila ML, Amiri N, Pullenayegum E, Blanchette V, Imbach P, Kühne T, & Intercontinental Cooperative ITP Study Group. Long term outcomes after splenectomy in children with immune thrombocytopenia: an update on the registry data from the Intercontinental Cooperative ITP Study Group. Haematologica.2020;105:2682–5.

19 Lee GM. Preventing infections in children and adolescents with asplenia. Hematology Am Soc Hematol Educ Program. 2020;2020:328–35.

20 Bride KL, Vincent T, Smith-Whitley K, Lambert MP, Bleesing JJ, Seif AE, et al. Sirolimus is effective in relapsed/refractory autoimmune cytopenias: results of a prospective multi-institutional trial. Blood. 2016;127:17–28.

21 Wang D, Cassady K, Zou Z, Zhang X, Feng Y. Progress on the efficacy and potential mechanisms of rapamycin in the treatment of immune thrombocytopenia. Hematology. 2022:1282–9.

22 Carcao M, Silva M, David M, Klaassen RJ, Steele M, Price V, et al. IVMP+IVIG raises platelet counts faster than IVIG alone: results of a randomized, blinded trial in childhood ITP. Blood Adv. 2020; 4(7):1492–500.

23 Barnes C, Blanchette V, Canning P, Carcao M. Recombinant FVIIa in the management of intracerebral haemorrhage in severe thrombocytopenia unresponsive to platelet-enhancing treatment. Transfus Med. 2005;15:145–50.

24 Lim J, Kim Y, Min S, Kim S, Lee Y, Lee J. Epidemiology and viral etiology of pediatric immune thrombocytopenia through Korean public health data analysis. J Clin Med. 2021;10:1356.

25 Jones N, Koletzko S, Goodman K, Bontems P, Cadranel S, Casswall T, et al. Joint ESPGHAN/NASPGHAN guidelines for the management of Helicobacter pylori in children and adolescents (Update 2016). J Pediatr Gastroenterol Nutr. 2017;64:991–1003.

26 Kato S, Shimizu T, Toyoda S, Gold B, Ida S, Ishige T, et al. The updated JSPGHAN guidelines for the management of Helicobacter pylori infection in childhood. Pediatr Int. 2020;62:1315–31.

27 Fuentes S, Chrétien B, Dolladille C, Alexandre J, Dumont A, Nguyen A, et al. An updated list of drugs suspected to be associated with immune thrombocytopenia based on the WHO pharmacovigilance database. Blood. 2022;140:922–7.

28 Tangye S, Al-Herz W, Bousfiha A, Cunningham-Rundles C, Franco J, Holland S, et al. Human inborn errors of immunity: 2022 update on the classification from the International Union of Immunological Societies Expert Committee. J Clin Immunol 2022:43:1473–507.

29 Gámez-Díaz L, Grimbacher B. Immune checkpoint deficiencies and autoimmune lymphoproliferative syndromes. Biomed J. 2021;44:400–11.

30 Carcao MD, Blanchette VS, Stephens D, He L, Wakefield CD, Butchart S, et al. Assessment of thrombocytopenic disorders using the Platelet Function Analyzer (PFA-100). Br J Haematol. 2002;117:961–4.

31 Frelinger AL, Grace RF, Gerrits AJ, Carmichael SL, Forde EE, Michelson AD. Platelet function in ITP, independent of platelet count, is consistent over time and is associated with both current and subsequent bleeding severity. Thromb Haemost. 2018;118(1):143–51.
32 Bacci M, Ferretti A, Marchetti M, Alberelli MA, Falanga A, Lodigiani C, et al. Autoimmune disorders of platelet function: systematic review of cases of acquired Glanzmann thrombasthenia and acquired delta storage pool disease. Blood Transfus. 2022;20:420–32.
33 Konkle BA. Acquired disorders of platelet function. Hematology Am Soc Hematol Educ Program. 2011;2011:391–6.
34 Lambert MP. Platelets in liver and renal disease. Hematology Am Soc Hematol Educ Program. 2016;2016:251–5.
35 Saini A, Hartman ME, Gage BF, Said A, Gazit AZ, Eghtesady P, et al. Incidence of platelet dysfunction by thromboelastography–platelet mapping in children supported with ECMO: a pilot retrospective study. Front Pediatr. 2016;3:116.
36 Revel-Vilk S, Szer J, Zimran A. Hematological manifestations and complications of Gaucher disease. Expert Rev Hematol. 2021;14(4):347–54.
37 Mittelman M, Zeidman A. Platelet function in the myelodysplastic syndromes. Int J Hematol 2000;71:95–8.
38 Marin Oyarzún CP, Heller PG. Platelets as mediators of thromboinflammation in chronic myeloproliferative neoplasms. Front Immunol. 2019;10:1373.
39 Chotsampancharoen T, Sripornsawan P, Duangchu S, McNeil E. Clinical course and outcome of childhood acquired platelet dysfunction with eosinophilia. Acta Haematol. 2018;139:28–32.
40 Arepally, G. Heparin-induced thrombocytopenia. Blood. 2017;129(21):2864–72.
41 Vakil N, Kanaan A,Donovan J. Heparin-induced thrombocytopenia in the pediatric population: a review of current literature. J Pediatr Pharmacol Ther 2012;17:12–30.
42 Arepally GM, Padmanabhan A. Heparin-induced thrombocytopenia A focus on thrombosis. Arterioscler Thromb Vasc Biol. 2021;41:141–52.
43 Cuker A, Gimotty P, Crowther M, Warkentin T. Predictive value of the 4Ts scoring system for heparin-induced thrombocytopenia: a systematic review and meta-analysis. Blood. 2012;120:4160–7.
44 Marchetti M, Zermatten M, Bertaggia Calderara D, Aliotta A, Alberio L. Heparin-induced thrombocytopenia: a review of new concepts in pathogenesis, diagnosis, and management. J Clin Med. 2021;10:683.
45 Cuker A, Arepally G, Chong B, Cines D, Greinacher A, Gruel Y, et al. American Society of Hematology 2018 guidelines for management of venous thromboembolism: heparin-induced thrombocytopenia. Blood Adv. 2018;2:3360–92.

Published online: December 5, 2024

Blanchette VS, Brandão LR, Carcao MD, Kumar R, Rand ML, Revel-Vilk S (eds): SickKids Handbook of Pediatric Thrombosis and Hemostasis, ed 3, rev. and ext. Basel, Karger, 2024, pp 117–144 (DOI: 10.1159/000538192)

Hemophilia

Samantha C. Gouw[a] Ester Zapotocka[b] Vanessa Bouskill[c, d]
Janaina B.S. Ricciardi[e] Manuel D. Carcao[d, f]

[a]Amsterdam UMC, University of Amsterdam, Emma Children's Hospital, Pediatric Hematology, Amsterdam, The Netherlands; [b]Department of Pediatric Hematology/Oncology, University Hospital Motol, 2nd Faculty of Medicine, Charles University, Prague, Czech Republic; [c]Department of Nursing, Hospital for Sick Children, Toronto, ON, Canada; [d]Child Health Evaluative Sciences, Research Institute, Hospital for Sick Children, Toronto, ON, Canada; [e]Hemophilia Treatment Center 'Cláudio Luiz Pizzigatti Corrêa', University of Campinas-UNICAMP, Campinas, SP, Brazil; [f]Division of Haematology/Oncology, Department of Pediatrics, University of Toronto, Toronto, ON, Canada

Introduction

Hemophilia is an X-linked recessive bleeding disorder caused by deficiency of factor VIII (FVIII) in hemophilia A or factor IX (FIX) in hemophilia B. Pathogenic variants in the *F8* or *F9* genes, both located on the long arm of the X chromosome, are detectable in most cases of hemophilia. During normal hemostasis, activated FVIII and activated FIX form an enzymatic complex with factor X (tenase complex) leading to generation of activated factor X, which ultimately leads to a "thrombin burst" and the formation of a fibrin-platelet thrombus at sites of vessel injury (see Chapter 2). In general, an equivalent deficiency of FVIII or FIX leads to a clinically similar phenotype. In contrast, deficiency of factor XI (previously termed "hemophilia C") is genetically and clinically distinct and is discussed further in Chapter 10. Similarly, "acquired hemophilia" is a pathogenically unrelated autoimmune disorder, the management of which is discussed in Chapter 11.

Hemophilia occurs in all racial groups with an estimated incidence of approximately 1/4,000 males for hemophilia A and 1/25,000 for hemophilia B [1]. As these are X-linked disorders, males are predominantly affected, whereas carrier females can vary from being completely asymptomatic to having significant bleeding issues. The variation in factor levels of heterozygous females is very wide, with most having levels that fall within the normal range but some females having low factor levels and now are being referred to as having mild, moderate, or even severe hemophilia according to their factor levels [2]. Very occasionally females may have extremely low FVIII/FIX levels through one of a variety of mechanisms, e.g., skewed X-inactivation, homozygosity, compound heterozygosity, or chromosomal abnormalities such as Turner syndrome. Confirmation of a carrier status generally requires genetic testing although clues to carrier status in at-risk females (e.g., mothers or sisters of boys with hemophilia) include having bleeding

Table 1. Classification of hemophilia

	FVIII/FIX level	Clinical phenotype (untreated)
Severe	<0.01 IU/mL (<1%)	Recurrent mucocutaneous, deep soft tissue, and joint bleeds, often with minimal or no identifiable trauma (spontaneous); progression to severe arthropathy due to recurrent hemarthroses; postsurgical bleeding can be life-threatening.
Moderate	0.01–0.05 IU/mL (1–5%)	Prolonged bleeding following trauma or surgery; phenotype may be similar as severe hemophilia, especially in individuals with FVIII/IX levels of 0.01–0.03 IU/mL (1–3%); spontaneous (joint) bleeding uncommon, especially in individuals with FVIII/IX levels of 0.03–0.05 IU/mL (3–5%).
Mild	0.06–0.40 IU/mL (6–40%)	Bleeding after surgery or trauma. May be clinically silent in the absence of hemostatic challenge.

FIX, factor IX; FVIII, factor VIII.

symptoms, having an abnormally elevated activated partial thromboplastin time (aPTT), having low FVIII or FIX levels (only seen in about 30% of carriers) or having a reduced ratio of FVIII to von Willebrand factor (VWF) level (usually below 85%) in the case of carriers of hemophilia A [3]. Of note, normal coagulation tests do not exclude carrier status.

Hemophilia is traditionally classified according to the baseline factor level as mild, moderate, or severe (Table 1) [4]. The clinical phenotype of hemophilia is generally in keeping with baseline factor levels. Consequently, prior to the advent of prophylactic factor concentrate infusion (prophylaxis), severely and most moderately affected individuals experienced frequent spontaneous bleeding, particularly into joints, muscles, and soft tissues leading to hemophilic arthropathy and in some cases early death. In contrast, many persons with mild hemophilia usually only bleed after trauma or surgery and as such rarely develop joint disease and are likely able to have a life span no different from the general nonhemophilic population [5].

Recurrent joint bleeding, the hallmark of severe hemophilia, results in chronic synovitis with destruction of cartilage and bone, ultimately leading to painful, disabling arthropathy and reduced health-related quality of life (shown in Fig. 1). The increasing implementation of prophylaxis has ameliorated this clinical phenotype.

General Management Principles

Hemostatic Management

The mainstay of treatment of persons with congenital hemophilia has traditionally been intravenous factor replacement therapy. Started in the 1970s, the routine use of clotting factor concentrates (CFCs) has dramatically changed the prognosis of hemophilia (see Chapter 1). As explained later, significant developments have occurred in the availability and characteristics of factor products and more recently in the advent of nonfactor replacement therapies. Persons with hemophilia are treated either on demand, i.e., only in case of bleeding or surgery, or with prophylaxis, i.e., regular treatment in order to prevent bleeding and arthropathy.

In addition, adjuvant therapies help to minimize or avoid the need for factor replacement in persons with milder forms of hemophilia and have proven to be of benefit.

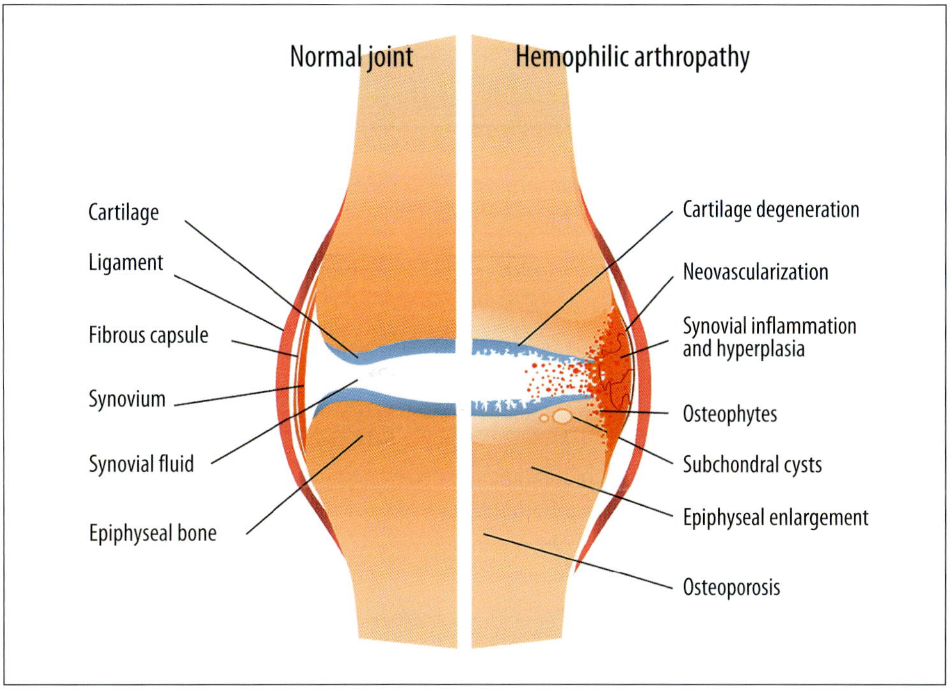

Fig. 1. Schematic representation of a healthy joint (left) and hemophilic arthropathy (right). Reprinted with permission from Elsevier (Pulles et al. [76]). Copyright 2017.

Factor Replacement Therapy

Therapeutic products containing FVIII or FIX can be broadly divided into those which are plasma derived and those manufactured using recombinant technology. Recombinant products can be subclassified according to production techniques, half-lives, possibly the variant FVIII molecule from which the product was derived (i.e., full length or B-domain deleted/truncated FVIII). Until one decade ago, all recombinant FVIII (rFVIII) products (and plasma-derived FVIII products) had virtually identical pharmacokinetics (PK) while there was only one recombinant FIX (rFIX) product which also showed similar PK to plasma derived FIX.

In the last 10 years, a variety of extended half-life (EHL) rFVIII and rFIX products have been developed. The older products are now referred to as standard half-life products (SHL). The newer EHL products were primarily developed to decrease the frequency of prophylactic infusions.

Several technologies have been used to prolong the half-life of FVIII/FIX concentrates.

The first is fusion to either albumin or the Fc portion of immunoglobulin G1 [6]. The Fc portion allows binding to the neonatal Fc receptor in endothelial cell lysosomes and subsequently inhibits lysosomal degradation of the fusion proteins and leads to their recycling back into the circulation.

The second is pegylation which involves the covalent attachment of polyethylene glycol (PEG) to the protein (FVIII or FIX) [7, 8]. PEG creates a hydrophilic cloud around the molecule thereby retarding proteolytic degradation and inhibiting receptor-mediated clearance. The EHL rFVIII products using the above technologies show a half-life prolongation of approximately 1.5-fold

Table 2. Current extended half-life FVIII and FIX clotting factor concentrates

Product	Technology	Manufacturer	$T_{1/2}$ vs. native FVIII/FIX	Recommended clotting factor assay
Extended half-life FIX				
rFIX-Fc (Alprolix)	Fusion protein with Fc fragment of IgG1	Sanofi/Sobi	3-fold	One-stage clotting assay (with selected aPTT reagents) or chromogenic assay
rFIX-FP (Idelvion)	Fusion protein with albumin	CSL-Behring	>5-fold	One-stage clotting assay (with selected aPTT reagents), not chromogenic assay
N9-GP (Rebinyn/Refixia)	Site-specific glycopegylation (40 kDa PEG)	Novo Nordisk	>5-fold	One-stage clotting assay (with selected aPTT reagents) or chromogenic assay
Extended half-life FVIII				
FVIII-Fc (Eloctate/Elocta)	B domain deleted FVIII fused to a monomeric Fc fragment of IgG	Sanofi/Sobi	1.5- to 1.7-fold	One-stage clotting assay (with selected aPTT reagents) and chromogenic assay (but consider overestimation by chromogenic assay)
BAY-94-9027 (Jivi)	Site-specific Pegylation (60 kDa PEG) of a B domain deleted FVIII	Bayer	1.4- to 1.6-fold	One-stage clotting assay (with selected aPTT reagents) and chromogenic assay
BAX 855 (Adynovate/ Adynovi)	Controlled Pegylation (20 kDa branched chain PEG) of a full-length FVIII	Takeda	1.4- to 1.6-fold	One-stage clotting assay or chromogenic assay
N8-GP (Esperoct)	Single site-specific glycopegylation (40 kDa PEG) of a B domain truncated FVIII	Novo Nordisk	1.6-fold	One-stage clotting assay (not with silica-based aPTT reagents) and chromogenic assay

aPTT, activated partial thromboplastin time; FIX, factor IX; FVIII, factor VIII; PEG, polyethylene glycol; $T_{1/2}$, half-life. The one-stage clotting assay factor VIII activity results can be affected by the used aPTT reagent and the reference standard [14–16]. Adapted and updated from Carcao [16]. Used with permissions of John Wiley & Sons-Books (Carcao [16]), permission conveyed through Copyright Clearance Center, Inc.

(Table 2). A third technology was the creation of a modified single chain FVIII, with increased binding affinity for VWF [9]. However, the prolongation of half-life was relatively limited.

A new EHL rFVIII – BIVV001 (efanesoctocog alfa) employs several technologies to extend the half-life of FVIII [10]. Attached to the rFVIII are both an Fc molecule along with two XTEN polypeptides composed of natural hydrophilic amino acids. The rFVIII in efanesoctocog is engineered to bind to a small part of the VWF molecule (D'D3) in such a way that efanesoctocog no longer binds to endogenous VWF causing it to no longer be cleared with VWF. These modifications result in a half-life 4-fold longer than that of SHL FVIII and may enable once weekly therapy for persons with hemophilia A with higher through levels. The product was recently approved by the FDA with the name Altuviiio.

In the case of rFIX, the 3 EHL rFIX CFCs show a half-life prolongation of 3- to 5-fold (Table 2) [11–13].

EHL rFVIII and rFIX CFCs offer the possibility of reducing the frequency of infusions. EHL

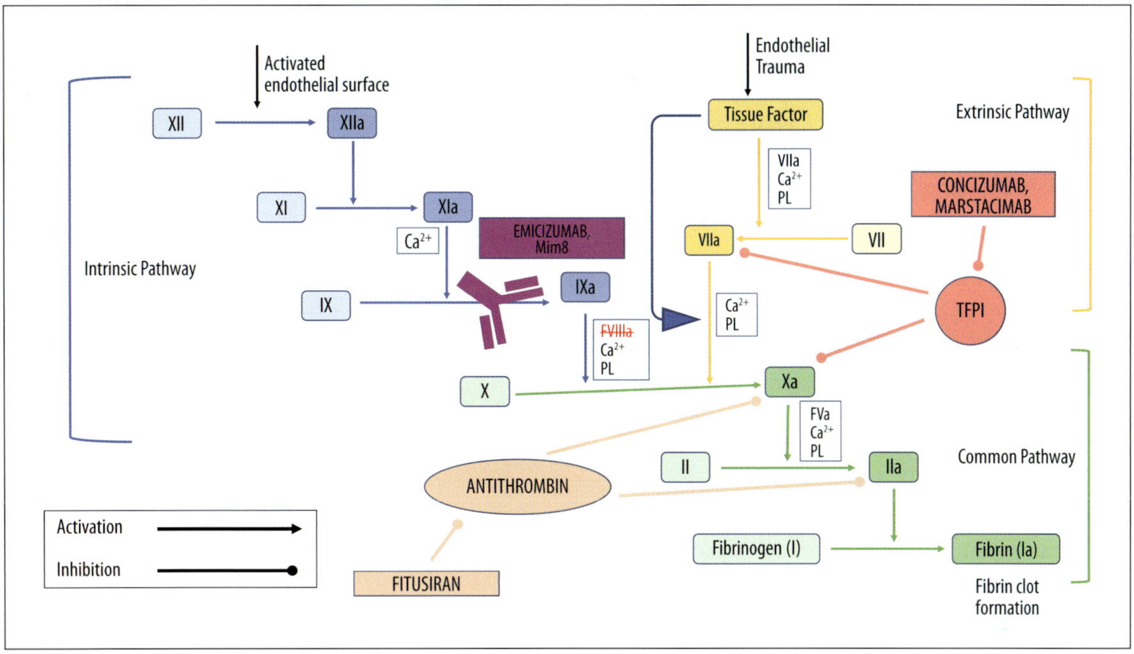

Fig. 2. Targets for nonfactor therapies in hemophilia. Originally published by and used with permission from Dove Medical Press Ltd. (Regling et al. [18]).

rFIX products may be for the most part given once per week, while EHL rFVIII CFCs with more modest prolongation of half-life need to be given generally twice weekly. Alternatively, the EHL rFVIII/IX CFCs provide the potential for maintaining higher trough (predose) factor levels for the same infusion frequency.

Until the advent of EHL CFCs, most laboratories evaluated factor levels post-CFC infusion using clot-based assays; these rely upon a coagulation contact pathway activator (ellagic acid, silica or kaolin) and a calibrator (factor-specific or standard). Many of the factor levels with EHL CFCs are not correctly measured by clot-based assays. Instead, chromogenic assays provide more reliable results [14, 15]. Table 2 includes the appropriate assay for measuring FVIII/FIX activity levels for each CFC type [14, 16, 17].

Non-Factor Therapies

Figure 2 illustrates the targets of current and future nonfactor therapies in the coagulation cascade [18, 19]. These therapies are used prophylactically to prevent bleeding and are not effective for on demand treatment or treatment of breakthrough bleeds.

Currently, one nonfactor therapy, emicizumab is licensed for use in hemophilia A in much of the world. This humanized bispecific monoclonal antibody functions by mimicking FVIII, binding and bridging activated FIX (FIXa) and FX (Table 3). By doing so, emicizumab can be used in children with hemophilia A, importantly including those with inhibitors to FVIII. Emicizumab is used as prophylaxis and has been shown to reduce annualized bleeding rates (ABRs) and improve target joints compared to on demand treatment and compared to FVIII prophylaxis in both non-inhibitor and inhibitor study cohorts [20].

Table 3. Main differences between activated factor VIII (FVIIIa) and Emicizumab

	FVIIIa	Emicizumab
Sites of interaction	Multiple sites	Single site
Affinity for FIXa and FX	High affinity	Low affinity
Specificity of binding	Specific for FIXa and FX	No distinction between zymogen and enzyme (binds both FIX and FIXa, and FX and FXa)
Cofactor activity	Full cofactor activity • Bridges FIXa to FX • Promotes phospholipid binding • Stabilizes FIXa active site	Partial cofactor activity • Bridges FIXa to FX
Rate limiting step	Concentration of FVIIIa (Enzyme [FIXa] and substrate [FX] are in excess)	Concentration of enzyme (FIXa) and substrate (FX) (Emicizumab is in excess)
On/off mechanism	Yes	No
Level of self-regulation	High	Low

FIX, factor IX; FIXa, activated factor IX; FX, factor X; FXa, activated factor X. Used with permissions of Elsevier Science & Technology Journals (Lenting et al. [22]), permission conveyed through Copyright Clearance Center, Inc.

Emicizumab has several clinical advantages over intravenous SHL or EHL FVIII CFCs. Emicizumab provides a steady-state level of protection (unlike the peaks and troughs in factor levels seen with FVIII infusions). Based on thrombin generation data, emicizumab has been suggested to provide a level of protection equivalent to that of FVIII levels of 0.20 IU/mL (20%) (with a 95% confidence interval between 0.12 and 0.28 IU/mL) [21]. Emicizumab significantly decreases the burden of care of hemophilia given that it is injected subcutaneously and its very long half-life (approximately 4 weeks) enabling once weekly to once monthly administration. However, although likely sufficient for most children for most activities, the protection provided by emicizumab may be insufficient for those engaging in higher risk sport/physical activities.

If a breakthrough bleed on emicizumab prophylaxis occurs, FVIII CFC can be administered safely. The administration of FVIII to children on emicizumab does not seem to increase the risk of thrombosis. FVIIIa has a higher binding affinity to FIXa as well as to FX than emicizumab; therefore, FVIIIa will preferentially bind to FIXa and FX and temporarily displace the emicizumab [22]. Children with inhibitors to FVIII who sustain a breakthrough bleed while on emicizumab require treatment with recombinant activated factor VII (rFVIIa). It is recommended to avoid treatment with activated prothrombin complex concentrate (aPCC) during emicizumab use. When persons on emicizumab are given aPCC (containing large amounts of both FIXa and FX – the substrates for emicizumab), a synergistic effect on thrombin generation causes increased risk of thrombosis and thrombotic microangiopathy [23]. Only in very rare situations should aPCC be given to persons on emicizumab and then only in lower doses (≤50 IU/kg) for no more than 24 h with close monitoring for signs of intravascular coagulation.

Another FVIII mimetic (Mim8) is currently under evaluation in phase 3 trials. Preliminary data suggests that it may be more potent with higher peak thrombin levels in comparison to emicizumab [24].

In addition to these FVIII-mimicking products, there are also procoagulant/anticoagulant rebalancing therapies being studied in phase 3 clinical trials [18, 19]. These therapies target natural anticoagulants such as tissue factor pathway inhibitor (TFPI), antithrombin, and proteins C and S, thereby creating a procoagulant state to balance the anticoagulant state created by the deficiency of FVIII/FIX in hemophilia A/B. These therapies, also administered subcutaneously, will offer children with hemophilia B the potential of a subcutaneous therapy as emicizumab cannot be used in hemophilia B.

Anti-TFPI human monoclonal antibodies currently being studied are concizumab and marstacimab. Both molecules are monoclonal antibodies directed against TFPI, and the dosing regimens have varied from daily to weekly.

Concizumab has been approved in Canada, and is administered subcutaneously. In the phase 3 study conducted in participants with hemophilia A/B with inhibitors, at least 12 years of age, the reported median ABR was 0.0 (interquartile range 0.0–3.3) [25].

Marstacimab is currently still under investigation. It is administered subcutaneously once weekly. In a phase 2 study of adults with severe hemophilia A/B with or without inhibitors treated with different dose regimens, median ABRs ranged from 0.0 (interquartile range 0.0–0.0) to 2.5 (interquartile range 0.0–5.0) [26].

Another rebalancing therapy makes use of small interfering RNAs (siRNAs). Fitusiran is a siRNA which reduces hepatic synthesis of antithrombin; as antithrombin inhibits thrombin, the effect of less antithrombin is enhanced hemostasis [19]. In this setting, hemostasis is proportional to antithrombin levels; lower antithrombin levels lead to better hemostasis but may increase thrombotic risk. Fitusiran is administered subcutaneously on a weekly to every 2-month regimen. Adults with severe hemophilia A/B without inhibitors in a phase 3 trial had median ABR of 0.0 (interquartile range 0.0–3.4) [19, 27].

The biggest concern with rebalancing agents is the concern of overcompensating for the hemophilia state leading to thrombotic events. Thrombotic events in trials of concizumab and fitusiran led to temporary halting of studies and adoption of risk mitigation strategies to reduce risk of thrombotic events. These risk mitigation strategies have generally consisted of using lower doses of FVIII, FIX, or bypassing agents in the event of breakthrough bleeds. In the case of fitusiran, it also involves targeting antithrombin levels to no lower than 0.15–0.20 IU/mL (15–20%). So far, these strategies have appeared successful [19].

Prophylaxis

Prophylaxis refers to the regular administration of hemostatic agents with the goal of preventing bleeding in people with hemophilia while allowing them to lead active lives and achieve quality of life comparable to nonhemophilic individuals [28]. Prophylaxis is now considered standard of care for all persons with a severe hemophilia phenotype [28]. Prophylaxis ideally should be started as early as possible to prevent bleeds from occurring as sometimes even one bleed may lead to joint damage. Prior to the availability of emicizumab, primary prophylaxis was defined as regular continuous treatment commenced before 3 years of age, prior to the onset of joint disease (determined by physical exam and/or imaging studies), and after no more than one clinically evident joint bleed. In contrast, secondary prophylaxis referred to regular prophylaxis commenced after ≥2 joint bleeds, but before the onset of joint disease, while tertiary prophylaxis referred to prophylaxis commenced after established joint disease to retard the progression of arthropathy. Shorter-term regular treatment (e.g., weeks to months) to reduce the risk of bleed recurrence following severe bleeding is termed intermittent (or periodic) prophylaxis [28, 29]. Nowadays with emicizumab and hopefully in the future with other nonfactor therapies which are all administered subcutaneously, prophylaxis may be able to be commenced at much younger ages than in the past with intravenously administered CFCs. A newer definition for primary prophylaxis may be needed for such prophylaxis commenced perhaps even at birth.

Currently, prophylaxis may be initiated with SHL or EHL rFVIII or rFIX CFCs or with emicizumab (in the case of hemophilia A). In a shared decision-making process, the pros and cons of the different options should be weighed [30]. Pros of CFC prophylaxis are long-term experience and possibility of tailoring the intensity of prophylaxis to the individual needs, while cons are the need for frequent intravenous infusions and inhibitor development against FVIII. For nonfactor therapy, the pros are convenient subcutaneous administration, only once every 1–4 weeks, allowing early start of prophylaxis and stable steady-state levels without troughs. Cons of nonfactor therapy are less knowledge on long-term adverse events, need for intravenous treatment when breakthrough bleeds occur; in this scenario, it is unlikely that the child could be treated at home as parents would not be trained in intravenous factor administration. Overall, the benefit of infrequent, subcutaneous injections in very young children is likely to offset the potential disadvantages and cause most young children to be commenced on emicizumab prophylaxis or prophylaxis with other nonfactor therapies once available rather than prophylaxis with CFCs.

With CFC prophylaxis, young children can be commenced on more, or less intensive regimens. Prior to the advent of EHL CFCs, to fully protect a child from bleeding would require up to every other day FVIII and twice per week FIX. To do such frequent infusions in young children would often require the insertion of central venous access devices (CVADs). To avoid CVADs, clinicians would often commence young children on less frequent infusions (e.g., once weekly) and then escalate the prophylaxis in those who experienced excessive bleeding. EHL products allow for significantly less frequent (in case of EHL rFIX) or slightly less frequent (in case of EHL rFVIII) infusion prophylaxis schedules thereby reducing the need for CVADs. Of course, with subcutaneously administered nonfactor therapies, there is no need for CVADs.

Prophylaxis with CFCs has often been tailored to individuals' perceived prophylaxis needs (based on individual PK parameters, timing and levels of physical activity, levels of other procoagulant and anticoagulant factors).

As alluded to earlier, there are a lot of differences between prophylaxis with CFCs versus prophylaxis with nonfactor therapies. There are substantial interpatient differences in PK of CFCs. This greatly impacts on designing effective prophylaxis regimens for individual children with hemophilia. With CFC prophylaxis, clinicians will often aim to not allow factor levels to fall below some arbitrary level; in the past, this was usually 0.01 IU/mL (1%), but over this past decade this has risen to 0.03 IU/mL (3%) or even higher. It is recognized that in general if FVIII or IX levels are kept at greater than 0.03–0.05 IU/mL (3–5%); this will result in less bleeding than if factor levels are allowed to drop to 0.01 IU/mL (1%) or less [28]. Given considerable interpatient variation, determining a child's individual PK may allow for tailoring of dosage and frequency to ensure that "the right amount of factor is given to the right person" without wastage. Determining individual PK parameters in the past was achieved through classical PK testing involving up to 10 blood samples obtained over 3–4 days with a washout period of at least 72 h for FVIII and 96 h for FIX, but now population PK programs and Bayesian forecasting allow for much more limited blood sampling (as little as two time points) and without a washout [31].

With SHL products, the timing of prophylactic administration was more important to avoid troughs occurring when a child would be most active; hence, morning administration of factor was most effective. With EHL CFCs and especially with nonfactor therapies, morning administration is less important.

Prophylaxis with emicizumab has consisted of a standard regimen involving the injection on a monthly basis of 6 mg/kg (given as either 1.5 mg/kg/week, 3 mg/kg every 2 weeks or 6 mg/kg every 4 weeks). It is likely that in the next few years emicizumab and other nonfactor therapies will also become more individualized. Consequently, less intensive (lower dose) and more intensive (higher dose) regimens may also be developed for nonfactor therapies – the former may permit greater use of these products in developing countries.

Of note, it is important to emphasize that, regardless of the prophylactic regimen, good adherence to prophylaxis is key to success. Long-term studies on lifelong prophylaxis with SHL CFCs have unfortunately shown that such prophylaxis does not completely prevent arthropathy in all persons with hemophilia. Furthermore, also many persons with moderate or even mild hemophilia have also been shown to develop joint damage. With newer EHL CFCs and nonfactor therapies such as emicizumab, perhaps less long-term joint damage will be seen.

Adjuvant Therapy

There are several pharmacologic agents that can be useful for achieving or maintaining hemostasis, either alone or in combination with CFCs.

Antifibrinolytic Agents

The antifibrinolytic agents ε-aminocaproic acid and tranexamic acid inhibit the binding of plasminogen/plasmin to fibrin thereby slowing fibrin dissolution at the site of clot formation. Antifibrinolytic agents are particularly useful to control bleeding from mucosal surfaces (e.g., epistaxis, gum bleeding, heavy menstrual bleeding), but are contraindicated in the setting of macroscopic hematuria due to the potential for ureteric or intrarenal clot formation and obstruction. They can be administered topically (e.g., as a mouth wash), orally, or intravenously (see Appendix III). Both agents are generally well tolerated, although dose-related gastrointestinal upset is common (particularly with ε-aminocaproic acid), and rapid intravenous infusion can cause dizziness, tachycardia and hypotension.

DDAVP

Desmopressin (1-deamino-8-D-arginine vasopressin, DDAVP) is a synthetic analogue of the antidiuretic hormone (vasopressin) which elevates plasma VWF and FVIII levels and increases platelet adhesiveness via VWF-independent mechanisms which are not fully understood (see Appendix III). DDAVP may avoid the need for CFC in some children with mild hemophilia A; however, individual responses vary and should be formally assessed with a test dose prior to therapeutic administration. Clinically meaningful responses are generally not seen in children with a baseline FVIII level of <0.05–0.10 IU/mL (5–10%) [32]. It has been suggested that age is a predictor of response to DDAVP, as children tend to respond less well to DDAVP and if retested at an older age, responses may improve [32]. DDAVP does not affect the FIX level.

Topical Hemostatic Agents

Topical hemostatic agents (e.g., fibrin glues) are biological products that can be applied directly to a bleeding site to achieve or maintain hemostasis (see Appendix III). In some centers, such agents are used routinely for hemostatic support of dental procedures, circumcision, or orthopedic surgery, to reduce the requirement for CFC.

Management of Bleeding Episodes

Initial Assessment

Despite the considerable advances in hemophilia care, bleeds still occur in persons with hemophilia – both in those on prophylaxis and even more so those not on prophylaxis including in most persons with mild/moderate hemophilia. Appropriate management depends not only upon the hemophilia subtype and site of bleeding, but also the severity of the bleed, identifiable precipitants (e.g., trauma), age, adequacy of venous access, presence or absence of inhibitors, previous history of bleeding at the same site (e.g., target joint), and the timing of onset in relation to prophylactic therapy. Minor bleeds may respond to local hemostatic measures, with or without antifibrinolytic agents, and may not require CFC. Similarly, DDAVP-responsive children with mild hemophilia A can often be managed without factor replacement. Children/families who are able to infuse CFCs at home should be advised to not wait to treat but to treat as expeditiously as possible (the "factor first" principle). When possible, this should occur in the home setting. Other important initial considerations include the applicability of basic first aid measures (e.g., ice, direct pressure, splinting etc.), and appropriate analgesia. There are specific types of bleeds for which more may be required (see Specific Sites of Bleeding below).

Dosing

Although it is practical to construct dosing regimens based on the site of bleeding, it must be highlighted that the assessment of bleed severity is subjective. In children without inhibitors, the required dose of factor replacement therapy can be estimated from the suggested target factor levels for any given bleed (Table 4). While such a guideline can be very useful as a quick reference, therapy must always be tailored to individual circumstances and local resources and requires a degree of clinical judgment. On average, for all FVIII concentrates 1 IU/kg of infused FVIII increases the plasma FVIII:C level by 0.02 IU/mL (2%). FIX has a larger volume of distribution (due to diffusion of FIX into extravascular tissues) as compared with FVIII. For plasma-derived FIX. the infusion of 1 U/kg increases the FIX:C level by 0.01 IU/mL (1%); recovery is slightly less with BeneFIX (0.7% rise per U/kg administered) and more with some of the EHL rFIXs – N9-GP (Rebinyn, Refixia) and FIX-FP (Idelvion) [33].

Most minor bleeds can be effectively managed with one or two doses of CFCs, and monitoring of factor levels is usually not necessary. More significant bleeds (including joint bleeds) should be treated more aggressively with a more prolonged course of CFC. Following the initial infusion of factor, repeated doses are given at a frequency dependent on the PK of the factor and on the clinical situation. Hence while SHL FVIII may need to be given every 8–12 h in the initial treatment of severe bleeds, the same bleeds may be treated with SHL FIX every 12–24 h. When treating bleeds with EHL CFCs, less frequent infusions are required. It should be highlighted that, in general, the half-life of infused FVIII/FIX products is shorter in young children as compared to adolescents and adults and is especially short in the immediate postsurgical period [34]. Where stable factor levels are required for several days, a continuous infusion may be more practical and cost-effective [35]. An inhibitor should be considered if the response to therapy is suboptimal. Postdose factor levels and aPTT testing should be done to determine if the laboratory response to therapy is appropriate.

DDAVP should always be considered as an alternative to CFC in children with mild hemophilia A who are known to respond to this agent [28], and especially in those carrying pathogenic variants known to have a higher risk for development of inhibitors. For details on dosing of DDAVP, see Appendix III. An intranasal preparation of DDAVP has been available which facilitates home treatment. Currently, there is difficulty in procuring this product. Doses can be repeated every 24 h, but the hemostatic response diminishes with repeated use because of depletion of endothelial FVIII/VWF [36]. Consequently, most centers will limit dosing with DDAVP to 2 or 3 consecutive days.

Specific Sites of Bleeding

Acute Hemarthrosis

All synovial joints are potentially at risk for bleeding in hemophilia; however, the most frequently

Table 4. Management of bleeding episodes

Site of bleed	Peak level desired, IU/mL	Treatment duration, days	Supportive care
Oral mucosa	>0.30	1	Antifibrinolytic agent (oral or mouth wash) Consider further topical measures (e.g., fibrin sealant)
Epistaxis	>0.30	1	Antifibrinolytic agent Local measures Consider ENT consultation
Joint	0.40–0.60	1–2[a]	Early physiotherapy is important. Splinting may be useful
Superficial/mild muscle	0.40–0.60	2–3[a]	Early physiotherapy is important to avoid contracture, loss of function, rebleeding
Iliopsoas of deep/ severe muscle	Initial: 0.80–1.00 Maintenance: 0.30–0.60	1–2 3–5	 Early physiotherapy important to avoid contracture, loss of function, rebleeding
Genitourinary (hematuria)	0.40–0.50	3–5	Avoid antifibrinolytic therapy, factor therapy may not be required in mild cases. Maintain good urine output.
Gastrointestinal	Initial: 0.80–1.00 Maintenance: 0.50	1–3 4–14	Antifibrinolytic agent Antifibrinolytic agent, monitor hemoglobin, consider gastroenterology consultation
Central nervous system/ intracranial bleeding	Initial: 0.80–1.00 Maintenance: 0.30–0.50	1–7 8–14	
Surgery (minor)	Preop: 0.50–0.80 Postop: 0.30–0.50	 1–5	Antifibrinolytic agent Antifibrinolytic agent
Surgery (major)	Preop: 0.80–1.00 Postop: 0.60–0.80 Postop: 0.40–0.60 Postop: 0.30–0.50	 1–3 4–6 7–14	Antifibrinolytic agent Antifibrinolytic agent Antifibrinolytic agent Antifibrinolytic agent

Note that there is no difference in desired factor levels needed between hemophilia A and B. Of course, doses and frequency of dosing will differ between hemophilia A and hemophilia B and between different factor concentrates (standard and extended half-life). For patients on emicizumab or other nonfactor therapies, guidelines need to be adapted according to more recent studies and recommendations. Adapted from Chapter 7 of the 2020 WFH guidelines [28]. Used with permissions of John Wiley & Sons-Books (Srivastava et al. [28]), permission conveyed through Copyright Clearance Center, Inc. [a]May be longer if response is inadequate. ENT, ear, nose and throat.

affected are the six large hinge joints (ankles, knees, elbows), and, to a lesser extent, the four ball-and-socket joints (hips, shoulders). Bleeding causes synovial inflammation and hypertrophy, the precursor to hemophilic arthropathy increasing susceptibility to mechanical damage; thus, early recognition and treatment of bleeds are paramount. Older children may describe an unpleasant tingling sensation or stiffness prior to the onset of overt pain, swelling, or redness; however, in young children and infants' reluctance to weight bear, pain on passive movement, or swelling that is warm to touch may be the only clues that there is a bleed. The affected limb may be held in an antalgic (partially flexed) position, and there can be some associated muscle spasms. It may not always be possible to differentiate clinically between a bleed within a joint (hemarthrosis) and bleeding into the surrounding soft tissue; however, assessment of range of movement can be useful in this regard. Although evaluation of bleeds has relied mainly on clinical examination, more recently, point of care ultrasound (POCUS) has been used to objectively discern if a joint bleed has occurred. POCUS may also be used following a bleed on a regular basis to track the response to therapy [37]. Septic arthritis can also occur, albeit uncommonly, in children with hemophilia, and should be considered when there is associated fever, constitutional symptoms, severe pain, poor response to hemostatic therapy, or when laboratory testing shows neutrophilia and/or elevated inflammatory markers.

Hemostatic treatment should be commenced at the first suspicion of bleeding (Table 4). Although factor replacement is the most effective way to relieve pain following hemarthrosis, analgesic medication should also be used when necessary. Therapy should be continued until full resolution of symptoms (typically 1–3 days); many clinicians will advocate for even longer therapy due to the higher risk of rebleeding into the affected area. Persistence of symptoms beyond 3 days is unusual and should prompt careful reevaluation, including exclusion of a new inhibitor.

Routine diagnostic imaging during the assessment of an uncomplicated acute hemarthrosis is generally not needed; however, there are specific circumstances in which directed radiological investigation can be useful. Table 5 summarizes the indications, advantages, and disadvantages of the diagnostic imaging modalities [38]. Plain radiographs (X-rays) may be indicated to exclude an associated fracture if there is a history of significant trauma. Ultrasound may be useful for investigation of hip pain as hip joint bleeding may not be readily distinguished from other bleeds in this region (e.g., iliopsoas bleeding); it is also useful for assessment of bleeding into the shoulder joint. Magnetic resonance imaging (MRI) can detect subtle changes such as ligamentous injury or early joint degeneration and may be useful when the response to standard therapy appears suboptimal. It should be emphasized that these imaging studies should only be done after factor replacement has been administered.

Involvement of a physiotherapist to supervise rehabilitation following acute hemarthrosis is recommended by current consensus guidelines [28]. Initially, the affected joint should be rested entirely. This is part of the RICE (Rest, Ice, Compression, and Elevation) approach. Use of bracing (such as a splint) can be useful and may be the only way to effectively immobilize and protect the joint in a young child; nonweight-bearing movement is recommended for several days. It has been recognized that prolonged rest can lead to muscle imbalance directly affecting strength and so an expanded concept known as the POLICE approach (Protection, Optimum Loading, Ice, Compression and Elevation) has been consolidated [39]. Isotonic exercises should be commenced once pain and swelling have subsided. Isometric exercises can be performed even within bracing. Resistance exercises and weight-bearing should be reintroduced gradually, with a rehabilitation program tailored to the individual [40].

Muscle Bleeding, Including Iliopsoas Bleeding

Muscle bleeds are common in hemophilia and usually involve the large muscles of the thighs, calves, and forearms. They are usually trauma-related (from direct impact or strain injury); however, the precipitating event may not always be recognized by the child/family. Pain on contraction of the affected muscle is the key finding; however, swelling, bruising, and focal tenderness are also common. Neurovascular compromise

Table 5. Comprehensive musculoskeletal approach

Tool	Purpose	Advantages	Disadvantages
Structure and functional score – Hemophilia Joint Health score	First line tool to evaluate structure, every 1–2 years if negative findings, every 3–6 months otherwise	Systematization of musculoskeletal assessment and routine clinical follow-up may optimize the diagnostic workflow	Insensitive to very early structural damages
Plain radiography (X-rays)	Detect fractures when trauma is part of clinical history or monitor advanced arthropathy	Widespread availability	Poor sensitivity to detect and monitor for early arthropathic changes
Ultrasound and POCUS (point of care ultrasound)	Acute bleed: assess for the presence of intraarticular fluid/muscle hematoma and monitor its evolution and location. Assess musculoskeletal structures (synovium, subclinical synovitis, tendons, cartilage/osteochondral interface, muscles) Evaluation of markers of disease activity and degenerative changes	Low cost, easy access, no need for sedation, noninvasive, no radiation. Power Doppler to measure synovial vascularity. Real-time technique with shorter exam time. Follow-up exam may influence treatment decisions	Operator dependent. Unable to penetrate deep tissues and visualize central aspect of the cartilage
Computed tomography (CT)	Useful to confirm iliopsoas hemorrhage and monitor patient recovery. Provide more detailed evaluation of a pseudotumor	More readily available than MRI; able to identify joint structures in more detail	Exposure to radiation. Need for anesthesia in young children. Expensive
Magnetic resonance imaging (MRI)	Allows visualization of early arthropathic changes (hemarthrosis, effusions, synovial hypertrophy, hemosiderin deposits, small focal cartilage defects). Provides detailed information about more advanced changes (erosions, subchondral cysts, cartilage destruction)	Gold standard for identifying early changes in joint structure	Need for sedation in young children. Difficult to investigate multiple joints. Need for anesthesia. Expensive. Limited availability and high-cost. Imperfect reference standard for assessment of synovial hypertrophy with severe hemosiderin deposition

Adapted and modified from Seuser et al. [72] and Lobet et al. [38].

distal to the bleeding site must be specifically excluded, particularly in the setting of anterior forearm or calf bleeds (see Compression of Vital Structures below). Management of muscle bleeding requires appropriate CFC therapy (Table 4), rest, elevation, graduated physiotherapy, and education to reduce the risk of recurrence [28]. Compression, ice, and splinting may be useful in some circumstances. Delayed recognition or treatment of muscle bleeding can lead to long-term sequelae such as contracture, loss of function, and neurovascular compromise.

Recognition of iliopsoas bleeding is particularly important due to the frequency of serious complications associated with bleeding at this site. The iliopsoas muscle group is a deep structure, and bleeding may produce diffuse pain (involving the hip, groin, thigh, lower abdomen, flank, or lower back), which is difficult to localize. Consequently, iliopsoas muscle bleeds are difficult to differentiate from hip bleeds and other bleeds or even nonbleeds (e.g., appendicitis). Iliopsoas bleeding should be suspected when a child presents with a partially flexed hip joint, and pain on passive extension. Altered sensation in the distribution of the femoral nerve may also be observed.

Ultrasound imaging can be quite useful for the assessment of muscle bleeds (i.e., location, volume/size, progression), and is recommended for confirmation of iliopsoas bleeding. Treatment with replacement CFC is required until there is full resolution of symptoms and physical findings. Resumption of physical activities should be gradual and under guidance of experienced clinician to prevent rebleeding at the same site of muscle fiber remodeling.

Mucosal Bleeding

Prolonged oral mucosal bleeding is common in toddlers with moderate/severe hemophilia and may be the first symptom of hemophilia. The lip frenulum is a particularly susceptible site for traumatic bleeding. Oral bleeding is often manifested by a "stop-start" pattern in children with hemophilia; this can continue for days if not appropriately managed. Initial oral bleeding should be managed with antifibrinolytic therapy and cold packs – ice packs and cool teething rings can be helpful – and the child should be encouraged to eat soft, cold foods for 2–3 days to minimize the risk of recurrence. In older children, antifibrinolytic agents can also be used as a mouthwash which is then swallowed. If the bleeding continues or recurs over the next day, additional treatment to raise the factor level for 2–3 days is recommended. DDAVP is usually sufficient to manage oral mucosal bleeding in responsive children with mild hemophilia A.

Epistaxis is not frequent in hemophilia but can occur. Minor epistaxis can usually be managed with local pressure for at least 10 min applied to the anterior nares, compressing Kiesselbach's plexus, a web of local arteries within the anteroinferior part of the nasal septum responsible for most nose bleeds. Factor therapy is rarely required except for severe bleeding. Topical agents such as Vaseline or polysporin are useful to keep the nasal mucosa moist and prevent recurrence. Short-term use of topical steroids or topical estrogen preparations may also be useful; recurrent bleeding may respond to cauterization of mucosal blood vessels.

Heavy menstrual bleeding can occur in female carriers of hemophilia particularly in those with low factor levels. For further details, see Chapter 5 on management of bleeds in young women with bleeding disorders.

Compression of Vital Structures

Failure to recognize bleeding at sites adjacent to vital structures can result in rapid demise (e.g., the brain, airway, heart, or lungs), or severe and permanent loss of function (e.g., the spinal cord, eye, kidney, or peripheral neurovascular bundles). These are all medical emergencies, and rapid administration of CFCs is crucial. Factor administration should always be given before diagnostic imaging and consultation with the relevant surgical team.

Upper airway obstruction may result from bleeding into the tongue, retropharyngeal space, or soft tissues of the neck, and typically presents with stridor and progressive respiratory distress. Pain may be poorly localized, and in younger children, this clinical picture may be confused with croup. A history of neck injury or oropharyngeal trauma (including vigorous coughing or iatrogenic injury) should be sought, and hemostatic therapy should be administered prior to imaging studies.

Compartment Syndrome

Persons with hemophilia are at particular risk of compartment syndrome due to bleeding into the soft tissues of the wrist, anterior forearm, or calf. Severe pain, tense swelling, paresthesia, and cool digits with slow capillary refill are key findings. Paresis and loss of an arterial pulse are late findings, and the absence of these features does not exclude the diagnosis. The need for decompression fasciotomy may be averted if the condition is recognized early and quickly treated with CFCs in addition to elevation of the affected limb.

Intracranial Bleeding

The reported incidence of intracranial hemorrhage (ICH) in hemophilia is highest during the neonatal period (2.1%, see Management of the Newborn below), but remains a significant cause of mortality and long-term neurological morbidity in older children [41]. Suspected ICH is a medical emergency, and in all cases CFC should be provided immediately, without waiting for results of imaging (Table 4). Risk factors for ICH beyond the neonatal period include severe hemophilia, presence of inhibitors, absence of prophylaxis, previously confirmed ICH, head trauma, and an altered level of consciousness [42]. Younger age is also a risk factor for ICH; however, this is not a useful discriminator when trying to decide regarding the need for diagnostic imaging. Other concerning symptoms at presentation include headache, vomiting, seizures, and focal neurologic signs.

Computerized tomography (CT) scanning performed after CFC has been given, remains the imaging modality of choice for initial assessment; however, it must be highlighted that a negative scan does not completely exclude an ICH, and children/parents/caregivers should be advised to return for medical assessment if there are new or persistent neurologic symptoms. There is a paucity of evidence regarding the role of imaging in asymptomatic children presenting after minor head injury; however, it may be reasonable to defer CT in such cases, considering their clinical status and the timing of head injury in relation to their last prophylaxis dose [43].

Children with confirmed ICH require intensive correction of hemostasis in addition to standard life-support measures. Neurosurgical consultation should be sought immediately, and transfer to the nearest hemophilia treatment center (HTC) should be undertaken as soon as practical. Steady-state factor levels of around 0.80–1.20 IU/mL (80–120%) should be maintained for 10–14 days; continuous infusion may allow for efficient dose titration in this context. Following discharge from hospital, long-term prophylaxis to prevent ICH recurrence is recommended in all children. At a minimum for those children with mild or moderate hemophilia, prophylaxis should be maintained for at least 3–4 months which is the period with the highest risk of rebleeding.

Gastrointestinal Bleeding

The causes of gastrointestinal bleeding (i.e., hematemesis, hematochezia, or melena) in children with or without hemophilia are similar. The approach to management and diagnostic workup depends on the site, volume, and duration of bleeding; however, in all cases, appropriate CFC should be administered early (Table 4). Careful attention to pulse, blood pressure, and hemoglobin level is important as the degree of blood loss may initially be underestimated.

Macroscopic Hematuria

Hematuria in children with hemophilia is not an uncommon presentation. It is usually benign in nature. Precipitating causes may include urinary tract infection or kidney stones. Investigations should include a urine culture and blood urea and creatinine. Renal ultrasound may be useful if there are any concerns about urinary obstruction. Painless hematuria in children with hemophilia should be initially managed with vigorous hydration, with the primary aim to maintain adequate urine output. Admission and bed rest along with fluids may be required in selected cases. If there is pain, or persistent gross hematuria, treatment with CFC should be considered (Table 4). Antifibrinolytic therapy is contraindicated due to the potential for intrarenal or ureteric clots leading to urinary obstruction [28].

Management of Surgery and Other Invasive Procedures

Any surgery (or invasive procedure) in a child with hemophilia should only be undertaken following consultation with the child's HTC. There must be close liaison between the hematologist, surgeon, and anesthetist. Formulation of an appropriate management plan for surgery requires estimation of the anticipated bleeding risk; this is subjective and must consider both surgical and patient-specific risk factors. Important surgical considerations include the experience of the operator, the anatomical site (in particular its accessibility and location with respect to vital structures), and whether significant bleeding occurs in children without hemophilia undergoing the same procedure. Age of the child, relevant comorbidities, and inhibitor status are important patient-specific factors. Surgery in children with inhibitors should always be considered high risk.

The perioperative management plan should be clearly documented in the medical record, and should include the date and time of surgery, any required baseline laboratory tests, the timing of the preoperative loading dose, the dosing schedule during and after the procedure, the requirements for monitoring (e.g., factor levels), the requirement for adjuvant therapy, and the arrangements for follow-up on discharge. There should be adequate laboratory support for the monitoring of factor levels in the postoperative period. An inhibitor screen should be performed prior to any elective surgery. DDAVP may be adequate for responsive children with mild hemophilia A undergoing low-risk procedures and this needs to be considered to reduce the risk of inhibitor formation in this group (see Appendix III for dosing).

Factor replacement therapy for surgery can be given by intermittent boluses or by continuous infusion. In general, all children will get a preoperative dose of factor (or DDAVP). The aim will be to achieve protective levels of the deficient factor (Table 4). Further postoperative doses and the frequency and duration of these depend on the surgical procedure and on the PK of the factor being used and nowadays will also depend on whether the child is on nonfactor therapy. Younger children have a shorter half-life of FVIII/IX and need more frequent dosing [34].

Continuous infusion can provide a more constant factor level, thereby avoiding the supratherapeutic peaks and the subtherapeutic troughs that may accompany frequent bolus doses of CFCs [35]. Typically, a continuous infusion of factor is commenced at a dose of 3–5 IU/kg/h (for SHL FVIII) of factor immediately after a bolus dose of factor calculated to reach the target level. Lower doses for continuous infusion would be used for SHL FIX and for EHL rFVIII or rFIX. If using continuous infusion, factor levels should be monitored daily and the infusion rate adjusted accordingly. If the monitored factor levels are significantly below the desired factor level, a bolus dose of factor will be required, in addition to increasing the infusion rate, to achieve satisfactory factor levels in a timely manner. Reconstituted CFCs are reasonably stable for 24 h; still for reasons of sterility, the syringe and tubing needs changing every 8–24 h.

Continuous infusion should be only used under supervision of experienced physicians. Any treatment center using continuous infusion for management of children with hemophilia should develop and quality assure their own specific protocols.

Supportive Care

Comprehensive Care

Although treatment and particularly prevention of bleeding through prophylaxis forms the basis of modern hemophilia care, management of the disorder is complex and is best achieved through the input of a multidisciplinary team. HTCs typically have consisted of a physician experienced in the assessment and treatment of children with hematologic disorders, a nurse, a physiotherapist, a social worker, and/or psychologist. In addition, such centers often require input from other specialist teams, such as rheumatology, orthopedics, surgery, and dentistry, as well as access to specialized coagulation laboratories and radiology/imaging services. Genetic testing and consultation with a medical genetics service is important for carrier testing and counselling of at-risk individuals, and for prenatal diagnosis (see Chapter 21). With newer therapies that allow for more effective prophylaxis (e.g., EHL concentrates, emicizumab, and potentially other nonfactor therapies), the composition of HTCs is likely to change with a lower need for rheumatology and orthopedics but a greater need for access to specialized coagulation laboratory testing.

Home Care

The aim of hemophilia care is to support the child/families to be able to manage their hemophilia, to reduce the number of hospital admissions and to minimize absence from school or work. The goal for all children and their families is ultimately for this care to be delivered in the home, enabling optimal early treatment of bleeds and superior convenience and health-related quality of life. The team at the HTC is responsible for educating the child and their family about hemophilia and training them in the administration of CFCs/nonfactor therapies, so that the goal of home therapy can be realized. Appropriate education of the family empowers families to be proactive and alert to detect signs of bleeds in their children. Children and adolescents should be involved in a continuing educational process to be able to assume full responsibility for self-care as they transition into adulthood. This has also traditionally involved teaching the child to be able to infuse themselves thus giving them some independence and a greater sense of being able to self-manage their hemophilia.

It is essential that the core team continues to maintain a close clinical relationship with children on home therapy to ensure that all bleeds are managed optimally.

Vaccinations

Although obvious, it still should be stated that children with hemophilia still need regular pediatric care, and this includes vaccinations. All children with hemophilia should be vaccinated according to the recommended schedule in their country. Whenever possible, the subcutaneous route of vaccination is preferable, but using a small (25 or 27 gauge) needle and application of local pressure for at least 10 min allows for the intramuscular route as well. In the past, vaccination against blood borne infections (hepatitis B) was more critical given the use of plasma-derived factor concentrates, whereas now this is less of a concern.

Routine Clinic Visits

The routine clinic visit provides an opportunity to review the status of the child with hemophilia, facilitates ongoing education of the family, and identifies any need for intervention, should it be required. Typically, a clinic visit involves reviewing the child's bleeding frequency and treatment schedule using the child's (electronic often using smart phone apps or paper diary) records [28]. For children on prophylaxis, causes of breakthrough bleeds, their timing in relation to the prophylactic schedule, and response to treatment should be ascertained. This review may reveal inadequate prophylaxis dosing or frequency, poor compliance, or suggest the development of an inhibitor. Practicalities of venous access are reviewed and managed as required. The clinician typically takes the opportunity to encourage physical activity, provide advice, as well as reminders about protective equipment and compliance with treatment that reduce the transient risks of bleeding associated with physical activity. Reminders of the importance of good oral hygiene and the wearing of a medic-alert bracelet/necklace are usually provided. Immunization status should be checked and where relevant, advice provided about timing. A thorough clinical examination is performed, and joint health documented ideally using a tool such as the Hemophilia Joint Health Score [44]. Regular musculoskeletal assessments can help to identify functional musculoskeletal issues that may be optimized with physical therapy exercises. Furthermore, such musculoskeletal assessments may identify musculoskeletal issues despite a lack of reported bleeds which may lead to changes in prophylaxis or recommendations regarding the child's activities. Routine blood tests such as inhibitor screening are performed at regular intervals [28].

Venous Access

Prior to the availability of EHL concentrates and more recently emicizumab, children with moderate or severe hemophilia were likely to require frequent intravenous infusions of CFCs for the treatment or prevention of bleeding. In all children, but especially in very young children, this was difficult and often required the insertion of CVADs (in most cases port-a-caths); CVADs are prone to several acute and chronic complications such as infections and line-associated thrombosis. Line-associated clots in children with hemophilia are often asymptomatic and usually are not treated with anticoagulation [45]. These complications are a reason why, in young children, the placement of a CVAD should always be viewed as a temporary measure, with a plan for early removal once the child/family are able to administer treatment either through peripheral venous access or subcutaneously (if switched to a subcutaneously administered product).

Pain Management

Bleeding in children with hemophilia often causes pain, especially when blood is accumulating in a confined space such as a joint cavity. While the primary treatment of the bleed with CFC or DDAVP is of the utmost importance (see above), there may be a need for analgesics to control pain in the short-term. Measures such as ice packs, immobilization, and simple analgesia with acetaminophen help in reducing pain. When simple analgesia is not sufficient, the addition of oral opiates may be considered for short periods. Acetylsalicylic acid (Aspirin) and other medications that inhibit platelet function (e.g., nonsteroidal anti-inflammatory drugs (NSAIDs)) are best avoided. However, in persons with chronic hemophilic arthropathy, short-term use of NSAIDs, in particular the selective COX-2 inhibitors (e.g., celecoxib, meloxicam, etoricoxib), may be indicated [28].

Dental Care

Prevention of dental problems is an essential component of care for persons with hemophilia. Good dental hygiene avoids periodontal disease and associated procedures which may be associated with risk of bleeding. Children with hemophilia should be reviewed by a dentist at least annually. Should dental procedures be required, close liaison between the HTC and the dentist is necessary to ensure appropriate management of bleeding risk. Local hemostatic measures, including topical antifibrinolytic agents or sealants, can reduce the requirement for CFC therapy. For minor procedures, antifibrinolytic therapy alone may suffice. Antifibrinolytic agents when used should be continued for 5–7 days to assist in maintenance of the thrombus (see Appendix III for doses). For more extensive dental procedures including nerve blocks raising the factor level to

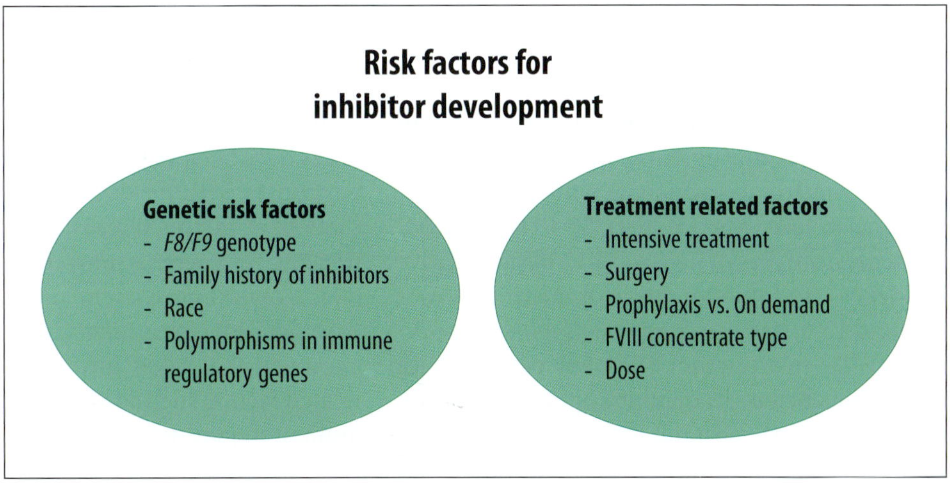

Fig. 3. Risk factors for inhibitor development. FVIII, factor VIII.

at least 0.50 IU/mL (50%) is advised to prevent bleeding. For many persons with mild hemophilia A, this may be achieved with DDAVP. For persons with hemophilia B, moderate-severe hemophilia A, or those with a suboptimal DDAVP response, CFC therapy will be required. Depending on the extent of the dental procedure(s), ongoing factor therapy may be required for several days to allow proper wound healing and prevent rebleeding. Given the constant level of protection provided by emicizumab, many children on this agent may not need any additional therapy when undergoing minor dental procedures.

Complications of Hemophilia

Inhibitors

Children with hemophilia are at risk of developing neutralizing alloantibodies ("inhibitors") against FVIII or FIX following exposure to CFCs. Inhibitors present a significant management challenge for persons with hemophilia, as their presence reduces or abolishes the therapeutic response to factor replacement. The strength of the inhibitory effect is measured in the laboratory using the Bethesda assay, in which one Bethesda unit (BU) corresponds to the amount of patient plasma inhibitor required to neutralize 50% of the FVIII/FIX activity in 1:1 mix of normal pooled plasma and patient plasma following a 2-h incubation at 37 °C [46]. The currently accepted cut-off value for confirmation of an inhibitor is ≥0.6 BU using the Nijmegen modification of the Bethesda assay documented on two separate occasions within a 4-week period, with clinically significant inhibitors being associated with <66% expected recovery of the factor as measured 10–15 min after the dose [29]. It is well recognized that some children whose inhibitor level falls below 0.6 BU can still exhibit suboptimal FVIII/FIX recovery, half-life, and/or clinical response, consistent with persistent inhibitory activity [47].

A "low-responder" inhibitor is defined as a level persistently ≤5 BU, while >5 BU at any time is considered a "high responder" and corresponds to the inhibitor level at which treatment with even very high doses of CFC becomes futile. In some children, the high responder status only becomes apparent following re-exposure to products containing FVIII/FIX, resulting in a sudden increase in inhibitor due to anamnesis [29].

Risk Factors for Inhibitor Development

In severe hemophilia A, the cumulative incidence of inhibitor development is around 25–40% [48]. For these children, the risk of inhibitor development is highest during the first 50 exposure days (EDs) to factor replacement, with the risk decreasing to less than 1% after 50 EDs. In mild/moderate subtypes of hemophilia, the cumulative incidence of inhibitor development is lower (around 13%), but the risk persists with the number of EDs to treatment [49]. For persons with hemophilia B, the risk of inhibitor development is around 10% with most inhibitors occurring within the first 10 EDs to FIX replacement [50].

Many factors influence the risk of inhibitor formation, and these include nonmodifiable genetic factors and potentially modifiable environmental factors (shown in Fig. 3). The strongest known risk factor for the development of inhibitors is the underlying pathogenic variant. Null variants, i.e., those inducing a complete deficit of any production of circulating FVIII/FIX polypeptide (such as large deletions) having the highest risk and nonnull variants (such as missense variants) having the lowest risk [51]. In nonsevere hemophilia A, certain missense variants are associated with an increased inhibitor risk (e.g., Arg593 > Cys) [49]. Other nonmodifiable constitutional factors that influence the risk include family history of inhibitors, ethnicity, and potentially polymorphisms in certain immune response genes and HLA class II alleles [52, 53]. The predictive value of any one specific factor outside of specific gene variants and a positive family history for development of an inhibitor is weak.

Environmental modifiers that have been suggested to influence inhibitor risk include both treatment related (e.g., the type of product, dosing regimen) and immune system activating risk factors (so-called "danger" signals, a term reflecting the release of inflammatory substances from damaged tissue). The significance of these modifiers is still yet to be fully determined with conflicting evidence published for modifiers such as the role of specific types and classes (recombinant vs. plasma-derived) of factor concentrates [54, 55]. The incidence of inhibitors with EHL CFCs is still being evaluated, but so far, no major differences have been seen with these products in comparison to SHL products [56]. While it is likely that not all factor concentrates have equal immunogenicity, there is currently insufficient evidence regarding current products on which to base definitive treatment decisions. A treatment approach that takes into consideration patient-related factors such as a history of inhibitor development in family members and the wishes of the child/family following discussion of the risks and benefits of available CFCs is recommended.

Regarding treatment-related factors, dosing regimens, in particular "peak" treatment moments, defined as episodes of infusions with CFCs to provide hemostatic cover for surgery or severe bleeds (e.g., ICH) for at least 3 consecutive days, have been shown to be related to increased inhibitor formation [48]. The clinician, can, where possible, try to minimize the child's exposure to these potential risk factors by measures such as postponement of elective surgery and avoidance of excessive treatment for relatively minor bleeds in very young children who have as yet not received 50 EDs to FVIII.

Children with hemophilia B who develop inhibitors are at risk of severe complications including anaphylactic reactions after exposure to FIX. An anaphylactic reaction may the first sign of inhibitor development [57]. During immune tolerance therapy (ITI), nephrotic syndrome may occur [58]. It is recommended that children who develop anaphylaxis to FIX are treated with rFVIIa and not aPCC, which contains FIX which may elicit anaphylaxis.

If a child with hemophilia develops an inhibitor, three main issues need to be considered:

1. how to treat bleeds
2. how to prevent bleeds
3. if/how/when to attempt to eradicate the inhibitor.

Management of Bleeds in Children with Inhibitors

Minor bleeding in children with inhibitors may still be effectively controlled with local hemostatic measures and antifibrinolytic therapy. When such measures fail, or are deemed inadequate for the type of bleeding, the treatment options include high-dose CFC therapy or alternative agents, so called bypassing agents, which achieve hemostasis by "bypassing" the normal requirement for the FVIII:FIX complex. There are two types of bypassing agents in common usage to date: plasma-derived aPCCs and rFVIIa.

The treatment of bleeds in a child with inhibitors depends on the inhibitor level, the severity of bleeding, the child's previous therapeutic response and whether the child is treated prophylactically with bypassing agents, emicizumab or in the future other nonfactor therapies. High-dose factor replacement is generally only feasible when the inhibitor level is ≤3 BU. Optimization of therapy using this approach requires some knowledge of an individual's FVIII/FIX recovery and half-life, such that dose and frequency can be adjusted accordingly.

Bypassing therapy is required when high-dose CFC is considered insufficient or is contraindicated due to a previous allergic reaction. In most settings, either bypassing agent can be used, but if contemplating commencing ITI, then rFVIIa is favored over aPCC, because aPCC contains small amounts of FVIII which may contribute to an anamnestic response. The hemostatic response to rFVIIa and aPCC varies between individuals, and individual responses to either agent can vary over time [59]. There is no standardized laboratory test to quantify the activity of a bypassing agent in vivo. Therefore, apart from indirect measurements of overall hemostatic potential (such as thromboelastography or a thrombin generation assay), assessment of response to a bypassing agent must be based on clinical symptoms (especially reduction in pain) and clinical examination (e.g., swelling, range of motion). Often, families will have a supply of one or both bypassing agents at home, allowing early treatment at the first sign of bleeding (ideally within first 2 h of first symptom). If a child is on regular prophylaxis with either agent, breakthrough bleeds can be managed initially with additional doses of the same agent. Failure to respond to one bypassing agent should prompt consideration of a switch to the other agent. In some instances, bleeding may be refractory to either agent, and use of both agents in sequential fashion is appropriate in this context [59, 60]; however, close monitoring for thrombosis or consumptive coagulopathy (platelet count, fibrinogen, D-dimer, etc.) is required [59]. Combination treatment should be reserved only for HTCs with extensive experience in managing children with inhibitors.

Previous studies have shown that effective hemostasis is achieved in >90% of mild–moderate bleeding episodes after 2–3 doses of 90 µg/kg rFVIIa administered at 2–3 hourly intervals, and that a single dose of 270 µg/kg is equally effective in this context [61]. To avoid product wastage, the dose is always rounded to the nearest whole vial. Children have faster drug clearance and this needs to be taken into consideration when planning a course of treatment [62]. Comparative studies have shown that the clinical efficacy of a single dose of aPCC at 75–100 IU/kg is equivalent to that of two doses of rFVIIa 90–120 µg/kg for joint bleeding [63]. Due to the risk of thrombosis, the maximum daily dose of aPCC should not exceed 200 IU/kg. Furthermore, antifibrinolytic therapy can be used in combination with rFVIIa, while antifibrinolytic therapy is generally not recommended in combination with aPCC.

Now with the availability of emicizumab in many parts of the world, most children with inhibitors to FVIII at least in more affluent countries are on emicizumab (see below) as a prophylactic agent. The use of aPCC is contraindicated in children on emicizumab due to the high risk of thrombosis and thrombotic microangiopathy. Therefore, rFVIIa is the agent of choice for man-

8

aging bleeds in children on emicizumab; for the most part, the regimens used in children on emicizumab are similar to the rFVIIa regimens used for those not on emicizumab although there is generally a reluctance to use the 270 μg/kg high dose. With emicizumab, the duration of treating bleeds can generally be reduced.

Prevention of Bleeds (Prophylaxis) in Children with Inhibitors

Prophylactic therapy is now considered standard of care for all persons with severe phenotype hemophilia [28]. However, for persons with inhibitors, particularly high-titer inhibitors, prophylaxis with FVIII or FIX concentrates is ineffective.

Emicizumab is the prophylactic agent of choice for children with hemophilia A and inhibitors. Emicizumab prophylaxis is effective against bleeding and is superior to bypassing agents [23, 64]. The superior bleed prevention and its convenience of administration (subcutaneous delivery) have rendered emicizumab prophylaxis the preferred therapy, especially for children with high-titer inhibitors. If emicizumab is unavailable, prophylaxis with bypassing agents (rFVIIa or aPCC) is a potential (although much less effective) alternative.

If, When, and How to Eradicate Inhibitors

Eradication of inhibitors by ITI therapy has several benefits; it enables regular treatment with conventional FVIII or FIX products including regular prophylaxis; this leads to improved quality of life and, despite the very high cost of ITI, to reduced costs of future care [65]. Yet ITI has only been successful in 60%–70% of persons with hemophilia A and high-titer inhibitors and in less than 50% of persons with hemophilia B and high-titer inhibitors. Furthermore, it generally takes 1 year or more to achieve success [66]. In addition to the extreme difficulty of frequent intravenous infusions to young children with hemophilia, ITI in hemophilia B may be associated with other severe complications including nephrotic syndrome and anaphylaxis.

In the past prior to the availability of emicizumab, different ITI regimens were used – these can be broadly classified as high dose/high frequency – usually daily doses of 100–200 IU/kg and low dose/low frequency – usually 3 days per week of 25–50 IU/kg [66]. There has been no consensus on what the best product type is for ITI. Some data suggest better outcomes with plasma-derived VWF-containing FVIII products [67], but there is no definitive evidence regarding this matter [68]. Customarily most centers have started ITI with the same product on which the inhibitor developed but have sometimes switched to a plasma-derived VWF-containing FVIII product if the child failed ITI with a VWF-free product. Now with emicizumab being widely used in children with hemophilia A and inhibitors, much has changed with respect to ITI including whether to not to even attempt ITI given that bleeds can be effectively prevented with emicizumab. Still many clinicians would advocate one attempt at ITI in order to allow future treatment of bleeds and surgery to be done with FVIII concentrates rather than rFVIIa. Even if ITI is still attempted in the era of emicizumab, most clinicians would opt for less-intensive ITI regimens (lower dose/frequency) to reduce treatment burden and cost and to avoid CVADs [69, 70]. Of note, even if clinicians are advocating for ITI, children/families may be unwilling to undertake ITI because of the treatment burden.

Chronic Complications

Synovitis

Following a joint bleed, the synovial lining of the joint becomes inflamed (referred to as acute synovitis), which results in an increased risk of recurrent bleeding. Acute synovitis should be managed with rest and prophylactic factor replacement. With repeated bleeding into the same joint, the synovium becomes chronically inflamed and synovial hypertrophy develops, which is evident clinically by persistent swelling, and can be demonstrated with imaging such as MRI or ultrasound. This condition referred to as chronic synovitis makes the joint more susceptible to recurrent bleeding. The joint becomes a "target joint", a term used when three or more spontaneous bleeds occurs into a single joint within a consecutive 6-month period [28]. To break the cycle of recurrent bleeding, the child needs to be placed on more intense prophylaxis and often also benefits from the use of an NSAID (selective COX-2 inhibitor) along with physiotherapy [28, 71]. Usually, these measures will lead to resolution of the target joint. Very infrequently synovectomy (radioisotopic or arthroscopic, depending on local resources and expertise) may be indicated in persistent cases [71].

Arthropathy
Chronic synovitis leads to localized destruction of cartilage and bone, resulting in loss of joint mobility, pain, and significant functional impairment. The problem is further compounded by wasting and contracture of surrounding muscle groups, producing a fixed flexion deformity, and osteoporosis of long bones due to lack of use. Plain radiographs will not detect arthropathy at an early stage. MRI is the best modality for imaging, but it has its limitations (Table 5). Instead, ultrasound which is more readily available and can detect chronic synovitis as well as peripheral destruction of joint structures may be a more preferred imaging modality [72].

Once arthropathy occurs, the major goals of therapy are to relieve pain and to limit progression of arthropathy. Good adherence to prophylaxis becomes of utmost important to prevent further bleeds that will worsen the joint arthropathy. Specific COX-2 inhibitors and splinting can be useful for analgesia (see Pain Management above). A tailored physiotherapy program to maintain joint mobility and muscle strength prior to the onset of fixed deformity is important. When arthropathy is at an advanced stage, bracing, orthotics and mobility aids can facilitate independent functioning and resumption of normal daily activities. Options for surgical intervention include arthroscopic joint debridement, alignment osteotomy, arthrodesis, or joint replacement. Fortunately, arthropathy is now quite uncommon in children with hemophilia who are commenced on prophylaxis at a young age.

Pseudotumors
Pseudotumors, a rare complication of hemophilia, result from repeated and unresolved soft tissue bleeding, usually into a muscle. The hematoma becomes encapsulated and calcified, and the mass progressively enlarges and may destroy surrounding bone and tissue. The most affected areas are the pelvis and the long bones in the legs and arms. Initial therapy should involve intensive factor replacement; however, other treatments including aspiration, embolization, radiotherapy, or surgery should be considered. These lesions are highly vascular; thus, surgical intervention should only be undertaken at an HTC with appropriate multidisciplinary support [28, 73].

8

Management of the Newborn with Suspected or Possible Hemophilia

Hemophilia may be suspected in a newborn male due to the presence of unusual bleeding symptoms, a known family history of hemophilia, or both. A general overview of bleeding in the neonate is provided in Chapter 3. Newborns with hemophilia are particularly prone to intra- and extracranial bleeding, and this risk is affected by mode of delivery, being highest for instrumental assisted (forceps or vacuum) vaginal delivery and lowest for elective cesarean section or uncomplicated vaginal delivery [74]. In addition to neurologic sequelae (ICH), loss of blood into the scalp or subgaleal space (extracranial bleeding) can be substantial. For this reason, instrumental delivery should be avoided in potentially affected infants (male fetus of a known or possible carrier) [28].

At delivery, such infants suspected of potentially having hemophilia should have blood collected ideally from the umbilical cord or a peripheral vein for urgent factor assays, bearing in mind that results must be interpreted with reference to age-specific ranges (in normal newborns FIX is reduced). For a complete review of age-appropriate coagulation developmental reference ranges, refer to Appendix II. Intramuscular vitamin K (or any other intramuscular injections) should be withheld pending these results (oral vitamin K can be given if there is likely to be significant delay). Factor replacement therapy should be available for use in the event of bleeding; however, due to the lack of efficacy data and the unknown risk of inhibitor development, current guidelines do not support the routine use of prophylactic CFC therapy in neonates without additional risk factors (such as prematurity or traumatic delivery).

Iatrogenic hemorrhage is a genuine risk in newborns with hemophilia, and arterial puncture for blood sampling should be avoided. Prolonged pressure is usually adequate for achieving hemostasis following heel prick for newborn screening or following venipuncture. Antifibrinolytic agents can be used, if needed. Infants with nonspecific symptoms such as respiratory distress or poor perfusion should be investigated for occult bleeding (head, thorax, abdomen), and the threshold for diagnostic imaging should be low [75]. In addition, the newly diagnosed infant must be referred to an HTC so that timely follow-up can be arranged.

If a newborn suspected to have hemophilia appears to have an ICH, they should be rapidly treated with appropriate CFC prior to imaging confirmation of an ICH. When a male fetus is found to have an ICH in a setting where there is no family history of hemophilia, an urgent aPTT should be performed. If the aPTT is prolonged, strong suspicion should be had for the presence of hemophilia (either A or B). If consanguinity exists in the child's parents, then type 3 VWD should also be considered. Although factor assays (FVIII, FIX, and VWF) should be rapidly performed, the child should be treated even prior to factor assay results being available. There are two approaches to this. The standard approach is to give plasma which will contain both FVIII and FIX but in low amounts. Another approach is to recognize that hemophilia A is much more common than hemophilia B and hence a rFVIII concentrate could be administered followed by an immediate repeat aPTT. If the aPTT corrects with administration of FVIII concentrate it indicates that the child has hemophilia A, while if it does not correct it indicates hemophilia B and the child could then get an immediate dose of a FIX concentrate followed by a repeat aPTT.

Future Directions

Gene Therapy

A potentially curative treatment has been developed for adults with severe hemophilia A and B, without inhibitors, specifically liver directed gene therapy using adeno-associated virus (AAV) vectors. Recently, for hemophilia the first two gene therapies were granted market authorization in Europe, and it is expected that several other gene therapy treatments will be approved also.

However, several obstacles remain before the real potential of this treatment can be realized in children. As current gene therapy options target liver cells, it is expected that the gene therapy effect will diminish as the liver grows considerably in children making current gene therapy not suitable for young children.

Conclusions

Modern hemophilia care has undergone considerable transformation in recent decades, largely due to the availability of safe, high-purity factor concentrates both of plasma-derived and recombinant origin for treatment and prevention of bleeding. In countries with unrestricted access to factor concentrates, the prognosis for persons with hemophilia has improved dramatically. Furthermore, newer products, mainly agents with EHL and nonfactor replacement therapy options, offer more convenient prophylaxis. Yet, inhibitor development is still a challenging complication facing hemophilia treaters in such countries, and ongoing research regarding inhibitor prevention and management is warranted. The involvement of an experienced multidisciplinary team cannot be understated. Future research will determine the role of gene therapy for clinical use. In the meanwhile, efforts should be directed to narrowing the gaps in diagnosis and availability of safe, effective treatments for persons with hemophilia living in resource constrained countries as compared to countries that are not resource constrained with respect to care for all persons with hemophilia.

Acknowledgements

Our special thanks go to Jeremy D. Robertson, Julie A. Curtin, and Victor Blanchette who were the authors of the chapter in the first or second editions of this Handbook, which presented a valuable background for this chapter edition.

Conflict of Interest Statement

Samantha C. Gouw received an unrestricted research grant from Sobi. Vanessa Bouskill has received research support from Takeda, NovoNordisk, Roche, Bayer, Pfizer, and Sanofi/Genzyme. Ester Zapotocka has received honoraria from NovoNordisk, Roche, Takeda, and Sobi. Janaina B.S. Ricciardi reports no conflicts of interest. Manuel Carcao has received research support from Bayer, Bioverativ/Sanofi, Novartis, Novo Nordisk, Pfizer, Roche and Shire/Takeda and has received honoraria for speaking/participating in advisory boards from Bayer, Bioverativ/Sanofi, LFB, Novo Nordisk, Pfizer, Roche, and Shire/Takeda.

Author Contributions

All authors substantially contributed to drafting of the chapter, revised it critically, and provided final approval of the published version.

Abbreviations

AAV	Adeno-associated virus
ABR	Annualized bleeding rate
aPCC	Activated prothrombin complex concentrate
aPTT	Activated partial thromboplastin time
BU	Bethesda unit
CT	Computed tomography
CFC	Clotting factor concentrate
COX	Cyclooxygenase
CVAD	Central venous access device
DDAVP	1-Deamino-8-D-arginine vasopressin (desmopressin)
ED	Exposure day
EHL	Extended half-life
FVIII	Factor VIII
FVIIIa	Activated factor VIII
FIX	Factor IX
FIXa	Activated factor IX
HTC	Hemophilia treatment center
ICH	Intracranial hemorrhage
ITI	Immune tolerance induction
IU	International unit
MRI	Magnetic resonance imaging
NSAID	Nonsteroidal anti-inflammatory drug
PK	Pharmacokinetics
PEG	Polyethylene glycol
POCUS	Point of care ultrasound
rFVIIa	Recombinant activated factor VII
rFVIII	Recombinant factor VIII
rFIX	Recombinant factor IX
RNA	Ribonucleic acid
siRNA	Small interfering RNA
SHL	Standard half-life
TFPI	Tissue factor pathway inhibitor
VWF	von Willebrand factor

References

1 Iorio A, Stonebraker JS, Chambost H, Makris M, Coffin D, Herr C, et al. Establishing the prevalence and prevalence at birth of hemophilia in males: a meta-analytic approach using national registries. Ann Intern Med. 2019;171(8):540–6.

2 van Galen KPM, d'Oiron R, James P, Abdul-Kadir R, Kouides PA, Kulkarni R, et al. A new hemophilia carrier nomenclature to define hemophilia in women and girls: communication from the SSC of the ISTH. J Thromb Haemost. 2021; 19(8):1883–7.

3 Labarque V, Perinparajah V, Bouskill V, Stain AM, Wakefield C, Manuel C, et al. Utility of factor VIII and factor VIII to von Willebrand factor ratio in identifying 277 unselected carriers of hemophilia A. Am J Hematol. 2017;92(6):E94–6.

4 Blanchette VS, Srivastava A. Definitions in hemophilia: resolved and unresolved issues. Semin Thromb Hemost. 2015; 41(8):819–25.

5 Hassan S, Monahan RC, Mauser-Bunschoten EP, van Vulpen LFD, Eikenboom J, Beckers EAM, et al. Mortality, life expectancy, and causes of death of persons with hemophilia in the Netherlands 2001–2018. J Thromb Haemost. 2021;19(3):645–53.

6 Young G, Mahlangu J, Kulkarni R, Nolan B, Liesner R, Pasi J, et al. Recombinant factor VIII Fc fusion protein for the prevention and treatment of bleeding in children with severe hemophilia A. J Thromb Haemost. 2015;13(6):967–77.

7 Santagostino E, Kenet G, Fischer K, Biss T, Ahuja S, Steele M. PROTECT VIII Kids: BAY 94-9027 (PEGylated Recombinant Factor VIII) safety and efficacy in previously treated children with severe haemophilia A. Haemophilia. 2020; 26(3):e55–65.

8 Mullins ES, Stasyshyn O, Alvarez-Román MT, Osman D, Liesner R, Engl W, et al. Extended half-life pegylated, full-length recombinant factor VIII for prophylaxis in children with severe haemophilia A. Haemophilia. 2017;23(2): 238–46.

9 Stasyshyn O, Djambas Khayat C, Iosava G, Ong J, Abdul Karim F, Fischer K, et al. Safety, efficacy and pharmacokinetics of rVIII-SingleChain in children with severe hemophilia A: results of a multicenter clinical trial. J Thromb Haemost. 2017;15(4):636–44.

10 von Drygalski A, Chowdary P, Kulkarni R, Susen S, Konkle BA, Oldenburg J, et al. Efanesoctocog alfa prophylaxis for patients with severe hemophilia A. N Engl J Med. 2023;388(4):310–8.

11 Carcao M, Zak M, Abdul Karim F, Hanabusa H, Kearney S, Lu MY, et al. Nonacog beta pegol in previously treated children with hemophilia B: results from an international open-label phase 3 trial. J Thromb Haemost. 2016;14(8): 1521–9.

12 Fischer K, Kulkarni R, Nolan B, Mahlangu J, Rangarajan S, Gambino G, et al. Recombinant factor IX Fc fusion protein in children with haemophilia B (Kids B-LONG): results from a multicentre, non-randomised phase 3 study. Lancet Haematol. 2017;4(2):e75–82.

13 Kenet G, Chambost H, Male C, Lambert T, Halimeh S, Chernova T, et al. Long-acting recombinant fusion protein linking coagulation factor IX with albumin (rFIX-FP) in children. Results of a phase 3 trial. Thromb Haemost. 2016;116(4): 659–68.

14 Gray E, Kitchen S, Bowyer A, Chowdary P, Jenkins PV, Murphy P, et al. Laboratory measurement of factor replacement therapies in the treatment of congenital haemophilia: a United Kingdom Haemophilia Centre Doctors' Organisation guideline. Haemophilia. 2020;26(1):6–16.

15 Müller J, Goldmann G, Marquardt N, Pötzsch B, Oldenburg J. Extended half-life factor VIII/factor IX products: assay discrepancies and implications for hemophilia management. Hamostaseologie. 2020;40(suppl 01):S15–20.

16 Carcao M. Changing paradigm of prophylaxis with longer acting factor concentrates. Haemophilia. 2014;20(suppl 4):99–105.

17 Müller J, Miesbach W, Prüller F, Siegemund T, Scholz U, Sachs UJ. An update on laboratory diagnostics in haemophilia A and B. Hamostaseologie. 2022; 42(4):248–60.

18 Regling K, Callaghan MU, Sidonio R Jr. Managing severe hemophilia A in children: pharmacotherapeutic options. Pediatric Health Med Ther. 2022;13:27–35.

19 Nogami K, Shima M. Current and future therapies for haemophilia-beyond factor replacement therapies. Br J Haematol. 2023;200(1):23–34.

20 Callaghan MU, Negrier C, Paz-Priel I, Chang T, Chebon S, Lehle M, et al. Long-term outcomes with emicizumab prophylaxis for hemophilia A with or without FVIII inhibitors from the HAVEN 1–4 studies. Blood. 2021;137(16): 2231–42.

21 Schmitt C, Adamkewicz JI, Xu J, Petry C, Catalani O, Young G, et al. Pharmacokinetics and pharmacodynamics of emicizumab in persons with hemophilia A with factor VIII inhibitors: HAVEN 1 study. Thromb Haemost. 2021;121(3): 351–60.

22 Lenting PJ, Denis CV, Christophe OD. Emicizumab, a bispecific antibody recognizing coagulation factors IX and X: how does it actually compare to factor VIII? Blood. 2017;130(23):2463–8.

23 Oldenburg J, Mahlangu JN, Kim B, Schmitt C, Callaghan MU, Young G, et al. Emicizumab prophylaxis in hemophilia A with inhibitors. N Engl J Med. 2017;377(9):809–18.

24 Østergaard H, Lund J, Greisen PJ, Kjellev S, Henriksen A, Lorenzen N, et al. A factor VIIIa-mimetic bispecific antibody, Mim8, ameliorates bleeding upon severe vascular challenge in hemophilia A mice. Blood. 2021;138(14):1258–68.

25 Matsushita T, Shapiro A, Abraham A, Angchaisuksiri P, Castaman G, Cepo K, et al. Phase 3 trial of concizumab in hemophilia with inhibitors. N Engl J Med. 2023;389(9):783–94.

26 Mahlangu J, Luis Lamas J, Cristobal Morales J, Malan DR, Teeter J, Charnigo RJ, et al. Long-term safety and efficacy of the anti-tissue factor pathway inhibitor marstacimab in participants with severe haemophilia: phase II study results. Br J Haematol. 2023;200(2):240–8.

27 Srivastava A, Rangarajan S, Kavakli K, Klamroth R, Kenet G, Khoo L, et al. Fitusiran prophylaxis in people with severe haemophilia A or haemophilia B without inhibitors (ATLAS-A/B): a multicentre, open-label, randomised, phase 3 trial. Lancet Haematol. 2023;10(5): e322–32.

28 Srivastava A, Santagostino E, Dougall A, Kitchen S, Sutherland M, Pipe SW, et al. WFH guidelines for the management of hemophilia, 3rd edition. Haemophilia. 2020;26(suppl 6):1–158.

29 Blanchette VS, Key NS, Ljung LR, Manco-Johnson MJ, van den Berg HM, Srivastava A, et al. Definitions in hemophilia: communication from the SSC of the ISTH. J Thromb Haemost. 2014;12(11):1935–9.
30 Mancuso ME, Male C, Kenet G, Kavakli K, Königs C, Blatný J, et al. Prophylaxis in children with haemophilia in an evolving treatment landscape. Haemophilia. 2021;27(6):889–96.
31 Collins PW, Björkman S, Fischer K, Blanchette V, Oh M, Schroth P, et al. Factor VIII requirement to maintain a target plasma level in the prophylactic treatment of severe hemophilia A: influences of variance in pharmacokinetics and treatment regimens. J Thromb Haemost. 2010;8(2):269–75.
32 Seary ME, Feldman D, Carcao MD. DDAVP responsiveness in children with mild or moderate haemophilia A correlates with age, endogenous FVIII:C level and with haemophilic genotype. Haemophilia. 2012;18(1):50–5.
33 Poon MC, Lillicrap D, Hensman C, Card R, Scully MF. Recombinant factor IX recovery and inhibitor safety: a Canadian post-licensure surveillance study. Thromb Haemost. 2002;87(3):431–5.
34 Ljung RC, Knobe K. How to manage invasive procedures in children with haemophilia. Br J Haematol. 2012;157(5):519–28.
35 Batorova A, Holme P, Gringeri A, Richards M, Hermans C, Altisent C, et al. Continuous infusion in haemophilia: current practice in Europe. Haemophilia. 2012;18(5):753–9.
36 Leissinger C, Carcao M, Gill JC, Journeycake J, Singleton T, Valentino L. Desmopressin (DDAVP) in the management of patients with congenital bleeding disorders. Haemophilia. 2014;20(2):158–67.
37 Nguyen S, Lu X, Ma Y, Du J, Chang EY, von Drygalski A. Musculoskeletal ultrasound for intra-articular bleed detection: a highly sensitive imaging modality compared with conventional magnetic resonance imaging. J Thromb Haemost. 2018;16(3):490–9.
38 Lobet S, Hermans C, Lambert C. Optimal management of hemophilic arthropathy and hematomas. J Blood Med. 2014;5:207–18.
39 Stephensen D, Bladen M, McLaughlin P. Recent advances in musculoskeletal physiotherapy for haemophilia. Ther Adv Hematol. 2018;9(8):227–37.
40 Lobet S, Timmer M, Königs C, Stephensen D, McLaughlin P, Duport G, et al. The role of physiotherapy in the new treatment landscape for haemophilia. J Clin Med. 2021;10(13):2822.
41 Zwagemaker AF, Gouw SC, Jansen JS, Vuong C, Coppens M, Hu Q, et al. Incidence and mortality rates of intracranial hemorrhage in hemophilia: a systematic review and meta-analysis. Blood. 2021;138(26):2853–73.
42 Andersson NG, Auerswald G, Barnes C, Carcao M, Dunn AL, Fijnvandraat K, et al. Intracranial haemorrhage in children and adolescents with severe haemophilia A or B – the impact of prophylactic treatment. Br J Haematol. 2017;179(2):298–307.
43 Traivaree C, Blanchette V, Armstrong D, Floros G, Stain AM, Carcao MD. Intracranial bleeding in haemophilia beyond the neonatal period – the role of CT imaging in suspected intracranial bleeding. Haemophilia. 2007;13(5):552–9.
44 Feldman BM, Funk SM, Bergstrom BM, Zourikian N, Hilliard P, van der Net J, et al. Validation of a new pediatric joint scoring system from the International Hemophilia Prophylaxis Study Group: validity of the hemophilia joint health score. Arthritis Care Res (Hoboken). 2011;63(2):223–30.
45 Price VE, Carcao M, Connolly B, Chait P, Daneman A, Temple M, et al. A prospective, longitudinal study of central venous catheter-related deep venous thrombosis in boys with hemophilia. J Thromb Haemost. 2004;2(5):737–42.
46 Verbruggen B, Novakova I, Wessels H, Boezeman J, van den Berg M, Mauser-Bunschoten E. The Nijmegen modification of the Bethesda assay for factor VIII:C inhibitors: improved specificity and reliability. Thromb Haemost. 1995;73(2):247–51.
47 Dardikh M, Albert T, Masereeuw R, Oldenburg J, Novakova I, van Heerde WL, Verbruggen B. Low-titre inhibitors, undetectable by the Nijmegen assay, reduce factor VIII half-life after immune tolerance induction. J Thromb Haemost. 2012;10(4):706–8.
48 Gouw SC, van den Berg HM, Fischer K, Auerswald G, Carcao M, Chalmers E, et al. Intensity of factor VIII treatment and inhibitor development in children with severe hemophilia A: the RODIN study. Blood. 2013;121(20):4046–55.
49 Eckhardt CL, van Velzen AS, Peters M, Astermark J, Brons PP, Castaman G, et al. Factor VIII gene (F8) mutation and risk of inhibitor development in nonsevere hemophilia A. Blood. 2013;122(11):1954–62.
50 Male C, Andersson NG, Rafowicz A, Liesner R, Kurnik K, Fischer K, et al. Inhibitor incidence in an unselected cohort of previously untreated patients with severe haemophilia B: a PedNet study. Haematologica. 2021;106(1):123–9.
51 Gouw SC, van den Berg HM, Oldenburg J, Astermark J, de Groot PG, Margaglione M, et al. F8 gene mutation type and inhibitor development in patients with severe hemophilia A: systematic review and meta-analysis. Blood. 2012;119(12):2922–34.
52 Astermark J, Donfield SM, Gomperts ED, Schwarz J, Menius ED, Pavlova A, et al. The polygenic nature of inhibitors in hemophilia A: results from the Hemophilia Inhibitor Genetics Study (HIGS) Combined Cohort. Blood. 2013;121(8):1446–54.
53 Lessard S, He C, Rajpal DK, Klinger K, Loh C, Harris T, Dumont J. Genome-wide association study and gene-based analysis of participants with hemophilia A and inhibitors in the my life, our future research repository. Front Med (Lausanne). 2022;9:903838.
54 Peyvandi F, Mannucci PM, Garagiola I, El-Beshlawy A, Elalfy M, Ramanan V, et al. A randomized trial of factor VIII and neutralizing antibodies in hemophilia A. N Engl J Med. 2016;374(21):2054–64.
55 Gouw SC, van der Bom JG, Ljung R, Escuriola C, Cid AR, Claeyssens-Donadel S, et al. Factor VIII products and inhibitor development in severe hemophilia A. N Engl J Med. 2013;368(3):231–9.
56 Prezotti ANL, Frade-Guanaes JO, Yamaguti-Hayakawa GG, Ozelo MC. Immunogenicity of current and new therapies for hemophilia A. Pharmaceuticals (Basel). 2022;15(8):911.
57 Recht M, Pollmann H, Tagliaferri A, Musso R, Janco R, Neuman WR. A retrospective study to describe the incidence of moderate to severe allergic reactions to factor IX in subjects with haemophilia B. Haemophilia. 2011;17(3):494–9.

58 Astermark J, Holstein K, Abajas YL, Kearney S, Croteau SE, Liesner R, et al. The B-Natural study – the outcome of immune tolerance induction therapy in patients with severe haemophilia B. Haemophilia. 2021;27(5):802–13.
59 Teitel J, Berntorp E, Collins P, D'Oiron R, Ewenstein B, Gomperts E, et al. A systematic approach to controlling problem bleeds in patients with severe congenital haemophilia A and high-titre inhibitors. Haemophilia. 2007;13(3): 256–63.
60 Seaman CD, Ragni MV. Sequential bypassing agents during major orthopedic surgery: a new approach to hemostasis. Blood Adv. 2017;1(17):1309–11.
61 Young G, Shafer FE, Rojas P, Seremetis S. Single 270 microg kg(-1)-dose rFVIIa vs. standard 90 microg kg(-1)-dose rFVIIa and APCC for home treatment of joint bleeds in haemophilia patients with inhibitors: a randomized comparison. Haemophilia. 2008;14(2):287–94.
62 Sørensen B, Dargaud Y, Kenet G, Lusher J, Mumford A, Pipe S, et al. On-demand treatment of bleeds in haemophilia patients with inhibitors: strategies for securing and maintaining predictable efficacy with recombinant activated factor VII. Haemophilia. 2012;18(2):255–62.
63 Astermark J, Donfield SM, DiMichele DM, Gringeri A, Gilbert SA, Waters J, et al. A randomized comparison of bypassing agents in hemophilia complicated by an inhibitor: the FEIBA NovoSeven Comparative (FENOC) study. Blood. 2007;109(2):546–51.
64 Young G, Liesner R, Chang T, Sidonio R, Oldenburg J, Jiménez-Yuste V, et al. A multicenter, open-label phase 3 study of emicizumab prophylaxis in children with hemophilia A with inhibitors. Blood. 2019;134(24):2127–38.
65 Oldenburg J, Austin SK, Kessler CM. ITI choice for the optimal management of inhibitor patients – from a clinical and pharmacoeconomic perspective. Haemophilia. 2014;20(suppl 6):17–26.
66 Hay CR, DiMichele DM. The principal results of the International Immune Tolerance Study: a randomized dose comparison. Blood. 2012;119(6):1335–44.
67 Escuriola Ettingshausen C, Vdovin V, Zozulya N, Svirin P, Andreeva T, Benedik-Dolničar M, et al. Immune Tolerance Induction (ITI) with a pdFVIII/VWF concentrate (octanate) in 100 patients in the Observational ITI (ObsITI) study. TH Open. 2022;6(2):e124–34.
68 van Velzen AS, Peters M, van der Bom JG, Fijnvandraat K. Effect of von Willebrand factor on inhibitor eradication in patients with severe haemophilia A: a systematic review. Br J Haematol. 2014; 166(4):485–95.
69 Hart DP, Alamelu J, Bhatnagar N, Biss T, Collins PW, Hall G, et al. Immune tolerance induction in severe haemophilia A: a UKHCDO inhibitor and paediatric working party consensus update. Haemophilia. 2021;27(6):932–7.
70 Carcao M, Escuriola-Ettingshausen C, Santagostino E, Oldenburg J, Liesner R, Nolan B, et al. The changing face of immune tolerance induction in haemophilia A with the advent of emicizumab. Haemophilia. 2019;25(4):676–84.
71 Hanley J, McKernan A, Creagh MD, Classey S, McLaughlin P, Goddard N, et al. Guidelines for the management of acute joint bleeds and chronic synovitis in haemophilia: a United Kingdom Haemophilia Centre Doctors' Organisation (UKHCDO) guideline. Haemophilia. 2017;23(4):511–20.
72 Seuser A, Djambas Khayat C, Negrier C, Sabbour A, Heijnen L. Evaluation of early musculoskeletal disease in patients with haemophilia: results from an expert consensus. Blood Coagul Fibrinolysis. 2018;29(6):509–20.
73 Rodriguez-Merchan EC. Hemophilic pseudotumors: diagnosis and management. Arch Bone Jt Surg. 2020;8(2):121–30.
74 Davies J, Kadir RA. Mode of delivery and cranial bleeding in newborns with haemophilia: a systematic review and meta-analysis of the literature. Haemophilia. 2016;22(1):32–8.
75 Moorehead PC, Chan AKC, Lemyre B, Winikoff R, Scott H, Hawes SA, et al. A practical guide to the management of the fetus and newborn with hemophilia. Clin Appl Thromb Hemost. 2018;24(9_suppl):29s-41s.
76 Pulles AE, Mastbergen SC, Schutgens RE, Lafeber FP, van Vulpen LF. Pathophysiology of hemophilic arthropathy and potential targets for therapy. Pharmacol Res. 2017;115:192–9.

Chapter 9

Published online: December 5, 2024

Blanchette VS, Brandão LR, Carcao MD, Kumar R, Rand ML, Revel-Vilk S (eds): SickKids Handbook of Pediatric Thrombosis and Hemostasis, ed 3, rev. and ext. Basel, Karger, 2024, pp 145–163 (DOI: 10.1159/000538200)

von Willebrand Disease

Rungrote Natesirinilkul[a] Lara Lobianco e Souza[b] Chris Barnes[c]
Victor S. Blanchette[b, d] Paula D. James[e]

[a]Department of Pediatrics, Faculty of Medicine, Chaing Mai University, Chiang Mai, Thailand; [b]Division of Haematology/Oncology, Research Institute, Hospital for Sick Children, Toronto, ON, Canada; [c]Division of Haematology, Royal Children Hospital, Melbourne, VIC, Australia; [d]Department of Pediatrics, University of Toronto, Toronto, ON, Canada; [e]Department of Medicine, Queen's University, Kingston, ON, Canada

Introduction

von Willebrand disease (VWD) is the most common inherited coagulation factor bleeding disorder in human subjects. It is estimated that up to 1% of all people are affected with VWD, although only about 1/1,000 are symptomatic [1] and only 1/10,000 are likely to be followed in a bleeding disorders' clinic. A deficiency or dysfunction of von Willebrand factor (VWF) results in defective primary hemostasis due primarily to absent or abnormal platelet adhesion and secondarily to reduced hemostasis associated with decreased levels of circulating factor VIII coagulant (FVIII:C). Despite its frequency, most individuals with VWD manifest a milder bleeding phenotype than those with severe forms of hemophilia. Type 1 VWD, a partial quantitative defect, and most forms of type 2 VWD (qualitative defects in VWF) are associated almost exclusively with mucocutaneous bleeding. Type 3 VWD, a rare but severe quantitative defect, and type 2N VWD are associated with significant (hemophilia-like) bleeding, including hemarthrosis.

In children, in the absence of a family history of the disease, milder forms of VWD may never be diagnosed or not diagnosed until there is a significant bleeding challenge (dental procedures, surgery, or menarche). Furthermore, incomplete penetrance and variable expressivity complicate the diagnosis especially in children who have not yet had hemostatic challenges. Laboratory testing is required to make the diagnosis and to delineate the subtype of VWD. Treatment depends on the clinical severity, disease responsiveness, and magnitude of bleeding/bleeding risk.

Pathophysiology of VWD

Dr. Erik von Willebrand reported the first family of patients with VWD from Finland in 1926. He noted an autosomal pattern of inheritance in a family with multiple individuals who had signifi-

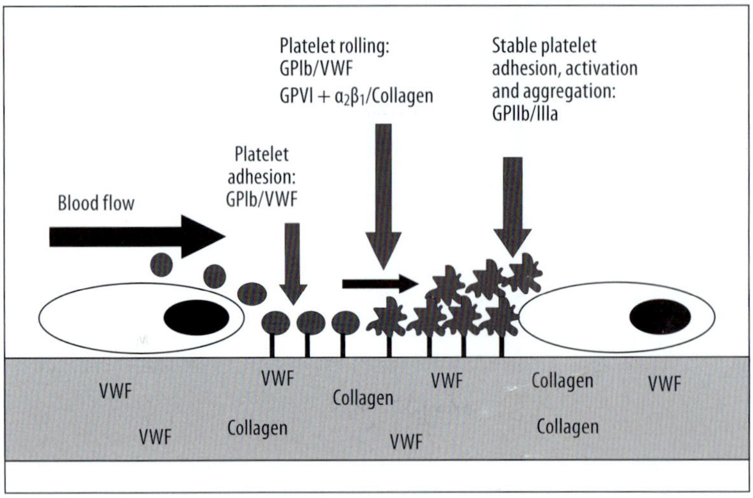

Fig. 1. An area of endothelial cell loss with the sequence of events involved in the primary hemostatic event, platelet plug formation. The platelets initially adhere transiently to subendothelial VWF through the GPIb-IX-V receptor. This contact significantly slows the movement of platelets that continue to roll across the subendothelium, maintaining an interaction with VWF and collagen through the GPIb-IX-V and platelet collagen receptors, respectively. Eventually, these contacts reach a threshold that signals the event of platelet activation. Platelets then adhere stably to the damaged vessel wall and undergo an aggregation response through a platelet GPIIb/IIIa receptor-mediated event [2]. Reproduced with kind permission from Lillicrap [3]. GP, glycoprotein; VWF, von Willebrand factor.

cant bleeding with a prolonged bleeding time despite a normal platelet count. It later became apparent that although FVIII:C was also reduced, a distinct protein (VWF) was diminished, dysfunctional, or absent in those with the bleeding disorder.

In the mid-1980s, the *VWF* gene was identified on the short arm of chromosome 12. The 178 kb gene is made up of 52 exons and codes for a 2,813 amino acid protein made of a signal peptide of 22 amino acids, a large propeptide of 741 amino acids, and the mature VWF, a protein consisting of 2,050 amino acids. During its biosynthesis, the protein undergoes modifications that result in the production of a VWF protein arranged into multimers that vary in size from dimers to multimers of up to 20 million daltons (Da) in size. VWF is produced in megakaryocytes and endothelial cells and stored in platelet α granules and Weibel-Palade bodies [2]. Further research into the protein suggests three distinct hemostatic functions of VWF, as follows: (1) to facilitate platelet adhesion to injured endothelium by binding to glycoprotein (GP) Ib-IX-V receptors on platelets and as well to collagen (Fig. 1) (see Chapter 2); (2) to assist platelet aggregation through binding to the activated GPIIb-IIIa (αIIbβ3) receptor at high shear (Fig. 1) (see Chapter 2); and (3) to carry FVIII in the circulation and protect it from degradation by protein C [3]. VWD can be caused by disorders of VWF production, assembly, secretion, or clearance (Fig. 2).

Clinical Presentations

The VWF Scientific and Standardization Committee (SSC) of the International Society on Thrombosis and Hemostasis (ISTH) published the generally accepted classification of VWD in 2006 [4]. In 2021, the American Society of Hematology (ASH)/ISTH/National Hemophilia Foun-

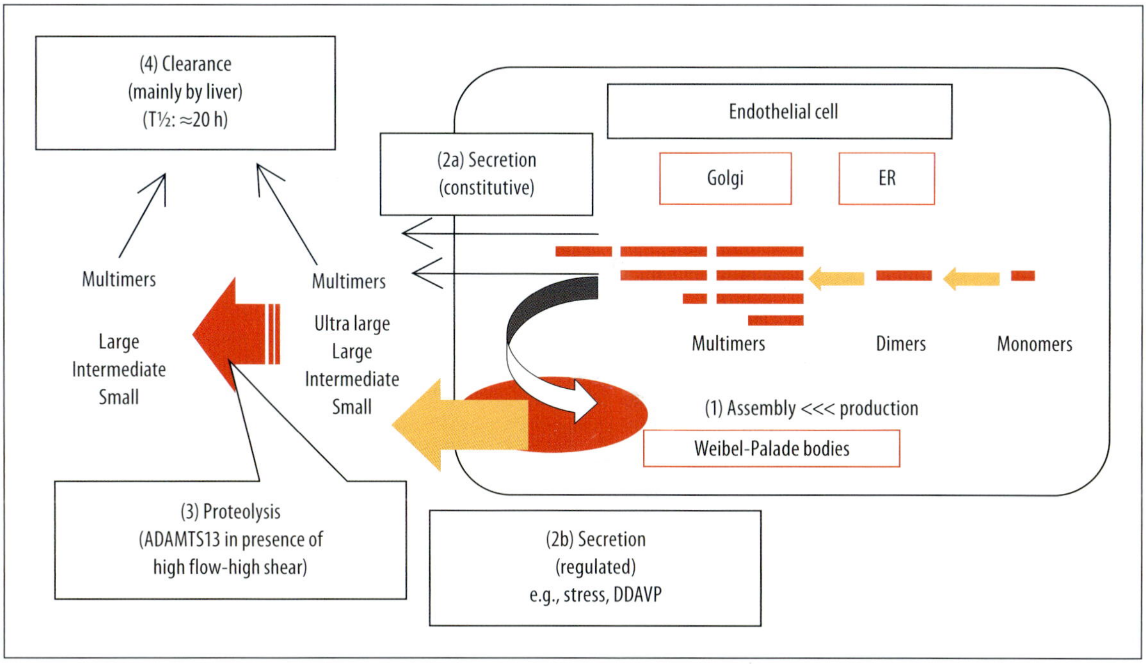

Fig. 2. VWD can be related to disorders of VWF production/assembly (1); secretion (2); proteolysis (3); or clearance (4). ADAMTS13, a disintegrin and metalloproteinase with a thrombospondin type 1 motif, member 13; DDAVP, 1-deamino-8-D-arginine vasopressin (desmopressin); ER, endoplasmic reticulum; T½, half-life.

dation (NHF) and the World Federation of Hemophilia (WFH) published a new evidence-based guideline for the diagnosis and management of VWD [5] (Tables 1 and 2).

Type 1 VWD

Type 1 VWD is the most common form of VWD accounting for approximately 75% of cases. Inheritance is autosomal dominant, but incomplete penetrance and variable expressivity can obscure positive family histories. Patients with type 1 VWD may present with mucocutaneous bleeding, including excessive epistaxis, bruising, and heavy menstrual bleeding, or may have prolonged bleeding after dental procedures or surgery. Clinically, there is a broad range of severity.

Type 2 VWD

Type 2 VWD accounts for approximately 25% of cases. There are four subtypes of type 2 VWD: 2A, 2B, 2M, and 2N, each having a different pathophysiological etiology and specific diagnostic findings (see Diagnosis). Clinically, children with types 2A, 2B, and 2M VWD present with increased mucocutaneous bleeding, similar to those with type 1 VWD. Children with type 2N present with a bleeding pattern more similar to that of mild-to-moderate hemophilia A [6]. Bleeding in type 2 VWD is often worse than in type 1 VWD, and one particularly frequent and problematic type of bleeding in adults with type 2 VWD is gastrointestinal bleeding secondary to angiodysplasia. In general, severe bleeding, such as intracranial hemorrhage (ICH), is rare in type 2 VWD cases but has been reported.

Table 1. Clinical and epidemiological features of the subtypes of VWD

	Type 1 VWD	Type 2 VWD	Type 3 VWD
Proportion	75% of cases	25% of cases	<1% of cases (1 in 1–3 million); increased with consanguinity
Inheritance pattern	AD with incomplete penetrance and variable expressivity	AD (2A, 2B, 2M) AR (2N)	AR
Clinical features	Mucocutaneous bleeding; wide range of severity correlates with amount of functional VWF in the circulation	Increased mucocutaneous bleeding (2A, 2B, 2M); mild/moderate hemophilia-like bleeding (2N); severe bleeds (e.g., ICH) reported but rare	Severe mucocutaneous bleeding and hemophilia-like bleeding; bleeding can lead to severe arthritis and chronic disability; ICH and other severe bleeds, although still rare, more commonly reported

AD, autosomal dominant; AR, autosomal recessive; ICH, intracranial bleeding; VWD, von Willebrand disease; VWF, von Willebrand factor.

Table 2. Classification of VWD

Type		Basis of defect	Description
1		Quantitative	Partial deficiency of VWF
	C	Quantitative	Partial deficiency with increased clearance of VWF
2	A	Qualitative	Decreased VWF-dependent platelet adhesion and deficiency of high-molecular-weight VWF multimers
	B	Qualitative	VWF shows increased affinity for platelet GPIb
	M	Qualitative	Decreased VWF-dependent platelet adhesion without a deficiency of high-molecular-weight VWF multimers
	N	Qualitative	Markedly decreased binding affinity of VWF for FVIII
3		Quantitative	Severe deficiency of VWF

FVIII, factor VIII; GPIb, glycoprotein Ib; VWD, von Willebrand disease; VWF, von Willebrand factor.

Type 3 VWD

Type 3 VWD is the most severe bleeding phenotype, due to severe deficiency of VWF (<0.05 IU/mL). This autosomal recessive condition is very rare, occurring in only 1–3 per million people. Its highest incidence is in regions where consanguinity is common. In addition to severe mucocutaneous bleeding, there can be repeated bleeding into muscles and joints. As in hemophilia, hemarthrosis in type 3 VWD may lead to severe arthritis, which may result in chronic disability. ICH and other severe bleeds, although still rare, are more commonly reported in type 3 VWD cases than in type 1 or type 2 VWD.

Table 3. Nonspecific laboratory investigations (and some potential findings)

Complete blood count	-Normocytic anemia from acute and excessive blood loss -Microcytic anemia, suggestive iron deficiency if the blood loss is chronic -Thrombocytopenia can be seen in type 2B VWD
aPTT	-Normal in most persons with VWD -Exceptions are severe forms of VWD that result in very low level of FVIII:C (e.g., type 3 VWD, type 2N VWD, and severe forms of types 1 and 2 VWD)
Bleeding time	-Often prolonged but not considered a good screen for VWD due to its low sensitivity and specificity (see Chapter 4) -No longer available in most centers
PFA-100®/200®	-Validated as an in vitro method for assessing primary hemostatic defect in children -More sensitive (80%) than the bleeding time as a screen for VWD, its use remains controversial and many centers prefer to do specific testing for VWD rather than only rely on the PFA-100®/200® as a screening test -The collagen/ADP closure time is more specific than the collagen/epinephrine in cases with VWD

ADP, adenosine 5′-diphosphate; aPTT, activated partial thromboplastin time; FVIII:C, factor VIII coagulant; PFA, platelet function analyzer; VWD, von Willebrand disease.

9

Diagnosis

The diagnosis of VWD is based on the patient's bleeding history, a family history of bleeding, and laboratory investigations that are consistent with a quantitative or a qualitative abnormality of VWF.

Personal and Family History of Bleeding

Obtaining a history of bleeding in the child being investigated as well as in his/her family is important in making the diagnosis (see Chapter 4). Ideally, the history is taken objectively, with a focus on both unprovoked bleeding and the response to bleeding challenges (surgeries, tooth extractions, etc.). In pediatrics, the Pediatric Bleeding Questionnaire (PBQ) or the International Society on Thrombosis and Hemostasis Bleeding Assessment Tool (ISTH-BAT) can be used to identify children with increased bleeding (see Chapter 4, Appendix I) [5, 7, 8]. For adolescent girls, a detailed menstrual history is important. Clinical estimation of menstrual blood loss can be done using the Pictorial Blood Loss Assessment Chart (PBAC) (see Appendix I) as an objective measure of heavy menstrual bleeding. This is recommended and may be implemented prospectively to monitor the degree of bleeding during menses [9]. Originally published in 1990, the PBAC scoring system was revalidated in 2021 with modern sanitary protection products [10] (see Appendix I). Similarly, as a more objective measure of the severity of epistaxis, the Katsanis epistaxis score can be used [11] (see Appendix I).

A family history of abnormal bleeding is also important, although it may not always be present. Dominant types of VWD may be present in each generation, with multiple people affected. Both type 2N and type 3 VWD are autosomal recessive conditions, so a family history of bleeding may be absent, but consanguinity may be noted.

The 2021 VWD guideline panel recommends the use of a validated Bleeding Assessment Tool (BAT) in the primary care setting and suggests its use in tertiary care settings to document bleeding severity [5]. A self-administered ISTH-BAT (Self-BAT) has been reported to be reliable and as effective as the expert-administered version [12]. In

Table 4. VWD laboratory investigations

	Type 1	Type 2				Type 3
		2A	2B	2M	2N	
VWF:Ag	↓	↓	↓	↓	↓/N	↓↓↓
Platelet-dependent VWF activity	↓	↓↓	↓↓	↓↓	↓/N	↓↓↓
FVIII:C, IU/mL	↓/N	↓/N	↓/N	↓/N	0.05–0.4	0.05–0.1
Platelet-dependent VWF activity/ VWF:Ag ratio	N	<0.7	<0.7	<0.7	N	N/A
Multimers	N	abN	abN	N	N	Absent
RIPA	N	↓	↑	↓	N	Absent
Genetic testing for *VWF*	NRS	NRS	S (exon 28)	NRS	S (exon 18–24)	S

↓, slightly reduced; ↓↓, moderately reduced; ↓↓↓, extremely reduced; abN, abnormal; Ag, antigen; FVIII:C, factor VIII coagulant; IU, international unit; mL, milliliter; N, normal; N/A, not applicable; NRS, not routinely suggested; RIPA, ristocetin-induced platelet agglutination; S, suggested; VWD, von Willebrand disease; VWF, von Willebrand factor.

addition, the ISTH-BAT can be used to longitudinally follow bleeding symptoms over time [13]. The use of a BAT in the pediatric setting was shown to improve provider knowledge, skill, and confidence in taking a bleeding history [14]. However, the use of a BAT in the pediatric population should be carefully interpreted as children may not have been exposed to hemostatic challenges. Additionally, the score saturates with recurrent severe bleeding symptoms (i.e., one nosebleed requiring cautery scores the same as 10 nosebleeds requiring cautery) [15].

Laboratory Investigations

Some nonspecific laboratory investigations including complete blood count (CBC), activated partial thromboplastin time (aPTT), bleeding time, and platelet function analyzer (PFA) 100®/200® can suggest VWD (Table 3).

Specific VWD Testing

An accurate diagnosis of VWD requires performing specific coagulation tests. Initial tests to investigate the possibility of VWD have traditionally included the VWF:Antigen (VWF:Ag) level, a measure of platelet-dependent VWF activity (i.e., VWF Mutant GlycoProtein Ib Assay [VWF:GPIbM], VWF Recombinant GlycoProtein Ib Assay [VWF:GPIbR], or VWF Ristocetin Cofactor Assay [VWF:RCo]) and a FVIII:C level. A guide to interpretation of these tests is detailed below and is presented in Table 4. The 2021 VWD guideline panel suggests the use of the newer assays (i.e., VWF:GPIbM or VWF:GPIbR) over the VWF:RCo due to a lower coefficient of variation and better accuracy in specific patient groups, such as individuals of African descent [4, 16–19].

The results of VWD testing can be influenced by both preanalytic and patient-related factors that should be considered during interpretation. Care must be taken to ensure that the blood draw is not traumatic and that samples are not shaken or agitated as this may initiate clotting and result in both VWF and FVIII being consumed. Samples should be tested within 4 h of collection to minimize the degradation of FVIII. If this is not feasible, plasma should be separated promptly at room temperature, and the plasma should be centrifuged thoroughly to remove platelets and then frozen at −40 °C or lower and transported to a reference laboratory for testing.

In addition, VWF levels are affected by a number of physiological parameters. Blood type affects VWF levels; individuals who are of type O blood will have VWF levels that are 20–25% lower than non-O blood type individuals [20]. Other parameters that might affect VWF levels include states of high estrogen levels (e.g., pregnancy or use of oral contraceptive pills), stress (including struggling or crying in children at the time of phlebotomy), very recent exercise, and acute illnesses, all of which increase VWF levels; in contrast, hypothyroidism decreases levels of VWF from reduced production.

VWF:Ag Assay
This is an immunoassay used to measure the concentration of VWF in blood plasma. Testing methods include enzyme-linked immunoassay (ELISA) or latex immunoassay. VWF:Ag is usually reported in international units (IU)/deciliter (dL), or IU/milliliter (mL).

Platelet-Dependent von Willebrand Activity Level
The VWF:RCo was previously the most commonly used test to assess the ability of VWF to bind GPIbα. This assay measures the ability of a patient's plasma to agglutinate platelets when exposed to high doses of the antibiotic ristocetin. The rate of ristocetin-induced agglutination is related to the concentration and functional activity of the plasma VWF. Newer assays have been developed to evaluate VWF-GPIbα interactions, e.g., GPIbR, GPIbM, and are currently suggested in the new guideline [5].

Ristocetin-Induced Platelet Agglutination
Ristocetin-induced platelet agglutination (RIPA) is utilized as a screen for type 2B VWD. In this test, different concentrations of ristocetin (typically a high dose, e.g., 1.5 mg/mL, and a low dose, e.g., 0.5 mg/mL) are added to a patient's platelet-rich plasma (PRP) in an aggregometer, and RIPA is measured. Most forms of VWD will show reduced agglutination to ristocetin. An exception is type 2B VWD in which even a low dose of ristocetin (0.5 mg/mL) will cause platelet agglutination due to a gain-of-function variant in VWD

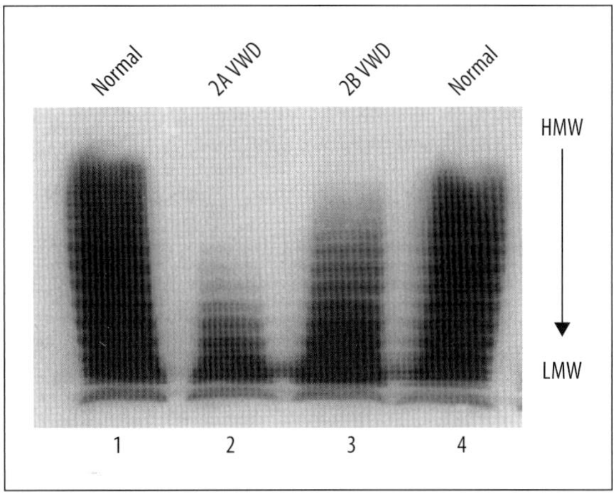

Fig. 3. Example of VWF multimer analysis. Plasma VWF multimer patterns in normal plasma (lanes 1 and 4; showing normal multimer pattern), type 2A plasma (lane 2; showing severely reduced HMW multimers), and type 2B plasma (lane 3; showing mildly reduced HMW multimers). HMW, high-molecular-weight; LMW, low molecular weight; VWD, von Willebrand disease; VWF, von Willebrand factor.

type 2B leading to a VWF with hyperresponsiveness to platelets. A similar hyperresponsiveness to ristocetin occurs in platelet-type VWD in which a defect in platelets causes them to bind VWF much more avidly (see below for details on platelet-type VWD). Genetic testing is a reliable way of distinguishing the two conditions [5].

Collagen-Binding von Willebrand Activity Level
VWF:collagen binding (VWF:CB) activity is used to assess VWF adhesive activity with collagen as it occurs at the subendothelial matrix at the injury site. VWF:CB also measures the binding between collagen and high-molecular-weight (HMW) VWF multimers [21].

Factor VIII Coagulant Assay
FVIII:C measures the cofactor function of FVIII in plasma. The test is most commonly used to diagnose hemophilia; however, in VWD, the level of FVIII:C in the circulation indicates the ability

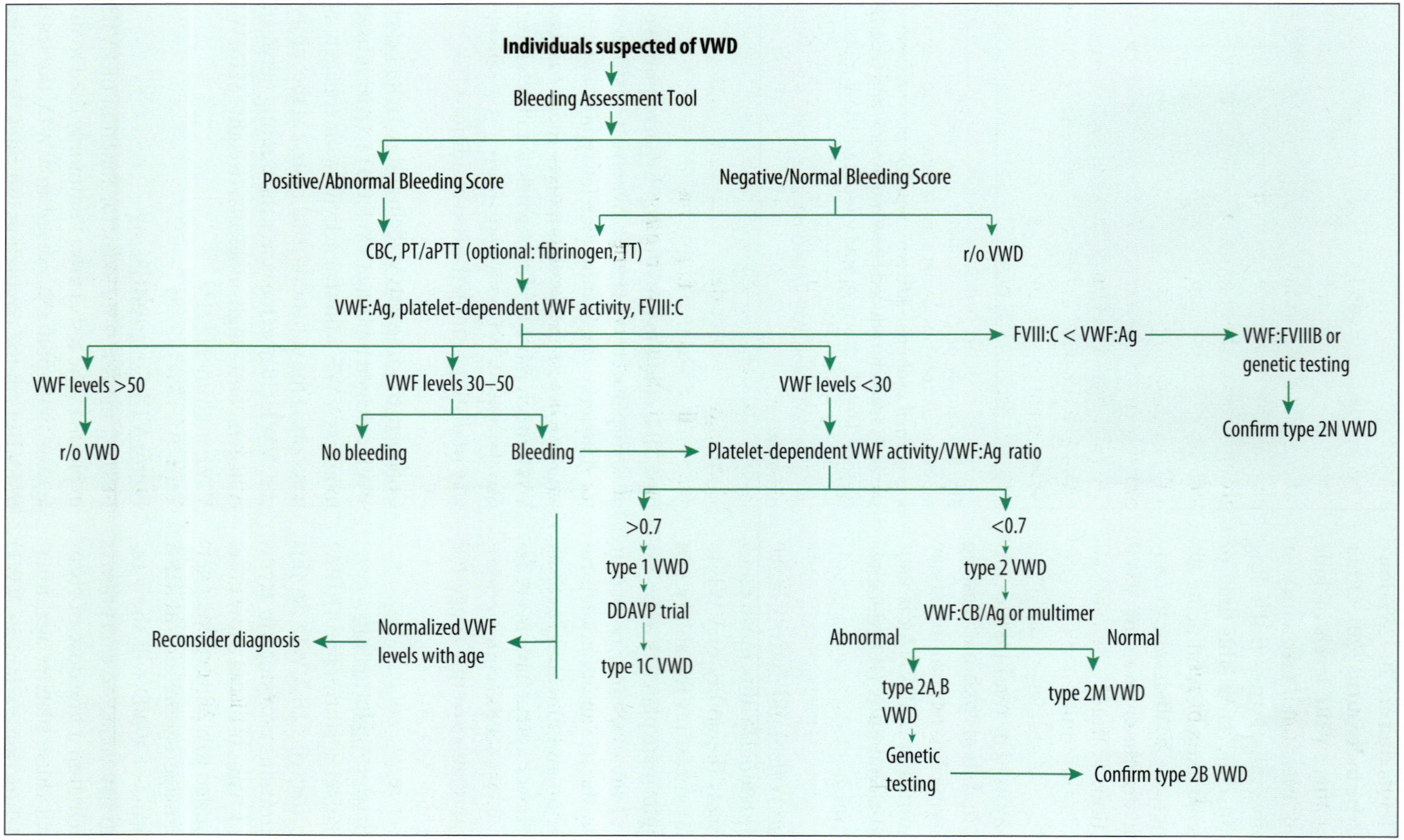

Fig. 4. An overall algorithm addressing the diagnosis of VWD. The algorithm says VWF level 30 to 50 for simplicity; this refers to VWF levels of 0.30 to 0.50 IU/mL, with the caveat that the lower limit of the normal range as determined by the local laboratory should be used if it is <0.50 IU/mL. Modified and reproduced with kind permission from James et al. [5]. CBC, complete blood count; FVIII:C, factor VIII coagulant; PT/aPTT, prothrombin time/activated partial thromboplastin time; TT, thrombin time; VWD, von Willebrand disease; VWF, von Willebrand factor; VWF:Ag, von Willebrand factor:antigen; VWF:CB, von Willebrand factor:collagen binding; VWF:FVIIIB, von Willebrand factor:factor VIII binding.

of VWF to bind to, and maintain FVIII in the circulation. FVIII:C activity is measured by a variety of methods, most commonly in an automatic one-stage clotting assay based on the aPTT.

VWF Multimers

These can be analyzed in cases of suspected type 2 VWD. This qualitative assay uses gel electrophoresis to show the variable concentrations of the different sized VWF multimers that are detected with radiolabeled antibodies applied to the gel (Fig. 3). Another method utilizes Western blot with immunofluorescence for multimer detection. Type 2A, 2B, and platelet-type VWD show abnormal patterns with deficiency of the HMW VWF multimers [22]. However, VWF multimer analysis is available in a limited number of specialized laboratories and requires a high level of expertise. Therefore, the 2021 VWD guideline panel suggests using either the VWF:CB/VWF:Ag ratio to further investigate individuals suspected of having type 2A, 2B, or 2M VWD [5].

Genetic Variant Analysis

This is not part of routine diagnostic testing for VWD, as it is limited by the size and complexity of the *VWF* gene [23]. Approximately 35% of patients with type 1 VWD have no identifiable variant in the promoter, coding region, or splice sites of the *VWF* gene, suggesting that there may be other genes that affect VWF production and clearance, or that variants are located in other regions of the *VWF* gene that are not routinely analyzed. Despite these challenges, there are a number of situations in which genetic testing can confirm the diagnosis when coagulation tests are not able to provide a definitive diagnosis. This includes type 2N disease (caused by variants in exons 18–24), type 2B, or 2M VWD (caused by variants in exon 28), and for prenatal diagnosis of type 3 VWD cases as mentioned above. See Chapter 21 for further consideration regarding genetic counseling and testing. The summary of approach and investigations for a definite diagnosis of VWD is shown in Fig. 4 [5].

Type 1 VWD

The diagnosis of type 1 VWD is often challenging due to the lack of a definitive cutoff that separates normal from abnormal VWF:Ag and platelet-dependent VWF activity levels, the impact of blood group type on these levels, and the variability in test results in the same individual over time [24]. VWF:Ag cutoff levels that have been proposed to differentiate normal from type 1 VWD range between 0.3 and 0.5 IU/mL [25]. Borderline results should be repeated at least once for confirmation before making a diagnosis. We suggest that a laboratory diagnosis of type 1 VWD requires at least two VWF:Ag or von Willebrand factor activity (VWF:Act) levels of <0.5 IU/mL in patients with bleeding manifestations or two VWF:Act levels of <0.3 IU/mL in patients regardless of bleeding symptoms [5]. An individual with VWF levels between 0.3 and 0.5 IU/mL but no bleeding could be designated as "low-VWF" [26]. Children in this category should be followed over time to see if bleeding symptoms develop. In an asymptomatic child with a positive family history, we advocate waiting (i.e., until 3 years of age or older) for specialized laboratory testing unless there is a need for surgery or procedures. The value of the FVIII/VWF ratio to distinguish girls who are carriers of hemophilia A from those with VWD has been shown and would be low in the former but increased in the latter [27].

In general, the lower the VWF levels in a patient, the more severe is the disease phenotype and the less likely the patient is to respond to desmopressin (1-deamino-8-D-arginine vasopressin; DDAVP) (see below). However, there is no consensus on what constitutes a severe form of type 1 VWD.

Type 1C VWD

Although not included in the 2006 classification, type 1C VWD is now well described and deserves mention due to its particular clinical/treatment implications. This disorder, which comprises approximately 15% of cases of type 1 VWD, is due

9

to increased VWF clearance. The initial report of expedited clearance of VWF showed a cohort with a specific VWF gene variant, R1205H, called the Vicenza variant [28]. Since then, other variants that result in increased clearance have been described. Typical laboratory findings include low VWF:Ag and proportionately low platelet-dependent VWF activity with a low or normal FVIII:C level. A high VWF propeptide/VWF:Ag ratio is very helpful in diagnosis; unfortunately, the VWF propeptide test is not widely available [29]. There may be persistence of larger than normal size VWF multimers. Practically, a DDAVP challenge test is most helpful, as patients with type 1C VWD show an exaggerated response to DDAVP at 1 h post administration but have a marked reduction at the 4-h mark due to accelerated clearance. Therefore, the new guideline suggests to use DDAVP challenge test with 1- and 4-h post-transfusion blood tests to confirm the diagnosis of type 1C VWD. In addition, identification of missense variants known to cause type 1C VWD in exons 26, 27, and 37 can confirm this condition.

Type 2 VWD

In patients with a combination of low VWF levels and a reduced VWF activity-to-antigen ratio (<0.7), type 2 VWD should be considered and additional testing performed. When type 2 VWD is suspected, it can be useful to assess VWF multimers by gel electrophoresis (Fig. 3). Recently published data show increased VWF clearance as a common mechanism underlying type 2 VWD, which can be identified by a DDAVP challenge (as above for type 1C) and/or the identification of causative missense variants [30].

Decreased HMW VWF Multimers Suggest Type 2A or Type 2B VWD

In type 2A VWD, the HMW VWF multimers are missing due to an inability to make these forms or because of premature degradation by a disintegrin and metalloproteinase with thrombospondin type 1 motif, member 13 (ADAMTS13). Similarly, type 2B VWD patients do not show the HMW forms as these spontaneously bind to platelets and are cleared from the circulation.

To differentiate type 2B VWD from type 2A VWD, RIPA testing or genetic testing may be performed. Under normal conditions, the addition of ristocetin to PRP induces platelet agglutination in RIPA. This activity is generally reduced in most VWD patients (including patients with types 2A and 2M VWD). In contrast, in type 2B VWD, there is hyperresponsiveness to low-dose ristocetin (abnormal RIPA test) due to enhanced binding of VWF to platelet GPIb-IX-V receptors (gain-of-function variant). This increased binding of VWF to platelets results in increased clearance of VWF-platelet complexes, loss of HMW VWF multimers, and often (but not always) thrombocytopenia [31]. Thrombocytopenia, if present, can result in such patients being mislabeled as having immune thrombocytopenia (ITP). In some patients, thrombocytopenia may only be seen during states of stress (bleeding states or surgery) or pregnancy. The severity of the thrombocytopenia appears to correlate most with bleeding symptomology.

Normal VWF Multimers Suggest Type 2M

Type 2M VWD is a disorder characterized by loss-of-function variants on the VWF binding site for collagen. Laboratory test results in type 2M VWD are similar to those in type 2A VWD with the exception that in type 2M VWD, the VWF multimer distribution and VWF:CB/VWF:Ag are normal, whereas HMW VWF multimers and VWF:CB/VWF:Ag are reduced in type 2A VWD.

Type 2N VWD Can Mimic Hemophilia A

The diagnosis of type 2N VWD can be challenging, and cases may be misdiagnosed as having mild/moderate hemophilia A or as being hemophilia carriers. VWF:Ag and platelet-dependent VWF activity may be slightly low, borderline, or normal. The diagnosis of type 2N VWD should be suspected when the FVIII:C level is disproportionately low relative to the VWF:Ag level or when there is consanguinity suggesting an autosomal recessive inheritance. An ELISA-based FVIII binding assay can be done to determine if VWF has decreased binding to FVIII to confirm the diagnosis; however, the binding assay is not generally available except in research laboratories. Alternatively, confirmation by genetic testing can be done (see below). Type 2N VWD should be considered in cases labeled as having mild/moderate hemophilia A in whom a hemophilia variant cannot be identified or in those patients thought to have hemophilia but who do not respond well to a recombinant or plasma-derived FVIII concentrate that does not contain VWF.

Type 3 VWD

Type 3 VWD is diagnosed when the VWF:Ag and platelet-dependent VWF activity levels are <0.05 IU/mL. The FVIII:C is usually between 0.01 and 0.10 IU/mL, VWF multimers are absent, and there can be a history of consanguinity. Type 3 VWD is caused by the inheritance of two mutant alleles – one from each parent – and thus a patient with type 3 VWD is either homozygous or compound heterozygous for VWD variants. The parents of the affected individual each carry one mutated allele and may or may not have low VWF levels (i.e., they may or may not have type 1 VWD). Genetic testing may be pursued for prenatal counseling in families with an affected child who are planning to have additional children.

Platelet-Type VWD

Platelet-type VWD is an autosomal dominant disorder that is caused by a gain-of-function variant in the *GP1BA* gene (found on short arm of chromosome 17) that codes for the α-subunit of the GPIb receptor on platelets. This bleeding disorder is characterized by an increased affinity of the platelet GPIb-IX-V receptor complex for VWF. This results in macrothrombocytopenia, platelet clumping on a blood smear, and increased platelet agglutination to low-dose ristocetin. Mild-to-moderate bleeding in affected patients is due to the increased loss of VWF multimers from the circulation. Platelet-type VWD can be mistaken for type 2B VWD, as both show increased agglutination of PRP to low-dose ristocetin. Genetic testing can be used to differentiate platelet-type VWD from type 2B VWD.

Acquired von Willebrand Syndrome

Acquired von Willebrand Syndrome (AVWS) is increasingly being diagnosed in children particularly in the settings of high-flow high-shear cardiac lesions (aortic stenosis, patent ductus arteriosus, pulmonary hypertension, and more recently, usage of left ventricular assist devices). In adults, AVWS is also reported in association with malignancies, lymphoproliferative disorders, and autoimmune disorders, but in children, this is seldom seen. Details of the diagnosis and management of AVWS are outlined in Chapter 11.

Management

Prevention of bleeding is important for patients with VWD. Patients should be advised to avoid acetylsalicylic acid (ASA) or ASA-containing medications, and other antiplatelet medications, e.g., other nonsteroidal anti-inflammatory drugs (NSAIDs). Protective gear, such as helmets for bike riding, should be recommended. In addition, optimal dental care is important, as the increased mucocutaneous bleeding can result in patients avoiding routine brushing/flossing, leading to dental caries and the need for dental extractions over time [32]. Despite these preventative measures, medical therapies are often needed to prevent/control bleeding in patients with VWD.

In general, treatment for patients with VWD is given to prevent operative bleeding or bleeding associated with invasive procedures, to manage bleeding during childbirth or miscarriage, and in the event of excessive mucosal bleeding such as heavy menstrual bleeding or epistaxis. Many practical reviews of VWD treatment have been published [33, 34]. Medical therapies for prevention/control of bleeding in VWD can be divided into two types: nonspecific adjunctive therapies that provide hemostatic support (antifibrinolytic agents, estrogens, and fibrin sealants) and treatments that directly increase levels of VWF and FVIII:C by DDAVP, VWF/FVIII concentrates, and cryoprecipitate in situations where VWF/FVIII concentrates are not available.

Nonspecific Adjunctive Therapies

Antifibrinolytic Agents

Two antifibrinolytic agents, tranexamic acid and epsilon-amino caproic acid are available to prevent/treat bleeding, in particular mucosal bleeding, for patients with VWD. Their mechanism of action is inhibition of plasminogen activation. They are generally safe and well tolerated but are contraindicated in patients with an elevated risk of thrombosis, patients with clinical disseminated intravascular coagulation, and in patients with gross hematuria. The elimination of these drugs is renal, so doses should be adjusted in renal impairment [35]. Antifibrinolytic treatment should continue for up to 10 days after a procedure depending on the procedure and the inherent risk of bleeding. Dosing of antifibrinolytic agents is detailed below.

Tranexamic Acid

10–30 mg/kg intravenous (IV) (maximum 1 g) prior to procedure and every 8 h postoperatively until oral tolerance is achieved [35]. By mouth, 25 mg/kg/dose (maximum 1.5 g/dose) can be given three to four times daily. Tranexamic acid is available in 500 mg tablets. For young children, the IV solution can be given by mouth, or alternatively, the tablets can be crushed [35]. The IV solution can also be applied topically in cases of circumcision, different types of surgical procedures, and epistaxis, as can a crushed tablet combined with water to make a paste [36]. Anecdotal reports raised a concern of using tranexamic acid in patients who were at risk of thrombosis and who have hematuria due to the risk of developing acute renal failure secondary to thrombotic obstruction of the collecting system of the kidney. However, recent systematic reviews show that tranexamic acid does not increase risk of venous and arterial thrombosis [37]. Moreover, using tranexamic acid does not increase the risk of acute renal failure in patients who have gross hematuria; however, this treatment should be considered on a case-by-case basis [38].

EACA

Loading dose of 100-200 mg/kg IV/per oral (PO) (maximum loading dose 10 g); maintenance dose of 50-100 mg/kg per dose every 4-6 h for 5-7 days (maximum 30 g/day). EACA is available in suspension (250 mg/mL) and 500 and 1,000 mg tablets.

Estrogens

In women with heavy menstrual bleeding, estrogens can be given to regulate menstrual cycles to decrease menstrual blood loss. Standard oral contraceptive pills that contain estrogen can be used (see section on heavy menstrual bleeding below and see Chapter 5).

Fibrin Sealants

Fibrin sealants, also known as fibrin glues, contain both fibrinogen and thrombin, which are mixed at the time of application. They can be applied directly (i.e., topically) to sites of bleeding during surgery. These agents, both recombinant and virally inactivated plasma derived, e.g., Tisseel® and Evicel®, are commercially available in some countries, and guidelines for administration are detailed in the product inserts and should be followed. Although antibodies to bovine thrombin have been reported with the use of some fibrin sealants, their clinical implications are less clear.

Treatments That Directly Increase Levels of VWF and FVIII:C

DDAVP

DDAVP is a synthetic form of vasopressin that acts to stimulate the release of VWF from Weibel-Palade bodies in endothelial cells. DDAVP is often sufficient treatment for mild bleeds or to prevent bleeding associated with dental procedures and minor surgeries in patients with type 1 or some forms of type 2 VWD. Because DDAVP can exacerbate thrombocytopenia in type 2B VWD, it is generally contraindicated in this condition. It is not beneficial for type 3 VWD cases.

It is important to know a patient's responsiveness to DDAVP, as approximately 20% of patients with type 1 VWD are considered nonresponders. A DDAVP challenge test should be done following diagnosis of type 1 or type 2 VWD with the exception of type 2B. This is provided that a child is old enough (generally at least 3 years of age) to undergo a DDAVP challenge. In this test, a dose of 0.3 μg/kg of DDAVP (some centers use a maximum dose of 20 μg) is given IV or subcutaneously (SC), and the response is assessed. Response to DDAVP is classified according to peak FVIII:C and platelet-dependent VWF:Act levels at 1 h. In addition, a 4-h sample is important to detect those patients with accelerated clearance of VWF (i.e., type 1C VWD). A complete response following a dose of DDAVP is defined as achieving platelet-dependent VWF activity and FVIII:C levels of ≥0.5 IU/mL at 4 h and at least >2 times the baseline VWF activity level [39], whereas a partial response is defined as achieving platelet-dependent VWF activity and FVIII:C levels of >0.3 IU/mL [33].

As the response to DDAVP has been shown to improve with age, children assessed to be DDAVP nonresponders at a young age (<10 years of age) should undergo a repeat DDAVP challenge test at an older age, perhaps 5 years after the initial DDAVP challenge.

DDAVP can be administered SC, intranasally, or IV. Standard DDAVP dosing is 0.3 μg/kg IV/SC (some centers will not give doses >20 μg). The pharmacokinetics of SC-administered DDAVP are similar to that of IV DDAVP [40]. Intranasal dosing usually consists of administering 300 μg (one 150-μg puff into each nostril) for older children and adults (≥50 kg) and 150 μg (1 puff into 1 nostril) for younger children (<50 kg). Intranasal dosing is associated with greater variability in absorption as well as in time to peak activity levels. Furthermore, decreased absorption of intranasal DDAVP may occur in patients experiencing epistaxis, in those with nasal anatomical or inflammatory conditions, or in young uncooperative children [41]. Consequently, although intranasal administration of DDAVP may be useful in certain circumstances (e.g., control of heavy menstrual bleeding), it may be less reliable in other situations.

The side effects of DDAVP are generally mild and transient and include tachycardia, flushing, and headache. An important but rare side effect of DDAVP is seizures, which can occur because of the antidiuretic properties of DDAVP that can lead to fluid overload and consequent hyponatremia. For this reason, DDAVP should generally be limited to once daily administration and should be used with extreme caution in very young children (<3 years), in elderly patients, or in those receiving IV fluids. In all three groups, fluid intake should be restricted for 12–24 h following administration, and patients on IV solutions should only receive isotonic solutions (e.g., normal saline) in the 24 h following DDAVP administration. With repeated exposure to DDAVP, stores of VWF become reduced. Consequently, after multiple consecutive doses, the hemostatic effect is diminished in many patients (a phenomenon known as "tachyphylaxis"). A study by Castaman et al. [42] showed a 30% fall in response to DDAVP after the second day of DDAVP administration. Consequently, most centers will limit use of DDAVP to no more than two or three consecutive doses [43]. If clinically significant tachyphylaxis occurs, one option is to use an alternating combination of a VWF concentrate and DDAVP.

Table 5. Initial dosing recommendations for VWF-containing concentrate replacement for prevention or management of bleeding

	Major surgery/bleeding	Minor surgery/bleeding	Uncomplicated surgery
Types of surgery	Cardiothoracic surgery Cesarean section Craniotomy Hysterectomy Open cholecystectomy Prostatectomy Tonsillectomy Adenoidectomy Dental extractions that are surgically complexed[b] (i.e., extraction of mandibular wisdom teeth)	Biopsy: breast, cervix, liver Central line placement Laparoscopic procedures Gingival surgery Circumcision Complicated dental extractions[b] (i.e., extraction of primary or secondary dentition for 3 or more teeth per one procedure or maxillary wisdom teeth)	Cardiac catherization Cataract surgery Endoscopy (without biopsy) Lacerations Simple dental extraction[b] (i.e., extraction of primary dentition for 1–2 teeth per one procedure)
Loading dose	40–60 IU/kg[a]	30–60 IU/kg[a]	30–60 IU/kg[a]
Maintenance dose	20–40 IU/kg[a] every 8–24 h	20–40 IU/kg[a] every 12–48 h	N/A
Duration of treatment	7–14 days	1–5 days	N/A
Monitoring	Frequent platelet-dependent VWF activity and FVIII:C trough and peak levels	Platelet-dependent VWF activity and FVIII:C trough and peak level, at least once	N/A
Therapeutic goal	Trough platelet-dependent VWF activity and FVIII:C >0.50 IU/mL for at least 3 days		N/A
Safety parameters	-Do not exceed platelet-dependent VWF activity and FVIII:C 1.5 IU/mL -May alternate with DDAVP for latter part of treatment		N/A

FVIII:C, factor VIII coagulant; IU, international unit; N/A, not applicable; VWF, von Willebrand factor. [a]Dosing is in platelet-dependent VWF activity per kg body weight from Nichols et al. [53]. [b]Regional mandibular blocks are contraindicated in persons with von Willebrand disease undergoing invasive dental procedures. Buccal infiltrations or intraligamentary single-tooth anesthesia and techniques to protect soft tissue should be used instead [58–60].

VWF/FVIII Concentrates

When the DDAVP response is insufficient or its use contraindicated, VWF-containing concentrates can be used. There are several plasma-derived VWF-containing concentrates. These are differentiated by the ratio of VWF to FVIII. Haemate-P (Humate-P®) has a VWF:FVIII ratio of 2.5:1, Wilate® has a ratio of 1:1, whereas Fandhi®/Alphanate® has a ratio of 0.5:1. All these products undergo one or more viral inactivation steps to minimize the risk of blood-borne infections. See Table 5 for dosing of VWF-containing concentrates.

Plasma-derived VWF-containing concentrates are generally well tolerated with minimal complications or side effects. Although the product is virally inactivated, a small theoretical risk of transmitting infection persists. For this reason, individuals with VWD who are hepatitis A and/or B antibody negative should be immunized prophylactically. There have been a small number of thromboembolic events reported in individuals who are treated with VWF-containing concentrates, mainly in those with other risk factors. Anti-VWF antibodies to VWF are rare but have been reported in individuals with type 3 VWD – particularly those with large deletion variants [44].

Recently, a recombinant form of VWF (rVWF) has been developed. Published results from phase III study in adults in 2015 and the recent ones in 2022 showed the recombinant product to be safe and hemostatically effective in persons with severe VWD [45, 46]. The study also demonstrated that the rVWF induced a sustained stability of endogenous FVIII, which led to postulation that coadministration of rFVIII may only be needed in the initial infusion when treating a bleed, but this needs additional study.

In the updated guideline on management of VWD in 2021, long-term prophylactic treatment is recommended for patients with a history of frequent and severe bleeding [47]. Although the indications for prophylaxis include recurrent gastrointestinal bleeding, hemarthrosis, epistaxis, and heavy menstrual bleeding, the median dose and the frequency of VWF/FVIII concentrate used for prophylaxis varied across studies [48]. A recent systematic review provided evidenced that long-term prophylaxis decreases spontaneous bleeding, epistaxis, and hospitalization [49]. Additionally, long-term prophylaxis in persons with VWD who had recurrent hemarthrosis reduced joint bleeds [50] and preserved joint status if it was introduced before the age of 5 years [51]. Unlike for hemarthrosis, regular prophylaxis for gastrointestinal bleeding was less effective (49% versus 86%) [50, 52].

Cryoprecipitate

Cryoprecipitate is a blood product that contains VWF, FVIII, fibrinogen, and factor XIII (FXIII). Cryoprecipitate is screened for human immunodeficiency virus and hepatitis B and C but is not virally inactivated. In patients with VWD, it should only be used if the response to DDAVP is insufficient and plasma-derived virus-inactivated FVIII/VWF or recombinant VWF concentrates are not available. Cryoprecipitate is dosed at 1 unit per 5–10 kg body weight and should be infused over 10–30 min. In most developed countries, cryoprecipitate is no longer used in the management of VWD due to the higher risk of transmission of infection.

Perioperative Management

Prior to someone with VWD undergoing invasive surgical procedures, a plan for hemostatic management should be developed. Ideally surgery in individuals with VWD, particularly in those with more severe forms of VWD, should only be performed in centers with expertise in the management of persons with VWD. Specific treatment plans should be based on prior laboratory testing, including the response to DDAVP or to VWF-containing concentrates.

Depending on the extent of the invasive procedure and the person's known response to DDAVP, either DDAVP or VWF-containing concentrates may be used. DDAVP should be given 1 h prior to dental/surgical intervention and can be given daily for up to 2 or at most 3 consecutive days. A general recommendation for dosing of VWF-containing concentrates for surgery is to aim to raise FVIII:C and VWF to adequate levels to allow for perioperative hemostasis [53]. However, when rVWF is used, the measurement of FVIII:C and VWF after administration of rVWF at 12–24 h prior to the surgery can be done to see the response in that individual. Coadministration of rFVIII should be considered if the target FVIII:C level in the circulation is not achieved [54].

Management of Heavy Menstrual Bleeding in VWD

Management of heavy menstrual bleeding can be considered in both the acute and chronic settings. This subject has been reviewed, and a consensus guideline has been published by an international expert panel [55]. For a complete discussion of this topic, see Chapter 5.

Management of Epistaxis

Epistaxis is one of the most frequent types of bleeding in children with VWD and occurs in all forms of VWD, particularly during the school age years. Although VWD itself predisposes to epistaxis, concomitant trauma to the nose (as caused by nose picking), mucosal dryness (as seen in dry climates or in dry seasons), and rhinitis can contribute to the occurrence of epistaxis. Given its frequency, quantifying the severity of epistaxis in any individual with VWD calls for the use of validated epistaxis scoring tools. The Katsanis score was developed to quantify the severity of epistaxis on the basis of five characteristics: frequency; duration; amount; involvement of one or both nostrils; and a measure of what proportion of a child's life has been affected by epistaxis [11] (see Appendix I). More recently developed bleeding severity scores have also incorporated semiquantitative definitions of epistaxis severity.

When managing epistaxis in children with VWD, two issues need to be addressed. The first is the immediate management of epistaxis in a child who is currently bleeding. For this, appropriately applied pressure for 5–10 min to the soft part of the nostrils in order to compress the vessels (Kiesselbach's plexus) in the anterior nares may stop bleeding. In situations where it is not stopped, then tranexamic acid +/− DDAVP (intranasal, SC, or IV) or a VWF-containing concentrate may be required. For those patients who require such therapy, there may be a role for nasal packing by someone experienced in doing so, i.e., an ear, nose, and throat specialist, an emergency department physician, or an individual experienced with nasal packing. The second major issue is the prevention of epistaxis in children suffering from recurrent epistaxis. For this, local measures may be useful: regular humidification of the nasal mucosa and reducing trauma to the nose by discouraging nose picking, and lubrication of the nose by application of various creams or ointments (e.g., Vaseline, Polysporin) to the anterior nares twice daily. One study showed the benefit of Premarin cream applied daily for 3 consecutive days to be useful in reducing the frequency of epistaxis [56]. Finally, for some affected individuals, particularly those with type 3 VWD with frequent severe episodes of epistaxis, regular prophylaxis with a VWF-containing concentrate may be indicated.

Prophylaxis in VWD

Recent studies suggest VWF prophylaxis to be safe and efficacious in reducing bleeding; however, it is not known which regimen should be used [50, 57]. We recommend that prophylaxis be considered in any person with VWD who has repeated severe bleeds (e.g., joint bleeds, epistaxis requiring transfusions or treatment with a VWF-containing concentrate, heavy menstrual bleeding leading to severe anemia or requiring treatment with a VWF-containing concentrate) or who suffers a major life-threatening bleed, e.g., ICH or gastrointestinal bleed with a significant drop in hemoglobin. Although there is no consensus on the ideal prophylaxis regimen, the escalating dose prophylaxis regimen suggested by Abshire et al. [57] is a reasonable approach. This approach starts with once per week dosing, generally using 50 platelet-dependent VWF activity IU/kg, and then escalating to twice per week and finally to 3 times/week or every other day if unacceptable bleeding continues. For prophylaxis for heavy menstrual bleeding, escalation prophylaxis commences with 50 platelet-dependent VWF activity IU/kg given on day 1 of menstruation and then escalates to the same dose given on both days 1 and 2 and finally to the same dose given on the first 3 days of menstruation.

Conclusion

VWD is a common bleeding disorder with a wide spectrum of clinical severity. Clinical suspicion is often based on the individual's history and/or a family history of mucocutaneous bleeding. Laboratory investigations are needed to confirm the diagnosis and the specific VWD subtype. Many therapies are available, and treatment strategies must take into account the pathophysiology of the individual's VWD and its responsiveness to therapy as well as the expected severity of the bleed/bleeding challenge.

Acknowledgements

Our special thanks go to Vicky R. Breakey and Manuel D. Carcao who were the authors of this chapter in the first and second editions of this Handbook, which provided a valuable background for this updated chapter. The authors express their appreciation for the thoughtful comments provided by Margaret L. Rand for this edition.

Conflict of Interest Statement

Rungrote Natesirinilkul reports receiving consultancy and speaker fees from Sanofi-Genzyme, Novo Nordisk, Pfizer, Roche, Takeda, Grifols, and Novartis. He is a recipient of research grants from Novo Nordisk Access to Insight Grant, Roche and World Bleeding Disorder Registry-Research Support Program (WBDR-RSP) of the World Federation of Hemophilia. Lara Lobianco e Souza has no conflicts of interest to declare. Chris Barnes has no conflicts of interest to declare. Victor S. Blanchette reports receiving consultancy and speaker fees from Bayer HealthCare, Sanofi-Genzyme, Novo Nordisk, Pfizer, Roche, Takeda, and Spark Therapeutics. He is a recipient of research grants from Sanofi-Genzyme, Bayer HealthCare, and Takeda and serves as a member of Data Safety Monitoring Boards for Octapharma and Takeda. He is Chair of a nonprofit organization, the International Prophylaxis Study Group (IPSG). Paula D. James reports receiving research funding from Bayer and has done consultant work for Band Therapeutics and Star Therapeutics.

Author Contributions

Rungrote Natesirinilkul drafted the chapter, critically revised the chapter, and approved the final version. Lara Lobianco e Souza critically revised the chapter and approved the final version. Chris Barnes critically revised the chapter and approved the final version. Victor S. Blanchette critically revised the chapter and approved the final version. Paula D. James drafted the chapter, critically revised the chapter, and approved the final version.

Abbreviations

ADAMTS13	A disintegrin and metalloproteinase with a thrombospondin type 1 motif, member 13
aPTT	Activated partial thromboplastin time
ASA	Acetylsalicylic acid
ASH	American Society of Hematology
AVWS	Acquired von Willebrand syndrome
BAT	Bleeding Assessment Tool
CBC	Complete blood count
Da	Dalton
DDAVP	1-Deamino-8-D-arginine vasopressin (desmopressin)
EACA	Epsilon-aminocaproic acid (Amicar)
ELISA	Enzyme-linked immunosorbent assay
FVIII	Factor VIII
FXIII	Factor XIII
FVIII:C	Factor VIII coagulant
GP	Glycoprotein
HIV	Human immunodeficiency virus
HMW	High-molecular-weight
ICH	Intracranial hemorrhage
ISTH	International Society on Thrombosis and Haemostasis
ITP	Immune thrombocytopenia
IU	International unit
IV	Intravenous
NHF	National Hemophilia Foundation
NSAIDs	Nonsteroidal anti-inflammatory drugs
PBAC	Pictorial Blood Loss Assessment Chart
PBQ	Pediatric Bleeding Questionnaire
PFA-100®/200®	Platelet function analyzer-100®/200®
PO	Per oral
PRP	Platelet-rich plasma
RIPA	Ristocetin-induced platelet agglutination
SC	Subcutaneous
SSC	Scientific and Standardization Committee
VWD	von Willebrand disease
VWF	von Willebrand factor
VWF:Act	von Willebrand factor activity
VWF:Ag	von Willebrand factor antigen
VWF:CB	von Willebrand factor collagen binding assay
VWF:RCo	von Willebrand factor activity (ristocetin cofactor assay)
WFH	World Federation of Hemophilia

References

1 Bolton-Maggs PH, Lillicrap D, Goudemand J, Berntorp E. von Willebrand disease update: diagnostic and treatment dilemmas. Haemophilia. 2008;14 Suppl 3:56–61.

2 Hough C, Notley C, Mo A, Videl B, Lillicrap D. Heterogeneity and reciprocity of FVIII and VWF expression, and the response to shear stress in cultured human endothelial cells. J Thromb Haemost. 2022;20(11):2507–18.

3 Lillicrap D. The basic science, diagnosis, and clinical management of von Willebrand disease. In: Schulman S, editor. Treatment of Hemophilia. 2nd ed. Montréal (QC): World Federation of Hemophilia; 2008. vol 35. p. 1–18.

4 Sadler JE, Budde U, Eikenboom JC, Favaloro EJ, Hill FG, Holmberg L, et al; Working Party on von Willebrand Disease Classification. Update on the pathophysiology and classification of von Willebrand disease: a report of the Subcommittee on von Willebrand Factor. J Thromb Haemost. 2006;4(10): 2103–14.

5 James PD, Connell NT, Ameer B, Di Paola J, Eikenboom J, Giraud N, et al. ASH ISTH NHF WFH 2021 guidelines on the diagnosis of von Willebrand disease. Blood Adv. 2021;5(1):280–300.

6 Seidizadeh O, Peyvandi F, Mannucci PM. Von Willebrand disease type 2N: an update. J Thromb Haemost. 2021;19(4): 909–16.

7 Bowman M, Riddel J, Rand ML, Tosetto A, Silva M, James PD. Evaluation of the diagnostic utility for von Willebrand disease of a pediatric bleeding questionnaire. J Thromb Haemost. 2009;7(8): 1418–21.

8 Rodeghiero F, Tosetto A, Abshire T, Arnold DM, Coller B, James P, et al; ISTH/SSC Joint VWF and Perinatal/ Pediatric Hemostasis Subcommittees Working Group. ISTH/SSC bleeding assessment tool: a standardized questionnaire and a proposal for a new bleeding score for inherited bleeding disorders. J Thromb Haemost. 2010; 8(9):2063–5.

9 Higham JM, O'Brien PM, Shaw RW. Assessment of menstrual blood loss using a pictorial chart. Br J Obstet Gynaecol. 1990;97(8):734–9.

10 Spence M, de Repentigny K, Bowman M, Hopman W, Thibeault L, James P. Validation of the pictorial blood loss assessment chart using modern sanitary products. Haemophilia. 2021;27(5): e632–5.

11 Katsanis E, Luke KH, Hsu E, Li M, Lillicrap D. Prevalence and significance of mild bleeding disorders in children with recurrent epistaxis. J Pediatr. 1988;113(1 Pt 1):73–6.

12 Deforest M, Grabell J, Albert S, Young J, Tuttle A, Hopman WM, et al. Generation and optimization of the self-administered bleeding assessment tool and its validation as a screening test for von Willebrand disease. Haemophilia. 2015; 21(5):e384–8.

13 Lavin M, Christopherson P, Grabell J, Abshire T, Flood V, Haberichter SL, et al. Longitudinal bleeding assessment in von Willebrand disease utilizing an interim bleeding score. J Thromb Haemost. 2022;20(10):2246–54.

14 Duran J, Lasky JL 3rd, Rodgers C. Use of a pediatric bleeding questionnaire in the screening of Von Willebrand disease in young females at Menarche in the primary care setting. J Pediatr Health Care. 2016;30(5):408–13.

15 Sidonio RF, Lavin M. Diagnostic pitfalls and conundrums in type 1 von Willebrand disease. Hematology Am Soc Hematol Educ Program. 2022;2022(1): 618–23.

16 Flood VH, Gill JC, Christopherson PA, Bellissimo DB, Friedman KD, Haberichter SL, et al. Critical von Willebrand factor A1 domain residues influence type VI collagen binding. J Thromb Haemost. 2012;10(7):1417–24.

17 Roberts JC, Flood VH. Laboratory diagnosis of von Willebrand disease. Int J Lab Hematol. 2015;37(Suppl 1):11–7.

18 Stufano F, Baronciani L, Pagliari MT, Franchi F, Cozzi G, Garcia-Oya I, et al. Evaluation of an heterogeneous group of patients with von Willebrand disease using an assay alternative to ristocetin induced platelet agglutination. J Thromb Haemost. 2015;13(10):1806–14.

19 Favaloro EJ, Mohammed S. Towards improved diagnosis of von Willebrand disease: comparative evaluations of several automated von Willebrand factor antigen and activity assays. Thromb Res. 2014;134(6):1292–300.

20 Jenkins PV, O'Donnell JS. ABO blood group determines plasma von Willebrand factor levels: a biologic function after all? Transfusion. 2006;46(10): 1836–44.

21 Favaloro EJ. Utility of the von Willebrand factor collagen binding assay in the diagnosis of von Willebrand disease. Am J Hematol. 2017;92(1):114–8.

22 Haberichter SL. von Willebrand factor propeptide: biology and clinical utility. Blood. 2015;126(15):1753–61.

23 James P, Lillicrap D. The role of molecular genetics in diagnosing von Willebrand disease. Semin Thromb Hemost. 2008;34(6):502–8.

24 Abildgaard CF, Suzuki Z, Harrison J, Jefcoat K, Zimmerman TS. Serial studies in von Willebrand's disease: variability versus "variants". Blood. 1980;56(4): 712–6.

25 Dutt T, Burns S, Mackett N, Benfield C, Lwin R, Keenan R. Application of UKHCDO 2004 guidelines in type 1 von Willebrand Disease – a single centre paediatric experience of the implications of altered or removed diagnosis. Haemophilia. 2011;17(3):522–6.

26 Lavin M, O'Donnell JS. How I treat low von Willebrand factor levels. Blood. 2019;133(8):795–804.

27 Labarque V, Perinparajah V, Bouskill V, Stain AM, Wakefield C, Manuel C, et al. Utility of factor VIII and factor VIII to von Willebrand factor ratio in identifying 277 unselected carriers of hemophilia A. Am J Hematol. 2017;92(6):E94–6.

28 Casonato A, Pontara E, Sartorello F, Cattini MG, Sartori MT, Padrini R, et al. Reduced von Willebrand factor survival in type Vicenza von Willebrand disease. Blood. 2002;99(1):180–4.

29 Sanders YV, Groeneveld D, Meijer K, Fijnvandraat K, Cnossen MH, van der Bom JG, et al; WiN study group. von Willebrand factor propeptide and the phenotypic classification of von Willebrand disease. Blood. 2015;125(19): 3006–13.

30 Seidizadeh O, Baronciani L, Pagliari MT, Cozzi G, Colpani P, Cairo A, Siboni SM, Biguzzi E, Peyvandi F. Genetic determinants of enhanced von Willebrand factor clearance from plasma. J Thromb Haemost. 2023;21(5):1112–22.

31 Flood VH. New insights into genotype and phenotype of VWD. Hematology Am Soc Hematol Educ Program. 2014; 2014(1):531–5.
32 Carcao MD, Seary ME, Casas M, Winter L, Stain AM, Judd P. Dental disease in type 3 Von Willebrand disease: a neglected problem. Haemophilia. 2010; 16(6):943–8.
33 Mannucci PM. Treatment of von Willebrand's Disease. N Engl J Med. 2004; 351(7):683–94.
34 Rodeghiero F, Castaman G, Tosetto A. How I treat von Willebrand disease. Blood. 2009;114(6):1158–65.
35 Carter G, Goss A, Lloyd J, Tocchetti R. Tranexamic acid mouthwash versus autologous fibrin glue in patients taking warfarin undergoing dental extractions: a randomized prospective clinical study. J Oral Maxillofac Surg. 2003;61(12): 1432–5.
36 Ker K, Beecher D, Roberts I. Topical application of tranexamic acid for the reduction of bleeding. Cochrane Database Syst Rev. 2013;7:CD010562.
37 Chornenki NLJ, Um KJ, Mendoza PA, Samienezhad A, Swarup V, Chai-Adisaksopha C, et al. Risk of venous and arterial thrombosis in non-surgical patients receiving systemic tranexamic acid: A systematic review and meta-analysis. Thromb Res. 2019;179: 81–6.
38 Lee SG, Fralick J, Wallis CJD, Boctor M, Sholzberg M, Fralick M. Systematic review of hematuria and acute renal failure with tranexamic acid. Eur J Haematol. 2022;108(6):510–7.
39 Connell NT, James PD, Brignardello-Petersen R, Abdul-Kadir R, Ameer B, Arapshian A, et al. von Willebrand disease: proposing definitions for future research. Blood Adv. 2021;5(2):565–9.
40 Lusher JM. Pharmacology and pharmacokinetics of desmopressin in haemostatic disorders. Drug Invest. 1990;2 (Suppl 5):25–31.
41 Leissinger C, Carcao M, Gill JC, Journeycake J, Singleton T, Valentino L. Desmopressin (DDAVP) in the management of patients with congenital bleeding disorders. Haemophilia. 2014;20(2):158–67.
42 Castaman G, Lethagen S, Federici AB, Tosetto A, Goodeve A, Budde U, et al. Response to desmopressin is influenced by the genotype and phenotype in type 1 von Willebrand disease (VWD): results from the European Study MCMDM-1VWD. Blood. 2008;111(7):3531–9.
43 Neff AT, Sidonio RF Jr. Management of VWD. Hematology Am Soc Hematol Educ Program. 2014;2014(1):536–41.
44 James PD, Lillicrap D, Mannucci PM. Alloantibodies in von Willebrand disease. Blood. 2013;122(5):636–40.
45 Gill JC, Castaman G, Windyga J, Kouides P, Ragni M, Leebeek FW, Obermann-Slupetzky O, Chapman M, Fritsch S, Pavlova BG, Presch I, Ewenstein B. Hemostatic efficacy, safety, and pharmacokinetics of a recombinant von Willebrand factor in severe von Willebrand disease. Blood. 2015;126(17):2038–46.
46 Leebeek FWG, Peyvandi F, Escobar M, Tiede A, Castaman G, Wang M, et al. Recombinant von Willebrand factor prophylaxis in patients with severe von Willebrand disease: phase 3 study results. Blood. 2022;140(2):89–98.
47 Connell NT, Flood VH, Brignardello-Petersen R, Abdul-Kadir R, Arapshian A, Couper S, et al. ASH ISTH NHF WFH 2021 guidelines on the management of von Willebrand disease. Blood Adv. 2021;5(1):301–25.
48 Franchini M, Seidizadeh O, Mannucci PM. Prophylactic management of patients with von Willebrand disease. Ther Adv Hematol. 2021;12: 20406207211064064.
49 El Alayli A, Brignardello Petersen R, Husainat NM, Kalot MA, Aljabiri Y, et al. Outcomes of long-term von Willebrand factor prophylaxis use in von Willebrand disease: A systematic literature review. Haemophilia. 2022;28(3): 373–87.
50 Abshire TC, Federici AB, Alvárez MT, Bowen J, Carcao MD, Cox Gill J, et al; VWD PN. Prophylaxis in severe forms of von Willebrand's disease: results from the von Willebrand Disease Prophylaxis Network (VWD PN). Haemophilia. 2013;19(1):76–81.
51 Berntorp E, Petrini P. Long-term prophylaxis in von Willebrand disease. Blood Coagul Fibrinolysis. 2005;16 Suppl 1:S23–6.
52 Chornenki NLJ, Ocran E, James PD. Special considerations in GI bleeding in VWD patients. Hematology Am Soc Hematol Educ Program. 2022;2022(1): 624–30.
53 Nichols WL, Hultin MB, James AH, Manco-Johnson MJ, Montgomery RR, Ortel TL, et al. von Willebrand disease (VWD): evidence-based diagnosis and management guidelines, the National Heart, Lung, and Blood Institute (NHLBI) Expert Panel report (USA). Haemophilia. 2008;14(2):171–232.
54 Peyvandi F, Mamaev A, Wang JD, Stasyshyn O, Timofeeva M, Curry N, et al. Phase 3 study of recombinant von Willebrand factor in patients with severe von Willebrand disease who are undergoing elective surgery. J Thromb Haemost. 2019;17(1):52–62.
55 James AH, Kouides PA, Abdul-Kadir R, Dietrich JE, Edlund M, Federici AB, et al. Evaluation and management of acute menorrhagia in women with and without underlying bleeding disorders: consensus from an international expert panel. Eur J Obstet Gynecol Reprod Biol. 2011;158(2):124–34.
56 Ross CS, Pruthi RK, Schmidt KA, Eckerman AL, Rodriguez V. Intranasal oestrogen cream for the prevention of epistaxis in patients with bleeding disorders. Haemophilia. 2011;17(1):164.
57 Abshire T, Cox-Gill J, Kempton CL, Leebeek FW, Carcao M, Kouides P, et al. Prophylaxis escalation in severe von Willebrand disease: a prospective study from the von Willebrand Disease Prophylaxis Network. J Thromb Haemost. 2015;13(9):1585–9.
58 Kaplovitch E, Dounaevskaia V. Treatment in the dental practice of the patient receiving anticoagulation therapy. J Am Dent Assoc. 2019;150(7):602–608.
59 Kumbargere Nagraj S, Prashanti E, Aggarwal H, Lingappa A, Muthu MS, Kiran Kumar Krishanappa S, et al. Interventions for treating post-extraction bleeding. Cochrane Database Syst Rev. 2018; 3(3):CD011930.
60 Srivastava A, Santagostino E, Dougall A, Kitchen S, Sutherland M, Pipe SW, et al. WFH guidelines for the management of eemophilia, 3rd edition. Haemophilia. 2020;26 Suppl 6:1–158.

Published online: December 5, 2024

Blanchette VS, Brandão LR, Carcao MD, Kumar R, Rand ML, Revel-Vilk S (eds): SickKids Handbook of Pediatric Thrombosis and Hemostasis, ed 3, rev. and ext. Basel, Karger, 2024, pp 164–187 (DOI: 10.1159/000538215)

Rare Inherited Coagulation Factor Deficiencies

Joel Livingston[a] Victor S. Blanchette[b] Muhammad Faisal Khanani[c] Shoshana Revel-Vilk[d, e]

[a]Paediatric Hematology, Stollery Children's Hospital, The University of Alberta, Edmonton, AB, Canada; [b]Division of Hematology/Oncology, The Hospital for Sick Children, University of Toronto, Toronto, ON, Canada; [c]Pediatric Hematology, Tawam Hospital Al Ain, Abu Dhabi, United Arab Emirates; [d]Pediatric Hematology/Oncology Unit and Gaucher Unit, Shaare Zedek Medical Center, Jerusalem, Israel; [e]Faculty of Medicine, Hebrew University, Jerusalem, Israel

Introduction

Rare inherited coagulation disorders other than factor VIII (FVIII) and factor IX (FIX) deficiencies and von Willebrand disease present clinical challenges in both diagnosis and management. These conditions have variable correlations between the circulating coagulation factor level and the clinical bleeding phenotype. In addition, due to the rarity of these disorders, clinical management guidelines are sparse or lacking depending on the condition. In this chapter, we review the clinical features, laboratory findings, and treatment options for rare congenital coagulation bleeding disorders including deficiencies in factors I (fibrinogen), II (prothrombin), V (FV), VII (FVII), X (FX), XI (FXI), XIII (FXIII), plasminogen activator inhibitor type 1 (PAI-1) deficiency, α2-antiplasmin (α2-AP) deficiency and combined deficiencies of the vitamin K-dependent coagulation factors and of FV and FVIII (Table 1). The physiologic expected functional activity level for each coagulation factor must be considered when diagnosing these disorders, and results must be compared with age-matched normal ranges (see Appendix II).

An algorithm for diagnosing coagulation disorders in children with bleeding symptoms is available in Chapter 4. A carefully taken family history with an emphasis on abnormal bleeding symptoms and presence of consanguinity are important points to consider in children referred for evaluation of a possible underlying rare inherited coagulation disorder. Most of these conditions can be suspected through disturbances in the screening coagulation tests, i.e., prothrombin time (PT)/international normalized ratio (INR), activated partial thromboplastin time (aPTT), and fibrinogen activity levels, except FXIII deficiency and inherited deficiencies of the fibrinolytic pathway where abnormalities in screening coagulation tests are absent (see Chapter 4, Fig. 1). Importantly, mild (heterozygous) deficiencies can be masked by other factors. For example, a slightly reduced FXI level may be missed on the basis that the aPTT may be normal if a patient has a high FVIII level.

Table 1. Genetics, epidemiology, and management options for rare congenital factor deficiencies

Factor	Estimated prevalence	Gene/chromosome	Hemostatic level	Half-life of transfused factor	Recovery (%rise/ IU/kg given)	Factor replacement therapy	Bleeding-factor level correlation
Fibrinogen Afibrinogenemia Hypofibrinogenemia Dysfibrinogenemia	 Extremely rare Rare Rare	*FGA, FGB, FGG* Chromosome 4	0.5 g/L	2–4 days	0.017 g/L per mg/kg administered (50 mg/kg will increase the fibrinogen level by 0.8 g/L)	Plasma-derived, pathogen-inactivated fibrinogen concentrate; cryoprecipitate; FP/FFP	Strong
Prothrombin	Extremely rare	*F2* Chromosome 11	0.2–0.3 IU/mL	3-4 days	1.6%	PCCs; FP/FFP	Strong
FV	1:1,000,000	*F5* Chromosome 1	0.15–0.2 IU/mL	16–36 h	1%	FP/FFP	Poor
FV + FVIII combined	1:1,000,000	*LMAN1* Chromosome 18 *MCFD2* Chromosome 2	As for individual factors	As for individual factors	As for individual factors	FP/FFP + FVIII concentrate	Weak
FVII	1:500,000	*F7* Chromosome 13	0.15–0.2 IU/mL	4–6 h	1%	Recombinant FVIIa; plasma-derived, pathogen-inactivated FVII concentrate; PCCs; FP/FFP	Poor
FX	1:1,000,000	*F10* Chromosome 13	0.15–0.2 IU/mL	40–60 h	1.5%	Plasma-derived, pathogen-inactivated FX concentrate; PCCs; FP/FFP	Strong
FXI	Depends on ethnicity[a]	*F11* Chromosome 4	0.15–0.3 IU/mL	40–70 h	2%	FP/FFP; plasma-derived, pathogen-inactivated FXI concentrate	No association
FXIII	1:2,000,000	*F13A1* Chromosome 6 *F13B* Chromosome 1	0.1–0.2 IU/mL	11–14 days	1.7%	Recombinant FXIII[b]; plasma-derived, pathogen-inactivated FXIII concentrate; cryoprecipitate; FP/FFP	Strong

The information provided in this table reflects the opinion of the authors based on available published literature. FV, factor V; FVII, factor VII; FVIII, factor VIII; FX, factor X; FXI, factor XI; FXIII, factor XIII; FP/FFP, frozen plasma/fresh frozen plasma; PCC, prothrombin complex concentrate. [a]Common in Ashkenazi Jews. [b]Recombinant FXIII provides replacement only for subunit A (not subunit B).

10

The severe forms of these disorders require genetic variants in two alleles. As for all rare autosomal recessive diseases, rare inherited coagulation disorders are seen more frequently in ethnic groups with high consanguinity rates and occasionally in groups that tend to marry within the group, e.g., Ashkenazi Jewish, Amish, and Gypsy communities. Individuals with genetic variants in one allele (heterozygotes) are generally asymptomatic, and screening coagulation tests may be normal or abnormal depending on the circulating functional activity level of the deficient coagulation factor and functional activity levels of other coagulation factors.

Recommendations for therapy will be made throughout this chapter according to published data and the authors' clinical experience for each deficiency. A general prescriptive hierarchy should be followed based upon the safety of replacement products with regard to blood-borne pathogens: recombinant products are the first choice for treatment, followed by pathogen-inactivated and plasma-derived concentrates (see Appendix III). As a last choice, due to a potential risk of transmission of a blood-borne pathogen, blood products such as frozen plasma/fresh frozen plasma (FP/FFP) or cryoprecipitate that are ideally pathogen inactivated can be considered (details on pathogen-inactivated blood products are provided in Appendix III). For some rare factor deficiencies (e.g., a2-AP deficiency), there are no good sources of replacement, and in such cases, antifibrinolytic agents are widely used.

It is the responsibility of the prescribing physician to discuss with the affected individual or the parents/guardians of young children the potential risks, benefits, and alternatives to any recommended therapy or therapies taking into consideration the various therapeutic options available locally and after consultation with the information in relevant product monographs.

The diagnosis and management of acquired rare coagulation factor deficiencies are beyond the scope of this chapter (see Chapter 11).

Fibrinogen Disorders

Fibrinogen is a dimeric soluble molecule, composed of three pairs of polypeptide chains (α, β, and γ chains); it is the precursor of insoluble fibrin that is required for the formation of the hemostatic plug in association with platelets (see Chapter 2). In vivo, thrombin catalyzes the conversion of fibrinogen to fibrin. Other fibrinogen functions include a role in platelet aggregation and fibrinolysis. Its diversity of functions in physiologic pathways that are part of the hemostatic system explain the variety of symptoms from bleeding to thrombotic phenotypes seen within the inherited fibrinogen disorders [1].

The normal plasma fibrinogen concentration is approximately 1.5–4 g/L. Fibrinogen is produced in the liver, and its production may be increased up to 20-fold, designating it as an acute-phase reactant. It has a half-life of approximately 3–4 days. Based on clinical and laboratory findings, four types of congenital fibrinogen disorders are recognized: (1) afibrinogenemia (+/− thrombotic phenotype), (2) hypofibrinogenemia (severe, moderate, mild, and hypofibrinogenemia with fibrinogen storage disease), (3) dysfibrinogenemia (+/− thrombotic phenotype), and (4) hypodysfibrinogenemia (severe, moderate, and mild) [1]. Quantitative fibrinogen deficiencies result from variants affecting fibrinogen synthesis or processing, whereas qualitative defects are caused by variants leading to abnormal polymerization, crosslinking, or assembly of the polypeptide chains [1].

Afibrinogenemia

Afibrinogenemia is a rare congenital bleeding disorder transmitted as an autosomal recessive trait with variable penetrance. Its incidence is estimated to be 1 in 1,000,000 births, with a higher incidence in consanguineous families [2]. Afibrinogenemia is associated with homozygous or compound heterozygous variants and is diagnosed when the circulating fibrinogen level is undetectable [1].

Affected individuals may be diagnosed early in life because of prolonged bleeding from the umbilical stump (~85% of cases). However, the diagnosis may be delayed, occurring only following a significant hemostatic challenge such as surgery or trauma. Other systems may also be affected, and affected individuals may experience skin and musculoskeletal bleeds, intracranial hemorrhage (ICH), hemorrhage in the gastrointestinal and genitourinary tracts, as well as antepartum or postpartum hemorrhage and first-trimester miscarriage. Thromboembolic events may occur before and after fibrinogen replacement therapy in affected individuals; therefore, close observation and monitoring are strongly recommended.

Hypofibrinogenemia

The inheritance pattern in cases with hypofibrinogenemia is autosomal dominant, and affected individuals are usually heterozygous for fibrinogen variants with fibrinogen levels of ~0.5 g/L [3]. Affected individuals frequently have a mild bleeding phenotype or are asymptomatic. Typically, diagnosis is delayed, occurring only following a significant hemostatic challenge such as surgery or injury. Among bleeding symptoms, heavy menstrual bleeding (HMB) and intramuscular hemorrhage are most common, followed by gastrointestinal bleeding. A few hypofibrinogenemic variants lead to intrahepatic accumulation of fibrin, resulting in liver disease (fibrinogen storage disease) [4].

Dysfibrinogenemia and Hypodysfibrinogenemia

Qualitative disorders include dysfibrinogenemia (decreased functional and normal antigenic fibrinogen levels) and hypodysfibrinogenemia (discrepant decrease of functional and antigenic fibrinogen levels). Affected individuals can present clinically with either a hemorrhagic or thrombotic disorder (up to 20%). The inheritance pattern is autosomal dominant. Abnormal fibrinogen may result in thrombosis due to its incapacity to bind to thrombin, resulting in accumulation of thrombin and leading to the development of an abnormal cross-linked fibrin network resistant to plasmin, or due to its abnormal binding to platelets [1].

Diagnosis

Global screening tests, such as PT/INR, aPTT, and thrombin time (TT), require the production of a fibrin clot as an endpoint and, therefore, may be prolonged in affected individuals with hypofibrinogenemia or afibrinogenemia (see Chapter 4, Fig. 1). These global tests may be normal in affected individuals with fibrinogen levels of >0.5 g/L and in cases of qualitative fibrinogen disorders.

Among the multiple laboratory methods for the measurement of fibrinogen, the most accurate is the Clauss method [4]. This assay involves adding a high concentration of thrombin to platelet-poor plasma and determining fibrinogen concentration using a reference curve prepared by testing dilutions of standardized reference platelet-poor plasma.

A stepwise procedure is recommended for diagnosing congenital fibrinogen disorders [4]. The first step includes aPTT, PT/INR, a functional assessment of the fibrinogen level by the Clauss method, and an antigenic measurement of circulating fibrinogen, which is generally only available in a reference coagulation laboratory. If an antigenic measurement is not available, PT-derived fibrinogen (PT-Fg) (indirect measurement based on the change in light transmission or scatter from a PT curve)/Clauss ratio assay may be used [4]. The TT and reptilase time are prolonged in all the severe forms of fibrinogen disorders: congenital afibrinogenemia and individuals with

10

severe hypofibrinogenemia, dysfibrinogenemia, or hypodysfibrinogenemia, and the results of these screening tests do not distinguish between quantitative and qualitative fibrinogen disorders.

Genetics

The three fibrinogen chains (α, β, and γ) are encoded by *FGA*, *FGB*, and *FGG* genes on chromosomes 4q31.3, 4q31.3, and 4q32.1, respectively. Genotyping can be of benefit in confirming the diagnosis and facilitating family screening. For cases with dysfibrinogenemia, the genotype may correlate with the clinical phenotype, particularly in the case of thrombotic variants [4].

Management

Antifibrinolytic agents may be sufficient for mild bleeding or minor surgery in affected individuals with hypofibrinogenemia/afibrinogenemia or hemorrhagic dysfibrinogenemia (dosing recommendations are provided in Appendix III) [5]. Replacement therapy should be considered for severe bleeding or major surgery [5]. Plasma-derived fibrinogen concentrates are available in many countries and are the preferred treatment option; where unavailable, cryoprecipitate or FP/FFP can also provide a source of fibrinogen (see Appendix III). The recommended pediatric doses for fibrinogen concentrates are described in Table 2. Doses are targeted to achieve a trough fibrinogen activity level of ≥1 g/L (children with life-threatening hemorrhage may require 200 mg/kg initially), and continuous infusions have also been anecdotally described. The plasma half-life of fibrinogen is approximately 3–4 days, thereby allowing every other day replacement therapy. If a fibrinogen concentrate is unavailable, cryoprecipitate can be used. One unit of cryoprecipitate from a single donor contains approximately 300 mg of fibrinogen (see Appendix III). The dose is 1 unit of cryoprecipitate per 5–10 kg to raise the fibrinogen concentration by 0.5–1 g/L. FP/FFP can also be used at a dose of 15–25 mL/kg and should be pathogen inactivated if available [6].

Long-term prophylaxis with weekly infusions of fibrinogen concentrate to maintain trough activity >0.5 g/L is recommended based on the history of severe bleeding or if fibrinogen activity is <0.1 g/L. Long-term prophylaxis is suggested following ICH [7].

HMB may be managed with oral contraceptives, a levonorgestrel intrauterine device, replacement therapy, and/or antifibrinolytic agents [7] (see Chapter 5). For pregnancy, fibrinogen levels should be maintained at or above 0.5 g/L during the first and second trimesters, at or above 1 g/L in the late third trimester and at or above 1.5 g/L during labor and delivery (for 3 days) [7]. The risk of thromboembolic events associated with afibrinogenemia and fibrinogen replacement therapy should be kept in mind when caring for affected individuals with fibrinogen defects.

For cases with a dysfibrinogenemia variant not previously associated with bleeding or thrombosis and with no personal or family history of bleeding or thrombosis, routine thromboprophylaxis should be considered after surgery and delivery; fibrinogen replacement is only indicated if there is abnormal bleeding [5, 8]. There is no standard antithrombotic therapy in affected individuals who develop thrombotic events, although using fibrinogen concentrate to balance the anticoagulant treatment is a common practice [7, 9].

Prothrombin Deficiency

Prothrombin (FII) deficiency is among the rarest of all congenital bleeding disorders, occurring in approximately 1 in 1–2 million births [2]. Prothrombin is a vitamin K-dependent glycoprotein whose activated form is thrombin, a pivotal enzyme responsible for cleaving fibrinogen to fibrin, and subsequently contributing to the formation of a stable fibrin thrombus (see Chapter 2). The plasma half-life of prothrombin is approximately 60 h. The inheritance of prothrombin deficiency is autosomal recessive; two phenotypes

Table 2. Dosing and therapeutic target levels for the rare coagulation factor deficiencies[a]

Concentrate, trade name[b]	Dosing[c]
Fibrinogen RiaSTAP® (CSL Behring) Haemocomplettan® P (CSL Behring) CLOTTAFACT® (LFB, France) FibCLOT® (LFB, France) Fibryga® (Octapharma AG, trade name in the US: Fibryna™)	*Bleeding*: 50–100 mg/kg, with smaller doses repeated, if necessary, at 2–4 days. Higher and more frequent doses may be required in children. Therapeutic target: • Major bleeding: plasma fibrinogen level of 1.5 g/L for 7 days • Minor bleeding: plasma fibrinogen level of 1 g/L for 5 days *Surgery*: Dose (mg/kg): (target level [g/L] – measured level [g/L])/product general recovery** (g/L/mg/kg) **RiaSTAP®/Haemocomplettan® P: 0.017; CLOTTAFACT®/FibCLOT®: 0.023 For example: target level 1 g/L, measured baseline level 0.2 g/L, body weight 20 kg; • For RiaSTAP®/HAEMOCOMPLETTAN® P the dose: (1–0.2 g/L)/0.017 = 47.1 mg/kg; 47.1 × 20 kg = 942 mg • For CLOTTAFACT®/FibCLOT® the dose (1–0.2 g/L)/0.023 = 34.8 mg/kg; 34.8 × 20 kg = 696 mg If the initial level is unknown, the initial dosing can be 70 mg/kg Therapeutic target: plasma fibrinogen levels of 1 g/L until hemostasis is achieved and above 0.5 g/L until wound healing is complete *Prophylaxis*: 50–100 mg/kg once per week, adjusted to maintain trough plasma fibrinogen level >0.5 g/L
FVII FVII concentrate (BPL, UK) Factor VII NF (Baxalta)	*Bleeding*: 10–40 IU/kg every 4–6 h until hemostasis is achieved *Surgery*: 10–40 IU/kg every 4–6 h immediately before surgery and every 4–6 h for the duration of surgery and until hemostasis is achieved (for up to 10 days) Alternative dose: 30–40 IU/kg twice per day (for up to 10 days) *Prophylaxis:* 10–30 IU/kg, three times a week, adjusted to maintain clinical response. The dose of FVII replacement therapy and frequency of injection for prophylaxis should be based on clinical response and adapted to each affected individual.
Recombinant FVIIa NovoSeven® (Novo Nordisk)	NovoSeven® dosing in FVII deficiency is different from dosing in other approved indications. Dosing for hemophilia patients with inhibitors is detailed in Chapter 8 *Bleeding*: 15–30 µg/kg every 4–6 h until hemostasis is achieved *Surgery:* 15–30 µg/kg immediately before surgery and every 4–6 h for the duration of surgery and until hemostasis is achieved *Prophylaxis*: 20–40 µg/kg, three times a week, adjusted to maintain clinical response (prophylaxis is not an FDA- and EMA-approved indication). The dose of FVII replacement therapy and frequency of injection for prophylaxis should be based on clinical response and adapted to each individual

10

Table 2 (continued)

Concentrate, trade name[b]	Dosing[c]
FX Coagadex® (Bio Products Laboratory)	*Bleeding:* Children <12 years: 30 IU/kg. Adults/adolescents ≥12 years: 25 IU/kg. Repeat daily until hemostasis is achieved. Postoperative bleeding: Dose to target FX levels of 0.5 IU/mL *Surgery:* Dose (IU): desired FX increase (target level [IU/mL] – measured level [IU/mL])/0.02 (IU/kg) Preoperative bleeding prophylaxis: dose to target FX levels of 0.7–0.9 IU/mL *Prophylaxis*: Children <12 years: 40 IU/kg twice weekly. Adults/adolescents ≥12 years: 25 IU/kg twice weekly. Monitor trough blood levels of FX targeting ≥0.05 IU/mL and adjust dosage to clinical response and trough levels. Do not exceed a peak level of 1.2 IU/mL.
FXI - Hemoleven® (LFB, France) - FXI concentrate (BPL, UK)	FXI concentrates should be utilized with caution, as the literature demonstrates a 10% risk of arterial and venous thromboembolic events after replacement therapy in these patients (see text for further details) *Bleeding*: 10–15 IU/kg *Surgery:* Dose (IU): desired FXI increase (target level [IU/mL] – measured level [IU/mL])/0.02 (IU/kg); For example: target level 0.3 IU/mL, measured level 0.05 IU/mL, BW 20 kg; dose: (0.3–0.05 IU/mL)/0.02 = 12.5 IU/kg; 12.5 × 20 kg = 250 IU Therapeutic target: • Major surgery: plasma XI level of ~0.45 IU/mL for 7 days • Minor surgery: plasma XI level of ~0.3 IU/mL for 5 days
FXIII Fibrogammin® (CSL Behring) Corifact® (CSL Behring)	*Bleeding:* 10–20 IU/kg. Daily for severe hemorrhage and extensive hematoma until bleeding has stopped. *Surgery:* up to 35 IU/kg to obtain normal FXIII levels. Required efficacy should be maintained by repeated injection until the wound has healed completely. *Prophylaxis*: 20–40 IU/kg, approximately once a month. Should be guided by the most recent trough FXIII activity level to maintain a trough FXIII activity level of approximately 0.05–0.2 IU/mL. Interval should be shortened if spontaneous hemorrhage develops.
Recombinant FXIII NovoThirteen® (Novo Nordisk) Tretten® (Novo Nordisk)	*Prophylaxis:* 35 IU/kg once a month. Dose adjustment, based on FXIII activity levels, can be considered necessary when the prevention of bleeding is not appropriately covered. This dose adjustment should be based on FXIII activity levels. Suggest maintaining FXIII trough level >0.1 IU/mL. This product is not indicated in patients with FXIII-B subunit deficiency

Table 2 (continued)

Concentrate, trade name[b]	Dosing[c]
PCCs	For treatment and/or prevention of bleeding in patients with congenital factor II, FVII, FX, and familial vitamin K deficiency. The recommended dose of PCCs depends on the amount of each factor in the specific product. It should be emphasized that not only is there a marked difference in factor content between the different commercial preparations, but factor content can also vary between product lots produced by the same manufacturer. (Note: Some PCCs do not contain an acceptable concentration of FVII for clinical use in patients with FVII deficiency)

EMA, European Medicines Agency; FVII, factor VII; FX, factor X; FXI, factor XI; FXIII, factor XIII; FDA, Food and Drug Administration; PCCs, prothrombin complex concentrates. [a] The information provided in this table reflects the opinion of the authors alone based on available published literature and information received from the following manufacturers of coagulation factor concentrates listed in the table. Of note, it is the responsibility of the prescribing physician to discuss with the patient and the parent/guardian of young children the potential risks, benefits, and alternatives to any recommended therapy or therapies taking into consideration the various therapeutic options available locally, and after consultation with the information in relevant product monographs. [b] The trade name list is *not* complete. Readers should refer to the local reference for products available in their country. [c] In general, dosing regimen should be individualized based on body weight, laboratory values, and the affected individual's clinical condition. See text for further data.

10

can be distinguished: (1) true hypoprothrombinemia (type I deficiency), characterized by concomitantly low levels of the zymogen antigen; and (2) dysprothrombinemia (type II deficiency), characterized by normal or near-normal synthesis of a dysfunctional protein [2].

Clinical Features

Symptoms usually correlate with the level of the functional protein [10]. The complete absence of prothrombin seems to be incompatible with life. Affected individuals who are homozygous or compound heterozygous may present with moderate to severe bleeding symptoms as early as the neonatal period. The most common manifestations include easy bruising, gingival bleeding, HMB, epistaxis or bleeding after surgery, dental extraction, or postpartum hemorrhage [2]. Hemarthrosis, umbilical cord bleeding, and ICH are also described in severe cases. Affected individuals with prothrombin levels >0.3 IU/mL may remain asymptomatic [6].

Diagnosis

Low prothrombin activity typically prolongs both the aPTT and PT/INR (see Chapter 4, Fig. 1), whereas the TT is normal. Functional and antigenic assays are required for the diagnosis of type I or type II deficiency.

Genetics

The *F2* gene resides on chromosome 11p11.2 with more than 40 variants described.

Management

Affected individuals with an FII activity >0.2 IU/mL usually do not require replacement therapy, but antifibrinolytic agents may be considered (dosing recommendations are provided in Appendix III) [2]. Antifibrinolytic agents may also be sufficient to control mild bleeding episodes or for minor procedures in affected individuals with an FII activity <0.2 IU/mL [5].

No purified prothrombin concentrates are available, making prothrombin complex concentrates (PCCs) and FP/FFP the mainstay of treatment [6]. Severe bleeding episodes can be treated

Table 3. Categories of clinical bleeding severity based on the European Network of Rare Bleeding Disorders

Severity of bleeding	Definition
Asymptomatic	No recorded bleeding
Grade I	Bleeding events resulting from trauma or related to the use of antiplatelet or anticoagulant medication
Grade II	Spontaneous minor bleeding, including mucocutaneous bleeding such as bruising, ecchymosis, minor wounds, oral cavity bleeding, epistaxis, and heavy menstrual bleeding
Grade III	Spontaneous major bleeding, including intracranial hemorrhage, hemarthrosis, intramuscular bleeding, gastrointestinal bleeding, and umbilical cord bleeding

Modified from Peyvandi et al. [13].

with FP/FFP at 15–25 mL/kg, which should result in an increase in prothrombin levels by 0.25 IU/mL. For prophylaxis in high-risk surgical interventions, a loading dose of 15–25 mL/kg of FP/FFP followed by 3–6 mL/kg every 12–24 h may be adequate for hemostasis. PCCs are the preferred option when available and especially when volume overload is a concern (Table 2) [5]. PCC dosing for FII deficiency requires careful monitoring of coagulation profiles; dosing of 20–40 IU/kg before surgery with further doses of 10–20 IU/kg every 48 h has been previously proposed [6].

Long-term prophylaxis for cases with a personal or family history of severe bleeding or with FII activity <0.01 IU/mL should be considered using PCC 20–40 IU/kg or FP/FFP 15–25 mL/kg once a week and adjusted to maintain trough FII activity >0.1 IU/mL [5]. The use of PCCs may be associated with thrombotic risk, in particular in affected individuals requiring prophylaxis; therefore, the evaluation of the antigen level is extremely important to ascertain the type of deficiency as it has been reported that dysfunctional FII (type II deficiency) could be associated with a thrombotic disorder [6].

HMB is reported to be frequent; when severe, it may be controlled using a prophylactic PCC regimen [7]. For delivery in women with an FII activity <0.2 IU/mL in the third trimester, PCC 20–40 IU/kg once in established labor or before cesarean section aimed to achieve an FII activity of 0.2 IU/mL is recommended [7]. Further PCC 10–20 IU/kg at 48 h to maintain an FII activity >0.2 IU/mL for at least 3 days should be considered. FP/FFP 15–25 mL/kg is an alternative if a PCC is unavailable [5].

FV Deficiency

FV deficiency is inherited in an autosomal recessive manner with a prevalence of ~1 in 1 million births [2, 11]. The bleeding phenotype of FV deficiency is variable; heterozygotes are usually asymptomatic, whereas homozygotes/compound heterozygotes exhibit a broad array of signs and symptoms ranging from minimal to severe bleeding. The half-life of FV ranges from 16–36 h. The variable phenotype may result from the availability of small amounts of FV in platelets in some affected individuals with congenital FV deficiency; in addition, reduced plasma levels of total and free tissue factor pathway inhibitor decrease the FV requirement for minimal thrombin generation in FV-deficient plasmas to <0.01 IU/mL [12]. For the 50 subjects with FV deficiency studied by the European Network of Rare Bleeding Disorders (EN-RBD), FV levels (IU/mL; 95% CI) for asymptomatic subjects and those with grade I, II, and III bleeding (Table 3) were 0.12 (0–0.34), 0.06 (0–0.28), 0 (0–0.23), and 0 (0–0.19), respectively [12]. The majority of severe cases are characterized by extremely low FV activity and antigen levels (<0.01 IU/mL) (Table 4).

Clinical Features

Individuals with severe FV deficiency are likely to present with clinical bleeding at an early age from skin and mucosal surfaces, including neonatal umbilical stump and nipple bleeding, epistaxis, gum bleeding, and subcutaneous hematomas [11]. However, milder cases may present in later childhood and adulthood with mucocutaneous and soft tissue bleeding, such as ecchymosis, easy bruising, petechiae, epistaxis, hemoptysis, hematemesis, melena, hemarthrosis, hematuria, and HMB. Cases with very low FV levels are at risk for bleeding into joints and muscles and ICH.

Diagnosis

Screening laboratory tests reveal prolongation of the PT/INR and aPTT, with normal TT and fibrinogen activity levels (see Chapter 4, Fig. 1). Measurement of FV activity is required for confirmation after excluding other causes of factor deficiencies, including liver disease or acquired antibodies to coagulation factors, such as lupus anticoagulants. Combined FV and FVIII deficiency should also be excluded (see below).

Genetics

The *F5* gene is located on the long arm of chromosome 1q24.2, spans 25 exomes, and is composed of six domains (A1, A2, A3, B, C1, and C2). Missense variants are most commonly identified (61.5%) and frequently occur at domains A2 and C2, whereas an additional 20% of variants occur at the B domain (https://f5-db.eahad.org/) [11].

Management

For mild episodes of bleeding and minor procedures, antifibrinolytic agents may be sufficient (dosing recommendations are provided in Appendix III) [6]. Currently, no FV concentrate is available for therapy, and FP/FFP remains the mainstay of treatment for moderate to severe FV deficiency when experiencing bleeding or undergoing invasive procedures. An initial preoperative dose (FP/FFP, 15–25 mL/kg) is recommended for major surgery, with additional FP/FFP (10 mL/kg every 12 h) to maintain FV levels >0.15–0.2 IU/mL until wound healing [7]. In neonates, when it is impossible to achieve adequate trough levels due to the volume of FP/FFP required, plasma exchange may be required. Platelet transfusions may be considered for unresponsive bleeding and are recommended for affected individuals with FV inhibitors [7].

For cases with a personal or family history of severe bleeding and FV activity of less than 0.05 IU/mL, short-term or long-term prophylaxis should be considered [7]. The prophylaxis dose is FP/FFP 20 mL/kg, at least twice weekly, adjusted to maintain the desired clinical response.

HMB is common and may be managed with oral contraceptives, antifibrinolytic agents, a levonorgestrel intrauterine device, and replacement therapy [7] (see Chapter 5). For delivery in women with FV activity of less than 0.20 IU/mL, FP/FFP 15–25 mL/kg once in established labor or before cesarean section, to achieve an FV activity 0.2–0.4 IU/mL is recommended [5]. Further FP/FFP 10 mL/kg at 12-hourly intervals to maintain an FV activity >0.2 IU/mL for at least 3 days is also recommended.

Combined FV and FVIII Deficiency

Combined FV and FVIII deficiency is an extremely rare condition (1:1,000,000 births) and unique among rare bleeding disorders as the condition results from an abnormality in the FV and FVIII intracellular transport pathway due to defects in the chaperone proteins, specifically lectin mannose-binding protein 1 (LMAN1) and multiple coagulation factor deficiency protein 2

Table 4. Proposed ISTH classification based on the association between coagulant factor activity and clinical bleeding severity

Coagulant factor	Laboratory phenotype/coagulant activity		
	Severe	Moderate	Mild
Fibrinogen	Undetectable	0.1–1 g/L	>1 g/L
Prothrombin	Undetectable	≤0.1 IU/mL	>0.1 IU/mL
Factor V	Undetectable	<0.1 IU/mL	≥0.1 IU/mL
Factor V + Factor VIII	<0.2 IU/mL	0.2–0.4 IU/mL	>0.4 IU/mL
Factor VII	<0.1 IU/mL	0.1–0.2 IU/mL	>0.2 IU/mL
Factor X	<0.1 IU/mL	0.1–0.4 IU/mL	>0.4 IU/mL
Factor XI	Not applicable	Not applicable	Not applicable
Factor XIII	Undetectable	<0.3 IU/mL	≥0.3 IU/mL

Modified from Peyvandi et al. [13]. ISTH, International Society on Thrombosis and Haemostasis.

(MCFD2) [2, 6]. MCFD2 plays a primary role in the export of FV and FVIII from the endoplasmic reticulum, whereas LMAN1 plays an indirect role through its interaction with MCFD2. This rare autosomal recessive condition is more common in Mediterranean countries and in individuals of Middle Eastern Jewish descent. Parents and children of a person with combined deficiency of FV and FVIII have normal FV and FVIII levels.

Clinical Features

The most commonly reported clinical symptom other than excessive bleeding after invasive procedures is mucosal bleeding. Hemarthrosis, typical in hemophilia A, occurs in less than one third of these affected individuals. The dual deficiency is not additive, thus bleeding symptoms are comparable to those observed in individuals with a single factor deficiency. Affected individuals with activity levels <0.2 IU/mL are most likely to experience spontaneous major bleeding, whereas those with levels >0.4 IU/mL are mainly asymptomatic [13] (Table 4).

Diagnosis

Screening coagulation tests reveal prolongation of both the PT/INR and aPTT (see Chapter 4, Fig. 1). Specific factor analyses reveal decreased FV and FVIII levels of approximately 0.05–0.2 IU/mL.

Genetics

The *LMAN1* and *MCFD2* genes are located on chromosome 18q21 and chromosome 2p21, respectively.

Management

Treatment is dependent on the level of each factor, the type of bleeding episode, or the nature of the procedure [7]. Treatment of bleeding episodes requires a source of both FV and FVIII; replacement of FV is achieved through the use of FP/FFP (see above), and replacement of FVIII through the use of desmopressin or FVIII concentrates (recombinant or plasma-derived FVIII products; see Chapter 8 and Appendix III). Due to the shorter half-life of FVIII (approximately 10–14 h) relative to FV (approximately 16–36 h), FP/FFP should not be administered to maintain the FVIII level, as it may lead to volume overload [5]. Therefore, for major bleeding events and surgical procedures, replacement of FVIII should be guided by protocols utilized for hemophilia A treatment, whereas FV replacement should be administered as FP/FFP every 12 h, targeting a minimal activity level of 0.25 IU/mL. Antifibrinolytic agents may be used for mild bleeding episodes or low-risk surgical procedures (dosing recommendations are provided in Appendix III) [5]. Routine long-term prophylaxis is rarely required but has been suggested in cases of recurrent severe hematomas or hemarthroses [7].

HMB is common and may be managed with oral contraceptives, antifibrinolytic agents, a levonorgestrel intrauterine device, and replacement therapy (see Chapter 5). For delivery in women with FV activity <0.2 IU/mL, FP/FFP 15–25 mL/kg once in established labor or before cesarean section to achieve FV activity 0.3–0.4 IU/mL is recommended [5]. Additional FP/FFP 10 mL/kg once every 12 h to maintain FV activity >0.2 IU/mL for at least 3 days should be considered. If the FVIII activity is <0.5 IU/mL in the third trimester, replacement with recombinant FVIII is recommended [5].

FVII Deficiency

Among the rare congenital bleeding disorders, FVII deficiency is the most frequent; the true incidence is difficult to determine due to individuals with few or no clinical symptoms and mild deficiencies [6]. FVII has the shortest half-life of the procoagulant factors, approximately 4–6 h. The incidence of clinically significant FVII deficiency (homozygous or compound heterozygous forms) is estimated to be one per 500,000 births, with no racial or ethnic group predilection, with the exception that it is more common in societies with a higher degree of consanguinity [2]. More recent data suggest that FVII deficiency might be much more prevalent than previously reported [14].

Clinical Presentation

FVII deficiency exhibits a clinically variable bleeding pattern ranging from severe life-threatening or organ-specific hemorrhage, such as ICH, gastrointestinal, and hemarthrosis, to minor mucocutaneous bleeding symptoms such as epistaxis. The International Registry on Congenital FVII Deficiency reports a poor association between the clinical bleeding phenotype and circulating FVII activity levels, more significant bleeding manifestations among females, and frequent surgery-related bleeding, which may often serve as the diagnostic trigger in previously asymptomatic individuals [15]. A potentially significant FVII deficiency is considered ≤0.25 IU/mL [16]. However, bleeding is uncommon with FVII levels >0.1 IU/mL, and spontaneous bleeding is unusual with FVII levels >0.2 IU/mL. Even so, severe bleeding has been reported in some rare cases with FVII activity >0.2 IU/mL [10] (Table 4). In general, those who presented with bleeding have a higher likelihood of further bleeding; thus, a personal and family history is important to estimate the bleeding phenotype in individual cases [16]. For 203 subjects with FVII deficiency studied by the EN-RBD, FVII levels (IU/mL; 95% CI) for asymptomatic subjects and those with grade I, II, and III bleeding (Table 3) were 0.25 (0.15–0.35), 0.19 (0.08–0.3), 0.13 (0.02–0.25), and 0.08 (0–0.21), respectively [12].

Diagnosis

FVII deficiency is characterized by an isolated prolongation of the PT/INR (see Chapter 4, Fig. 1). Liver disease and vitamin K deficiency must be excluded. An FVII activity assay is commonly available and has been standardized to reduce the variability of interlaboratory determinations, particularly of low to very low plasma FVII levels.

Genetics

Molecular diagnosis is available, with a broad spectrum of variants characterized in the *FVII* gene, located on chromosome 13 (https://f7-db.eahad.org/) [14]. Of note, the gene for FVII is adjacent to the gene for FX on chromosome 13, and large deletions may cause minor deficiency of both factors. Affected individuals with moderate

10

and severe disease are either homozygotes or compound heterozygotes for an FVII variant. However, phenotype-genotype correlations can be challenging as even individuals homozygous for the same variant do not always present with the same bleeding severity, most likely due to some polymorphisms that cause altered expression of FVII in the circulation.

Management

Replacement therapy for affected individuals with FVII deficiency should be individualized and is dependent on the bleeding history, severity of the deficiency, site of bleeding, type of intervention required (i.e., major or minor surgery), and the presence of comorbidities [16]. It is recommended that affected individuals with FVII deficiency should be considered at a higher risk for bleeding if the FVII activity is <0.1 IU/mL or if there is a coexisting coagulopathy or a personal history of bleeding [5]. Antifibrinolytic agents may be sufficient to provide hemostatic cover for surgery in affected individuals with low bleeding risk, for treatment of mild bleeding, or the provision of hemostatic cover for minor surgery for those with higher bleeding risk (dosing recommendations are provided in Appendix III). However, for the provision of hemostatic cover for major surgical procedures in affected individuals with a higher risk for bleeding or more significant bleeds, FVII replacement is recommended [5]. The minimal FVII level required to prevent excess bleeding during surgery is not clearly defined; recommendations range for FVII trough levels of >0.08, 0.1–0.2, and >0.2 IU/mL, reflecting interpatient differences and the hemostatic requirements of each surgical procedure [7].

Recombinant activated FVII (rFVIIa), if available, is the replacement product most often used, although it does not represent the deficient protein, i.e., nonactivated FVII. Consequently, certain features, such as the short in vivo half-life and the increased clearance in young children, influence the treatment plan. The recommended dose is a bolus of 15–30 μg/kg every 4–6 h until hemostasis is achieved [7]; it is important to note that these doses are significantly lower than those used in hemophilia patients with inhibitors (Table 2). The plasma half-life of rFVIIa has been estimated around 3 h, although the biological effect may be more prolonged because of interstitial redistribution of rFVIIa [5]. Longer half-life of rFVIIa concentrates are under development but not yet licensed for commercial use [6].

If rFVIIa is unavailable, other alternatives exist, including plasma-derived, pathogen-inactivated FVII concentrates, PCCs containing FVII and FP/FFP (Table 2). Plasma-derived, pathogen-inactivated FVII concentrate 10–40 IU/kg every 4–6 h has a similar efficacy to rFVIIa, with an estimated plasma half-life of 5–6 h; however, a theoretical chance of transmission of blood-borne agents exists, depending upon the specific viral inactivation processes utilized, e.g., vapor heat treatment or nanofiltration (see Appendix III for details about pathogen reduction techniques). FP/FFP, 10–20 mL/kg, continues to be used in developing countries. The most significant associated challenges are blood volume overload, inability to achieve and maintain hemostatic FVII levels, and a relatively higher risk for transmission of blood-borne infections.

Thrombotic episodes, such as deep vein thrombosis, have been reported in 3–4% of affected individuals with FVII deficiency, particularly in those requiring surgery and replacement treatment, but "spontaneous" thromboembolic events may also occur [14]. PCCs contain other vitamin K-dependent factors in higher concentrations than FVII, potentially increasing the risk for thrombosis [14].

Long-term prophylaxis is recommended for affected individuals with a personal history/family history of severe bleeding or an FVII level <0.01 IU/mL [7]. A long-term prophylaxis regimen of rFVIIa 20–40 μg/kg three times a week, adjusted to maintain the desired clinical response, has been suggested [5]. Alternatively, plasma-derived FVII can be used usually at a dose of 20–30 IU/kg every 2 days.

HMB is common and may be managed with oral contraceptives, antifibrinolytic agents, and a levonorgestrel intrauterine device (see Chapter 5). For women with severe FVII deficiency (<0.03 IU/mL), rFVIIa or pathogen-inactivated FVII concentrate on the first days of menses may be needed [7]. The management of FVII deficiency during pregnancy is not well established, with a range of treatment options reported, including the use of FP/FFP, rFVIIa for labor and delivery, and antifibrinolytic agents during the peripartum period. For pregnant women with FVII activity <0.2 IU/mL (in the third trimester), who require cesarean delivery or who have a history of bleeding, rFVIIa 15–30 μg/kg every 4–6 h for at least 3 days should be considered. For all other women with FVII deficiency, rFVIIa 15–30 μg/kg should be given only in response to abnormal bleeding [5].

Monitoring of replacement therapy in FVII deficiency is achieved via the FVII activity assay. Routine bedside monitoring may be accomplished with screening of the PT/INR in some cases as normalization of these screening coagulation tests approximately correlates with hemostatic FVII levels.

FX Deficiency

FX is a vitamin K-dependent glycoprotein that plays a crucial role in the coagulation cascade as it is the initial common pathway proenzyme. FX deficiency is the most severe rare coagulation disorder; it is inherited as an autosomal recessive condition estimated to occur in 1:1,000,000 births [2]. Still, frequencies are 8 to 10 times higher in countries with a high frequency of consanguineous families [17]. Two subclassifications exist: type I (proportionally low functional activity and antigen levels) and type II (low coagulant activity and near-normal antigen levels) [17].

Clinical Features

FX deficiency results in a variable bleeding tendency with a relatively strong correlation between baseline FX activity and bleeding manifestations [10] (Table 4). Neonates with severe deficiency may present with ICH, bleeding following circumcision, prolonged bleeding from the umbilical stump, umbilical stump separation at 7–14 days, and gastrointestinal bleeding. Moderately affected individuals may be recognized only after hemostatic challenges, such as surgery or trauma, or may only present at the onset of menses with HMB. Affected individuals with levels >0.4 IU/mL are largely asymptomatic [13]. The most common bleeding symptoms reported in affected individuals with all levels of severity of FX deficiency are epistaxis and HMB [2]. For the 34 subjects with FX deficiency studied by the EN-RBD, FX levels (IU/mL; 95% CI) for asymptomatic subjects and those with grade I, II, and III bleeding (Table 3) were 0.56 (0.29–0.83), 0.4 (0.14–0.67), 0.25 (0–0.52), and 0.1 (0–0.39), respectively [12].

Diagnosis

Screening tests reveal prolongation of both the PT/INR and aPTT (see Chapter 4, Fig. 1). The diagnosis of FX deficiency may be confirmed by quantifying plasma FX:C through serial dilutions with FX-deficient plasma. The corresponding degrees of prolongation may be influenced by differences in sensitivity between types of thromboplastin [17].

Genetics

The *F10* gene is located on chromosome 13q34. The majority of reported genetic alterations are missense variants, duplications, and partial deletions, with most affected individuals usually being compound heterozygotes (https://f10-db.eahad.org/).

Management

The preferred option for the treatment and prevention of bleeding episodes is a plasma-derived,

10

pathogen-inactivated FX concentrate [7] (Table 2). If an FX concentrate is unavailable, daily infusions of PCCs 20–30 (FIX) IU/kg or FP/FFP (10–20 mL/kg) are necessary when prolonged hemostatic coverage is required to maintain an FX level >0.2 IU/mL. Affected individuals should be closely monitored to avoid FII, FVII, and FIX levels accumulating above 1.5 IU/mL [5]. Antifibrinolytic agents may be used for mild bleeding episodes or minor surgery (dosing recommendations are provided in Appendix III) [5].

Long-term prophylaxis is recommended for cases with a personal or family history of severe bleeding or with FX activity <0.02 IU/mL (Table 2). Alternatively, PCC 20–30 IU/kg twice or three times a week, adjusted to maintain trough FX activity >0.02 IU/mL, can be used [5].

HMB is common and may be managed with oral contraceptives, antifibrinolytic agents, a levonorgestrel intrauterine device, and replacement therapy (see Chapter 5). Women with severe FX deficiency may experience miscarriage, placental abruption, premature delivery, and postpartum hemorrhage. For pregnant women (or women wishing to conceive) who have severe FX deficiency and a history of recurrent bleeding or adverse pregnancy outcomes, FX concentrate to maintain trough levels >0.2 IU/dL until the end of pregnancy is suggested. For delivery in women with FX activity <0.3 IU/mL in the third trimester who have a history of bleeding and all those who require cesarean section, FX concentrate or PCC 20–40 IU/kg to achieve an FX activity >0.4 IU/mL is recommended. Consideration should be given to maintaining FX activity at 0.3 IU/mL for at least 3 days [5].

FXI Deficiency

The major biological function of activated FXI (FXIa) is the activation of FIX (see Chapter 2). Another function of FXIa is sustaining thrombin generation initiated by the tissue factor/FVIIa complex. The proenzyme FXI is produced in the liver and circulates in the plasma as a complex with high-molecular-weight kininogen. FXI deficiency is inherited as an autosomal trait. Homozygotes/compound heterozygotes or heterozygotes are identified by severe or partial deficiency of FXI coagulant levels, respectively; homozygotes/compound heterozygotes generally have levels of <0.15 IU/mL, whereas heterozygotes have levels >0.15 but <0.7 IU/mL. Parents and children of a severely affected person will have partial FXI deficiency. FXI deficiency is a coagulopathy found predominantly, but not exclusively, in individuals of Ashkenazi Jewish descent, with incidences of the heterozygous state as high as 8–9% in this population; 1 in 450 individuals will be homozygous/compound heterozygous. Outside this at-risk population, homozygous/compound heterozygous FXI deficiency occurs in approximately 1:1,000,000 [2, 6]. For the 125 subjects with FXI deficiency studied by the EN-RBD, FXI levels (IU/mL; 95% CI) for asymptomatic subjects and those with grade I, II, and III bleeding (Table 3) were 0.26 (0.14–0.39), 0.26 (0.13–0.38), 0.25 (0.11–0.39), and 0.25 (0.09–0.41), respectively [12].

Clinical Presentation

FXI deficiency is generally associated with a mild bleeding tendency that most commonly manifests as delayed bleeding after injury, trauma, surgery, dental extractions, and childbirth. Easy bruising is common. Spontaneous bleeding, except for HMB, is rare even in affected individuals with severe FXI deficiency. Bleeding symptoms are very heterogeneous, with no correlation with baseline FXI activity levels [10]. Some affected individuals with very low FXI levels may not bleed following trauma, whereas others may exhibit major and/or clinically significant bleeding, including ICH [18].

Injury/surgery-related bleeding occurs particularly when it involves tissues containing activators of fibrinolysis, such as the oral cavity, nose, oral-pharyngeal area, and urinary tract (e.g., associated with adenoidectomy/tonsillectomy, extraction of molar/wisdom teeth, prostatectomy). It has been shown that the reduced resistance to fibrinolysis is due to different mechanisms, including defective thrombin-activatable fibrinolysis inhibitor [6]. Bleeding is less common at other sites of trauma/surgery, for example, during orthopedic surgery, appendectomy, circumcision, or cutaneous lacerations.

Diagnosis

Affected individuals with congenital FXI deficiency most often manifest with an isolated prolongation of the aPTT (see Chapter 4, Fig. 1). A normal aPTT may not detect a partial deficiency (FXI activity = 0.2–0.6 IU/mL) [19]. Confirmation of the disorder requires demonstrating reduced levels of coagulant FXI in a clotting assay on two or more occasions and the absence of an alternative cause for the laboratory abnormality (e.g., liver disease, lupus anticoagulant, etc.). Determination of FXI antigen levels is necessary only in rare cases of a qualitative deficiency. Family studies are recommended to provide additional evidence of an inherited condition.

Because affected individuals with severe FXI deficiency can remain asymptomatic until unmasked by an injury, it is suggested that all affected individuals of Ashkenazi Jewish descent who require surgery be screened with an aPTT [20] and, if prolonged, an FXI activity assay should be performed to rule out a deficiency state. FXI activity in healthy term neonates has a broad range and increases throughout the initial year of life. Therefore, the diagnosis of FXI at birth requires comparing test results with neonatal reference ranges and confirmation with retesting at an older age, generally 6 months or beyond (see Appendix II).

Genetics

The *FXI* gene is located on chromosome 4q35 with more than 400 different variants described (https://f11-db.eahad.org/). Genetic testing for *FXI* gene variants is not required as part of the routine diagnostic evaluation. However, testing in high-prevalence populations with well-characterized variants (e.g., individuals of Ashkenazi Jewish ancestry) may be appropriate in cases with borderline FXI levels and a severe bleeding phenotype and in cases with very low levels ≤0.01 IU/mL, allowing accurate identification of those with a null variant, which confers a greater risk of inhibitor development, which might affect management (e.g., use of a bypassing agent rather than factor replacement) [21].

Management

As FXI levels do not correlate with the risk for bleeding, important aspects to be considered when assessing the need for treatment include the personal and family history of bleeding, and the severity of the presenting bleeding episode or the anticipated hemostatic challenge associated with the planned procedure. Prior to planned surgery, several factors should be considered, including deciding whether the procedure is clearly indicated, the type and site of surgery, the previous bleeding history, exclusion of other bleeding abnormalities and cessation of antiplatelet agents and/or other nonsteroidal anti-inflammatory drugs (NSAIDs), if utilized.

For high-risk surgical procedures associated with high levels of local fibrinolysis (e.g., neurosurgery, ophthalmic surgery, tonsillectomy/adenoidectomy, surgery of the genitourinary tract, prostatectomy, and removal of molar/wisdom teeth) in affected individuals with severe FXI deficiency, or for individuals with a prior history of significant clinical bleeding, preoperative and postoperative replacement therapy should be given [5].

In affected individuals with severe FXI deficiency undergoing surgeries not associated with fibrinolysis, e.g., orthopedic surgery, appendectomy, or dental extraction or for individuals without a prior history of significant clinical bleeding, oral antifibrinolytic agents alone starting the night before and continuing for 5–7 days are recommended (dosing recommendations are provided in Appendix III) [5]. Fibrin glue can be used as an adjunctive hemostatic agent. For urological procedures, flushing the bladder with antifibrinolytic-containing solutions can also be used. Antifibrinolytic agents are contraindicated in cases of gross hematuria due to the risk of mechanical obstruction secondary to ureteral clots.

Oral antifibrinolytic agents alone are usually sufficient to prevent postcircumcision bleeding [5]. Religious circumcision is usually performed on male Jewish infants at 8 days of age. In families with known FXI deficiency, FXI testing before circumcision is advisable. For neonates with low FXI levels (<0.3 IU/mL), our experience is to give oral antifibrinolytic agents, the first dose to be given at least an hour before and continue 1–2 days post-circumcision.

The standard therapy for replacement of FXI is FP/FFP (15–20 mL/kg to start) and should be pathogen inactivated if available; large volumes may be required in severely deficient affected individuals. Importantly, the commercially available pooled solvent detergent–FP/FFP has less variation in FXI content compared with single donor FP/FFP (mean FXI activity of 0.7–0.9 IU/mL) [2]. Virally inactivated, purified FXI concentrates are available in Europe; however, they may not be available in all countries. Where available, it is recommended that FXI concentrates be used, taking into consideration the recommendations in the product monograph and that dosing should be planned with the goal of not exceeding plasma FXI activity levels of >0.7 IU/mL due to the risk of promoting serious thrombotic events [7]. Replacement therapy commonly aims to increase the circulating FXI level to approximately 0.45 IU/mL for 7 days (major surgery) or 0.3 IU/mL for 5 days (minor surgery; Table 2). The plasma half-life of FXI is approximately 45 h; if prolonged coverage is required, bolus infusions may be given on alternate days in conjunction with monitoring peak and trough FXI levels to adjust dosing amount and frequency of FXI replacement. In affected individuals at high risk for thromboembolic complications, alternatives to FXI concentrate, i.e., FP/FFP, should be considered. It should also be noted that combining antifibrinolytic agents with FXI concentrate is associated with increased thrombosis risk and should probably be avoided [7]. Antifibrinolytic agents can, however, be combined safely with FP/FFP replacement therapy.

Antifibrinolytic agents are often sufficient to treat HMB. The decision for prophylactic therapy during labor and delivery needs to be individualized according to the baseline FXI level, bleeding history, and mode of delivery [5]. Currently, there is no consensus on the routine need for replacement therapy in affected individuals with severe FXI deficiency and vaginal delivery [7]. It is recommended that FXI concentrate (10–15 IU/kg), or FP/FFP (15–20 mg/kg) and antifibrinolytic agents be considered in females with FXI levels <0.15 IU/mL at established labor or prior to cesarean section. Women with FXI activity 0.15–0.7 IU/mL and a history of bleeding should consider prophylactic antifibrinolytic agents for ≥3 days.

Replacement therapy for affected individuals with inherited FXI deficiency developing inhibitors to FXI consists of using rFVIIa and/or antifibrinolytic agents during procedures and in the postoperative period according to the associated bleeding risk [7]. If unavailable, an activated prothrombin complex concentrate (aPCC), such as FEIBA NF® with regimens similar to those used for acquired hemophilia A, may be used (see Chapter 11).

FXIII Deficiency

FXIIIa plays a pivotal role in coagulation through the covalent linkage of fibrin to stabilize the fibrin polymer and of fibrin to α2-plasmin inhibitor, creating a fibrin web resistant to fibrinolysis via plasmin [22] (see Chapter 2). FXIII circulates in plasma as a tetrameric molecule (FXIII-A2B2) composed of two potentially active A subunits (FXIII-A) and two B subunits (FXIII-B). The FXIII-A represents the protransglutaminase that is converted by thrombin to the active transglutaminase, and the FXIII-B serves as a carrier and regulatory protein for the A subunit [23]. Bone marrow/placenta and liver cells produce FXIII-A and FXIII-B, respectively [24].

FXIII deficiency is transmitted as an autosomal recessive trait, and severely affected individuals have either homozygous or compound heterozygous variants. FXIII-A deficiency has an incidence of approximately 1:2,000,000 births; severe FXIII-B deficiency has only been documented in a few cases [2]. FXIII-A deficiency is divided into type I (quantitative defect) as a result of a production defect and type II (qualitative defect), which results from a normal or near-normal concentration of functionally defective subunit A. The absence of FXIII-B leads to a shorter plasma half-life of FXIII-A, thus FXIII-B deficiency causes a less severe phenotype due to the remaining 0.05–0.1 IU/mL FXIII activity present in the plasma. Parents and children of a severely affected person will have partial FXIII deficiency; such individuals are generally asymptomatic.

FXIII also plays a role in angiogenesis, extracellular matrix deposition, osteoblastic differentiation, wound healing, immune response, and tissue repair [22], thereby providing the pathophysiologic explanation for observed poor wound healing in a subgroup of affected individuals (approximately 20%) and recurrent spontaneous miscarriages in most women if not placed on FXIII replacement therapy.

Clinical Presentation

FXIII deficiency may be suspected in neonates with ICH and/or prolonged bleeding. Poor healing/prolonged bleeding from the umbilical stump is observed in more than 80% of severely deficient neonates and, therefore, almost pathognomonic and highly suggestive of FXIII deficiency [23]. Due to the autosomal recessive nature of the condition, it is not uncommon for the child to be the product of a consanguineous marriage. Other presentations may include delayed bleeding after surgery or trauma, recurrent spontaneous miscarriages, and non-neonatal ICH. ICH can reach incidences as high as 25–30% in some registries and is the main cause of death and disability among affected individuals with this condition. For the 33 subjects with FXIII deficiency studied by the EN-RBD, FXIII levels (IU/mL; 95% CI) for asymptomatic subjects and those with grade I, II, and III bleeding (Table 3) were 0.31 (0.11–0.51), 0.17 (0–0.37), 0.03 (0–0.24), and 0 (0–0.11), respectively [12].

Diagnosis

Standard screening tests of coagulation, including the PT/INR, aPTT, TT, and fibrinogen level are all normal even in cases of severe FXIII deficiency (see Chapter 4, Fig. 1). Historically, the urea clot solubility test was used to screen for FXIII deficiency [23]. It still has some value, but it is only sensitive to severe deficiencies (<0.05 IU/mL), and consequently, if a patient with severe FXIII deficiency has received any source of FXIII (e.g., FP/FFP), the test will be falsely normal.

Quantitative FXIII activity assays, i.e., ammonia release, amine incorporation, and isopeptidase assays, are recommended as first-line screening tests, whenever possible [23]. If FXIII activity is decreased, the deficiency subtype, FXIII-A or FXIII-B, is determined using an immunological FXIII antigen assay. Although assays for the measurement of the different FXIII subunits are available, some centers may only use the most frequently employed FXIII-A enzyme-linked immunosorbent assay (ELISA), thereby not complying with current recommendations and potentially missing the rarer FXIII-B subunit deficiency [23].

Genetics

Genetic analysis is an important tool for the diagnosis of FXIII deficiency. The *F13A1* gene is located on chromosome 6p25.1 and the *F13B* gene on chromosome 1q31.3 [23].

Management

The clinical severity of FXIII deficiency requires treatment with regular prophylaxis from the time of diagnosis for all affected individuals with severe disease (<0.01 IU/mL) and for all symptomatic affected individuals regardless of severity [7]. Regular prophylaxis is feasible as effective hemostatic levels of FXIII may be as low as 0.05 IU/mL, and the plasma half-life is 11–14 days. Accordingly, replacement material can be infused at intervals as long as every 20–30 days. Antifibrinolytic agents may be used for mild bleeding episodes or minor surgery (dosing recommendations are provided in Appendix III) [5].

There are four options for replacing FXIII: recombinant FXIII (rFXIII), plasma-derived, pathogen-inactivated FXIII concentrates, FP/FFP, and cryoprecipitate. The recommended dosages for rFXIII and pasteurized FXIII plasma concentrates are detailed in Table 2. If rFXIII or pasteurized plasma concentrates are unavailable, the recommended dose for FXIII replacement (every 20–30 days) is 10–20 mL/kg for FP/FFP or 1 unit of cryoprecipitate per 10 kg. For treatment of an acute bleeding episode, a single dose of FP/FFP of 2–3 mL/kg can be sufficient to raise the FXIII level to >0.05 IU/mL, often adequate to achieve initial hemostasis [6]. Compared with FP/FFP, which contains 1.2 ± 0.3 IU/mL (mean ± SD), cryoprecipitate has approximately 15–30% higher enrichment of FXIII (2.8 ± 1.5 IU/mL) [25]. Prophylaxis with a single dose of FFP at 10 mL/kg would last 4–6 weeks. Similarly, cryoprecipitate can be administered as 1 bag per 10–20 kg every 3–4 weeks [22].

HMB is common and may be managed with oral contraceptives, antifibrinolytic agents, a levonorgestrel intrauterine device, and replacement therapy (see Chapter 5). Severe FXIII-deficient women require prophylactic replacement therapy during pregnancy to prevent spontaneous abortion and miscarriage. The optimal dosing of FXIII in this clinical situation has not yet been standardized. The United Kingdom Haemophilia Centre Doctors' Organization guideline recommends that women on FXIII prophylaxis should be monitored closely throughout pregnancy with increasing prophylaxis frequency every 14–21 days to maintain FXIII activity >0.2 IU/mL [5]. For delivery, additional FXIII concentrate 10–40 IU/kg given once during established labor or before cesarean section, depending on the interval since the last prophylaxis infusion, is recommended [5]. An alternative weekly dosing regimen of 250 IU until week 22 and 500 IU from week 23 with the aim of FXIII levels >0.1 IU/mL, and a 1,000 IU dose at labor has also been recommended [7]. Antifibrinolytic agents for 5–7 days following a cesarean section are suggested.

Familial Deficiency of Vitamin K-Dependent Clotting Factors

Hereditary combined deficiency of FII, FVII, FIX, and FX is a very rare (incidence approximately 1:2,000,000) autosomal recessive bleeding disorder. The disorder also involves the vitamin K-dependent naturally occurring anticoagulants, proteins C, S, and Z, in addition to the vitamin K-dependent bone proteins [6, 26]. This combined deficiency results from a defective carboxylation step in the vitamin K-dependent factors. The diagnosis should be considered only after other more common causes of combined vitamin K deficiency, such as liver disease, vitamin K antagonist (i.e., warfarin) overdose, and malabsorption (inflammatory bowel disease or celiac disease), have been ruled out (see Chapter 11).

Clinical Features

Affected individuals may exhibit a severe bleeding phenotype that includes early ICH identical to that observed in hemorrhagic disease of the newborn period prior to routine vitamin K prophylaxis. Some cases also are associated with dysmorphic features (warfarin embryopathy like), developmental delay, skeletal defects, osteoporosis, and a high incidence of miscarriages. The severity of symptoms may be affected by diet, gut microflora, and genetic penetrance. Anecdotal cases of thrombosis likely due to associated deficiencies of protein C and protein S are reported.

Diagnosis

Screening laboratory tests reveal a prolonged PT/INR and aPTT (see Chapter 4, Fig. 1). Proportionally, the PT/INR is more prolonged than the aPTT. After excluding other causes of vitamin K deficiency, genotyping of *VKOR* complex and *GGCX* is strongly recommended. A vitamin K assay, if available, may be useful; however, final diagnosis requires genetic confirmation.

Genetics

This rare disease is caused by point variants in the vitamin K pathway genes, *GGCX* or *VKORC1* located on chromosome 2p11.2, and 16p11, respectively. Heterozygous cases are asymptomatic. A genotype-phenotype correlation for GGCX-related phenotype was suggested, which can help in genetic counseling and management [27].

Management

Administration of large doses of vitamin K is the current standard of care, however, bleeding symptoms may still be observed. Long-term prophylaxis should start at diagnosis with oral vitamin K1 (5–20 mg/day) or parenteral vitamin K1 (5–20 mg/week) [7]. Despite the generally acknowledged efficacy of vitamin K, a fixed therapeutic schedule does not exist, and intervals can be based on PT/INR values. Antifibrinolytic agents alone may be sufficient for mild bleeding or minor surgery (dosing recommendations are provided in Appendix III) [5]. For severe bleeding or major surgery, four-factor PCC (containing FII, FVII, FIX, and FX) at a dose of 20–30 FIX IU/kg with parental vitamin K1 5–20 mg is recommended. FP/FFP 15–25 mL/kg is an alternative if four-factor PCC is unavailable [6]. Three-factor PCC (containing FII, FIX, and FX) could also be successfully administered in vitamin K-dependent clotting factor deficiency [26]; however, most recent guidelines suggest using four-factor PCC.

HMB is common and may be managed with oral contraceptives, antifibrinolytic agents, a levonorgestrel intrauterine device, and replacement therapy (see Chapter 5). For delivery in women with activities of any of the vitamin K factors <0.2 IU/mL in the third trimester, four-factor PCC at a dose of 20–30 FIX IU/kg once in established labor or before cesarean section is recommended for at least 3 days. The risk of thrombosis must be considered [7]. Prenatal diagnosis of the combined deficiency is not indicated; instead, administration of oral vitamin K1 during the third trimester should be considered if the child is at risk of inheriting the deficiency.

PAI-1 Deficiency

PAI-1 is involved in the downregulation of the fibrinolytic pathway as an inhibitor of tissue plasminogen activator and urokinase plasminogen activator (see Chapter 2). The half-life of PAI-1 is short, ~10 min. In addition to the role of PAI-1 in the hemostatic system, recent studies document its importance in inflammation, atherosclerosis, tissue fibrosis, and cancer. While the true incidence of PAI-1 deficiency is not known, it is estimated to be rare. Most affected individuals with symptomatic PAI-1 deficiency have homozygous or double heterozygous PAI-gene abnormalities, resulting in no PAI-1 production or formation of a dysfunctional PAI-1 with reduced or absent activity. Affected individuals with heterozygous PAI-1 deficiency usually do not have increased bleeding.

Clinical Features

PAI-1 deficiency usually manifests as a mild to moderate bleeding phenotype with delayed bleeding after hemostatic challenges, including trauma, dental extractions, invasive medical interventions, HMB, and abnormal bleeding in pregnancy. Spontaneous bleeding episodes are rare. PAI-I deficiency has been found to be associated with impaired wound healing and spontaneous miscarriages [28].

Diagnosis

Screening tests with aPTT, PT/INR, fibrinogen, and TT are normal (see Chapter 4, Fig. 1). Diagnosis is challenging and requires a combination of a detailed bleeding history, laboratory evaluation, and a high index of suspicion. Both PAI-1 antigen and activity levels tests are needed, as the deficiency can be qualitative or quantitative [29, 30]. Affected individuals with PAI-1 activity assays <0.01 IU/mL in association with low antigen levels are most easily diagnosed, but those with dysfunctional proteins with normal antigen levels may be difficult to diagnose.

Genetics

PAI-1 is encoded by a gene (*SERPINE1*) localized on chromosome 7q21.3–22 [28]. Genetic testing for biallelic *SERPINE1* pathogenic variants can assist in diagnosis. Heterozygotes are asymptomatic.

Management

Therapy is mainly based on antifibrinolytic agents for prevention or control of bleeding (dosing recommendations are provided in Appendix III) [7]. Delayed bleeding following a surgical procedure is a hallmark of PAI-1 deficiency; the use of antifibrinolytic agents for several days before and after a procedure may be effective. FP/FFP (15–25 mL/kg) may be used to rapidly increase levels of PAI-1 prior to achieving a therapeutic level of antifibrinolytic agents [7]. Females with HMB may require initiation of antifibrinolytic agents a few days prior to the menstrual cycle [7, 31].

α2-AP Deficiency

α2-AP is a serine protease inhibitor that plays an integral role in inhibiting plasmin (see Chapter 2). As such, deficiency of α2-AP leads to an increase in plasmin that leads to increased fibrinolysis and bleeding. While the true incidence α2-AP deficiency is not known, it is estimated to be rare. Consanguinity is common in families with homozygous deficiency.

Clinical Features

Homozygous deficiency of α2-AP has been reported to cause significant bleeding, including post-trauma and postsurgical bleeding [28, 30]. Women with homozygous α2-AP deficiency may experience HMB and postpartum hemorrhage [7]. Individuals who are heterozygous for α2-AP deficiency may also experience increased bleeding but less so than homozygous individuals.

Diagnosis

Screening tests with aPTT, PT/INR, fibrinogen, and TT are normal (see Chapter 4, Fig. 1). Clot lysis time may be shorter in affected individuals [28]. However, to diagnose α2-AP deficiency, assays for α2-AP activity and antigen should be performed. Homozygotes or compound heterozygotes for α2-AP deficiency usually have activity levels <0.1 IU/mL. Heterozygotes typically have α2-AP activity levels from 0.35 to 0.7 IU/mL.

Genetics

The α2-AP gene *(SERPINF2)* is located on chromosome 17p. Genetic testing showing variants in *SERPINF2* may also be useful in the diagnosis [28].

Management

Antifibrinolytic agents are the mainstay of treatment for α2-AP deficiency (dosing recommendations are provided in Appendix III) [7]. In planned surgical procedures, including dental extraction, antifibrinolytic agents should be started before surgery and continued 7–10 days postprocedure [28].

Other Rare Factor Deficiencies

Deficiencies of other coagulation factors, such as factor XII (FXII) and plasminogen, were not discussed as they generally do not cause bleeding. Of note, FXII deficiency (at least in a mild form) is thought to be very common, particularly in persons of East Asian origin and is the most common reason for a prolonged aPTT in this population; it should always be tested for in settings of a prolonged aPTT with a normal PT/INR (see Chapter 4, Fig. 1).

Quebec platelet disorder, an autosomal dominant disorder caused by gain-of-function tandem duplication of the *PLAU* gene, is discussed in Chapter 6.

When all other bleeding disorders have been excluded, East Texas Bleeding Disorder (caused by variants in FV that ultimately lead to an excess of tissue factor pathway inhibitor) [32] and thrombomodulin defects have to be considered [33]. It is only recently that these conditions have been discovered. Genetic panels are leading to increased recognition of such rare bleeding disorders.

Conclusion

Diagnosis and treatment of rare severe bleeding disorders represent significant challenges to the treating physician as often inadequate information exists in the literature for these disorders due to their rarity. The diagnosis of a rare bleeding disorder should be considered in all children with unusual bleeding symptoms, and urgent diagnosis is required to institute appropriate care. Pediatricians caring for populations where consanguinity is common should have heightened awareness of these disorders. Neonatal ICH is one of the most severe bleeding events associated with a significant risk of morbidity and mortality and requires urgent evaluation, diagnosis, and treatment; the most common disorders in this clinical situation to consider include, but are not limited to, FXIII, FVII, FX deficiencies, and congenital afibrinogenemia. Management for each specific deficiency is outlined above and should include the involvement of a physician who has experience in this field. Collaboration with experts in reference centers familiar with the assessment and management of children and adolescents with severe rare inherited bleeding disorders is strongly recommended from an early stage in the assessment of neonates, children, and adolescents with a possible severe rare inherited bleeding disorder based on clinical signs/symptoms or results of laboratory tests. Prevention of bleeding is important. Affected individuals and families should be advised to avoid antiplatelet medications (such as acetylsalicylic acid/other NSAIDs). Protective gear, such as helmets for bike riding, are recommended. Optimal preventive dental care is important. In severe cases, an alert bracelet may be needed. Specific replacement therapy is available for only some of these conditions, whereas for others, nonspecific factor replacement is available (FP/FFP; cryoprecipitate; PCC). Particular issues are observed in females with rare bleeding disorders due to menstruation, pregnancy, and childbirth, and require careful management in conjunction with an obstetrician/gynecologist, ideally provided in the setting of a multidisciplinary Women's Bleeding Disorders Program (see Chapter 5). Genetic analysis, if available, is important for accurate diagnosis, management, improved genetic counseling, and the possibility of prenatal diagnosis (see Chapter 21). The potential role of new therapeutic modalities, such as nonreplacement therapies and gene therapy used already in hemophilia (see Chapter 8), is the subject of ongoing research and should also be explored in the management of individuals with rare and severe coagulation factor deficiencies [34, 35].

Acknowledgments

Our special thanks go to Frederico Xavier, who was an author of this chapter in the first and second editions of this Handbook, which provided a valuable background for this updated chapter. We would like to express our appreciation for the thoughtful comments provided by Alexandra Zabeida and Nancy Robitaille, who reviewed this chapter for the third edition.

Conflict of Interest Statement

Joel Livingston declares no conflict of interest. Victor Blanchette reports receiving consultancy and speaker fees from Bayer HealthCare, Sanofi-Genzyme, Novo Nordisk, Pfizer, Roche, Takeda, and Spark Therapeutics. He is recipient of research grants from Sanofi-Genzyme, Bayer HealthCare, and Takeda and serves as a member of Data Safety Monitoring Boards for Octapharma and Takeda. He is Chair of a nonprofit organization, the International Prophylaxis Study Group (IPSG). Muhammad Faisal Khanani declares no conflict of interest. Shoshana Revel-Vilk received grant/research support, honoraria, and advisory fees from Takeda, Pfizer, and Sanofi/Genzyme.

Author Contributions

Shoshana Revel-Vilk wrote the first draft of the chapter. Joel Livingston critically revised the chapter and approved the final version. Victor S. Blanchette critically revised the chapter and approved the final version. Muhammad Faisal Khanani critically revised the chapter and approved the final version.

Abbreviations

aPCC	Activated prothrombin complex concentrate
aPTT	Activated partial thromboplastin time
α2-AP	α2-Antiplasmin
ELISA	Enzyme-linked immunosorbent assay
EN-RBD	European Network of Rare Bleeding Disorders
FP/FFP	Frozen plasma (FP)/fresh frozen plasma (FFP)
FII	Factor II (prothrombin)
FV	Factor V
FVII	Factor VII
FVIII	Factor VIII
FIX	Factor IX
FX	Factor X
FXI	Factor XI
FXII	Factor XII
FXIII	Factor XIII
GGCX	γ-Glutamyl carboxylase
HMB	Heavy menstrual bleeding
ICH	Intracranial hemorrhage
INR	International normalized ratio
ISTH	International Society on Thrombosis and Haemostasis
LMAN1	Lectin mannose-binding protein 1
MCFD2	Multiple coagulation factor deficiency protein 2
NSAIDs	Nonsteroidal anti-inflammatory drugs
PAI-1	Plasminogen activator inhibitor type 1
PCC	Prothrombin complex concentrate
PT	Prothrombin time
PT-Fg	Prothrombin time-derived fibrinogen
rFVIIa	Recombinant activated factor VII
rFXIII	Recombinant factor XIII
TT	Thrombin time
VKOR	Vitamin K epoxide reductase

References

1 Litvinov RI, Pieters M, de Lange-Loots Z, Weisel JW. Fibrinogen and fibrin. Subcell Biochem. 2021;96:471–501.

2 Franchini M, Marano G, Pupella S, Vaglio S, Masiello F, Veropalumbo E, et al. Rare congenital bleeding disorders. Ann Transl Med. 2018;6(17):331.

3 de Moerloose P, Casini A, Neerman-Arbez M. Congenital fibrinogen disorders: an update. Semin Thromb Hemost. 2013;39:585–95.

4 Casini A, Undas A, Palla R, Thachil J, de Moerloose P; Subcommittee on Factor X and Fibrinogen. Diagnosis and classification of congenital fibrinogen disorders: communication from the SSC of the ISTH. J Thromb Haemost. 2018;16(9):1887–90.

5 Mumford AD, Ackroyd S, Alikhan R, Bowles L, Chowdary P, Grainger J, et al. Guideline for the diagnosis and management of the rare coagulation disorders: a United Kingdom Haemophilia Centre Doctors' Organization guideline on behalf of the British Committee for Standards in Haematology. Br J Haematol. 2014;167(3):304–26.

6 Menegatti M, Peyvandi F. Treatment of rare factor deficiencies other than hemophilia. Blood. 2019;133(5):415–24.

7 Shapiro A. The use of prophylaxis in the treatment of rare bleeding disorders. Thromb Res. 2020;196:590–602.

8 Ruiz-Saez A. Occurrence of thrombosis in rare bleeding disorders. Semin Thromb Hemost. 2013;39(6):684–92.

9 Casini A, de Moerloose P. How I treat dysfibrinogenemia. Blood. 2021;138(21):2021–30.

10 Saes JL, Verhagen MJA, Meijer K, Cnossen MH, Schutgens REG, Peters M, et al. Bleeding severity in patients with rare bleeding disorders: real-life data from the RBiN study. Blood Adv. 2020;4(20):5025–34.

11 Stoj KM, Pierro J. Factor V deficiency. In: StatPearls [Internet]. Treasure Island (FL): StatPearls Publishing; 2023 Jan. Available from: https://www.ncbi.nlm.nih.gov/books/NBK580494/ [updated 2023 Jan 23].

12 Peyvandi F, Palla R, Menegatti M, Siboni SM, Halimeh S, Faeser B, et al. Coagulation factor activity and clinical bleeding severity in rare bleeding disorders: results from the European Network of Rare Bleeding Disorders. J Thromb Haemost. 2012;10(4):615–21.

13 Peyvandi F, Di Michele D, Bolton-Maggs PH, Lee CA, Tripodi A, Srivastava A, et al. Classification of rare bleeding disorders (RBDs) based on the association between coagulant factor activity and clinical bleeding severity. J Thromb Haemost. 2012;10(9):1938–43.

14 Bernardi F, Mariani G. Biochemical, molecular and clinical aspects of coagulation factor VII and its role in hemostasis and thrombosis. Haematologica. 2021;106(2):351–62.

15 Lapecorella M, Mariani G; International Registry on Congenital Factor VIID. Factor VII deficiency: defining the clinical picture and optimizing therapeutic options. Haemophilia. 2008;14(6):1170–5.

16 Robinson KS. An overview of inherited factor VII deficiency. Transfus Apher Sci. 2019;58(5):569–71.

17 Peyvandi F, Auerswald G, Austin SK, Liesner R, Kavakli K, Alvarez Roman MT, et al. Diagnosis, therapeutic advances, and key recommendations for the management of factor X deficiency. Blood Rev. 2021;50:100833.

18 Barg AA, Levy-Mendelovich S, Budnik I, Mandel-Shorer N, Dardik R, Avishai E, et al. Pediatric severe factor XI deficiency: a multicenter study. Pediatr Blood Cancer. 2022;69(3):e29545.

19 Lewandowska MD, Connors JM. Factor XI deficiency. Hematol Oncol Clin North Am. 2021;35(6):1157–69.

20 Seligsohn U. Factor XI deficiency in humans. J Thromb Haemost. 2009;7(suppl 1):84–7.

21 Setty S, Reddell A, England A, Gomez K, Kadir R. The role of recombinant factor VIIa for obstetric block in women with severe factor XI deficiency. Haemophilia. 2011;17(6):906–9.

22 Mangla A, Hamad H, Kumar A. Factor XIII deficiency. In: StatPearls [Internet]. Treasure Island (FL): StatPearls Publishing; 2023 Jan. Available from: https://www.ncbi.nlm.nih.gov/books/NBK557467/StatPearls [updated 2022 Nov 30].

23 Karimi M, Peyvandi F, Naderi M, Shapiro A. Factor XIII deficiency diagnosis: challenges and tools. Int J Lab Hematol. 2018;40(1):3–11.

24 Dorgalaleh A, Assadollahi V, Tabibian S, Shamsizadeh M. Molecular basis of congenital factor XIII deficiency in Iran. Clin Appl Thromb Hemost. 2018;24(2):210–6.

25 Caudill JSC, Nichols WL, Plumhoff EA, Schulte SL, Winters JL, Gastineau DA, et al. Comparison of coagulation factor XIII content and concentration in cryoprecipitate and fresh-frozen plasma. Transfusion. 2009;49(4):765–70.

26 Napolitano M, Mariani G, Lapecorella M. Hereditary combined deficiency of the vitamin K-dependent clotting factors. Orphanet J Rare Dis. 2010;5:21.

27 De Vilder EY, Debacker J, Vanakker OM. GGCX-associated phenotypes: an overview in search of genotype-phenotype correlations. Int J Mol Sci. 2017;18(2):240.

28 Jain S, Acharya SS. Inherited disorders of the fibrinolytic pathway. Transfus Apher Sci. 2019;58(5):572–7.

29 Mehic D, Pabinger I, Ay C, Gebhart J. Fibrinolysis and bleeding of unknown cause. Res Pract Thromb Haemost. 2021;5(4):e12511.

30 Saes JL, Schols SEM, van Heerde WL, Nijziel MR. Hemorrhagic disorders of fibrinolysis: a clinical review. J Thromb Haemost. 2018;16(8):1498–509.

31 Mehta R, Shapiro AD. Plasminogen activator inhibitor type 1 deficiency. Haemophilia. 2008;14(6):1255–60.

32 Broze GJ Jr, Girard TJ. Factor V, tissue factor pathway inhibitor, and east Texas bleeding disorder. J Clin Invest. 2013;123(9):3710–2.

33 Mehic D, Tolios A, Hofer S, Ay C, Haslacher H, Downes K, et al. Thrombomodulin in patients with mild to moderate bleeding tendency. Haemophilia. 2021;27(6):1028–36.

34 Jain S, Acharya SS. Management of rare coagulation disorders in 2018. Transfus Apher Sci. 2018;57(6):705–12.

35 Arruda VR, Weber J, Samelson-Jones BJ. Gene therapy for inherited bleeding disorders. Semin Thromb Hemost. 2021;47(2):161–73.

Chapter 11

Published online: December 5, 2024

Blanchette VS, Brandão LR, Carcao MD, Kumar R, Rand ML, Revel-Vilk S (eds): SickKids Handbook of Pediatric Thrombosis and Hemostasis, ed 3, rev. and ext. Basel, Karger, 2024, pp 188–215 (DOI: 10.1159/000538216)

Acquired Bleeding Disorders

Riten Kumar[a, b] Markus Schmugge[c] Marie-Claude Pelland-Marcotte[d]
Manuel D. Carcao[e, f]

[a]Dana Farber/Boston Children's Cancer and Blood Disorders Center, Boston, MA, USA; [b]Harvard Medical School, Boston, MA, USA; [c]University Children's Hospital, University of Zurich, Zurich, Switzerland; [d]Centre Hospitalier Universitaire de Québec, Québec City, QC, Canada; [e]Department of Pediatrics, Hospital for Sick Children, Toronto, ON, Canada; [f]University of Toronto, Toronto, ON, Canada

Introduction

Acquired bleeding disorders encompass a heterogeneous group of conditions with varied and complex etiology and are typically encountered in hospitalized children with underlying infectious, cardiovascular, neoplastic, hepatic, and renal comorbidities. Diagnosis and management are often a challenge and rely on a detailed medical history, including family history, a careful physical examination, and selected laboratory investigations. The paucity of randomized controlled trials or prospective cohort studies makes it difficult to postulate evidence-based treatment guidelines for these children. Many of the recommendations made in this chapter have been extrapolated from the adult literature and expert opinion.

Disseminated Intravascular Coagulation

Disseminated intravascular coagulation (DIC) is a consumptive coagulopathy characterized by the dysregulated systemic activation of coagulation, with the simultaneous impairment of natural anticoagulant and fibrinolytic pathways. DIC results in the widespread deposition of fibrin, occlusion of small- to medium-sized blood vessels, and may eventually result in multiorgan failure. Concurrent consumption of platelets and clotting factors from the ongoing coagulation may result in profuse hemorrhage, thereby complicating the clinical picture and laboratory evaluation (Fig. 1). DIC rarely occurs in isolation and is usually secondary to an underlying pathology. The most common cause of DIC in children is sepsis. In addition, a wide spectrum of disorders, such as malignancy, trauma, and vascular anomalies, have also been implicated (Table 1). These conditions result in activation of the coagulation system by release of inflammatory cytokines (IL-1, IL-6, and

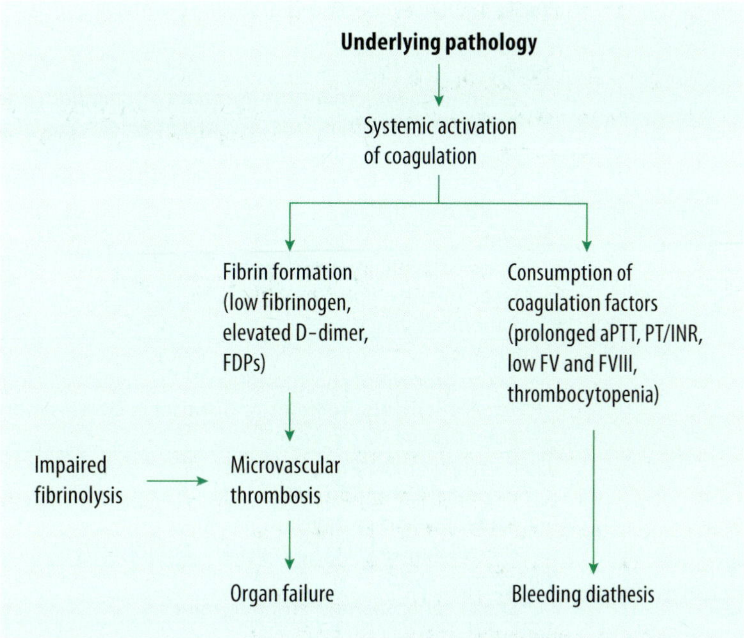

Fig. 1. Mechanism of disseminated intravascular coagulation. aPTT, activated partial thromboplastin time; FDPs, fibrin degradation products; FV, factor V; FVIII, factor VIII; PT/INR, prothrombin time/international normalized ratio.

tumor necrosis factor-alpha) leading to increased expression of tissue factor (TF) on endothelial cells and circulating monocytes, as well as by the exposure of blood to TF released from damaged tissue or tumor cells. TF activates downstream coagulation factors and thrombin generation through the extrinsic pathway. Bacterial lipopolysaccharides and neutrophil extracellular traps are also potent activators of coagulation.

Clinical Presentation

The clinical presentation of DIC is often complicated by the underlying pathology. DIC may be subclinical (compensated), manifesting as laboratory abnormalities alone; or clinically overt (decompensated), where laboratory abnormalities are associated with symptoms of bleeding and/or microvascular thrombosis. Bleeding, in the form of oozing from venipuncture sites, postoperative bleeding, petechiae, and ecchymosis has been reported in about 50% of children with DIC; whereas symptomatic thromboembolic event (TE) is seen in about 5% of children with DIC [1]. Untreated, clinically overt DIC may eventually progress to multiorgan failure.

Purpura fulminans, a particularly severe form of DIC, is characterized by skin infarction and necrosis. In older children, purpura fulminans is commonly associated with meningococcal and herpes zoster infection (where it is thought to result from acquired protein S and protein C deficiency). Neonatal purpura fulminans usually occurs in children with inherited severe protein C and rarely protein S deficiency (homozygotes and compound heterozygotes) (see Chapter 13). The Kasabach-Merritt phenomenon, a condition associated with DIC, is discussed in Chapter 12. DIC with enhanced fibrinolysis and increased risk of bleeding remains a major cause of morbidity and mortality in children with acute promyelocytic leukemia (APML) [2].

Diagnosis

No single laboratory test can accurately establish or rule out DIC. Scoring systems based on commonly available laboratory tests may be used [3].

Table 1. Clinical conditions associated with DIC

Sepsis
Gram-negative organisms (*Neisseria meningitidis, Haemophilus influenzae*)
Gram-positive organisms (group B *Streptococcus, Staphylococcus*)
Viral (COVID-19, Ebola, dengue fever, yellow fever)
Rickettsia (Rocky Mountain spotted fever, typhus)
Protozoan (malaria)
Trauma
Massive tissue injury/surgery
Head injury
Fat embolism
Malignancy
Acute promyelocytic, monoblastic, or myelocytic leukemia
Transient myeloproliferative disorder in Down syndrome
Solid tumors
Obstetric complications
Placental abruption
Amniotic fluid embolism
Pre-eclampsia (HELLP syndrome, hemolysis, elevated liver enzymes, low platelets)
Reaction to toxins
Snake venom, drugs, amphetamines
Vascular anomaly
Kaposiform hemangioendothelioma and tufted angioma (Kassabach-Merritt syndrome)
Large venous malformations (e.g., Klippel Trenaunay syndrome)
Miscellaneous
Acute hemolytic transfusion reaction
Transplant rejection
Severe allergic reaction
Extensive burn
Specific neonatal DIC
Sepsis
Perinatal asphyxia
Meconium aspiration syndrome
Necrotizing enterocolitis
Respiratory distress syndrome
Metabolic conditions (e.g., galactosemia)
Severe congenital protein C/protein S deficiency (purpura fulminans)

COVID-19, coronavirus disease 2019; DIC, disseminated intravascular coagulation; HELLP, hemolysis, elevated liver enzyme, low platelet levels.

Given the dynamic nature of DIC, repeated scores with clear trends are preferred over a single assessment.

Complete Blood Count (CBC) and Examination of a Peripheral Blood Smear

Thrombocytopenia from thrombin-induced platelet aggregation is seen in nearly 50% of cases with DIC. The peripheral blood smear may provide evidence in support of microangiopathic hemolysis in the form of fragmented red blood cells (RBCs) (schistocytes) and polychromasia reflecting an increase in reticulocytes (Fig. 2).

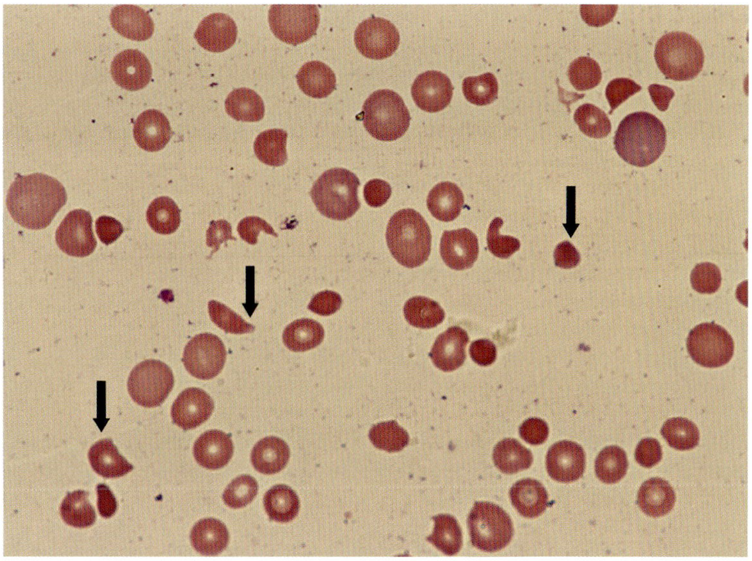

Fig. 2. Microangiopathic hemolytic anemia. Peripheral blood smear from a patient with microangiopathic hemolytic anemia showing helmet cells, schistocytes, and microspherocytes. Courtesy of William Brien, MD, FRCP, Division of Pathology and Laboratory Medicine, Hospital for Sick Children.

11

Coagulation Testing

A normal prothrombin time/international normalized ratio (PT/INR) and activated partial thromboplastin time (aPTT) should not be used alone to exclude DIC, as a prolonged PT/INR, and aPTT are reported in only 50–60% of cases. Factor V (FV) and factor VIII (FVIII) levels are both reduced in DIC (this may help differentiate DIC from coagulopathy of liver disease where FVIII levels are often elevated). There is elevation of fibrin degradation products (FDPs) including D-dimer, with reduced fibrinogen levels (fibrinogen is an acute phase reactant, and occasionally, fibrinogen levels may be normal or even elevated). The thrombin time (TT) may be prolonged secondary to low fibrinogen levels and/or interference of the high-molecular-weight FDPs on the thrombin used for the test. A reduction in plasma native anticoagulants (protein C, protein S, and antithrombin) has also been described.

International Society on Thrombosis and Haemostasis Algorithm

The International Society on Thrombosis and Haemostasis (ISTH) harmonized three national guidelines to recommend a standardized five-step algorithm to diagnose overt DIC [3]. This algorithm is based on laboratory tests that are available in most hospitals (Table 2). The presence of a condition known to predispose to DIC is a prerequisite for use of the algorithm. This algorithm has demonstrated a 91% sensitivity and 97% specificity in adults and reliably predicts mortality [4]. While not prospectively validated in children, retrospective pediatric data have shown that the ISTH DIC score is an independent predictor of both vasopressor use and mortality in children [5]. The score should be interpreted with caution in children younger than 6 months of age, since several coagulation parameters do not reach adult values until 6 months of age (see Appendix II). While further validation of the ISTH DIC score in children is warranted, when used, repeated scores with clear trends are preferred over a single evaluation.

Management

Given the paucity of relevant pediatric literature and prospective randomized studies, it is difficult to make evidence-based treatment recommendations regarding the management of DIC in children. The cornerstone for treatment of DIC re-

Table 2. ISTH diagnostic scoring system for overt (uncompensated) DIC

1. Risk assessment: Does the patient have an underlying disorder?
   If yes: proceed; if no: do not use this algorithm
2. Order global coagulation tests: platelet count, PT, fibrinogen, FDPs (D-dimers)
3. Score global coagulation results:
   - Platelet count (>100 × 10^9/L = 0; <100 × 10^9/L = 1; <50 × 10^9/L = 2)
   - Elevated fibrin-degradation products (no increase = 0; moderate increase = 2; strong increase = 3)
   - Prolonged PT (<3 s = 0; >3 but <6 s = 1; >6 s = 2)
   - Fibrinogen level (>1 g/L = 0; <1 g/L = 1)
4. Calculate score
5. Interpretation of score
   - If total score ≥5: compatible with overt DIC; repeat score daily
   - If total score <5: suggestive (not affirmative) for subclinical DIC; repeat in 1–2 days

Modified with permission from Taylor et al. [3]. DIC, disseminated intravascular coagulation; FDPs, fibrin degradation products; ISTH, International Society on Thrombosis and Haemostasis; PT, prothrombin time; s, seconds.

mains the aggressive management of precipitating conditions (e.g., antibiotic therapy for sepsis and early institution of all *trans* retinoic acid at the first suspicion of APML) [2]. The following general recommendations have been extrapolated from adult guidelines and should be individualized based on the child's presentation and clinical status [4, 6].

Blood Component Therapy

Transfusion of platelets and plasma products, i.e., fresh plasma (FP)/fresh frozen plasma (FFP), cryoprecipitate, should be based on symptoms of bleeding and not abnormal laboratory values. However, asymptomatic individuals who are thought to be at high risk of bleeding (e.g., postoperative, prior to invasive procedures, or diagnosis of APML) may be candidates for replacement therapy as well. Reasonable goals for such individuals are to maintain the platelet count >30–50 × 10^9/L, fibrinogen >1 g/L, and PT/aPTT <1.5 times the normal range. Cryoprecipitate or a plasma-derived, virus-inactivated fibrinogen concentrate, if available, may be considered in children with severe hypofibrinogenemia (<1 g/L) and active bleeding, which does not improve despite FP/FFP infusion (see Appendix III for dosing guidelines).

Anticoagulation

Children with DIC presenting with limb or life-threatening arterial thromboses, symptomatic venous TE, or purpura fulminans may be candidates for anticoagulation. Given its short half-life and reversibility, unfractionated heparin (UFH) (see Chapter 20 for dosing recommendations) is preferred over low molecular weight heparin (LMWH). TE with concurrent bleeding may warrant an initial trial of prophylactic doses of UFH (~10 units/kg/h). Anti-Xa level is the preferred assay to monitor UFH and should be closely followed given the increased risk of hemorrhage (see Chapter 20).

Recombinant Factor VIIa

Some data suggest a potential role of recombinant factor VIIa (rFVIIa) in adults with DIC and uncontrolled bleeding [7], but pediatric data are anecdotal and conflicting. However, in situations of significant bleeding despite replacement of blood components, rFVIIa may be used cautiously. Although the recommended dose for hemophilia patients with inhibitors is 90 μg/kg/dose every 2–3 h, the optimal dose in the setting of DIC is not known as no evidence-based data exist. If rFVIIa is considered, most experts consider using a lower dose of rFVIIa in DIC (15–30 μg/kg/dose repeated every 2–3 h based on clinical symptoms/signs). Treatment with rFVIIa may result in an increased risk of TE, including stroke, and potential risks and benefits should be discussed upfront with the patient/guardian.

Protein C Concentrate
Individuals with congenital severe protein C deficiency presenting with neonatal purpura fulminans require, in addition to anticoagulation, the replacement of protein C either with FP/FFP or human plasma-derived, viral-inactivated protein C concentrate (see Chapter 13).

Recombinant Human Activated Protein C
The use of activated protein C is not recommended in children with DIC [8].

Antifibrinolytic Agents
The use of antifibrinolytic agents is not recommended in children with DIC, with the exception of uncontrolled bleeding associated with marked hyperfibrinolysis (e.g., APML).

Other Agents
The use of antithrombin has not been systematically studied in children with DIC but may be considered if antithrombin plasma levels are low and treatment with UFH is contemplated. Recombinant, human-soluble thrombomodulin is being investigated in neonates and children with DIC, though a significant mortality benefit has not been demonstrated [9].

Thrombotic Microangiopathic Disorders

Thrombotic microangiopathic disorders (TMAs) are characterized by thrombosis in medium- and small-sized blood vessels with resulting thrombocytopenia, microangiopathic hemolytic anemia (MAHA), and end organ damage. Hemolytic-uremic syndrome (HUS) and thrombotic thrombocytopenic purpura (TTP) are the classic variants of this condition and are called primary TMAs. Secondary TMAs are triggered by a wide spectrum of conditions and systemic diseases like hematopoietic stem cell transplantation (HSCT), pregnancy, systemic lupus erythematosus (SLE), diabetes, hypertension, and various infections including COVID-19. A consensus on the classification, etiology, criteria for clinical response, and remission of HUS, congenital and immune-mediated TTP, and secondary TMAs has been recently published [10]. The last few years have also seen a paradigm shift in the management of these conditions with monoclonal antibody therapy (i.e., caplacizumab and eculizumab) emerging as frontline treatment options. An algorithm for diagnosis of TMA is presented in Figure 3.

11

Hemolytic Uremic Syndrome

HUS is defined by the simultaneous occurrence of thrombocytopenia, MAHA, and renal dysfunction. HUS remains the most common cause of acute and chronic renal failure requiring dialysis in children. Ninety percent of HUS is caused by shiga toxin (verotoxin) producing serotypes of *Escherichia coli* (STEC-HUS), the prototype being *E. coli* 0157:H7, although other serotypes and bacteria (including invasive pneumococcal infection) have also been implicated. The verotoxin causes direct injury to the vascular endothelium resulting in the activation of coagulation cascade with formation of platelet-fibrin thrombi and subsequent thrombo-occlusive injury to dependent organ systems, classically affecting the kidney, through ischemic injury to the intestines and central nervous system (CNS) has also been described. A prospective surveillance study estimated the incidence of STEC-HUS to be 0.7/100,000 children younger than 16 years of age, with nearly 70% of the cases occurring in children younger than 5 years [11].

Approximately 10% of pediatric HUS is classified as atypical HUS (aHUS) as it does not occur

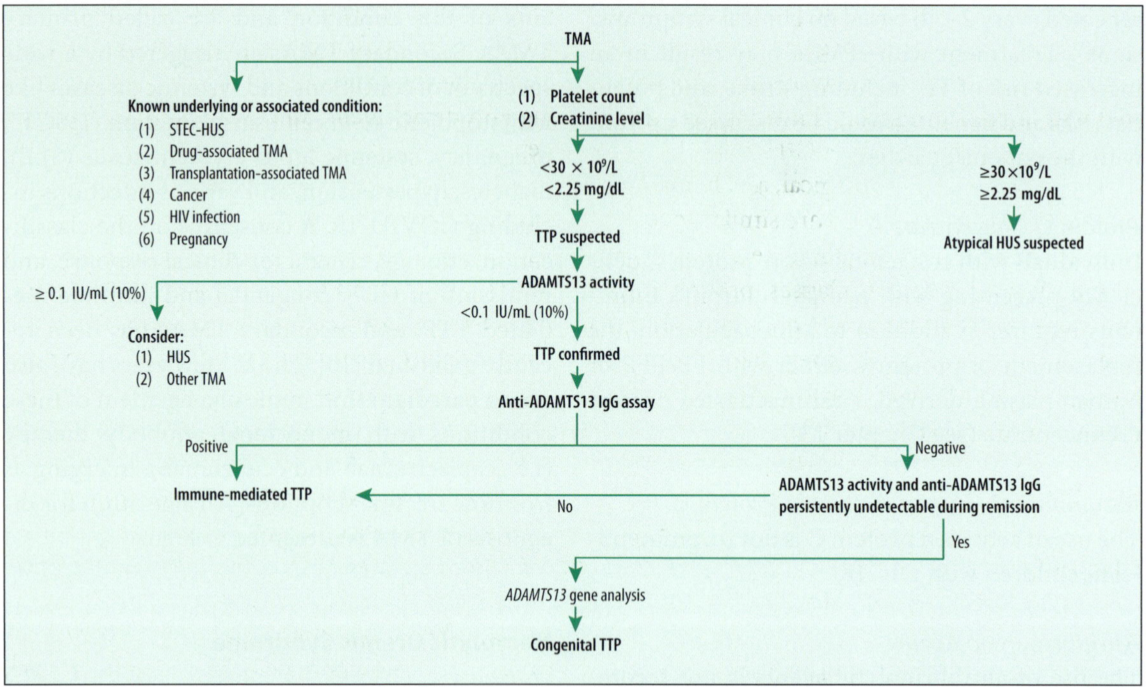

Fig. 3. Diagnostic algorithm for TMA. HUS, hemolytic uremic syndrome; STEC, Shiga toxin *Escherichia coli*; TMA, thrombotic microangiopathic disorder; TTP, thrombotic thrombocytopenic purpura. Reproduced with permission from Kremer Hovinga et al. [76].

after infection with verotoxin-producing bacteria. These are a heterogeneous group of disorders that typically occur secondary to inherited or acquired defects in complement regulation (particularly the alternate pathway of complement). The constitutively "over" active complement system damages the vascular endothelium resulting in platelet aggregation and subsequent thrombus formation in the kidneys and other organs [12, 13]. Putative variants have been identified in genes encoding complement regulators (*CFH*, *CFI*, *CFHRs*, *MCP/CD46*) as well as complement activators (*CFB*, *C3*). A novel subtype of aHUS characterized by both the deletion of *CFHR1* and *CFHR3*, in combination with complement factor H (CFH) autoantibody positivity has been described.

Clinical Presentation

The rate of STEC-HUS following *E. coli* 0157:H7 infection ranges from 8% to 18%. After ingestion of *E. coli*, there is usually an incubation period of 3–8 days after which symptoms typically start with watery diarrhea progressing to bloody diarrhea in about 48 h. Only 30% of children have concurrent fever. Pallor and oliguria or anuria eventually develops. Renal complications requiring dialysis are seen in 50–60% and acute hypertension in about 30% of children. Seizures, lethargy, irritability, and other neurological complications may be noted in 25–50% of children [11].

Bleeding, despite significant thrombocytopenia, is rare, and generally restricted to mucocutaneous symptoms such as petechiae and ecchymosis. Long-term renal sequelae of STEC-HUS include impaired renal function, hypertension, low glomerular filtration rate, and proteinuria. Severity of acute illness, neurological symptoms, and need for initial dialysis are thought to be associated with a poor prognosis. End-stage renal failure occurs only in 5% of STEC-HUS [14].

The acute renal, neurological, and hematological manifestations of aHUS are similar to STEC-HUS. In contrast, aHUS is characterized by familial inheritance, frequent relapses, progression to end-stage renal disease in 50% of cases, and a high rate of recurrence postkidney transplant (30–100%). The use of eculizumab has improved the outcome of children with aHUS and allowed for successful kidney transplantation in these children [15].

Diagnosis

CBC and Examination of a Peripheral Blood Smear

Anemia and moderate thrombocytopenia are present. A peripheral blood smear typically shows schistocytes, helmet cells, and polychromasia (Fig. 2), consistent with MAHA. Serum lactate dehydrogenase (LDH) is elevated, and serum haptoglobin is low. The direct antiglobulin test (Coombs') test is negative.

Coagulation Testing

PT/INR, aPTT, and fibrinogen are typically normal, which differentiates STEC-HUS from DIC.

Microbiological Testing

Stool culture for *E. coli* and direct evaluation of shiga toxin in stool through PCR should be carried out. Given that STEC-HUS is not always preceded by diarrhea, stool evaluation should be done even in the absence of diarrhea. Urine culture is recommended as STEC-HUS has been reported after urinary tract infections.

Renal Function Testing

Renal abnormalities include proteinuria, hematuria, and acute renal failure. Renal function needs to be closely monitored. Renal biopsy is not required for diagnosis. However, when performed, biopsy findings typically show thickening of arterioles and capillaries, endothelial swelling and detachment, and subendothelial protein deposition.

Atypical HUS

All children presenting with signs/symptoms of MAHA should undergo measurement of ADAMTS13 (a disintegrin and metalloproteinase with a thrombospondin type 1 motif, member 13) activity levels in addition to screening for Shiga toxin (to exclude TTP and STEC-HUS, respectively). If ADAMTS13 levels are normal (>10%) and the shiga toxin screen is negative, further evaluation for aHUS should be carried out (Fig. 3). We additionally recommended suspecting aHUS in a child with thrombotic microangiopathy when the following features are present: presentation before 6 months of age, insidious onset, previous episode of HUS or unexplained hemolytic anemia, family history of HUS and HUS post-transplantation [15, 16]. In a patient with suspected aHUS, measurement of plasma concentrations of C3, C4, CFH, CFH antibodies, complement factor I (CFI), and complement factor B (CFB) levels and surface expression of membrane cofactor protein / CD46 on mononuclear leukocytes is recommended. In addition, testing for susceptibility genes *CFH, CFI, CFHR1–5, MCP/CD46, DGKE,* and *CFB* C3 should be undertaken [15]; however, genetic testing is only informative in 50–60% of cases [12]. For details, the reader is referred to the published International consensus statement for the diagnosis and management of aHUS [15]. Consultation and multidisciplinary care with pediatric nephrology is highly recommended.

Management

General Guidelines

Fluid management should be directed to rapidly correct any evidence of volume depletion. Management of acute renal failure remains the cornerstone for therapy of STEC-HUS. Electrolyte management, antihypertensive therapy, and dialysis should be guided by a pediatric nephrologist. Peritoneal and hemodialysis are equally effective.

Blood Component Therapy

RBC concentrates and platelet transfusions should be reserved for children requiring surgical interventions including renal biopsy or in children with significant symptomatic anemia. Platelet transfusions carry a theoretical risk of exacerbating the microvascular thrombosis in STEC-HUS. FP/FFP are not indicated in children with STEC-HUS, though these products may have role in the management of aHUS (i.e., plasma exchange, see below). As bleeding risk seems to be low and platelet count in STEC-HUS mostly ranges $>50 \times 10^9$/L, peritoneal dialysis catheter and central venous catheter placement can be accomplished safely without the need for platelet transfusion support [17].

Antibiotics

Currently, antibiotics are not recommended with the exception of aHUS associated with invasive pneumococcal disease.

Anticoagulation

In the absence of symptomatic venous TE, anticoagulation is not recommended in STEC-HUS or aHUS. In cases with acute venous TE, UFH or LMWH (dose adjusted for abnormal renal function) may be used (see Chapter 20).

Miscellaneous

Strict isolation of hospitalized children to reduce person-to-person transmission is recommended as soon as the diagnosis is made. Antimotility agents are not recommended. Steroids and shiga toxin binding agent (Synsorb-PK) have not been found to be beneficial. Novel therapies, including vaccination, monoclonal shiga toxin antibody, and shiga toxin receptor analogs remain investigational. Eculizumab has been successfully used in refractory cases of STEC-HUS, though it has not been systematically evaluated in a randomized trial [18].

Atypical HUS

aHUS has a significantly higher mortality and recurrence rate compared with STEC-HUS. With the advent of the complement terminal pathway blocker eculizumab, there has been a paradigm shift in the management of aHUS. Historically, aggressive and early plasmapheresis was thought to be the only therapeutic modality available for children with aHUS. However, following the Food and Drug administration (FDA) approval of eculizumab in 2011, the recombinant monoclonal antibody directed against complement C5, where available, has become the standard of care for children with aHUS [15]. In prospective studies, treatment with eculizumab was shown to inhibit disease progression and reverse organ damage [19]. Of note, plasmapheresis may still be needed acutely in children with suspected aHUS (until TTP is ruled out and eculizumab can be procured). In cases where there is a delay or inability to obtain eculizumab, plasmapheresis may be initiated as per the published 2009 guidelines [20].

Dosing recommendations for eculizumab are weight based and may be obtained through the product monograph. Children receiving eculizumab should receive meningococcal, pneumococcal, and *Haemophilus influenzae* vaccination and prophylactic antibiotics for a minimum of 2 weeks. Duration of treatment with eculizumab remains unknown. Discontinuation of treatment after a 6–12 month course of eculizumab has been suggested in selected cases [21]. Close monitoring for relapse after withdrawal of eculizumab is needed. Resuming eculizumab promptly after relapse is effective in most cases.

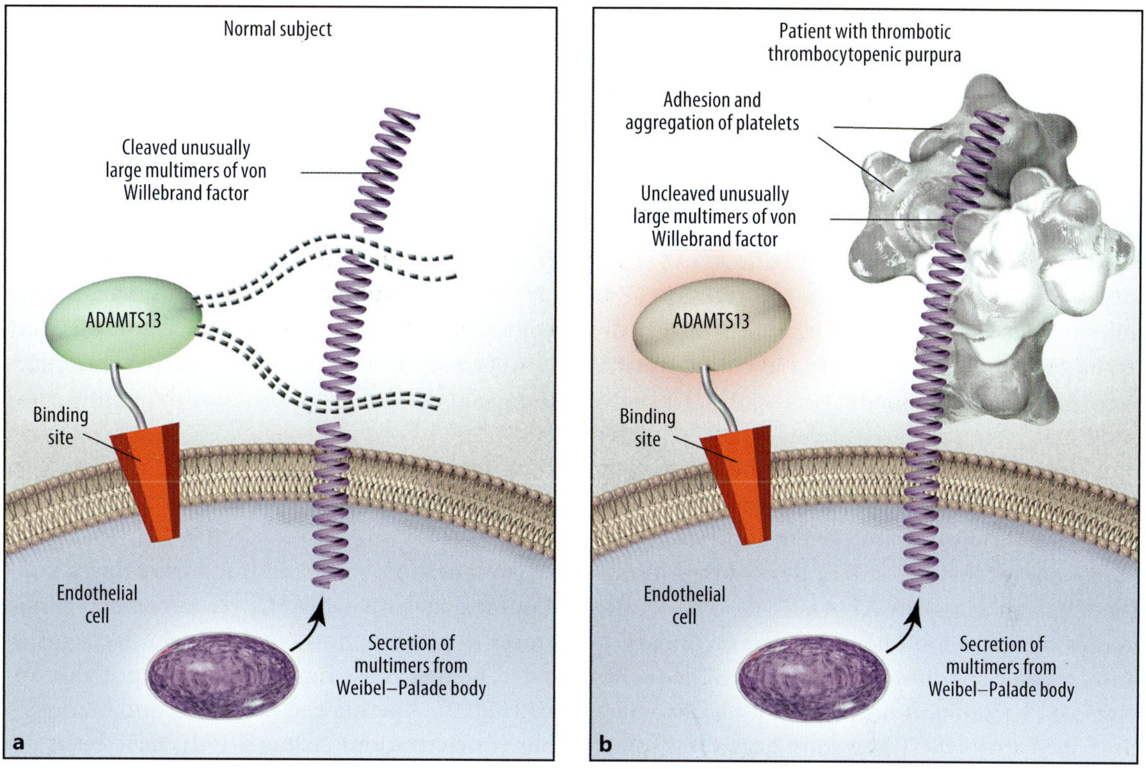

Fig. 4. Postulated mechanism of thrombotic thrombocytopenic purpura. **a** Normally ultra large von Willebrand factor (ULVWF) secreted by the Weibel-Palade bodies of the endothelial cells are cleaved by ADMTS13 (A disintegrin and metalloproteinase with a thrombospondin type 1 motif, member 13). **b** In thrombotic thrombocytopenic purpura (TTP), ADAMTS13 is deficient due to genetic defect (Upshaw-Schulman syndrome) or secondary to acquired inhibitors (immune-mediated TTP). In such subjects, there is formation of platelet-ULVWF microthrombi in terminal arterioles and capillaries resulting in symptoms of TTP. Reproduced with permission from Moake [23].

Thrombotic Thrombocytopenic Purpura

TTP has been historically characterized by the pentad of MAHA, thrombocytopenia, fever, neurological deficit, and renal impairment. The availability of appropriate therapy and urgency to treat may warrant a less stringent definition; the presence of thrombocytopenia and MAHA in the absence of an alternate etiology may be sufficient to make a presumptive diagnosis of TTP and initiate therapy [22]. TTP is rare, with an incidence of 1 in 4–11 million, with less than 5% of cases occurring in children.

ADAMTS13 and TTP

ADAMTS13 is a metalloprotease enzyme responsible for cleaving ultra large von Willebrand factor (ULVWF) into smaller inactive monomers. The gene for ADAMTS13 has been localized to chromosome 9q34. TTP is thought to result from either congenital (Upshaw-Schulman syndrome) or acquired (immune-mediated) deficiency of ADAMTS13. In the absence of the protease, platelets bind to the ULVWF resulting in the formation of platelet-von Willebrand factor (VWF) microthrombi (as opposed to platelet-fibrin microthrombi in HUS) in terminal arterioles resulting in thrombocytopenia and end-organ infarction (Fig. 4) [23]. Anemia secondarily occurs because of shearing of red cells travelling through these microthrombi resulting in fragmentation of red cells leading to production of schistocytes.

Upshaw-Schulman syndrome is a rare autosomal-recessive condition, often presenting in neonates who are homozygous or compound heterozygous for genetic variants in the *ADAMTS13* gene, with less than 0.1 IU/mL (10%) ADAMTS13 activity. Parents of such infants are usually asymptomatic, though they have low-normal ADAMTS13 activity (about 0.5 IU/mL). Upshaw-Schulman syndrome is rare with an estimated prevalence of 1–2/million [24]. The more common form of TTP is the immune-mediated form, which is typically encountered in adolescents and adults and occurs secondary to acquired inhibitors (IgG subclass) to ADAMTS13. These antibodies may develop idiopathically, secondary to autoimmune conditions, specifically SLE, or after viral and bacterial infections. TTP has also been described after HSCT and solid organ transplantation and with certain medications (i.e., cyclosporine, tacrolimus, clopidogrel, ticlopidine).

Clinical Presentation

The clinical presentation of TTP can be nonspecific and variable depending on the age of the patient and sites of microvascular thrombi. Upshaw-Schulman syndrome classically presents in the early neonatal period with Coombs' negative MAHA, thrombocytopenia, and severe hyperbilirubinemia, often warranting exchange transfusion. Thrombocytopenia may be severe, and bleeding symptoms including intraventricular hemorrhage have been described. Diagnosis is often delayed and is made after infants present with recurrent episodes of anemia and thrombocytopenia. Developmental delay has also been noted in these infants and is thought to be secondary to leukoencephalopathy and kernicterus. A "late-onset phenotype" of Upshaw-Schulman syndrome characterized by mild thrombocytopenia during childhood and exacerbations associated with pregnancy and infections has also been described [25].

Immune-mediated TTP typically occurs in previously healthy children and adolescents. CNS manifestations are present in 30–50%, including headache, altered mental status, intracranial hemorrhage, focal neurological deficiencies, seizures, and hemiparesis. General symptoms including fever, abdominal symptoms, nausea, and vomiting have also been described. Bleeding symptoms (e.g., petechiae, gingival bleeding, purpura, and epistaxis) are seen less frequently.

Diagnosis

CBC and Examination of a Peripheral Blood Smear

At presentation, most children have evidence of a Coombs' negative MAHA. A peripheral blood smear typically shows polychromasia, schistocytes, helmet cells, anisocytosis, and poikilocytosis (Fig. 2). Anemia can be severe, and hemoglobin concentrations below 5 g/dL have been described. Thrombocytopenia is often severe (typically more severe than in cases of HUS), with presenting platelet counts often less than 20×10^9/L. Serum LDH is elevated, and haptoglobin is low. Children diagnosed with immune-mediated TTP should be evaluated for SLE (antinuclear antibody and anti-dsDNA).

Coagulation Testing

PT/INR, aPTT, and fibrinogen are usually normal (this may help differentiate TTP from DIC). D-dimer levels may be elevated.

Renal Function Testing

Renal abnormalities including hematuria, proteinuria, and elevated creatinine have been described (renal abnormalities are typically less severe than in STEC HUS and aHUS).

PLASMIC Score

The PLASMIC (**P**latelet count; combined hemo**L**ysis variable; absence of **A**ctive cancer; absence

Table 3. The PLASMIC[a] diagnostic score

Parameter	Points
Platelet count <30 × 10^9/L	1
Combined hemolysis parameter – indirect bilirubin >2 mg/dL OR reticulocyte count >2.5% OR haptoglobin undetectable	1
No active cancer	1
No history of solid-organ or hematopoietic stem cell transplantation	1
MCV <90 fL	1
INR <1.5	1
Creatinine <2.0 mg/dL	1

Score <5: low risk for severe ADAMTS13 deficiency; close observation required. Score = 5: intermediate risk for severe ADAMTS13 deficiency; send ADAMTS13 testing, consider plasma infusion or total plasma exchange in high-risk cases. Score >5: high risk for severe ADAMTS13 deficiency; send ADAMTS13 testing and immediate total plasma exchange if high clinical suspicion for thrombotic thrombocytopenic purpura. Modified from with permission from Bendapudi et al. [26]. [a]See text for details.

of **S**tem-cell or solid-organ transplant; **M**CV; **I**NR; **C**reatinine) score is a clinical prediction tool that helps estimate the probability of ADAMTS13 activity <0.1 IU/mL (10%) and therefore helps identifying cases on whom ADAMTS13 testing should be performed, and facilitates rapid diagnosis and initiation of appropriate therapy (Table 3) [26].

ADAMTS13 Testing

ADAMTS13 activity and inhibitors to ADAMTS13 can be measured in specialized laboratories [10]. Obtaining a blood sample for measuring ADAMTS13 activity and inhibitors prior to initiation of plasmapheresis is important, though this should not delay initiation of therapy when there is high clinical suspicion of TTP. Patients with TTP classically have ADAMTS13 activity <0.1 IU/mL (10%); and higher levels should raise suspicion for an alternative diagnosis (such as aHUS).

Genetic Testing

ADAMTS13 gene sequencing may be pursued for children with suspected Upshaw-Schulman syndrome. Nearly 150 candidate variants in the *ADAMTS13* gene have been identified, with an evolving genotype-phenotype correlation. Variants in the highly conserved N-terminal domains are associated with lower ADAMTS13 activity and a more severe phenotype [25]. Sequence variation also can help to define childhood- and late onset type (mostly in pregnancy) of Upshaw-Schulman syndrome.

Management

Treatment guidelines and good practice statements for the clinical care for patients with TTP have been published [27, 28]. The following recommendations are extrapolated from these consensus guidelines.

Management of Upshaw-Schulman Syndrome

Blood Component Therapy

FP/FFP replacement remains the treatment modality of choice for infants with Upshaw-Schulman syndrome. Replacement of 10–15 mL/kg of FP/FFP is usually sufficient to achieve remission. Most infants will require FP/FFP infusion every 2–3 weeks to maintain normal platelet counts. Case reports have documented that plasma-derived FVIII concentrates with high AD-

AMTS13 content were also effective in replacing ADAMTS13 and thereby managing Upshaw-Schulman syndrome [29].

Novel Agents

New treatments focusing on substituting or supplementing plasma therapy with ADAMTS13 replacement have been explored for congenital TTP. These therapies involve using enzyme replacement to administer recombinant ADAMTS13 through intravenous infusion, thereby replenishing enzyme levels [30].

Management of Immune-Mediated (Acquired) TTP

Plasmapheresis

Plasmapheresis with plasma (FP/FFP) or cryosupernatant remains the cornerstone for management of immune-mediated TTP and has reduced the mortality from 90% to less than 10%. It is thought to act by replenishing ADAMTS13 as well as removing ULVWF multimers and ADAMTS13 antibodies. It should be initiated as soon as the diagnosis of TTP is seriously considered. Daily plasmapheresis (exchange volume: 40–60 mL/kg; or 1–2 times the plasma volume) until resolution of clinical symptoms and correction of thrombocytopenia is recommended [27, 28].

Blood Component Therapy

Plasmapheresis is superior to FP/FFP infusion for immune-mediated TTP. However, FP/FFP infusions may be a reasonable alternative until plasmapheresis is initiated [27]. There have been case reports of clinical deterioration and death after platelet transfusion. As such, platelet transfusion should be restricted for symptomatic bleeding or prior to invasive procedures [27].

Immunosuppressive Agents

Steroids (prednisone/prednisolone 1–2 mg/kg/day, divided every 12 h) are often used as initial therapy in conjunction with plasmapheresis. If platelet counts do not improve within 3–4 days, methylprednisolone (30 mg/kg/dose, every 24 h [maximum daily dose 1 g]) intravenously for 1–3 days followed by a rapid taper may be attempted. Retrospective and prospective nonrandomized studies have demonstrated that early use of rituximab (375 mg/m^2/dose [maximum dose 1 g] once a week × 4 doses) in adults with immune-mediated TTP is associated with fewer plasma exchanges, shorter inpatient stay, and fewer relapses. Lower doses of rituximab may also be effective [31]. While not confirmed in a randomized trial, both adult and pediatric consensus guidelines have suggested the use of upfront rituximab for management of immune-mediated TTP, in addition to plasma exchange and steroids [32]. It is also reasonable to consider treatment with rituximab in patients with relapsing/refractory TTP [27].

Cyclosporine, vincristine, and cyclophosphamide have all been used in patients with relapsing/refractory TTP. Paradoxically, cyclosporine has also been associated with post-transplant TTP. Antiplatelet agents are not indicated.

Novel Agents

Caplacizumab, an anti-VWF nanobody, directed against the A1 domain of VWF inhibits the interaction between ULVWF multimers and platelets. Adult studies have documented that the addition of caplacizumab to plasmapheresis and immunosuppression accelerates the time for platelet count normalization, reduces duration of hospitalization, and in-hospital mortality [33]. It was licensed by the FDA and European Medicines Agency for use in adults and children above the age of 12 years. It has a low toxicity profile, and it is now included in adult treatment guidelines for both incident and relapsed immune-mediated TTP [34]. Pediatric data on the use of caplacizumab are restricted to case reports (refer to drug monograph for dosing).

Recombinant human ADAMTS13, and small molecules that target the VWF-platelet interaction, including aptamers (ARC1779) are also being investigated for the management of immune-mediated TTP [30].

Splenectomy
Splenectomy acts by depleting B-cell reservoirs and may theoretically benefit patients with immune-mediated relapsing/refractory TTP. There have been no pediatric studies of splenectomy in TTP.

Transplant-Associated Thrombotic Microangiopathic Disorder

Transplant-associated thrombotic microangiopathic disorder (TA-TMA) is a complication of HSCT and is associated with a high mortality rate. In TA-TMA, complement dysregulation and endothelial injury lead to an increase in proinflammatory cytokines, procoagulant factors, and soluble adhesion molecules, which promote further endothelial damage and complement cascade activation. Nitric oxide depletion diminishes the vasodilatory properties of the vessel and leads to platelet aggregation and subsequent microthrombi development. Studies confirm the role of complement activation, indicated by significant increases in C3b and sC5b-9 [35].

Clinically, TA-TMA resides within a spectrum of transplant-associated endothelial cell activation syndromes, including capillary leak syndrome, engraftment syndrome, and idiopathic pneumonia syndrome. Diagnosis can be delayed and confounded by expected cytopenias and end organ toxicities. Risk factors in adults for TA-TMA include unrelated donor or haploidentical transplant, graft versus host disease (GVHD), fungal and bacterial infections.

Diagnostic criteria for TA-TMA have been published [36]. TA-TMA is diagnosed in HSCT recipients with ≥4 diagnostic markers present simultaneously: (1) LDH above normal for age; (2) schistocytes on blood smear; (3) de novo thrombocytopenia or >50% decrease in the platelet count or sudden increase in transfusion requirements; (4) de novo anemia or increased transfusion requirements; (5) hypertension >99% for age (<18 years); (6) proteinuria ≥30 mg/dL (on two separate measurements) or random urine protein/creatinine ratio of nephrotic range; and (7) elevated soluble terminal complement complex activity (plasma sC5b-9, normal range <244 ng/mL). Alternatively, TA-TMA is diagnosed based on histologic evidence of TMA on tissue sample.

TA-TMA may affect multiple organs. The kidneys are typically the primary site of microangiopathy, causing proteinuria, acute kidney injury, and hypertension. TA-TMA can also present as intestinal TMA with or without gut-GVHD, as pulmonary hypertension, posterior reversible encephalopathy syndrome with headache and/or seizures, and polyserositis. Most cases occur before day 100 post-HSCT (which may help distinguish it from other post-HSCT complications). Children may also present with multiple organ dysfunction syndrome, which is associated with high morbidity and mortality. The PLASMIC is not applicable in children with suspected TA-TMA [37].

Management
Therapy in TA-TMA should mainly address organ dysfunction and includes mainly supportive care measures. A reduction of cyclosporine or tacrolimus should be considered. Bleeding due to cytopenias and involvement of the gastrointestinal tract is frequent and correlates to worse outcome.

In case of bleeding symptoms, platelet transfusion, substitution of FP/FFP, and if necessary antifibrinolytic agents are therapy mainstays. Due to hepatic involvement, severe hypofibrinogenemia and low (<0.4 IU/mL) factor XIII (FXIII) levels may occur. In selected cases of TA-TMA

11

Table 4. Rebalanced hemostasis in chronic liver disease

Factors promoting bleeding	Factors promoting thrombosis
↓ Synthesis of factors II, V, VII, IX, X, XI, XIII	↓ Synthesis of protein C, protein S, and antithrombin
Hypofibrinogenemia/ Dysfibrinogenemia	↑ Factor VIII
	↑ von Willebrand factor
↓ Synthesis of TAFI and α_2-antiplasmin	↓ Synthesis of ADAMTS13
↓ Clearance of tPA	↓ Synthesis of plasminogen
↓ Thrombopoietin production	
Platelet sequestration in the spleen	
Platelet functional defects	

Modified from Lisman [38]. ADAMTS13, a disintegrin and metalloproteinase with a thrombospondin type 1 motif, member 13; TAFI, thrombin-activatable fibrinolysis inhibitor; tPA, tissue plasminogen activator.

with findings resembling veno-occlusive disease, the use of defibrotide may be cautiously considered [37].

Patients should be evaluated for complement C3, elevated sC5b-9, and antibodies against CFH. Plasmapheresis is indicated in patients with CFH antibodies. Although not FDA approved so far for TA-TMA, terminal complement inhibition with eculizumab has been shown to improve outcome in children, particularly in high-risk TA-TMA (i.e., nephrotic range proteinuria with proteinuria ≥30 mg/dL × 2; or random urine protein/creatinine ratio ≥2 mg/mg and elevated sC5b-9 >244 ng/mL at the time of TA-TMA diagnosis). In both children and adults, the drug has shown a better response rate compared with the use of plasmapheresis [37].

Coagulopathy of Chronic Liver Disease

The coagulopathy associated with chronic liver disease has historically been the prototype of acquired bleeding disorders. Studies underline a paradigm shift in this dogma and now recognize that chronic liver disease is associated with a "rebalanced state" of hemostasis, secondary to its simultaneous impact on procoagulant, anticoagulant, and fibrinolytic pathways (Table 4) [38]. This rebalanced state is more labile and may result in bleeding associated with invasive procedures, vitamin K deficiency, renal dysfunction, sepsis, and variceal bleeding resulting from local vasculopathy.

Conventional tests of hemostasis such as the PT/INR and aPTT, although significantly prolonged, do not predict the bleeding risk in chronic liver disease. Global tests of hemostasis such as thromboelastography (TEG) and rotational thromboelastometry (ROTEM) are being increasingly studied [39]. Studies have also indicated that the prolonged PT/INR does not protect patients with chronic liver disease from venous TE. In fact, the incidence of venous TEs in chronic liver disease is reported to be significantly higher than the general population; with portal vein thrombosis, deep venous thrombosis, and pulmonary embolism being the common thrombotic manifestations [40].

Clinical Presentation

The coagulopathy of chronic liver disease occurs in the setting of cirrhosis, for which common causes in young infants include biliary atresia, inborn errors of metabolism, familial cholestatic diseases, intestinal failure-associated liver disease, and idiopathic neonatal hepatitis. In older children and adolescents, causes of cirrhosis include autoimmune hepatitis, primary sclerosing cholangitis, and less commonly, chronic hepatitis B and C, nonalcoholic fatty liver disease, and cystic fibrosis liver disease.

While bruising, purpura, ecchymosis, epistaxis, and bleeding from gums may be seen in children with cirrhosis, it is often abnormal coagulation parameters tested prior to an invasive procedure that prompts a hematology consult. Bleeding from esophageal varices is primarily the result of a mechanical breach in the variceal wall resulting from increased intraluminal pressure and mural thinning related to increasing venous diameter. Variceal bleeding is unrelated to coagulopathy.

Diagnosis

CBC and Examination of a Peripheral Blood Smear

Mild to moderate thrombocytopenia may be present. The peripheral blood smear in advanced liver disease may show target cells.

Coagulation Testing

The PT/INR is typically prolonged secondary to impaired synthesis of coagulation factors and/or vitamin K deficiency resulting from cholestasis. The PT is used in both the Child-Pugh score for prognosis of chronic liver disease and the pediatric end-stage liver disease score for ranking of children awaiting transplant. aPTT and D-dimer levels may be normal to slightly prolonged, and fibrinogen levels may be low in chronic liver disease. While the PT/INR, aPTT, and platelet count do not predict bleeding in chronic liver disease, low fibrinogen levels have been associated in some, but not all, studies with periprocedural bleeding [40].

Global Hemostatic Assays

Global hemostatic assays including TEG and ROTEM are being increasingly studied in adults with chronic liver disease and are typically normal despite significant abnormalities in the PT/INR, aPTT, and platelet count and fibrinogen levels. Use of TEG and ROTEM prior to procedures is associated with decreased need for transfusion [39]. Lack of universal access to these assays, the absence of consensus on test thresholds used to trigger transfusion, and lack of validation in children are some limitations of these assays. Further studies are required before routine use of these assays in this cohort can be recommended.

Management

There are little data on the management of coagulopathy in children with chronic liver disease who present with variceal bleeding or during liver transplantation and liver biopsy. Management of variceal bleeding relies on vasoactive drugs to reduce variceal pressure and endoscopic occlusion of the varices with band ligation or sclerotherapy. The following recommendations for treatment of coagulopathy are based on adult consensus guidelines [40–43].

Blood Component Therapy

Using FP/FFP to simply correct abnormal coagulation labs (PT/INR and aPTT) is not recommended for most procedures. The large volume of plasma required to increase clotting factor levels and thereby correct the PT/INR may be associated with volume overload, increased portal pressure, and may paradoxically increase the risk of rebleeding from esophageal varices. Published recommendations from selected professional societies suggest no preprocedural correction of hemostatic labs based on PT/INR, aPTT, fibrinogen, or platelet counts for most procedures [41, 42]. Prior to high-risk procedures (e.g., cardiac and spinal surgeries), an individualized approach after careful consideration of risks and benefits is recommended.

In children with overt bleeding and a PT/INR >1.5 times the normal range, a reasonable approach is to administer an initial infusion of 15 mL/kg of FP/FFP (range 10–20 mL/kg) with a follow-up PT/

INR. Maintaining a platelet count greater than 50 × 10^9/L during clinically significant bleeding is recommended. Of note, the response to platelet transfusion may be markedly less than expected secondary to splenic sequestration of transfused platelets. Cryoprecipitate should be considered in children with hypo-/dysfibrinogenemia as evidenced by a fibrinogen activity level of <1.0 g/L and clinically significant bleeding (see Appendix III for cryoprecipitate dosing).

Vitamin K
Despite a paucity of evidence, it is reasonable to replace vitamin K in children with chronic liver disease and bleeding symptoms. We recommend intravenous vitamin K (0.3 mg/kg/dose [maximum dose 10 mg]) daily for 3 days.

Thrombopoietin Receptor Agonists
Adult randomized trials have documented that thrombopoietin receptor agonists (avatrombopag and lusutrombopag) can increase platelet counts before planned surgical procedures and thereby decrease the need for periprocedure platelet transfusion [40, 44]. Both agents are currently approved for use in adults with chronic liver disease. Romiplostim use has been reported anecdotally. Two pivotal trials of eltrombopag were complicated by a high risk of TE (particularly portal vein thrombosis). It may be reasonable to consider using thrombopoietin receptor agonists in patients scheduled to undergo high-risk procedures (spinal or cardiac surgeries) when there is sufficient time (1–2 weeks) to raise the platelet count.

Antifibrinolytic Agents
Antifibrinolytic agents have been shown to reduce the need for RBC transfusion in patients undergoing liver transplant without increasing the risk of TEs. Tranexamic acid or ε-aminocaproic may be considered for mucous membrane bleeding and have been reported for the management of bleeding from gastric antral vascular ectasia associated with cirrhosis (see Appendix III for dosing).

Recombinant Factor VIIa
While there is no evidence to support the use of rFVIIa in children with coagulopathy of liver disease, it might be considered if there is failure to control bleeding with standard therapy or where there are concerns of volume overload. The recommended dose of rFVIIa is unclear, but most experts would consider using a low dose of rFVIIa in chronic liver disease (15–30 μg/kg/dose repeated every 2–3 h based on the clinical situation). Treatment with rFVIIa may result in an increased risk of TEs and should be used only after discussing risks and benefits with the patient/guardian.

Prothrombin Complex Concentrates
Prothrombin complex concentrates (PCCs) are plasma-derived, viral-inactivated products containing factors II (FII), VII (FVII), IX (FIX), FX, protein C, protein S, and traces of antithrombin, heparin, and vitronectin (4-factor products). Given the high risk of TEs and very limited pediatric experience, PCCs should be used with extreme caution and only if bleeding cannot be controlled with any of the above-mentioned modalities. An initial dose of 20–25 IU/kg with a follow-up PT/INR in 30–60 min is recommended [40, 45] (see Appendix III).

Bleeding in Chronic Renal Failure

Bleeding is a common and serious complication in patients with chronic renal failure, though its incidence has decreased with the advent of improved dialysis techniques and routine use of erythropoietin for management of anemia. The pathophysiology of bleeding is thought to be multifactorial. Platelet dysfunction, abnormal platelet-endothelial interaction, the presence of uremic toxins, and anemia have been implicated as contributory factors (Table 5). In addition, thrombocytopenia may also be present, though platelet counts are rarely less than 100 × 10^9/L. Bleeding usually manifests as mucocutaneous

Table 5. Mechanisms affecting hemostasis in uremia

Mechanisms
Platelet dysfunction:
Reduction in dense granule content, intracellular ADP and serotonin, and release of platelet α-granule protein and β-thromboglobulin
Enhanced intracellular c-AMP
Defective cyclo-oxygenase activity
Abnormalities in mobilization of platelet calcium, arachidonic acid metabolism
Ex vivo platelet aggregation
Defects in platelet-vessel wall interaction:
Abnormal platelet adhesion
Altered von Willebrand factor
Increased formation of vascular prostacyclin (PGI_2)
Increased expression of nitric oxide
Uremic toxins
Anemia:
Altered blood rheology
Defective platelet diffusivity
Decreased release of ADP by erythrocytes
Erythropoietin deficiency
Drug treatment:
Anticoagulants, antiplatelet agents, NSAIDs, β-lactam antibiotics, third-generation cephalosporins

Modified with permission from Galbusera et al. [47]. ADP, adenosine 5′-diphospate; c-AMP, cyclic adenosine monophosphate; NSAIDs, nonsteroidal anti-inflammatory drugs.

11

bleeding including easy bruising, petechiae, epistaxis, and bleeding from venipuncture sites [46].

Diagnosis

Treatment is usually reserved for bleeding. However, laboratory evaluation may be helpful in predicting the risk of bleeding with invasive procedures.

CBC and Examination of a Peripheral Blood Smear

Mild to moderate thrombocytopenia is common. A peripheral blood smear may show a reduced mean platelet volume.

Coagulation Testing

aPTT, PT/INR, and TT are typically normal. A bleeding time was historically thought to be the best laboratory test for predicting bleeding in patients with uremia. However, the test has poor reproducibility and accuracy and is rarely performed. In vitro tests of platelet function, including platelet aggregation and closure times with the platelet function analyzer (PFA-100®/200®), have been investigated but need further validation for clinical application (see Chapter 4).

Renal Function Testing

Tests of renal function including glomerular filtration rate, serum creatinine, and blood urea nitrogen do not predict bleeding [46].

Management

Given the paucity of pediatric studies, the following recommendations are based on adult studies and consensus guidelines [47, 48].

Dialysis

Dialysis remains the cornerstone of management of renal failure and may help prevent bleeding. Although heterogeneous in nature, many studies show that dialysis can improve platelet function abnormalities and reduce the risk of hemorrhage. It is thought to work by removing uremic toxins from the circulation. In patients with active bleeding, peritoneal dialysis may be preferable over hemodialysis as heparin administration is not required.

Desmopressin
DDAVP (1-deamino-8-D-arginine vasopressin) remains the most common modality of treatment of acute bleeds. It is thought to act by increasing plasma concentration of FVIII and VWF. It has a quick onset of action (1 h) and may be given subcutaneously or intravenously. Major limitations of DDAVP remain tachyphylaxis associated with use of multiple doses, the need for fluid restriction, and risk of hyponatremia and seizures. DDAVP should be used with caution in very young children (≤3 years) (see Appendix III).

Correction of Anemia
Correction of anemia either through RBC transfusion (10–20 mL/kg), the use of erythropoietin (50 units/kg/day × 3 times a week intravenous or subcutaneous), or darbepoetin (0.45 μg/kg/dose once a week intravenous or subcutaneous) has been shown to correct coagulation parameters.

Cryoprecipitate
In both prospective and retrospective studies, cryoprecipitate has been shown to improve coagulation parameters. It has a quick onset of action and may be beneficial in acute bleeding.

Estrogen Therapy
Multiple adult studies have evaluated the role of estrogen although there are no pediatric data available. While its exact mechanism remains unclear, conjugated estrogen (minimum dose of 0.6 mg/kg injected intravenously over 30–40 min daily for 5 days) has been shown to improve clinical bleeding. Onset of action is within 6 h, and duration of action is approximately 14–21 days. Given easy access and good response to dialysis and DDAVP, estrogen therapy is rarely used to control bleeding and should be reserved as a last option for refractory bleeding.

Acquired Hemophilia

Acquired hemophilia is a rare but serious bleeding disorder characterized by the development of neutralizing autoantibodies (inhibitors) targeting specific epitopes of FVIII. It classically presents with the sudden onset of bleeding symptoms in a patient with no past or family history of a bleeding disorder. It is exceedingly rare in children with an estimated annual incidence of 0.045 per million [49]. Pediatric acquired hemophilia has been described in association with autoimmune conditions, infections, and antibiotic exposure, most commonly penicillin or penicillin-like medications [50]. Neonatal acquired hemophilia due to transplacental transfer of maternal autoantibodies has also been described.

Unlike congenital severe hemophilia where hemarthrosis is the characteristic bleeding manifestation, most patients with acquired hemophilia present with mucocutaneous, deep muscular, and/or retroperitoneal bleeding [51]. Significant local bleeding following venipuncture and intramuscular injections have also been described.

Diagnosis

Acquired hemophilia should be suspected in a child with a negative past and family history of bleeding who presents with a sudden onset of subcutaneous or mucocutaneous bleeding. Children diagnosed with acquired hemophilia should be evaluated for immune dysfunction, particularly SLE.

Coagulation Testing
Patients with acquired hemophilia have a prolonged aPTT, and a normal PT/INR and fibrinogen. Whenever applicable, heparin contamina-

tion could be ruled out by performing an anti-Xa level, by neutralization of heparin with a heparinase or by performing a TT and reptilase time (typically, heparin contamination results in a prolonged TT and a normal reptilase time).

A 1:1 mixing study helps differentiate between congenital factor deficiency and acquired antibodies. The aPTT in congenital factor deficiencies typically corrects after mixing the patient plasma in a 1:1 ratio with normal plasma. In cases of acquired hemophilia or lupus anticoagulant (LAC)/antiphospholipid antibodies, the aPTT remains prolonged after mixing. Unlike LAC/antiphospholipid antibodies, FVIII inhibitors are typically time and temperature sensitive, and therefore, incubated mixing studies must be performed at 37 °C for 1–2 h (see Chapter 13) [52].

Factor assays for factors VIII, IX, XI, and XII should be done to identify the specificity of inhibitors. In case of acquired FVIII inhibitors, the Nijmegen modification of the Bethesda assay is recommended for quantification of the inhibitor titer (see Chapter 8). Of note, in contrast to congenital hemophilia, bleeding symptoms in children with acquired hemophilia correlate poorly with the FVIII level and inhibitor titers.

Management

Given the rarity of acquired hemophilia in children, recommendations regarding management of bleeds and inhibitor eradication are extrapolated from adult data and based on expert opinion [53, 54]. Management of acquired hemophilia entails avoiding nonurgent therapeutic and diagnostic interventions, management during acute bleeding episodes, and eradication of the antibody. Given the risk of life-threatening bleeds, these children should be urgently referred to a comprehensive hemophilia/bleeding disorder center.

Bypassing agents are needed to manage acute bleeding events. Both rFVIIa and activated prothrombin complex concentrates (aPCCs) have been used with similar efficacy. Dosing of bypassing agents is identical to doses used in patient with congenital hemophilia and inhibitors (see Chapter 8). Additionally, porcine FVIII is approved by the FDA for use in adults with acquired hemophilia, though pediatric experience is limited. An initial dose of 200 units/kg is recommended, with titration of subsequent doses based on desired FVIII trough levels and individual clinical response [55]. There are reports of using emicizumab in patients with acquired hemophilia to prevent bleeding [56].

Despite the availability of emicizumab, it is still recommended that patients with acquired hemophilia should receive immunosuppressive agents to attempt to eradicate the inhibitors. Different approaches in adults have been used including steroids (usually 1–2 mg/kg/day, divided every 12 h for 4–6 weeks followed by taper), alone or combined with oral cyclophosphamide (1.5–2 mg/kg/day) for 1–2 months [54]. A systematic review published in 2007 showed that patients treated with rituximab (375 mg/m^2/dose [maximum dose 1 g] once a week × 4 doses) alone or in combination with other immunosuppressive agents reported a complete or partial response in 90% of cases [57]. Consequently, rituximab is now widely used in adults with acquired hemophilia and may be considered in children with acquired hemophilia.

Acquired von Willebrand Syndrome

Acquired von Willebrand Syndrome (AVWS) is rare in children, though its exact incidence is difficult to ascertain. In children, AVWS has been described in association with Wilms' tumor, hypothyroidism, SLE, congenital cardiac defects, extracorporeal membrane oxygenation (ECMO), and the use of left ventricular assist devices (LVADs). This is distinct from adults where 50–60% of AVWS is associated with lymphoproliferative and myeloproliferative disorders. While the exact pathophysiology of AVWS remains unclear, five distinct mechanisms have been proposed: (1) decreased production/impaired release of VWF (e.g., hypothyroidism, valproic acid); (2) increased clearance of the VWF-FVIII complex by circulating autoantibodies (e.g., SLE); (3) adsorption of VWF to tumor cells (e.g., Wilms tumor); (4) drug-mediated destruction of VWF multimers (e.g., ciprofloxacin); and (5) increased clearance of high-molecular-weight multimers in association with high flow/high shear cardiac defects (e.g., ECMO, LVAD, ventricular septal defects, patent ductus arteriosus, aortic stenosis) [58]. In ECMO and LVAD, AVWS develops shortly after implantation and persists as long as patients remain on support. Recovery from AVWS occurs rapidly after ECMO/LVAD explantation [59, 60]. AVWS has also been reported in the setting of idiopathic pulmonary hypertension where it is postulated that the narrowed pulmonary vasculature acts like a high flow/high shear lesion much like in cardiac defects [61]. Clinical manifestations of AVWS are identical to congenital von Willebrand disease (VWD), consisting of mainly mucocutaneous bleeding (see Chapter 9).

Diagnosis

An abrupt onset of bleeding symptoms in the presence of a known predisposing condition (e.g., VAD placement, hypothyroidism, etc.) should raise clinical suspicion for AVWS. In the absence of a clear etiology for AVWS, it is often difficult to distinguish congenital VWD from AVWS. The absence of a family history of bleeding and negative test results on parents may help. Consensus guidelines recommend that children with underlying conditions known to be associated with AVWS undergo testing prior to surgical interventions [62].

CBC and Examination of a Peripheral Blood Smear

A CBC and peripheral smear are usually normal, although in cardiac defect induced AVWS, mild thrombocytopenia can be seen because of platelet consumption.

Coagulation Testing

The PT/INR and fibrinogen are typically normal. The aPTT may be slightly prolonged based on the FVIII procoagulant activity (FVIII:C).

von Willebrand-specific testing typically reveals a low-to-normal VWF antigen (VWF:Ag) and FVIII:C. Functional assays of VWF activity (VWF:Act), including ristocetin cofactor activity, collagen binding activity, and VWF glycoprotein 1bM usually show a more marked decrease. VWF multimer analysis typically shows a decrease in high-molecular-weight multimers. An increased VWF propeptide/VWF:Ag ratio may be seen in AVWS caused by increased clearance. PFA-100®/200® is very sensitive to AVWS; closure times are usually markedly prolonged with both the collagen/epinephrine and collagen/ADP cartridges.

Management

The following recommendations are based on pediatric and adult consensus guidelines [62, 63]. Goals of management of AVWS include (1) management of acute bleeding symptoms and prevention of bleeding with invasive procedures and (2) treatment of the underlying disorder. Treatment of the underlying medical disorder, such as chemotherapy/surgery for Wilms' tumor; hormone replacement for hypothyroidism; surgical correction of the underlying cardiac defect; and ECMO/LVAD explantation usually results in rapid resolution of symptoms. Considerations for hemostatic and other immunomodulatory agents are as follows.

Desmopressin

DDAVP generally results in a rapid increase in plasma VWF:Ag and may be used to treat minor bleeds in selected cases. Response to DDAVP in AVWS is less predictable than congenital VWD, with significant heterogeneity noted across AVWS causes. Clinical efficacy of DDAVP is better in patients with AVWS secondary to malignancy or lymphoproliferative disease. Given the variable individual response, we recommend a trial of DDAVP when possible (including measurement of VWF:Ag, VWF:Act, and FVIII:C pre- and 1 and 4 hours post DDAVP administration). DDAVP should be used with caution in very young children (≤3 years) and those with seizure disorders (see Appendix III for dosing).

VWF Concentrates
Both plasma-derived and recombinant VWF concentrates may be used for prevention of bleeding before invasive procedures or as treatment for more serious bleeds (see Appendix III for dosing) [64]. A starting dose between 40 and 80 IU/kg can be used, depending on bleeding severity. Given the unpredictable response to VWF concentrates, we recommend measuring the VWF:Ag, VWF:Act, and FVIII:C preinfusion, 30 min, 4 h and 24 h postinfusion to establish the half-life of infused VWF concentrates. The initial recovery and subsequent measurements may be used to guide subsequent therapy.

Antifibrinolytic Agents
Antifibrinolytic agents such as tranexamic acid and ε-aminocaproic acid may be used as an adjunct to VWF concentrates and/or DDAVP. These are particularly useful in gastrointestinal bleeds and postprocedure bleeds (see Appendix III for dosing).

Recombinant Factor VIIa
rFVIIa (90 µg/kg/dose every 2–3 h) could be used for serious uncontrollable bleeds that do not respond to standard therapy, particularly in antibody-mediated AVWS. Caution should be exerted in children with high-flow high shear AVWS. Risk of TEs should be considered, and risks and benefits should be reviewed with patient/guardians.

Intravenous Immunoglobulin
Intravenous immunoglobulin (IVIG) (1 g/kg) is useful in AVWS associated with lymphoproliferative disorders, particularly monoclonal gammopathy of uncertain significance (MGUS-IgG). Its use has been reported in children with acute lymphoblastic leukemia and biclonal IgM gammopathy.

Plasmapheresis
Plasmapheresis can help to remove pathologic autoantibodies and restore hemostasis. It has been used mostly in patients with MGUS-IgM where IVIG is not effective.

11

Lupus Anticoagulant Hypoprothrombinemia Syndrome

LACs are a heterogeneous group of antibodies that are often diagnosed incidentally in children, tend to be transient, and result in an isolated prolongation of the aPTT. Antiphospholipid antibody syndrome is an acquired thrombophilia that presents with recurrent arterial and venous TE and/or fetal loss in combination with nontransient LAC (see Chapter 13). Lupus anticoagulant hypoprothrombinemia syndrome (LAHS) is a rare condition where LACs are associated with a bleeding diathesis. This is thought to result from the presence of non-neutralizing antiprothrombin antibodies; the subsequent rapid clearance of prothrombin antigen-antibody complexes eventually results in a prothrombin deficiency state.

Presentation and Diagnosis

Case reports of LAHS typically describe a sudden onset of bleeding in a child with SLE or in a previously healthy child following a viral infection (particularly adenovirus) [65]. Bleeding manifestations vary from mild mucocutaneous bleeds (epistaxis, gingival bleeding, and petechiae) to life-threatening gastrointestinal bleeds and hemarthrosis. Laboratory findings in LAHS include prolongation of both the PT/INR and aPTT with evidence of LAC, low prothrombin (FII) levels, and evidence of antiprothrombin antibodies (FII

IgG and IgM by ELISA). Since the antibodies are non-neutralizing, the mixing study for PT may show complete/near complete correction of the PT with mixing.

Management

The rarity of LAHS makes it difficult to formulate evidence-based guidelines. Children with LAHS presenting with moderate-to-severe bleeding symptoms should be managed with FP/FFP as a source of prothrombin; aPCCs have also been used. For severe life-threatening bleeding, rFVIIa may be considered. However, it should be recognized that the thrombotic risk is high in LAHS, and hence caution should be used particularly when aPCCs or rFVIIa are used. Shared decision making after careful review of risks and benefits of aPCCs and rFVIIa with patient/guardian is encouraged. In very severe life-threatening cases, plasmapheresis to remove antibodies may need to be considered.

Children (specifically older children and adolescents) with LAHS should be investigated for SLE. If signs of SLE, with moderate-to-severe bleeding symptoms are present, immunosuppressive therapy with prednisone/prednisolone at 1–2 mg/kg/day (divided every 12 h) should be promptly commenced. Referral to the rheumatology service for definitive management of SLE is recommended. Rituximab has been used in SLE presenting with LAHS with some success [66]. In patients without evidence of SLE or any other autoimmune disorder where the LAHS is thought to stem from a viral infection, the condition usually resolves spontaneously without immunosuppressive therapy. However, in case of clinically significant bleeding, a short course of corticosteroids (prednisone/prednisolone, 1–2 mg/kg/day [divided every 12 h] for 2 weeks) should be considered [65].

Coagulopathy of Massive Transfusion

The transfusion of large amounts of RBC concentrates may lead to dilutional coagulopathy and life-threatening bleeding. It can be exacerbated by hypocalcaemia (due to calcium chelation by the citrate used in blood products), acidosis, and hypothermia, as they delay clot formation and lead to a deficit in fibrinogen. In the setting of trauma, these impairments can be combined with acute coagulopathy due to the massive release of TF and endothelial dysfunction. Trauma-induced coagulopathy is often characterized by abnormalities of the fibrinolytic system, either in the form of fibrinolysis shutdown or hyperfibrinolysis, both of which are associated with increased mortality compared with physiologic fibrinolysis [67].

While several definitions of massive transfusion exist, it is usually recognized that the transfusion of more than 10 units of RBC concentrates in adults or the transfusion of 40 mL/kg/24 h; or >50% blood volume within 3 h in children increase the risk of dilutional coagulopathy [68].

Diagnosis

Coagulopathy of massive transfusion is characterized by thrombocytopenia, elevated PT/INR and aPTT, elevated TT, and reduced fibrinogen. Viscoelastic testing (ROTEM or TEG) may be helpful to diagnose coagulopathy of massive transfusion, notably to detect abnormalities of fibrinolysis [69].

Management

The goals of therapy should be to prevent bleeding, keep platelets above 50×10^9/L, and normalize PT/INR, aPTT, and TT to the extent possible. The blood bank should be notified early of the need for continuous blood products. To optimize tissue delivery of oxygen, hemoglobin should be ideally kept above 10 mg/dL. Early resuscitation should aim for a ratio of 1:1:1 replacement of RBCs, plasma, and platelets using standard doses (see Appendix III). Fibrinogen levels should be

Table 6. Most common causes of acquired factor deficiencies

Factor deficiency	Underlying causes	
	Reduced synthesis	Accelerated clearance/consumption Nonimmune (NI) or immune (I)
Fibrinogen	Severe liver disease Medication (e.g., asparaginase)	
Prothrombin (FII) and thrombin	Vitamin K antagonist therapy Vitamin K deficiency	Antiphospholipid antibodies (I) Autoimmune diseases (SLE, rheumatoid arthritis) (I) Lymphoproliferative disorders (I) Exposure to bovine thrombin (I)
Factor V	Liver disease	Exposure to topical fibrin glue or bovine thrombin preparations (I) Autoimmune disease (I) Malignancy (I)
Factor VII	Liver disease Vitamin K antagonist therapy Vitamin K deficiency	
Factor X	Severe liver disease Vitamin K antagonist therapy Vitamin K deficiency	Amyloidosis (NI) Burns (NI) Exposure to bovine thrombin preparations (I) Respiratory infections Malignancies: low-grade gastrointestinal lymphoma, gastric adenocarcinoma, adrenal cortical carcinoma (I)
Factor XI	Liver disease	Nephrotic syndrome Autoimmune diseases (SLE, rheumatoid arthritis, Crohn's disease) (I)
Factor XII	Liver disease	Nephrotic syndrome (NI)
Factor XIII	Liver disease Leukemia Medication (e.g., valproate, tocilizumab)	Surgery (NI) DIC, sepsis (NI) Inflammatory bowel disease (NI) Henoch-Schonlein purpura (NI) Thrombosis (NI) Autoimmune diseases (SLE, rheumatoid arthritis) (I) Malignancies (I) Medication (e.g., isoniazid, penicillin) (I) Monoclonal gammopathy of undetermined significance (I)

DIC, disseminated intravascular coagulation; SLE, systemic lupus erythematosus.

monitored, and deficiencies are corrected with cryoprecipitate/fibrinogen concentrates whenever fibrinogen levels fall below the 1.0 g/L. Efforts should be made to avoid acidosis and hypothermia, notably by warming the RBC concentrate before transfusion. Platelets and plasma should not be warmed. Potential side effects of transfusion should be serially monitored, including hyperkalemia, hypomagnesemia, and hypocalcemia, as well as fluid overload and pulmonary edema. Addition of antifibrinolytic agents should be considered for overt bleeding, especially mucocutaneous or postprocedural bleeding, although whether antifibrinolytic agents reduce mortality in children with trauma-induced coagulopathy remains unclear [70, 71].

Acquired Factor Deficiencies

Acquired factor deficiencies are rare during childhood. They may be due to reduced synthesis of procoagulant factors (e.g., liver disease, vitamin K deficiency), accelerated clearance of coagulation factors (e.g., DIC, surgery, nephrotic syndrome), or immune-mediated destruction of factors (e.g., autoimmune diseases, malignancies), as shown in Table 6 [72–74]. For example, SLE has been described in association with antibodies to a variety of coagulation factors, including antibodies directed against factors II, VIII, IX, XI, XII, and XIII [65]. Specific factor deficiencies have also been described notably following exposure to bovine thrombin (FII, FV), amyloidosis (FX), burns (FX), Henoch-Schonlein purpura (FXIII), and various medications (fibrinogen, vitamin K-dependent factors, FXIII) [75]. The management of acquired factor deficiencies varies based on the specific deficiency and the underlying cause. The management of neonatal vitamin K deficiency is discussed in Chapter 3.

Conclusion

In summary, acquired bleeding disorders are a heterogeneous group of disorders with symptoms ranging from mild mucocutaneous bleeding to life-threatening hemorrhage. A high index of suspicion and appropriate laboratory tests are key to making a diagnosis and instituting appropriate therapy. There is limited pediatric-specific evidence for the management of these conditions, and most recommendations have been extrapolated from the adult literature and expert opinion. Physicians who are not familiar with dealing with these entities should seek advice from reference centers familiar with the assessment and management of children with clinically significant acquired bleeding disorders. In selected cases, it may be appropriate to arrange transfer of care of a patient to a specialist treatment center.

Acknowledgements

The authors express their appreciation for the thoughtful comments provided by Dr. Christoph Licht (Toronto, Canada) and Dr. Johanna A. Kramer Hovinga (Bern, Switzerland). Our special thanks also go to Dr. MacGregor Steele who was an author of this chapter in the first and second editions of this Handbook, which provided a valuable background for this updated chapter/appendix.

Conflict of Interest Statement

Riten Kumar has served on an Advisory Board for Bayer and has received research funding from Bioverativ. Markus Schmugge and Marie-Claude Pelland-Marcotte report no relevant conflicts of interest. Manuel Carcao has received research support from Bioverativ/Sanofi, Novartis, Novo Nordisk, Pfizer, Roche, and Shire/Takeda; and has received honoraria for speaking/participating in advisory boards from Bayer, Bioverativ/Sanofi, CSL Behring, LFB, Novo Nordisk, Pfizer, Roche, and Shire/Takeda.

Author Contributions

Riten Kumar drafted the chapter, critically revised the chapter, and approved the final version. Markus Schmugge drafted the chapter, critically revised the chapter, and approved the final version. Marie-Claude Pelland-Marcotte drafted the chapter, critically revised the chapter, and approved the final version. Manuel Carcao drafted the chapter, critically revised the chapter, and approved the final version.

Abbreviations

ADAMTS13	A disintegrin and metalloproteinase with a thrombospondin type 1 motif, member 13
aHUS	Atypical hemolytic uremic syndrome
Anti-Xa	Anti-factor Xa
aPCC	Activated prothrombin complex concentrate
APML	Acute promyelocytic leukemia
aPTT	Activated partial thromboplastin time
AVWS	Acquired von Willebrand syndrome
CBC	Complete blood count

CFB	Complement factor B
CFH	Complement factor H
CFI	Complement factor I
CNS	Central nervous system
DDAVP	1-Deamino-8-D-arginine vasopressin (desmopressin)
DIC	Disseminated intravascular coagulation
ECMO	Extracorporeal membrane oxygenation
FDA	Food and Drug Administration
FDP	Fibrin degradation product
FFP	Fresh frozen plasma
FP	Frozen plasma
FII	Factor II (prothrombin)
FV	Factor V
FVII	Factor VII
FVIII	Factor VIII
FIX	Factor IX
FX	Factor X
FXI	Factor XI
FXII	Factor XII
FXIII	Factor XIII
GVHD	Graft versus host disease
HSCT	Hematopoietic stem cell transplantation
HUS	Hemolytic uremic syndrome
IgG	Immunoglobulin G
IgM	Immunoglobulin M
INR	International normalized ratio
ISTH	International Society on Thrombosis and Haemostasis
IVIG	Intravenous immunoglobulin
LAC	Lupus anticoagulant
LAHS	Lupus anticoagulant hypoprothrombinemia syndrome
LDH	Lactate dehydrogenase
LMWH	Low-molecular-weight heparin
LVAD	Left ventricular assist device
MAHA	Microangiopathic hemolytic anemia
MGUS	Monoclonal gammopathy of uncertain significance
PCC	Prothrombin complex concentrate
PFA-100®/200®	Platelet function analyzer-100®/200®
PT/INR	Prothrombin time/international normalized ratio
RBC	Red blood cell
rFVIIa	Recombinant activated factor VII
ROTEM	Rotational thromboelastometry
SLE	Systemic lupus erythematosus
STEC	Shiga toxin *Escherichia coli*
TAFI	Thrombin-activatable fibrinolysis inhibitor
TA-TMA	Transplant-associated thrombotic microangiopathic disorder
TE	Thromboembolism/thromboembolic event
TEG	Thromboelastography
TF	Tissue factor
TMA	Thrombotic microangiopathic disorder
TT	Thrombin time
TTP	Thrombotic thrombocytopenic purpura
UFH	Unfractionated heparin
ULVWF	Ultra large von Willebrand factor
VWD	von Willebrand disease
VWF	von Willebrand factor
VWF:Act	VWF activity
VWF:Ag	VWF antigen

11

References

1 Rajagopal R, Thachil J, Monagle P. Disseminated intravascular coagulation in paediatrics. Arch Dis Child. 2017;102(2):187–93.

2 Franchini M, Di Minno MN, Coppola A. Disseminated intravascular coagulation in hematologic malignancies. Semin Thromb Hemost. 2010;36(4):388–403.

3 Taylor FB Jr, Toh CH, Hoots WK, Wada H, Levi M; Scientific Subcommittee on Disseminated Intravascular Coagulation of the International Society on T, et al. Towards definition, clinical and laboratory criteria, and a scoring system for disseminated intravascular coagulation. Thromb Haemost. 2001;86(5):1327–30.

4 Levi M, Scully M. How I treat disseminated intravascular coagulation. Blood. 2018;131(8):845–54.

5 Slatnick LR, Thornhill D, Deakyne Davies SJ, Ford JB, Scott HF, Manco-Johnson MJ, et al. Disseminated intravascular coagulation is an independent predictor of adverse outcomes in children in the emergency department with suspected sepsis. J Pediatr. 2020;225:198–206.e2.

6 Wada H, Thachil J, Di Nisio M, Kurosawa S, Gando S, Toh CH, et al. Harmonized guidance for disseminated intravascular coagulation from the International Society on Thrombosis and Haemostasis and the current status of anticoagulant therapy in Japan: a rebuttal. J Thromb Haemost. 2013;11(11):2078–9.

7 Franchini M, Manzato F, Salvagno GL, Lippi G. Potential role of recombinant activated factor VII for the treatment of severe bleeding associated with disseminated intravascular coagulation: a systematic review. Blood Coagul Fibrinolysis. 2007;18(7):589–93.

8 Goldstein B, Nadel S, Peters M, Barton R, Machado F, Levy H, et al. ENHANCE: results of a global open-label trial of drotrecogin alfa (activated) in children with severe sepsis. Pediatr Crit Care Med. 2006;7(3):200–11.

9 Hirata N, Ngo DT, Phan PH, Ainai A, Phung TTB, Ta TA, et al. Recombinant human thrombomodulin for pneumonia-induced severe ARDS complicated by DIC in children: a preliminary study. J Anesth. 2021;35(5):638–45.

10 Scully M, Cataland S, Coppo P, de la Rubia J, Friedman KD, Kremer Hovinga J, et al. Consensus on the standardization of terminology in thrombotic thrombocytopenic purpura and related thrombotic microangiopathies. J Thromb Haemost. 2017;15(2):312–22.

11 Tarr PI, Gordon CA, Chandler WL. Shiga-toxin-producing Escherichia coli and haemolytic uraemic syndrome. Lancet. 2005;365(9464):1073–86.

12 Brodsky RA. Complement in hemolytic anemia. Blood. 2015;126(22):2459–65.

13 Riedl M, Fakhouri F, Le Quintrec M, Noone DG, Jungraithmayr TC, Fremeaux-Bacchi V, et al. Spectrum of complement-mediated thrombotic microangiopathies: pathogenetic insights identifying novel treatment approaches. Semin Thromb Hemost. 2014;40(4): 444–64.

14 Rosales A, Hofer J, Zimmerhackl LB, Jungraithmayr TC, Riedl M, Giner T, et al. Need for long-term follow-up in enterohemorrhagic Escherichia coli-associated hemolytic uremic syndrome due to late-emerging sequelae. Clin Infect Dis. 2012;54(10):1413–21.

15 Loirat C, Fakhouri F, Ariceta G, Besbas N, Bitzan M, Bjerre A, et al. An international consensus approach to the management of atypical hemolytic uremic syndrome in children. Pediatr Nephrol. 2016;31(1):15–39.

16 Noris M, Remuzzi G. Atypical hemolytic-uremic syndrome. N Engl J Med. 2009;361(17):1676–87.

17 Weil BR, Andreoli SP, Billmire DF. Bleeding risk for surgical dialysis procedures in children with hemolytic uremic syndrome. Pediatr Nephrol. 2010;25(9): 1693–8.

18 Lapeyraque AL, Malina M, Fremeaux-Bacchi V, Boppel T, Kirschfink M, Oualha M, et al. Eculizumab in severe Shiga-toxin-associated HUS. N Engl J Med. 2011;364(26):2561–3.

19 Legendre CM, Licht C, Muus P, Greenbaum LA, Babu S, Bedrosian C, et al. Terminal complement inhibitor eculizumab in atypical hemolytic-uremic syndrome. N Engl J Med. 2013;368(23): 2169–81.

20 Ariceta G, Besbas N, Johnson S, Karpman D, Landau D, Licht C, et al. Guideline for the investigation and initial therapy of diarrhea-negative hemolytic uremic syndrome. Pediatr Nephrol. 2009;24(4):687–96.

21 Genest DS, Patriquin CJ, Licht C, John R, Reich HN. Renal thrombotic microangiopathy: a review. Am J Kidney Dis. 2023;81(5):591–605.

22 George JN. How I treat patients with thrombotic thrombocytopenic purpura: 2010. Blood. 2010;116(20):4060–9.

23 Moake JL. Thrombotic microangiopathies. N Engl J Med. 2002;347(8):589–600.

24 van Dorland HA, Taleghani MM, Sakai K, Friedman KD, George JN, Hrachovinova I, et al. The international hereditary thrombotic thrombocytopenic purpura registry: key findings at enrollment until 2017. Haematologica. 2019;104(10): 2107–15.

25 Loirat C, Coppo P, Veyradier A. Thrombotic thrombocytopenic purpura in children. Curr Opin Pediatr. 2013;25(2): 216–24.

26 Bendapudi PK, Upadhyay V, Sun L, Marques MB, Makar RS. Clinical scoring systems in thrombotic microangiopathies. Semin Thromb Hemost. 2017; 43(5):540–8.

27 Zheng XL, Vesely SK, Cataland SR, Coppo P, Geldziler B, Iorio A, et al. Good practice statements (GPS) for the clinical care of patients with thrombotic thrombocytopenic purpura. J Thromb Haemost. 2020;18(10):2503–12.

28 Zheng XL, Vesely SK, Cataland SR, Coppo P, Geldziler B, Iorio A, et al. ISTH guidelines for the diagnosis of thrombotic thrombocytopenic purpura. J Thromb Haemost. 2020;18(10):2486–95.

29 Scully M, Gattens M, Khair K, Liesner R. The use of intermediate purity factor VIII concentrate BPL 8Y as prophylaxis and treatment in congenital thrombotic thrombocytopenic purpura. Br J Haematol. 2006;135(1):101–4.

30 Moroniti JJ, Vrbensky JR, Nazy I, Arnold DM. Targeted ADAMTS-13 replacement therapy for thrombotic thrombocytopenic purpura. J Thromb Haemost. 2023 Dec 22:S1538-7836 (23)00918-2.

31 Zwicker JI, Muia J, Dolatshahi L, Westfield LA, Nieters P, Rodrigues A, et al. Adjuvant low-dose rituximab and plasma exchange for acquired TTP. Blood. 2019;134(13):1106–9.

32 Lim W, Vesely SK, George JN. The role of rituximab in the management of patients with acquired thrombotic thrombocytopenic purpura. Blood. 2015; 125(10):1526–31.

33 Peyvandi F, Scully M, Kremer Hovinga JA, Cataland S, Knobl P, Wu H, et al. Caplacizumab for acquired thrombotic thrombocytopenic purpura. N Engl J Med. 2016;374(6):511–22.

34 Zheng XL. The standard of care for immune thrombotic thrombocytopenic purpura today. J Thromb Haemost. 2021;19(8):1864–71.

35 Jodele S, Davies SM, Lane A, Khoury J, Dandoy C, Goebel J, et al. Diagnostic and risk criteria for HSCT-associated thrombotic microangiopathy: a study in children and young adults. Blood. 2014; 124(4):645–53.

36 Jodele S, Dandoy CE, Sabulski A, Koo J, Lane A, Myers KC, et al. Transplantation-associated thrombotic microangiopathy risk stratification: is there a window of opportunity to improve outcomes? Transplant Cell Ther. 2022; 28(7):392.e1-e9.

37 Young JA, Pallas CR, Knovich MA. Transplant-associated thrombotic microangiopathy: theoretical considerations and a practical approach to an unrefined diagnosis. Bone Marrow Transplant. 2021;56(8):1805–17.

38 Lisman, T. How to assess hemostasis in patients with severe liver disease. Hematology Am Soc Hematol Educ Program. 2023;2023(1):267–273.

39 Janko N, Majeed A, Kemp W, Roberts SK. Viscoelastic tests as point-of-care tests in the assessment and management of bleeding and thrombosis in liver disease. Semin Thromb Hemost. 2020;46(6): 704–15.

40 Roberts, LN. How to manage hemostasis in patients with liver disease during interventions. Hematology Am Soc Hematol Educ Program. 2023;2023(1):274–80.

41 Northup PG, Garcia-Pagan JC, Garcia-Tsao G, Intagliata NM, Superina RA, Roberts LN, et al. Vascular liver disorders, portal vein thrombosis, and procedural bleeding in patients with liver disease: 2020 practice guidance by the American Association for the Study of Liver Diseases. Hepatology. 2021;73(1):366–413.

42 O'Shea RS, Davitkov P, Ko CW, Rajasekhar A, Su GL, Sultan S, et al. AGA clinical practice guideline on the management of coagulation disorders in patients with cirrhosis. Gastroenterology. 2021;161(5):1615–27.e1.

43 Simonetto DA, Singal AK, Garcia-Tsao G, Caldwell SH, Ahn J, Kamath PS. ACG clinical guideline: disorders of the hepatic and mesenteric circulation. Am J Gastroenterol. 2020;115(1):18–40.

44 Khemichian S, Terrault NA. Thrombopoietin receptor agonists in patients with chronic liver disease. Semin Thromb Hemost. 2020;46(6):682–92.

45 Liumbruno G, Bennardello F, Lattanzio A, Piccoli P, Rossetti G; Italian Society of Transfusion M, et al. Recommendations for the use of antithrombin concentrates and prothrombin complex concentrates. Blood Transfus. 2009;7(4):325–34.

46 Molino D, De Lucia D, Gaspare De Santo N. Coagulation disorders in uremia. Semin Nephrol. 2006;26(1):46–51.

47 Galbusera M, Remuzzi G, Boccardo P. Treatment of bleeding in dialysis patients. Semin Dial. 2009;22(3):279–86.

48 Hedges SJ, Dehoney SB, Hooper JS, Amanzadeh J, Busti AJ. Evidence-based treatment recommendations for uremic bleeding. Nat Clin Pract Nephrol. 2007; 3(3):138–53.

49 Collins PW, Hirsch S, Baglin TP, Dolan G, Hanley J, Makris M, et al. Acquired hemophilia A in the United Kingdom: a 2-year national surveillance study by the United Kingdom Haemophilia Centre Doctors' Organisation. Blood. 2007; 109(5):1870–7.

50 Franchini M, Zaffanello M, Lippi G. Acquired hemophilia in pediatrics: a systematic review. Pediatr Blood Cancer. 2010;55(4):606–11.

51 Knoebl P, Marco P, Baudo F, Collins P, Huth-Kuhne A, Nemes L, et al. Demographic and clinical data in acquired hemophilia A: results from the European Acquired Haemophilia Registry (EACH2). J Thromb Haemost. 2012; 10(4):622–31.

52 Pengo V, Tripodi A, Reber G, Rand JH, Ortel TL, Galli M, et al. Update of the guidelines for lupus anticoagulant detection. Subcommittee on Lupus Anticoagulant/Antiphospholipid Antibody of the Scientific and Standardisation Committee of the International Society on Thrombosis and Haemostasis. J Thromb Haemost. 2009;7(10):1737–40.

53 Baudo F, Collins P, Huth-Kuhne A, Levesque H, Marco P, Nemes L, et al. Management of bleeding in acquired hemophilia A: results from the European Acquired Haemophilia (EACH2) Registry. Blood. 2012;120(1):39–46.

54 Collins P, Baudo F, Knoebl P, Levesque H, Nemes L, Pellegrini F, et al. Immunosuppression for acquired hemophilia A: results from the European Acquired Haemophilia Registry (EACH2). Blood. 2012;120(1):47–55.

55 Kruse-Jarres R, St-Louis J, Greist A, Shapiro A, Smith H, Chowdary P, et al. Efficacy and safety of OBI-1, an antihaemophilic factor VIII (recombinant), porcine sequence, in subjects with acquired haemophilia A. Haemophilia. 2015;21(2):162–70.

56 Thomas VM, Abou-Ismail MY, Lim MY. Off-label use of emicizumab in persons with acquired haemophilia A and von Willebrand disease: a scoping review of the literature. Haemophilia. 2022;28(1): 4–17.

57 Franchini M. Rituximab in the treatment of adult acquired hemophilia A: a systematic review. Crit Rev Oncol Hematol. 2007;63(1):47–52.

58 Langer AL, Connell NT. Acquired von Willebrand syndrome. Hematol Oncol Clin North Am. 2021;35(6):1103–16.

59 Geisen U, Brehm K, Trummer G, Berchtold-Herz M, Heilmann C, Beyersdorf F, et al. Platelet secretion defects and acquired von Willebrand syndrome in patients with ventricular assist devices. J Am Heart Assoc. 2018;7(2):e006519.

60 Kalbhenn J, Schlagenhauf A, Rosenfelder S, Schmutz A, Zieger B. Acquired von Willebrand syndrome and impaired platelet function during venovenous extracorporeal membrane oxygenation: rapid onset and fast recovery. J Heart Lung Transplant. 2018;37(8):985–91.

61 Pelland-Marcotte MC, Humpl T, James PD, Rand ML, Bouskill V, Reyes JT, et al. Idiopathic pulmonary arterial hypertension—a unrecognized cause of high-shear high-flow haemostatic defects (otherwise referred to as acquired von Willebrand syndrome) in children. Br J Haematol. 2018;183(2):267–75.

62 Callaghan MU, Wong TE, Federici AB. Treatment of acquired von Willebrand syndrome in childhood. Blood. 2013; 122(12):2019–22.

63 Franchini M, Lippi G. Acquired von Willebrand syndrome: an update. Am J Hematol. 2007;82(5):368–75.

64 Gill JC, Castaman G, Windyga J, Kouides P, Ragni M, Leebeek FW, et al. Hemostatic efficacy, safety, and pharmacokinetics of a recombinant von Willebrand factor in severe von Willebrand disease. Blood. 2015;126(17):2038–46.

65 Sun Y, Nie W, Tian D, Ye Q. Lupus anticoagulant-hypoprothrombinemia syndrome in children: three case reports and systematic review of the literature. Lupus. 2023;32(10):1211–21.

66 Paschal RD, Neff AT. Resolution of Hypoprothrombinemia-Lupus Anticoagulant Syndrome (HLAS) after multidrug therapy with rituximab: a case report and review of the literature. Haemophilia. 2013;19(2):e62–5.

67 Napolitano LM. Hemostatic defects in massive transfusion: an update and treatment recommendations. Expert Rev Hematol. 2021;14(2):219–39.

68 Neff LP, Beckwith MA, Russell RT, Cannon JW, Spinella PC. Massive transfusion in pediatric patients. Clin Lab Med. 2021;41(1):35–49.

69 Drucker NA, Wang SK, Newton C. Pediatric trauma-related coagulopathy: balanced resuscitation, goal-directed therapy and viscoelastic assays. Semin Pediatr Surg. 2019;28(1):61–6.

70 Maeda T, Michihata N, Sasabuchi Y, Matsui H, Ohnishi Y, Miyata S, et al. Safety of tranexamic acid during pediatric trauma: a nationwide database study. Pediatr Crit Care Med. 2018;19(12): e637–42.

71 Thomson JM, Huynh HH, Drone HM, Jantzer JL, Tsai AK, Jancik JT. Experience in an urban level 1 trauma center with tranexamic acid in pediatric trauma: a retrospective chart review. J Intensive Care Med. 2021;36(4):413–8.

72 Lee G, Duan-Porter W, Metjian AD. Acquired, non-amyloid related factor X deficiency: review of the literature. Haemophilia. 2012;18(5):655–63.

73 Peyvandi F, Auerswald G, Austin SK, Liesner R, Kavakli K, Alvarez Roman MT, et al. Diagnosis, therapeutic advances, and key recommendations for the management of factor X deficiency. Blood Rev. 2021;50:100833.

74 Yan MTS, Rydz N, Goodyear D, Sholzberg M. Acquired factor XIII deficiency: a review. Transfus Apher Sci. 2018; 57(6):724–30.

75 Bomgaars L, Carberry K, Fraser C, West A, Teruya J. Development of factor V and thrombin inhibitors in children following bovine thrombin exposure during cardiac surgery: a report of three cases. Congenit Heart Dis. 2010;5(3): 303–8.

76 Kremer Hovinga JA, Coppo P, Lammle B, Moake JL, Miyata T, Vanhoorelbeke K. Thrombotic thrombocytopenic purpura. Nat Rev Dis Primers. 2017;3: 17020.

Published online: December 5, 2024

Blanchette VS, Brandão LR, Carcao MD, Kumar R, Rand ML, Revel-Vilk S (eds): SickKids Handbook of Pediatric Thrombosis and Hemostasis, ed 3, rev. and ext. Basel, Karger, 2024, pp 216–232 (DOI: 10.1159/000538190)

Hemostatic and Thrombotic Challenges in Vascular Anomalies

Soumitra Tole[a] Victoria Price[b] Denise Adams[c] Joao Guilherme Amaral[d] Manuel D. Carcao[e]

[a]Division of Paediatric Haematology/Oncology, Department of Paediatrics, Western University and Children's Hospital, London Health Sciences Centre, London, ON, Canada; [b]Division of Paediatric Hematology-Oncology, Department of Paediatrics, Dalhousie University, Halifax, NS, Canada; [c]Division of Oncology, Department of Pediatrics, Comprehensive Vascular Anomalies Program, Children's Hospital of Philadelphia, University of Pennsylvania Medical Center, Philadelphia, PA, USA; [d]Division of Interventional Radiology, Department of Diagnostic Imaging, The Hospital for Sick Children, University of Toronto, Toronto, ON, Canada; [e]Division of Haematology/Oncology, Department of Paediatrics, The Hospital for Sick Children, Toronto, ON, Canada

Introduction

Pediatric hematologists and oncologists are becoming increasingly involved in the management of patients with vascular anomalies – either in prescribing targeted medical therapies (e.g., sirolimus, trametinib, alpelisib, etc.) or in dealing with the hemostatic and thrombotic issues associated with vascular anomalies.

Vascular anomalies are a large heterogeneous group of disorders that are subdivided into either vascular tumors or malformations with a proposed classification by the International Society for the Study of Vascular Anomalies (Table 1).

Vascular tumors are proliferative endothelial vascular lesions that are generally solitary masses. The most common benign vascular tumors are hemangiomas. These can be infantile hemangiomas (IHs), the most classical form, or congenital hemangiomas (CHs). Unlike IHs, which classically only appear a few days to weeks after birth, CHs are fully formed at birth and may be noted on antenatal imaging. CHs are further subdivided into three types: noninvoluting CH (NICH), which, as the name suggests, does not involute and grow proportionally to the child; rapidly involuting CH (RICH), which regress spontaneously by 15 months of age; and partially involuting CH (PICH) which begin to involute but do not regress completely before stabilizing in size [1–3]. In addition, there are locally aggressive but benign vascular tumors such as Kaposiform hemangioendothelioma (KHE) and tufted angiomas (TAs) and malignant tumors such as angiosarcomas and epithelioid hemangioendothelioma.

Vascular malformations are thought to always be present at birth, although they may not be recognized. They grow progressively throughout life, although occasionally with episodes of accelerated growth, such as early on in life and around puberty. Vascular malformations are conditions in which vascular structures (arteries, veins, capillaries, or lymphatics) are not formed correctly but are "mal"formed. Vascular malformations can involve only one vascular tissue (arteriovenous malformations [AVMs], venous malformations [VMs], capillary malformations [CMs], or lymphatic malformations [LMs]) or can consist of a combination of these vascular channels, often in association with tissue overgrowth. This includes well-described conditions such as Klippel-Trenaunay syndrome (KTS; CM + VM +/− LM + limb overgrowth), Parkes-Weber (CM + AVM + limb overgrowth), and CLOVES (congenital lipomatous [fatty] overgrowth, vascular malformations, epidermal nevi, and spinal/skeletal abnormalities syndrome).

This classification of vascular anomalies has existed for quite some time [4, 5]. The last 10 years have witnessed an incredible transformation in the management of vascular anomalies, and this has coincided with a greater understanding of their pathophysiology and genetic derivation. It is now appreciated that vascular anomalies are caused by genetic variants (generally in endothelial cells) in genes involved in angiogenesis, growth, and differentiation of vascular structures. Most variants (90%) are somatic gain-of-function variants that occur sporadically during embryogenesis [6]. Only 10% of patients with vascular anomalies carry germline loss-of-function variants, including variants in *EPHB4*, *RASA1*, *glomulin*, *TIE2/TEK*, and *PTEN* genes (Fig. 1). Given that somatic variants cause 90% of vascular anomalies, most patients with vascular anomalies are mosaic, having both abnormal mutated cells representing the vascular anomaly and nonmutated cells in the rest of the body.

The genes involved in growth, differentiation, and angiogenesis comprise two different pathways that are referred to as pikopathies (phosphatidylinositol 3-kinase [PI3K] coded for by *PIK3CA/AKT/mTOR* and other genes that are involved in this pathway – *TIE2/TEK*, *PTEN*, and

Table 1. Classification of vascular anomalies

Vascular tumors
Benign
Infantile hemangioma
Congenital hemangiomas
RICH
NICH
PICH
Tufted angioma
Others
Locally aggressive
Kaposiform hemangioendothelioma
Others
Malignant
Angiosarcoma
Epithelioid hemangioendothelioma
Others
Vascular malformations
Simple
Capillary
Lymphatic
Venous
Arteriovenous
Arteriovenous fistula
Combined
Capillary-venous
Capillary-lymphatic
Lymphatic-venous
Capillary-venous-lymphatic
Capillary-arteriovenous
Capillary-lymphatic-arteriovenous
Others
Associated with other anomalies
Klippel-Trenaunay
Parkes-Weber
CLOVES
Proteus
Others
Provisionally unclassified vascular anomalies
MLT
CAT
PHOST
FAVA
Others

Adapted from the International Society for the Study of Vascular Anomalies Classification for vascular anomalies 2018 (https://www.issva.org/UserFiles/file/ISSVA-Classification-2018.pdf). CAT, cutaneovisceral angiomatosis with thrombocytopenia; CLOVES, congenital lipomatous overgrowth, vascular malformations, epidermal nevi, and spinal/skeletal abnormalities syndrome; FAVA, fibroadipose vascular anomaly; MLT, multifocal lymphangiomatosis with thrombocytopenia; NICH, noninvoluting congenital hemangioma; PHOST, PTEN hamartoma of soft tissue; PICH, partially involuting congenital hemangioma; RICH, rapidly involuting congenital hemangioma.

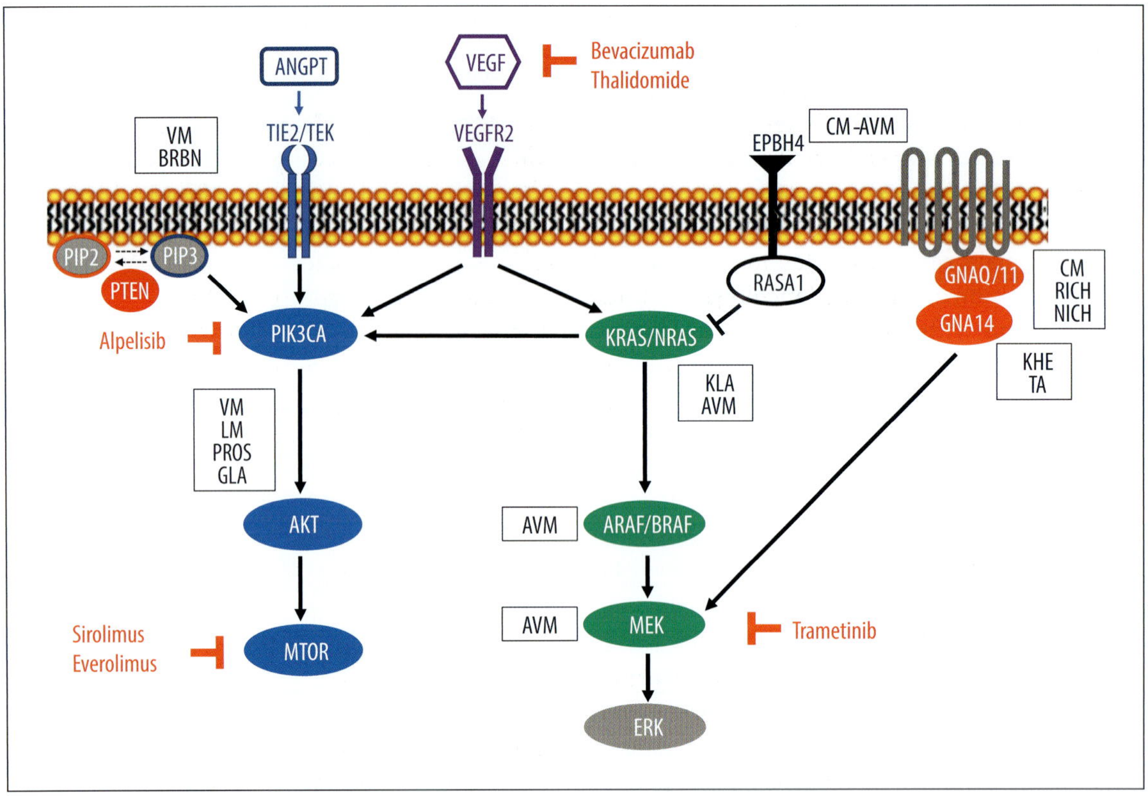

Fig. 1. Signaling pathways affected in vascular anomalies and targeted therapies. ANGPT, angiopoietin; AVM, arteriovenous malformation; BRBN, blue rubber bleb nevus syndrome; CM, capillary malformation; CM-AVM, capillary malformation-arteriovenous malformation; EPHB4, Ephrin B4; GLA, generalized lymphatic anomaly; KHE, kaposiform hemangioendothelioma; KLA, kaposiform lymphangiomatosis; LM, lymphatic malformation; NICH, noninvoluting congenital hemangioma; PROS, PIK3CA-related overgrowth syndrome; RICH, rapidly involuting congenital hemangioma; TA, tufted angioma; VEGF, vascular endothelial growth factor; VM, venous malformation.

TSC) and rasopathies (variants in RAS/*MAPK*/*ERK* genes) [7, 8] (Fig. 1).

Variants in the PIK3CA-AKT-mTOR pathway tend to result in solitary or complex LM or VM that are usually associated with variants in *AKT* or *PIK3CA*. Often overgrowth syndromes are associated with variants in *PIK3CA* or *AKT*. PIK3CA-related disorders include CLOVES, KTS, megalencephaly-CM-polymicrogyria syndrome, and other PIK3CA-related overgrowth syndromes – now designated by the term PROS: PIK3CA-related overgrowth spectrum. Gain-of-function variants in AKT are responsible for Proteus syndrome.

In contrast, most AVMs (intracranial and extracranial) are caused by variants in the RAS pathway, consisting of several genes, including *RAS*, *BRAF*, *MAP2K*, and *ERK*. Somatic variants in *GNA11* and *GNAQ* cause CMs often with tissue overgrowth, such as Sturge-Weber syndrome. These conditions seem to be associated with activation of extracellular signal-regulated kinase and are linked to rasopathies.

With the identification of these molecular pathways and genetic variants involved in the pathogenesis of vascular anomalies, there is an increasing recognition of the potential role of targeted medical therapies. This has seen a repurposing of drugs that are effective in the treatment of malignant tumors associated with variants in these pathways, and this has led to a greater role for pediatric hematologists/oncologists in the treatment of vascular tumors and malformations. There is a more in-depth discussion of management of vascular anomalies toward the end of this chapter.

Vascular anomalies may be associated with hemostatic and thrombotic disturbances. Kasabach-Merritt phenomenon (KMP) occurs in the setting of certain complex vascular tumors, KHE, and TAs. Additionally, most VMs have the potential to cause localized intravascular coagulation (LIC). Certain types of complex vascular anomalies can predispose to thromboembolic event (TE), including pulmonary embolism (PE), specifically CLOVES syndrome, and, to a lesser extent, KTS due to the presence of valveless ectatic embryonic veins. Last, certain types of vascular anomalies are characterized by thrombocytopenia. This is particularly the case in Kaposiform lymphangiomatosis (KLA) and multifocal lymphangiomatosis with thrombocytopenia (MLT), where thrombocytopenia is a diagnostic clue to both disorders.

The management of patients affected by vascular anomalies requires a large multidisciplinary team. The role of the pediatric hematologist/oncologist has become crucial and includes prescribing and managing side effects of targeted therapies, such as sirolimus, trametinib, and alpelisib, managing the associated hemostatic abnormalities, and prescribing anticoagulation to reduce LIC and reduce the likelihood of TE, especially in the perioperative setting.

Hemostatic Complications of Vascular Anomalies

Kasabach-Merritt Phenomenon

KMP is characterized by severe thrombocytopenia and hypofibrinogenemia with or without microangiopathic hemolytic anemia. KMP is typically seen in KHE and TA. TA and KHE are believed to be on the spectrum of the same disease, with TA being benign and KHE locally aggressive. TA and KHE are typically unifocal and involve the head and neck, extremities, and trunk but may be found in abdominal and thoracic cavities. Historically, bleeding-related mortality from KMP has been reported to be as high as 30%, but this appears to be improving with early recognition and treatment [9].

Pathophysiology

Thrombocytopenia occurs due to platelet trapping within the abnormal vascular structure, with subsequent activation and consumption of platelets [10]. In KHE and TA, endothelial cells express podoplanin that causes C-type lectin-like receptor 2 (CLEC2)-mediated platelet aggregation. In turn, platelet activation may stimulate tumor growth by promoting angiogenesis, causing further endothelium changes, leading to increased mechanical defects and platelet trapping, activation, and consumption. Additionally, with rapidly expanding lesions, a breech in the integrity of the endothelium exposes subendothelial collagen and tissue factor with activation of the coagulation cascade, leading to intralesional thrombus formation and fibrinolysis. Mechanical shearing of red blood cells due to abnormal blood flow caused by tortuous and/or partially thrombosed vasculature contributes to microangiopathic hemolytic anemia [11, 12].

Laboratory Findings

Severe thrombocytopenia ($<50 \times 10^9$/L) is the hallmark of the condition. Hypofibrinogenemia is less extreme compared with the degree of

12

thrombocytopenia. Additionally, elevated fibrinogen degradation products and D-dimers, and some degree of microangiopathic hemolytic anemia, can be seen.

Management

Coagulopathy

For managing thrombocytopenia, platelet transfusions should be reserved for active bleeding or prior to surgery. This is because platelet half-life is severely reduced to <24 h due to intralesional platelet trapping. Furthermore, platelets accumulate within the lesion and may cause painful swelling. Platelets release proendothelial growth factors that may stimulate further endothelial proliferation.

Fibrinogen activity should be maintained at >1 g/L using cryoprecipitate or fibrinogen concentrate in children with active bleeding or prior to operative interventions (Appendix III).

Antifibrinolytic agents may be helpful in the management of bleeding (see Appendix III for dosing) [13]. Due to the substantial risk of bleeding, the use of heparin is contraindicated.

Specific Treatment

There is no FDA-approved treatment for KMP. A consensus statement published in 2013 recommended corticosteroids and vincristine as first-line therapy [13]. Since then, several case reports, case series, and clinical trials have proved sirolimus to be an efficacious therapy for KHE/TA-associated KMP, leading to sirolimus now being widely accepted as first-line treatment [14–16]. A recent randomized controlled trial compared sirolimus + prednisone to sirolimus monotherapy in the management of KMP. Significantly more patients receiving the combination therapy achieved the primary outcome of a durable platelet count $>100 \times 10^9$/L at 4 weeks of therapy, suggesting consideration of sirolimus together with prednisone as initial treatment [17].

Corticosteroid dosing: oral prednisone 2 mg/kg/day divided twice daily or intravenous methylprednisolone 1.6 mg/kg/day and weaned when clinically stable and coagulopathy has resolved; usually, this constitutes 3–4 weeks [15]. For sirolimus dosing, see Table 2.

Antiplatelet agents may have a role given the underlying platelet activation and release of proangiogenic factors that drive the process. These agents have been used as single agents or in combination in various doses for varying lengths of time with mixed results [13].

Surgical excision is limited to those lesions that are small and can be completely excised. However, surgery is often not possible due to the risk of bleeding. Arterial embolization is reserved for organ and or life-threatening lesions, for cases refractory to first-line therapies, or possibly for a more rapid rescue of the consumptive coagulopathy [18].

KMP-Like Coagulopathy

KLA is a rare complex lymphatic anomaly that behaves aggressively, leading to significant morbidity and mortality [19, 20]. The thorax, spleen, bones, and retroperitoneum are the most frequently involved sites [21]. Aberrant lymphatic channels in the thoracic cavity with involvement of the pleura, pericardium, and lung parenchyma are particularly associated with effusions and hemorrhage.

Children present at an early age with cough or dyspnea and bleeding. The coagulopathy of KLA resembles KMP and includes severe hypofibrinogenemia, usually mild-moderate thrombocytopenia, and bleeding [22]. Like KMP, platelet trapping can also occur in KLA, suggesting a similar pathogenesis [23]. Biopsy may result in significant bleeding and worsening of coagulopathy. Of note, not all patients with KLA will develop coagulopathy.

In the absence of treatment, KLA is progressive and results in bleeding, effusions, and cardiopulmonary compromise. Given its rarity, there are no available guidelines for management. As platelet trapping occurs in KLA and may worsen coagulopathy, platelet transfusions should be

Table 2. Suggested dosing and monitoring for targeted therapies

	Usually starting dose	Monitoring	Adverse effects
Sirolimus	0.8 mg/m^2/dose given twice daily OR 2.5 mg/m^2/daily given as one dose Lower starting doses in neonates and infants due to reduced sirolimus metabolism Target level: 5–15 ng/mL	Lab monitoring every 1–3 months depending on phenotype and target sirolimus level including CBC; renal and liver function, cholesterol and triglycerides, D-dimers and fibrinogen Ferritin, albumin, total protein, and IgG levels useful in cases of recurrent bleeding or protein losing enteropathy	Common: Mouth sores (stomatitis) Acne Hyperlipidemia Headache Gastrointestinal discomfort Rare/life-threatening: Increased risk of infections Hyperglycemia Capillary leak syndrome Difficulty with wound healing Pneumonitis Leukopenia
Trametinib	0.025–0.035 mg/kg/dose once daily Children often begin with 0.5 mg daily Adults may start with 1 mg daily Available in 0.5 mg and 2 mg tablets Target levels generally not available; doses adjusted according to tolerance and adverse effects; most patients need no more than 0.5 mg or 1 mg/day total	Dermatology exams as needed Cardiac (ECHO, ECG) – every 3 months Ophthalmology (retinal evaluation) – every 3 months Lab monitoring similar to sirolimus but additionally includes CPK, lipase	Common: Acne and other rashes Paronychia Diarrhea Stomatitis Transaminitis Lymphedema Fatigue and arthralgias Headache Hypertension Rare/life-threatening: Visual impairment (retinal vein occlusion, retinal detachment) Gastrointestinal perforation Cardiac dysfunction Pneumonitis Rhabdomyolysis
Alpelisib	25 mg/day for <5 years 50 mg/day for 5–18 years 125 mg/day for ≥18 years Available in 50 mg, 125 mg, and 300 mg tablets Target levels generally not available; doses adjusted according to tolerance and adverse effects	Lab monitoring similar to trametinib every 1–3 months	Common: Alopecia Dry skin and other rashes Diarrhea Hyperglycemia Nausea Rare/life-threatening: Severe hyperglycemia Hypersensitivity reactions

CBC, complete blood count; CPK, creatine phosphokinase; ECG, electrocardiogram; ECHO, echocardiogram; IgG, immunoglobulin G.

Table 3. Clinical and laboratory features comparing Kasabach-Merritt phenomenon and VM-associated LIC

	Kasabach-Merritt phenomenon	VM-associated LIC
Lesion	Kaposiform hemangioendothelioma Tufted angioma	VM Combined slow-flow malformations
Age	Birth and infancy	Lifelong association
Main clinical features	Congenital lesion with rapid growth and pain Purpura, bruising High risk for bleeding	Often asymptomatic Pain with palpable phleboliths Risk for DIC and VTE with interventions
Main laboratory features	Severe thrombocytopenia Low fibrinogen Elevated D-dimers +/– microangiopathic hemolytic anemia	Elevated D-dimers Low fibrinogen +/– mild thrombocytopenia
Treatment	Steroids + sirolimus[a] Cryoprecipitate, fibrinogen concentrate Antifibrinolytic agents	Thromboprophylaxis – LMWH/DOAC Sirolimus

DIC, disseminated intravascular coagulation; DOAC, direct oral anticoagulant; LIC, localized intravascular coagulopathy; LMWH, low molecular weight heparin; VM, venous malformation; VTE, venous thromboembolism/thromboembolic event. [a]Vincristine is much less used due to side effects.

used with caution and reserved for patients with active bleeding. Hypofibrinogenemia should be corrected using cryoprecipitate or fibrinogen concentrates to maintain fibrinogen >1 g/L (Appendix III). Some experts suggest keeping fibrinogen >1.5 g/L for major procedures [24]. Red blood cell transfusions do not cause complications and should be used to treat symptomatic anemia. Sirolimus, steroids, and bisphosphonates have been reported to have success in stabilizing lymphatic overgrowth [25, 26]. For sirolimus dosing, see Table 2. More recently, variants in *NRAS* and *CBL* have been identified in patients with KLA, and the use of the MEK inhibitor trametinib has shown marked clinical improvements in respiratory function and normalization of hematologic parameters [20, 27, 28].

Localized Intravascular Coagulopathy

Definition

LIC is a consumptive coagulopathy associated with VM or mixed slow-flow malformations with a large venous component. The presence of LIC is proportional to VM size and is notably seen in PROS (with a significant VM component) such as CLOVES and KTS [29].

Pathophysiology

The exact pathophysiology of LIC is unclear but may be explained with Virchow's triad (abnormal blood flow, hypercoagulability, and endothelial injury). Dysplastic venous channels, abnormal endothelium, and persistent embryonal veins are hypothesized as potential contributors to the development of LIC. There is altered blood flow and stagnation within the lesion, and the presence of elevated D-dimers in LIC supports the presence of excessive thrombin generation and activation of the fibrinolytic pathway [30, 31].

Laboratory Findings

The term LIC is somewhat of a misnomer as there is systemic evidence of activation of the coagulation system as characterized by elevated D-dimers and decreased fibrinogen. Elevated D-dimers are seen in up to 40% of VM, with severe LIC seen in up to 10% of VM [31]. Thrombocytopenia is sometimes seen, but it is mild in comparison to that seen in KMP [30]. Associated acquired deficiencies of von Willebrand factor, factor VIII, antithrombin, and factor XIII have also been reported [11]. See Table 3 for a comparison of KMP and LIC.

Clinical Findings
LIC is frequently asymptomatic. However, chronic activation of the coagulation cascade can result in the development of intralesional thrombi, which may calcify, leading to the development of phleboliths – hard pebble-like structures. LIC can worsen with trauma, infection, or intervention, including sclerotherapy, embolization, and surgery. This usually presents with an exacerbation of pain – thought to be caused by distension of veins from thrombi. LIC-associated bleeding has been reported in 5–12% of cases of LIC in the setting of vascular malformations and is particularly associated with procedures [30, 32, 33]. Progression of LIC to disseminated intravascular coagulation (DIC) has been described in the context of surgery, particularly for patients with large lower extremity lesions [31]. Exacerbations of LIC are also associated with hormonal changes, e.g., during puberty and pregnancy [34].

Management
Treatment of LIC associated with VMs is focused on managing symptoms, primarily pain, and avoiding hemorrhagic and thrombotic complications. Compression therapy (commonly 20–30 mm Hg) can be helpful in extremity VMs and may decrease LIC by reducing venous stasis, decreasing the generation of phleboliths, and improving pain [35]. In children, the cost of frequently replacing garments every 4 to 6 months and compliance with wearing properly fitted compression garments can be challenging. Antiplatelet therapy, including acetylsalicylic acid and other nonsteroidal anti-inflammatory agents, has been used to alleviate pain with mixed results [36]. Short-term low-molecular-weight heparin (LMWH) is often used at either prophylactic dosing or therapeutic dosing to dampen LIC and treat pain associated with phleboliths [37]. In adults, the successful use of direct oral anticoagulants (DOACs) has also been reported [38]. These are likely to be increasingly used in children as well, although there are no data from clinical trials to support their use in the context of LIC.

Periprocedural anticoagulation may be used to prevent LIC-related bleeding and TE. As is the case with DIC, anticoagulation is thought to improve dysregulated coagulation by reducing thrombin generation, fibrinogen consumption, and platelet consumption. There are no evidence-based guidelines on the periprocedural management of patients with LIC. Consensus recommendations from the American Society of Pediatric Hematology/Oncology identified the presence of embryonal veins, venous ectasia, elevated D-dimers, hypofibrinogenemia, and thrombocytopenia as risk factors that would warrant the use of anticoagulation [12]. Depending on a patient's risk profile, they may get no periprocedural anticoagulation, only postprocedural anticoagulation for 2 weeks, or get both preprocedural (usually 2 weeks of preprocedure) and postprocedural anticoagulation (usually 2–4 weeks); see Table 4. Anticoagulation dosing and duration of anticoagulation remain unclear. A retrospective cohort study evaluating the use of this protocol in patients with VM undergoing sclerotherapy found no increase in the risk of bleeding and noted no TEs in children [22]. Fibrinogen should be maintained >1 g/L with the use of cryoprecipitate or fibrinogen concentrate (Appendix III).

Other Coagulopathies (Primarily Associated with Thrombocytopenia)

Congenital Hemangiomas

CHs are benign vascular tumors that are fully formed at birth and distinct from the more common IHs. CHs are frequently seen in the head, neck, liver, and upper extremities. Unlike IHs,

Table 4. Periprocedural thromboprophylaxis in children with LIC

Risk category	Recommendation
Low (meets all criteria)	
Normal PT/INR, aPTT, fibrinogen	Early ambulation
D-dimers <5 × normal	Compression stockings
No personal or family history of VTE	Post-procedure VTE prophylaxis as per the institutional policy
Average risk	
Mild features of LIC without significant venous ectasia	Early ambulation Compression stockings LMWH/DOAC[a] for 2 weeks post-procedure
High (meets at least 1 criterion)	
Venous ectasia	Early ambulation
Significant signs of LIC:	Compression stockings
Low fibrinogen (<1 g/L)	LMWH/DOAC[a] at least 2 weeks pre-operative and 2–4 weeks postprocedure
D-dimers >5 × normal	
Thrombocytopenia <150 × 10^9/L (without other reason)	Pre-procedure start with prophylactic dosing and repeat labs after 1 week
Positive personal or family history of VTE	Escalate LMWH dosing until fibrinogen level is >1 g/L

Reprinted from Ricci et al. [12], with permission from Elsevier and Brandão, L.: Periprocedural Anticoagulation Protocol. American Society of Pediatric Hematology Oncology with permission from the author. aPTT, activated partial thromboplastin time; DOAC, direct oral anticoagulant; INR, international normalized ratio; LIC, localized intravascular coagulopathy; LMWH, low molecular weight heparin; PT, prothrombin time; VTE, venous thromboembolism/thromboembolic event. [a]DOAC dosing for primary VTE prophylaxis is not well established in children.

CHs are negative for GLUT-1 (glucose transporter 1) staining on histopathology.

Hematological complications have primarily been described in CH, particularly RICH and PICH, where transient thrombocytopenia and hypofibrinogenemia, and occasional coagulopathy may be seen during the rapid involution phase, typically in the first weeks of life [2, 39]. Thrombocytopenia is usually mild with similarly modest increased D-dimers and decreased fibrinogen levels. This contrasts with the severe thrombocytopenia seen in KMP. Bleeding is not common, and hematologic abnormalities typically resolve within 2 weeks. Of note, bleeding has been described in RICH when there is superficial crusting and ulceration, lesions greater than 5 cm in size, and lesions with large venous lakes [2, 39, 40]. Hepatic RICH may also develop a transient coagulopathy secondary to central necrosis and thrombosis occurring with transition from fetal to postnatal circulation [41].

Thrombocytopenia and coagulopathy in RICH are usually self-resolving and do not require treatment, but deaths related to bleeding have been reported. Embolization may be required in cases with bleeding or in large tumors with significant arteriovenous shunting causing cardiac failure. Antifibrinolytic agents may be helpful and can also be used topically in superficial lesions [40]. While rarely necessary, platelet transfusions are well tolerated and do not worsen coagulopathy, as seen with KMP.

MLT/Cutaneovisceral Angiomatosis with Thrombocytopenia

MLT/cutaneovisceral angiomatosis with thrombocytopenia (CAT) is a newly identified multifocal disorder and is a "provisionally unclassified vascular anomaly" according to the most recent International Society for the Study of Vascular Anomalies classification. MLT/CAT is typically characterized by multiple and progressive red-brown lesions in the skin and gastrointestinal tract [42]. The lesions are GLUT-1 negative and express lymphatic markers LYVE-1 and D2-40 (podoplanin).

Thrombocytopenia presents early in infancy and typically ranges from 50 to 100 × 10^9/L [43]. It does not improve with time and may be exacerbated by concurrent infection or intervention. Coagulation testing and D-dimer and fibrinogen levels are typically normal. Bleeding complications are primarily related to gastrointestinal involvement. Some individuals may have significant bleeding resulting in iron deficiency anemia requiring intravenous iron infusions or red blood cell transfusions. Lesions involving the brain, lung, muscle, liver, and bone have occasionally been reported [44].

As MLT/CAT is a rare diagnosis, the preferred treatment strategy has not been established. While previous studies using steroids, vincristine, interferon, and thalidomide have not been successful, encouraging results with clinical improvement and an increase in platelet count have been reported with sirolimus (Table 2) [44]. As bleeding, including intracranial hemorrhage, can be seen in infancy in MLT/CAT, platelet transfusions to maintain platelet counts >30 × 10^9/L are suggested.

Bleeding in Vascular Malformations

Bleeding is often a complication of vascular malformations and may relate to either thrombocytopenia or hypofibrinogenemia (or both) as occurs in KMP, KLA, or MLT. It can also be related to structural involvement of the gastrointestinal tract as occurs in MLT or in blue rubber bleb nevus syndrome, a condition characterized by widespread VM throughout the skin and gastrointestinal tract [45]. In these conditions, severe anemia may necessitate iron infusions or red blood cell transfusions. VM that involves joints, particularly the knee, may be accompanied by bleeding into the joint, leading to joint damage and the development of chronic arthropathy. Sclerotherapy, surgical resection/synovectomy, or glue casting with surgical resection of VM around joints may reduce the occurrence of hemarthrosis with subsequent joint destruction [46–49].

Thrombotic Complications

TEs are particularly associated with large capillary-lymphatic-venous malformations (CLVMs) as seen in KTS and CLOVES. In these conditions, there are frequently persistent embryological veins such as the lateral vein of Servelle or a persistent sciatic vein. These vessels can be ectatic (meaning dilated), thereby leading to the pooling of blood. The rate of venous TE in KTS and CLOVES has been reported to be between 9% and 14% [50]. Importantly, the risk of TEs appears to be directly associated with the presence of aberrant vessels, as the study by Reis et al. [50] found that 94% of all PEs in patients with CLVM occurred in patients with venous ectasia. The mean age of PE was 15.5 years in patients with KTS and 16.6 years in patients with CLOVES. The risk of PE was significantly greater after surgery or sclerotherapy, with 64% occurring during the postoperative period. This is in keeping with previous studies in patients with KTS [51]. Interestingly, the use of an inferior vena cava filter did not appear to provide adequate protection against PE. Proteus syndrome, also characterized by CLVM and asymmetric overgrowth secondary to *AKT1* variants, also carries a similarly increased risk of venous TE [52]. Based on the above, it is recommended that all patients with CLVM receive periprocedural thromboprophylaxis (Table 4). The ideal time for prophylactic closure of ectatic veins remains unclear, but the risk of PE appears to increase significantly with adolescence. Given the strong association of PE with venous ectasia and surgery, proactive endovascular closure of ectatic and embryonic veins should be considered in all patients with these conditions, if a connection to the deep venous system is present [50]. In children who have had severe TE (e.g., massive PE, splanchnic vein thrombosis), long-term anticoagulation should be considered, at least until ectatic vessels are closed.

Management of Vascular Anomalies

The management of vascular anomalies is complex and involves a multidisciplinary team of hematologists/oncologists, dermatologists, radiologists, interventional radiologists, geneticists, pathologists, and surgeons (plastics, ear, nose, and throat, orthopedics, and general surgery). In addition, physiotherapists and occupational therapists are needed to deal with many of the orthopedic issues associated with limb vascular malformations (leg length discrepancies, joint damage, leg swelling with the need for compression garments, and orthotics). Genetic counsellors are also vital as many patients with vascular anomalies may be at risk of developing several types of cancers: Wilms tumor in the setting of CLOVES and other PROS conditions and different carcinomas in the setting of *PTEN* hamartoma syndromes. Furthermore, patients/families need guidance on the genetic transmissibility implications, if any, of vascular malformations. Medical photography is extremely helpful in providing objective assessment of any changes in the size and color of vascular anomalies. For the purposes of this chapter on hemostatic and thrombotic complications in vascular anomalies, there will only be a short synopsis of the main aspects of management.

Medical Management

IHs seldom require treatment as they will grow but usually will stabilize and then spontaneously regress over time. Indications for treatment of hemangiomas include life-threatening complications (airway obstruction, liver IH with high-output cardiac failure, and profuse bleeding), functional impairment (visual disturbance or difficulty with feeding), ulceration, associated structural anomalies (posterior fossa anomalies, hemangioma, arterial anomalies, cardiac anomalies, and eye anomalies [PHACES] or lower-body hemangioma, urogenital abnormalities/ulceration, myelopathy, bony deformities, anorectal malformations/arterial anomalies, and rectal anomalies [LUMBAR] syndrome), and risk of disfigurement [53]. Several therapies have been shown to be effective in the treatment of IH, including corticosteroids, interferon, vincristine, and beta-blockers [54, 55]. The serendipitous discovery that beta-blockers (initially propranolol and recently atenolol/nadolol) are effective in the treatment of GLUT-1 positive hemangiomas has led to them now being recommended as the first-line therapy for the treatment of IH [53, 55]. GLUT-1 negative CH does not respond to beta-blockers.

Unfortunately, beta-blockers are ineffective in locally aggressive vascular tumors (KHE or TA). Several therapies have been used for these complex lesions with varying results (e.g., corticosteroids, interferon, and vincristine). However, all these treatments have significant toxicities. Adams et al. [14, 15] proved in phase II clinical trial that sirolimus is an effective agent in the treatment of KHE as well as in the treatment of microcystic and mixed LMs. This revolutionized the management of patients with these vascular malformations, which up until then were primarily managed with palliative procedures by surgeons or interventional radiologists. From 2011 onward, many centers started incorporating medical therapies (initially only sirolimus and later other medical therapies) for such patients. See Table 2 for sirolimus dosing.

Several case series demonstrating the benefits of sirolimus in vascular malformations have since been published, typically showing a partial response. This is particularly the case for LMs and fibroadipose vascular anomalies; the response is less robust in VMs, whereas AVMs generally do not respond to sirolimus. Side effects from sirolimus include mouth sores, skin toxicity (acne), and hyperlipidemias and, as it is an immune-suppressing agent, there is concern that it may increase the risk of infections. Sirolimus targets many of the hemostatic and thrombotic manifestations in vascular malformations, including KMP in KHE and TA and LIC in VM. As well, the thrombocytopenia in MLT seems to respond to sirolimus. Most studies have shown that the median time to respond is less than 12 weeks, and in the prospective single-arm sirolimus study by Adams et al. [15, 56–58], 83% of patients showed a response by 6 months. In most cases, if a patient has shown no response to sirolimus after a 3–4-month trial, it is generally discontinued. One of the main issues with using sirolimus is the duration of use and whether patients can safely discontinue the medication without a rebound in the growth of the vascular malformation. Patients who demonstrate a clinical response typically are maintained on the medication for at least 2–3 years before attempting to wean off therapy. More recently, there has been recognition that much lower doses of sirolimus than traditionally used in the setting of transplantation can be efficacious in treating vascular anomalies. As such, in children without life-threatening complications, targeting the lowest effective trough dose to minimize toxicity is increasingly favored [59, 60]. Although many patients may respond to sirolimus, complete responses are uncommon, particularly in patients with complex vascular anomalies. The management of fever in a child on sirolimus depends on patient-specific factors. Children who appear unwell, have persistent fever, or have a history of severe infections or neutropenia should be evaluated immediately in the emergency department. There is no consensus guideline on the use of prophylaxis for *Pneumocystis jirovecii* (PJP) while taking sirolimus. As PJP has been previously reported in children with VA taking sirolimus, the use of PJP prophylaxis should be considered in children with the highest risk, including children under 2 years, those showing lymphopenia, and those taking concurrent high-dose steroids [61]. Some clinicians will hold sirolimus when patients receive live vaccinations (such as measles, mumps and rubella, and varicella [chicken pox]).

In the last few years, our understanding of the genetic pathways that underlie vascular anomalies has progressed very rapidly. Consequently, there has been increased use of other targeted medical therapies for vascular malformations that do not respond to sirolimus. Trametinib, a MEK inhibitor, has been found to be effective in treating extracranial AVMs and some complex lymphatic anomalies, such as KLA and central conducting lymphatic anomaly [62, 63]. Trametinib has also been shown to be effective in correcting the thrombocytopenia that occurs in KLA [27].

Another newer targeted medical therapy increasingly used in *PIK3CA*-related vascular anomalies is alpelisib – a direct PIK3CA antagonist. Venot et al. [64] demonstrated symptomatic and measurable radiologic improvement in 19 adults and children with PROS treated with alpelisib. A subsequent review of the EPIK-P1 study, a single-arm clinical trial of patients with PROS over the age of 2 years who received alpelisib as part of an expanded access program for compassionate use, confirmed these results. This led to conditional Food and Drug Administration approval for the use of alpelisib in adults and children above the age of 2 years with PROS. There is an ongoing phase 2 prospective, randomized, placebo-controlled trial of the efficacy and safety of alpelisib in children and adults with PROS (NCT04589650). No head-to-head trial comparing sirolimus to alpelisib has been undertaken;

12

where alpelisib has been used, it has usually been in patients who had previously been treated with sirolimus with no/minimal response.

In general, the effective dose for trametinib and alpelisib in vascular malformations tends to be lower than that used in cancer therapy. Traditional dosing based on cancer therapy results in excessive toxicity for many patients. The usual starting doses for these drugs are shown in Table 2.

The rapid recognition of targeted therapies in vascular anomalies is an exciting development in a field where patients have traditionally had few therapeutic options. However, there remain many questions about the use of these medications, including identifying patients who will respond, optimal response criteria, optimal duration of therapy, and long-term complications. Where possible, it is recommended that patients with complex vascular anomalies be referred to specialized centers and targeted therapies be administered as part of clinical trials.

Interventional Radiology

Interventional radiologists are extensively involved in managing patients with various types of vascular malformations.

LMs are cystic lesions that may present as macrocystic, microcystic, or mixed lesions. There is a significant benefit to drainage of macrocysts with the instillation of a sclerosing agent (e.g., sodium tetradecyl sulfate, doxycycline, bleomycin, OK432, ethanol, etc.), which leads to inflammation and fibrosis of the cyst, with subsequent sclerosis of the cyst. Bleomycin injection into microcystic lymphatic malformations has also been shown to be effective in reducing LM size [65].

Sclerotherapy with sodium tetradecyl sulfate, bleomycin, polidocanol, and ethanol is also occasionally effective in the treatment of VM, reducing both lesion size and pain symptoms.

Additionally, interventional radiologists perform embolizations for AVMs. The objective is to destroy the nidus of the AVM and not simply embolize the feeding vessel as it results in recurrence of the AVM. Liquid embolic agents, ethanol, and, more recently, bleomycin, have been used to treat AVMs. Occlusion of the venous outflow is another technique that helps to reduce blood flow through AVMs [66–68].

For complex lymphatic anomalies involving disorders of the central lymphatics, interventional radiologists can diagnose abnormalities with dynamic contrast magnetic resonance lymphangiography, perform lymphangiograms and then undertake therapeutic lymphatic embolizations to control leakage symptoms (e.g., plastic bronchitis, chylothorax, chylopericardium, protein losing enteropathy, chylous ascites, etc.), or potentially perform lymphatic recanalization to improve lymphatic drainage into the central venous system [69–71].

For patients with KTS and CLOVES, there is a role for proactive occlusion (coils)/ligation (surgical) and endovascular ablation (glue, mechanochemical, laser, and radiofrequency) of all embryonic or dilated and dysplastic veins that predispose patients to TE.

Surgical Management

Surgery has historically been a primary treatment option for vascular anomalies. However, with the availability of targeted medical therapies, the role of surgical treatment is being redefined. For solitary vascular malformations that could be completely resected without significant morbidity, surgical excision is still likely to be a preferred modality of therapy. Unfortunately, few lesions fulfill these criteria. Often surgery is not an option as the malformation may be too widespread, infiltrative, or involve or encircle critical vessels or organs making surgery hazardous or disfiguring. Partial surgical excision may sometimes be more detrimental than useful leading to various complications such as lymphatic fluid leakage and rapid growth of the remaining lesion in partially excised LMs. Nevertheless, surgery continues to play important roles, e.g., securing the airway and placement of tracheostomy tubes in head and neck malformations, debulking in patients with overgrowth syndromes, resecting intra-articular lesions to improve function, reconstruction surgery to improve cosmesis in lesions that have failed medical or interventional management, and obtaining biopsy tissue for pathologic and genetic testing.

Moreover, the combination of interventional and surgical therapies may offer the best outcomes in some cases, as is seen with intra-arterial embolization and surgical excision and reconstruction in AVMs or glue casting followed by surgical excision of VMs.

Conclusions

The management of patients with vascular anomalies requires a large multidisciplinary team for both the medical management as well as dealing with the significant hemostatic and thrombotic abnormalities that are common in children with vascular anomalies. These range from mild thrombocytopenia in certain hemangiomas to life-threatening consumptive coagulopathy in KLA and KHE with KMP. TEs are particularly associated with large VM, venous ectasia, and CLVM. Periprocedural anticoagulation is recommended for patients with venous ectasia or LIC. Sirolimus has been shown to improve hemostatic abnormalities and is a useful agent in treating many complex vascular anomalies. With a better understanding of the genetic pathways underlying vascular anomalies, we are entering the era of targeted therapies for vascular anomalies and, with it, an expanding role for pediatric hematologists/oncologists in the care of these patients.

Acknowledgments

We thank Ms. Alicia Koo (Toronto, Canada) for the critical review of the chapter.

Conflict of Interest Statement

D.A. reports being a consultant for Novartis and Nobias Therapeutics, participating in advisory boards for Novartis, and writing a chapter for UpToDate. M.C. reports having received research support from Bayer, Bioverativ/Sanofi, Novartis, Novo Nordisk, Pfizer, Roche, and Shire/Takeda and having received honoraria for speaking/participating in advisory boards from Bayer, Bioverativ/Sanofi, CSL Behring, LFB, Novo Nordisk, Pfizer, Roche, and Shire/Takeda.

Funding Sources

The authors received no funding.

Author Contributions

Soumitra Tole drafted the chapter, critically revised the chapter, and approved the final version. Victoria Price drafted the chapter, critically revised the chapter, and approved the final version. Joao Amaral critically revised the chapter and approved the final version. Denise Adams critically revised the chapter and approved the final version. Manuel Carcao drafted the chapter, critically revised the chapter, and approved the final version. The opinions expressed in the chapter are those of the named authors alone.

Abbreviations

AVM	Arteriovenous malformation
CM	Capillary malformation
CAT	Cutaneovisceral angiomatosis with thrombocytopenia
CH	Congenital hemangioma
CLOVES	Congenital lipomatous overgrowth, vascular malformations, epidermal nevi, and spinal/skeletal abnormalities syndrome
CLVM	Capillary-lymphatic-venous malformation
DIC	Disseminated intravascular coagulation
DOAC	Direct oral anticoagulant
IH	Infantile hemangioma
KHE	Kaposiform hemangioendothelioma
KLA	Kaposiform lymphangiomatosis
KMP	Kasabach-Merritt phenomenon
KTS	Klippel-Trenaunay syndrome

12

LIC	Localized intravascular coagulopathy
LMWH	Low-molecular-weight heparin
LM	Lymphatic malformation
LUMBAR	Lower-body hemangioma, urogenital abnormalities/ulceration, myelopathy, bony deformities, anorectal malformations/arterial anomalies, and rectal anomalies
MCAP	Megalencephaly-capillary malformation-polymicrogyria
MLT	Multifocal lymphangiomatosis with thrombocytopenia
NICH	Noninvoluting congenital hemangioma
PICH	Partially involuting congenital hemangioma
PI3K	Phosphatidylinositol 3-kinase
PE	Pulmonary embolism
PHACES	Posterior fossa anomalies, hemangioma, arterial anomalies, cardiac anomalies, and eye anomalies
PJP	*Pneumocystis jirovecii*
PROS	PIK3CA-related overgrowth spectrum
RICH	Rapidly involuting congenital hemangioma
TA	Tufted angioma
TE	Thromboembolism/thromboembolic event
VM	Venous malformation

References

1 Enjolras O, Mulliken JB, Boon LM, Wassef M, Kozakewich HP, Burrows PE. Noninvoluting congenital hemangioma: a rare cutaneous vascular anomaly. Plast Reconstr Surg. 2001;107(7):1647–54.
2 Berenguer B, Mulliken JB, Enjolras O, Boon LM, Wassef M, Josset P, et al. Rapidly involuting congenital hemangioma: clinical and histopathologic features. Pediatr Dev Pathol. 2003;6(6):495–510.
3 Nasseri E, Piram M, McCuaig CC, Kokta V, Dubois J, Powell J. Partially involuting congenital hemangiomas: a report of 8 cases and review of the literature. J Am Acad Dermatol. 2014;70(1):75–9.
4 Mulliken JB, Glowacki J. Classification of pediatric vascular lesions. Plast Reconstr Surg. 1982 Jul;70(1):120–1.
5 Mulliken JB, Glowacki J. Hemangiomas and vascular malformations in infants and children: a classification based on endothelial characteristics. Plast Reconstr Surg. 1982 Mar;69(3):412–22.
6 Queisser A, Seront E, Boon LM, Vikkula M. Genetic basis and therapies for vascular anomalies. Circ Res. 2021;129(1):155–73.
7 Dekeuleneer V, Seront E, Van Damme A, Boon LM, Vikkula M. Theranostic advances in vascular malformations. J Invest Dermatol. 2020;140(4):756–63.
8 Van Damme A, Seront E, Dekeuleneer V, Boon LM, Vikkula M. New and emerging targeted therapies for vascular malformations. Am J Clin Dermatol. 2020;21(5):657–68.
9 Ryan C, Price V, John P, Mahant S, Baruchel S, Brandao L, et al. Kasabach-Merritt phenomenon: a single centre experience. Eur J Haematol. 2010;84(2):97–104.
10 O'Rafferty C, O'Regan GM, Irvine AD, Smith OP. Kasabach-Merritt syndrome, kaposiform haemangioendothelioma and platelet blockade. Br J Haematol. 2015;171(1):11.
11 Adams DM. Special considerations in vascular anomalies: hematologic management. Clin Plast Surg. 2011;38(1):153–60.
12 Ricci KW, Brandao LR. Coagulation issues in vascular anomalies. Semin Pediatr Surg. 2020;29(5):150966.
13 Drolet BA, Trenor CC, 3rd, Brandao LR, Chiu YE, Chun RH, Dasgupta R, et al. Consensus-derived practice standards plan for complicated Kaposiform hemangioendothelioma. J Pediatr. 2013;163(1):285–91.
14 Hammill AM, Wentzel M, Gupta A, Nelson S, Lucky A, Elluru R, et al. Sirolimus for the treatment of complicated vascular anomalies in children. Pediatr Blood Cancer. 2011;57(6):1018–24.
15 Adams DM, Trenor CC, 3rd, Hammill AM, Vinks AA, Patel MN, Chaudry G, et al. Efficacy and safety of sirolimus in the treatment of complicated vascular anomalies. Pediatrics. 2016;137(2):e20153257.
16 Cashell J, Smink GM, Helm K, Xavier F. Kaposiform hemangioendothelioma with Kasabach-Merritt phenomenon in an infant: successful treatment with prednisolone, vincristine, and addition of sirolimus. Pediatr Blood Cancer. 2018;65(12):e27305.
17 Ji Y, Chen S, Zhou J, Yang K, Zhang X, Xiang B, et al. Sirolimus plus prednisolone vs sirolimus monotherapy for kaposiform hemangioendothelioma: a randomized clinical trial. Blood. 2022;139(11):1619–30.
18 Brill R, Uller W, Huf V, Muller-Wille R, Schmid I, Pohl A, et al. Additive value of transarterial embolization to systemic sirolimus treatment in kaposiform hemangioendothelioma. Int J Cancer. 2021;148(9):2345–51.
19 Ozeki M, Fujino A, Matsuoka K, Nosaka S, Kuroda T, Fukao T. Clinical features and prognosis of generalized lymphatic anomaly, kaposiform lymphangiomatosis, and Gorham-Stout disease. Pediatr Blood Cancer. 2016;63(5):832–8.
20 Perez-Atayde AR, Debelenko L, Al-Ibraheemi A, Eng W, Ruiz-Gutierrez M, O'Hare M, et al. Kaposiform lymphangiomatosis: pathologic aspects in 43 patients. Am J Surg Pathol. 2022;46(7):963–76.
21 Croteau SE, Kozakewich HP, Perez-Atayde AR, Fishman SJ, Alomari AI, Chaudry G, et al. Kaposiform lymphangiomatosis: a distinct aggressive lymphatic anomaly. J Pediatr. 2014;164(2):383–8.
22 Adams DM, Ricci KW. Vascular anomalies: diagnosis of complicated anomalies and new medical treatment options. Hematol Oncol Clin North Am. 2019;33(3):455–70.
23 Ji Y, Chen S, Peng S, Xia C, Li L. Kaposiform lymphangiomatosis and kaposiform hemangioendothelioma: similarities and differences. Orphanet J Rare Dis. 2019;14(1):165.
24 Ricci KW, Iacobas I. How we approach the diagnosis and management of complex lymphatic anomalies. Pediatr Blood Cancer. 2022;Suppl 3:e28985.

25 Wang Z, Li K, Yao W, Dong K, Xiao X, Zheng S. Successful treatment of kaposiform lymphangiomatosis with sirolimus. Pediatr Blood Cancer. 2015;62(7):1291–3.
26 Tole S, Price V, Pope E, Powell J, David M, Zwicker K, et al. Abnormal hemostasis in children with vascular anomalies, part I: thrombocytopenias among different vascular anomalies. Thromb Res. 2020;196:626–34.
27 Foster JB, Li D, March ME, Sheppard SE, Adams DM, Hakonarson H, et al. Kaposiform lymphangiomatosis effectively treated with MEK inhibition. EMBO Mol Med. 2020 Oct 7;12(10):e12324.
28 Chowers G, Abebe-Campino G, Golan H, Vivante A, Greenberger S, Soudack M, et al. Treatment of severe kaposiform lymphangiomatosis positive for NRAS mutation by MEK inhibition. Pediatr Res. 2022 Mar 4.
29 Koo KS, Dowd CF, Mathes EF, Rosbe KW, Hoffman WY, Frieden IJ, et al. MRI phenotypes of localized intravascular coagulopathy in venous malformations. Pediatr Radiol. 2015;45(11):1690–5.
30 Mazoyer E, Enjolras O, Laurian C, Houdart E, Drouet L. Coagulation abnormalities associated with extensive venous malformations of the limbs: differentiation from Kasabach-Merritt syndrome. Clin Lab Haematol. 2002;24(4):243–51.
31 Dompmartin A, Acher A, Thibon P, Tourbach S, Hermans C, Deneys V, et al. Association of localized intravascular coagulopathy with venous malformations. Arch Dermatol. 2008;144(7):873–7.
32 Enjolras O, Ciabrini D, Mazoyer E, Laurian C, Herbreteau D. Extensive pure venous malformations in the upper or lower limb: a review of 27 cases. J Am Acad Dermatol. 1997;36(2 Pt 1):219–25.
33 Ricci KW, Chute C, Hammill AM, Dasgupta R, Patel M. Retrospective study of hematologic complications in patients with slow-flow vascular malformations undergoing sclerotherapy. Pediatr Blood Cancer. 2020;67(10):e28277.
34 Hassanein AH, Mulliken JB, Fishman SJ, Alomari AI, Zurakowski D, Greene AK. Venous malformation: risk of progression during childhood and adolescence. Ann Plast Surg. 2012;68(2):198–201.
35 Dasgupta R, Patel M. Venous malformations. Semin Pediatr Surg. 2014;23(4):198–202.
36 Nguyen JT, Koerper MA, Hess CP, Dowd CF, Hoffman WY, Dickman M, et al. Aspirin therapy in venous malformation: a retrospective cohort study of benefits, side effects, and patient experiences. Pediatr Dermatol. 2014;31(5):556–60.
37 Adams DM, Brandao LR, Peterman CM, Gupta A, Patel M, Fishman S, et al. Vascular anomaly cases for the pediatric hematologist oncologists – an interdisciplinary review. Pediatr Blood Cancer. 2018;65(1).
38 Mack JM, Verkamp B, Richter GT, Nicholas R, Stewart K, Crary SE. Effect of sirolimus on coagulopathy of slow-flow vascular malformations. Pediatr Blood Cancer. 2019;66(10):e27896.
39 Baselga E, Cordisco MR, Garzon M, Lee MT, Alomar A, Blei F. Rapidly involuting congenital haemangioma associated with transient thrombocytopenia and coagulopathy: a case series. Br J Dermatol. 2008;158(6):1363–70.
40 Powell J, Blouin MM, David M, Dubois J. Bleeding in congenital hemangiomas: crusting as a clinical predictive sign and usefulness of tranexamic acid. Pediatr Dermatol. 2012;29(2):182–5.
41 Hsi Dickie B, Fishman SJ, Azizkhan RG. Hepatic vascular tumors. Semin Pediatr Surg. 2014;23(4):168–72.
42 North PE, Kahn T, Cordisco MR, Dadras SS, Detmar M, Frieden IJ. Multifocal lymphangioendotheliomatosis with thrombocytopenia: a newly recognized clinicopathological entity. Arch Dermatol. 2004;140(5):599–606.
43 Prasad V, Fishman SJ, Mulliken JB, Fox VL, Liang MG, Klement G, et al. Cutaneovisceral angiomatosis with thrombocytopenia. Pediatr Dev Pathol. 2005;8(4):407–19.
44 Droitcourt C, Boccara O, Fraitag S, Favrais G, Dupuy A, Maruani A. Multifocal lymphangioendotheliomatosis with thrombocytopenia: clinical features and response to sirolimus. Pediatrics. 2015;136(2):e517–22.
45 Ballieux F, Boon LM, Vikkula M. Blue bleb rubber nevus syndrome. Handb Clin Neurol. 2015;132:223–30.
46 Pireau N, Boon LM, Poilvache P, Docquier PL. Surgical treatment of intra-articular knee venous malformations: when and how? J Pediatr Orthop. 2016;36(3):316–22.
47 Chewning RH, Monroe EJ, Lindberg A, Koo KSH, Ghodke BV, Gow KW, et al. Combined glue embolization and excision for the treatment of venous malformations. CVIR Endovasc. 2018;1(1):22.
48 Laurian C, Masonni C, Wassef M, Houdart E, Toni F, Marteau V, et al. Surgical treatment of venous malformations of the knee: Treatment outcomes for 35 patients. J Pediatr Orthop. 2018;38(6):e325–31.
49 Uller W, El-Sobky S, Alomari AI, Fishman SJ, Spencer SA, Taghinia AH, et al. Preoperative embolization of venous malformations using n-butyl cyanoacrylate. Vasc Endovascular Surg. 2018;52(4):269–74.
50 Reis J, 3rd, Alomari AI, Trenor CC, 3rd, Adams DM, Fishman SJ, Spencer SA, et al. Pulmonary thromboembolic events in patients with congenital lipomatous overgrowth, vascular malformations, epidermal nevi, and spinal/skeletal abnormalities and Klippel-Trenaunay syndrome. J Vasc Surg Venous Lymphat Disord. 2018;6(4):511–6.
51 Oduber CE, van Beers EJ, Bresser P, van der Horst CM, Meijers JC, Gerdes VE. Venous thromboembolism and prothrombotic parameters in Klippel-Trenaunay syndrome. Neth J Med. 2013;71(5):246–52.
52 Cohen MM, Jr. Proteus syndrome: an update. Am J Med Genet C Semin Med Genet. 2005;137C(1):38–52.
53 Krowchuk DP, Frieden IJ, Mancini AJ, Darrow DH, Blei F, Greene AK, et al. Clinical practice guideline for the management of infantile hemangiomas. Pediatrics. 2019;143(1).
54 Perez Payarols J, Pardo Masferrer J, Gomez Bellvert C. Treatment of life-threatening infantile hemangiomas with vincristine. N Engl J Med. 1995;333(1):69.
55 Leaute-Labreze C, Hoeger P, Mazereeuw-Hautier J, Guibaud L, Baselga E, Posiunas G, et al. A randomized, controlled trial of oral propranolol in infantile hemangioma. N Engl J Med. 2015;372(8):735–46.
56 Triana P, Dore M, Cerezo VN, Cervantes M, Sanchez AV, Ferrero MM, et al. Sirolimus in the treatment of vascular anomalies. Eur J Pediatr Surg. 2017;27(1):86–90.

57 Hammer J, Seront E, Duez S, Dupont S, Van Damme A, Schmitz S, et al. Sirolimus is efficacious in treatment for extensive and/or complex slow-flow vascular malformations: a monocentric prospective phase II study. Orphanet J Rare Dis. 2018;13(1):191.
58 Tole S, Fantauzzi M, Cottingham D, Amaral JG, John PR, Lara-Corrales I, et al. The use of rapamycin to treat vascular tumours and malformations: a single-centre experience. Paediatr Child Health. 2021;26(1):e25–32.
59 Mizuno T, Fukuda T, Emoto C, Mobberley-Schuman PS, Hammill AM, Adams DM, et al. Developmental pharmacokinetics of sirolimus: implications for precision dosing in neonates and infants with complicated vascular anomalies. Pediatr Blood Cancer. 2017;64(8).
60 Shimano KA, Eng W, Adams DM. How we approach the use of sirolimus and new agents: medical therapy to treat vascular anomalies. Pediatr Blood Cancer. 2022;Suppl 3:e29603.
61 Russell TB, Rinker EK, Dillingham CS, Givner LB, McLean TW. Pneumocystis jirovecii pneumonia during sirolimus therapy for kaposiform hemangioendothelioma. Pediatrics. 2018;141(Suppl 5):S421–4.
62 Lekwuttikarn R, Lim YH, Admani S, Choate KA, Teng JMC. Genotype-guided medical treatment of an arteriovenous malformation in a child. JAMA Dermatol. 2019;155(2):256–7.
63 Edwards EA, Phelps AS, Cooke D, Frieden IJ, Zapala MA, Fullerton HJ, et al. Monitoring arteriovenous malformation response to genotype-targeted therapy. Pediatrics. 2020;146(3).
64 Venot Q, Blanc T, Rabia SH, Berteloot L, Ladraa S, Duong JP, et al. Targeted therapy in patients with PIK3CA-related overgrowth syndrome. Nature. 2018; 558(7711):540–46.
65 Chaudry G, Guevara CJ, Rialon KL, Kerr C, Mulliken JB, Greene AK, et al. Safety and efficacy of bleomycin sclerotherapy for microcystic lymphatic malformation. Cardiovasc Intervent Radiol. 2014;37(6):1476–81.
66 Do YS, Yakes WF, Shin SW, Lee BB, Kim DI, Liu WC, et al. Ethanol embolization of arteriovenous malformations: interim results. Radiology. 2005; 235(2):674–82.
67 Jin Y, Zou Y, Hua C, Chen H, Yang X, Ma G, et al. Treatment of early-stage extracranial arteriovenous malformations with intralesional interstitial bleomycin injection: a pilot study. Radiology. 2018;287(1):194–204.
68 Soulez G, Gilbert Md Frcpc P, Giroux Md Frcpc MF, Racicot Md Frcpc JN, Dubois J. Interventional management of arteriovenous malformations. Tech Vasc Interv Radiol. 2019;22(4):100633.
69 Krishnamurthy R, Hernandez A, Kavuk S, Annam A, Pimpalwar S. Imaging the central conducting lymphatics: initial experience with dynamic MR lymphangiography. Radiology. 2015;274(3): 871–8.
70 Chavhan GB, Amaral JG, Temple M, Itkin M. MR Lymphangiography in children: technique and potential applications. Radiographics. 2017;37(6):1775–90.
71 Ramirez-Suarez KI, Tierradentro-Garcia LO, Smith CL, Krishnamurthy G, Escobar FA, Otero HJ, et al. Dynamic contrast-enhanced magnetic resonance lymphangiography. Pediatr Radiol. 2022;52(2):285–94.

Published online: December 5, 2024

Blanchette VS, Brandão LR, Carcao MD, Kumar R, Rand ML, Revel-Vilk S (eds): SickKids Handbook of Pediatric Thrombosis and Hemostasis, ed 3, rev. and ext. Basel, Karger, 2024, pp 233–255 (DOI: 10.1159/000538201)

Diagnostic Approach to Thrombosis and Thrombophilia

Christine Sabapathy[a] Ali Amid[b] Riten Kumar[c] Laura Avila[d] Heleen van Ommen[e]

[a]Division of Hematology/Oncology, Department of Pediatrics, Montréal Children's Hospital, McGill University Health Centre, Montréal, QC, Canada; [b]Division of Hematology/Oncology, Department of Pediatrics, University of British Columbia, Vancouver, BC, Canada; [c]Dana Farber/Boston Children's Cancer and Blood Disorders Center, Harvard Medical School, Boston, MA, USA; [d]Division of Haematology-Oncology, Department of Paediatrics, The Hospital for Sick Children, Toronto, ON, Canada; [e]Department of Pediatric Hematology & Oncology, Erasmus University Medical Center Sophia Children's Hospital, Rotterdam, The Netherlands

Introduction

The term "thrombosis" refers to a thrombus within a blood vessel (arterial or venous [superficial or deep venous system]) or in a chamber in the circulatory system (e.g., the atrium). In 1856, Rudolf Virchow postulated three factors that contribute to venous thromboembolism (VTE): (1) impaired blood flow in vessels (stasis); (2) changes in the vessel wall (injury); and (3) alterations in the constitution of the blood (hypercoagulability).

While historically considered rare, VTE is being increasingly recognized in hospitalized children. Age distribution of pediatric VTE is bimodal with peaks noted during infancy and adolescence [1–3]. Similarly, children aged 1 year or less represent the greatest risk group for arterial thromboembolic events (ATEs) [4]. The vast majority of children with thromboembolic events (TEs) have associated underlying medical conditions. Increased awareness of thrombosis and continuing improvement in intensive care of critically ill children likely contribute to the increase in incidence of TEs [5].

Thromboembolism (TE) in children is associated with a direct mortality rate of 1.5%–2.2% and with significant morbidity, such as the development of post-thrombotic syndrome (PTS) (see Chapter 14), growth impairment of the involved limb or loss of organ function by arterial occlusion (see Chapter 15), and neurological and neurocognitive deficits in the setting of stroke (see Chapter 17).

The purpose of this chapter is to provide a clinical approach to the diagnostic and etiologic investigation of a child presenting with TE. The role of risk assessment models (RAMs) in identifying at-risk pediatric patients and the use of thromboprophylaxis measures will also be addressed. Assessment should start with a detailed personal and family history followed by a careful physical examination to determine the severity of the TE and to identify potential underlying conditions associated with an increased risk of thrombosis (Table 1). Imaging studies such as compression Doppler ultrasonography (DUS) identify elements to confirm the diagnosis and to evaluate the extent and severity of TE. Although no specific diagnostic laboratory tests for VTE are available, measurement of coagulation parameters, a complete blood count, and tests of renal and hepatic function are recommended as baseline investigations prior to initiating anticoagulation therapy. Investigation for an underlying hypercoagulable state, often referred to as a "thrombophilia workup," may be part of the laboratory evaluation of a child with thrombosis. The indications and recommended timing for a "thrombophilia workup" will be discussed later in this chapter.

Background

Risk Factors

TE in children usually occurs in the setting of one or more acquired or inherited prothrombotic risk factors and frequently represents secondary complications of an underlying disease (Table 1). The presence of a central venous and/or arterial catheter represents the single most important risk factor in the development of systemic VTE and ATE, respectively, in the pediatric population and accounts for more than 90% of systemic TEs in infants and more than half of TEs in all other age groups [3]. These "foreign" devices are often essential for supportive care of critically ill children. Rarely, TE may represent the primary manifestation of an unsuspected disorder, such as a tumor or a chronic inflammatory process.

TE occurring in the neonatal age group may be associated with maternal, perinatal, and/or neonatal conditions (Table 1). Severe congenital neonatal purpura fulminans is a rare life-threatening disorder affecting neonates and presents with cutaneous hemorrhage and necrosis resulting from microvascular thrombosis in the dermis as a result of an inherited homozygous (or compound heterozygous) deficiency of protein C and rarely protein S (see later) [6]. TE in neonates may involve specific vessel sites, such as renal vein thrombosis and portal vein thrombosis, the latter frequently associated with the presence of an umbilical venous catheter (see Chapter 16). The risk factors for cerebral sinovenous thrombosis (CSVT) and arterial ischemic stroke (AIS) in the neonatal period are distinct from those occurring later in life (see Chapter 17).

VTEs or ATEs are less frequent in toddlers as compared with preadolescents and are generally associated with a combination of identifiable risk factors such as presence of a central venous catheter (CVC), hematologic malignancy, congenital heart disease requiring cardiac catheterization or surgery, infection, or autoimmune disorders. Spontaneous TE in this age group is unusual and should raise the possibility of an undiagnosed disorder associated with an increased risk of TE.

TE in adolescents is more common, and as with younger children, may occur in association with an underlying disorder and/or its related treatment and/or the use of medications such as hormonal contraceptives [7].

Medical History

A detailed medical history should capture information about an underlying disease, ongoing treatments, and medications (Table 1). Past history of a TE including the type, location, and presence (or absence) of associated risk factors is important and may have a direct impact on the management including the duration of anticoagulation. Finally, information on symptoms of bleeding or bruising and a history of renal or hepatic problems should be obtained to assist in the assessment of hemorrhagic risk of anticoagulation.

Table 1. Clinical conditions associated with thrombosis in children

Age Newborn > infant/child < adolescent Maternal conditions: diabetes mellitus, arterial hypertension, antiphospholipid syndrome Perinatal/neonatal risk factors: prematurity, asphyxia (including meconium aspiration), sepsis, congenital heart disease, congenital diaphragmatic hernia, polycythemia
Cancer Tumor-related (e.g., hyperleukocytosis, vascular compression) Drug-related (e.g., corticosteroids, asparaginase, doxorubicin, trametinib, lenalidomide) Central venous catheter-related
Endovascular device placement Pacemakers Endovascular stents Central venous/arterial catheter Peritoneovenous shunts, ventriculoatrial shunts
Cardiac conditions Mechanical heart valves Congenital heart diseases Shunts (e.g., Blalock-Thomas-Taussig), surgical procedures (e.g., Fontan procedure) Heart failure secondary to cardiomyopathy, acquired myocarditis, and/or arrhythmia Extracorporeal device (e.g., extracorporeal membrane oxygenation, ventricular assist device)
Drugs Oral contraceptive, hormone replacement, or gender-affirming hormone therapy Corticosteroids Erythropoiesis-stimulating agents Thrombopoietin analogs Heparinoids (e.g., heparin-induced thrombocytopenia)
Hematological disorders Hyperviscosity syndrome (e.g., hyperleukocytosis, cyanotic congenital heart disease, hereditary hemorrhagic telangectasia/pulmonary arteriovenous malformations) Hemoglobinopathies (e.g., sickle cell disease, thalassemia) Myeloproliferative neoplasms (e.g., essential thrombocythemia, polycythemia vera) Inherited thrombophilia (protein C/S/antithrombin deficiency, factor V Leiden, prothrombin gene variant) Paroxysmal nocturnal hemoglobinuria
Infections/inflammatory Systemic (e.g., sepsis, human immunodeficiency virus, varicella) Localized (e.g., head/neck infection – Lemierre's syndrome, thrombophlebitis) Vasculitis (e.g., Kawasaki disease, systemic lupus erythematosus, Takayasu's, Alagille) Antiphospholipid syndrome Inflammatory bowel diseases (ulcerative colitis, Crohn's disease)
Prolonged immobilization Surgery Trauma Neurological diseases
Conditions with protein loss Nephrotic syndrome Protein-losing enteropathies Chylothorax

(Table continued on next page.)

Table 1 (continued)

Anatomical thrombophilia
Inferior vena cava anomalies
Paget-Schroetter syndrome (e.g., venous thoracic outlet syndrome)
May-Thurner syndrome (e.g., iliac vein compression)
Vascular malformations (e.g., *PIK3CA*-related overgrowth syndromes)
Others
Obesity
Previous thrombotic event
Positive family history of thrombosis

Family History

An accurate family history is important in assessing children presenting with TE. A positive family history of a TE is an independent risk factor for TEs. This risk increases with the number of relatives affected, younger age of a family member at the time of TE [8], and in the presence of a known thrombophilia trait [9]. A detailed family history should include information on parental consanguinity, VTE at any age, cardiovascular events such as myocardial infarction and AIS at a younger adult age, e.g., <40 years, and obstetric complications, particularly occurrence of recurrent miscarriage and/or known familial thrombophilia.

Physical Examination

Signs and symptoms of TE may be nonspecific, subtle, or even absent. Clinical manifestations depend on a variety of factors, including type of blood vessel affected (arterial vs. venous), the degree of vessel occlusion (occlusive vs. nonocclusive), and location of TE (Table 2).

The physical examination should include an assessment of the affected body part, most often a limb, plus a general physical examination, in order to identify underlying disorders or conditions that may be associated with TE. The clinical examination of an affected limb should record skin discoloration (i.e., pale, cyanotic), skin temperature (cold in arterial and warm in venous occlusion), presence of swelling, tenderness, presence of collaterals, and the degree of functional impairment. Presence of cutaneous lesions and/or scars may reflect the site of a previous catheter or of localized inflammatory/infectious processes. Rapid onset of cutaneous purpuric lesions after birth or during an acute infection represents the clinical manifestation of purpura fulminans, a life-threatening condition requiring urgent intervention.

In VTE, the outflow of blood from the organ/body part is compromised causing progressive stasis of blood and fluid accumulation in the interstitial compartment leading to swelling. Acute onset of swelling and pain represent the most frequent clinical presentation of VTE affecting a limb. In relation to arterial obstruction, ATE may present with signs of absent or diminished peripheral pulses, cool and pale extremities, or necrotic areas. Impaired arterial flow represents an urgent condition requiring rapid assessment and treatment (see Chapter 15). Similarly, VTE, when severe, may secondarily occlude arterial blood flow (*phlegmasia alba dolens*) and if not treated appropriately, progress to venous gangrene (*phlegmasia cerulae dolens*). Therefore, the assessment of perfusion and pulses is of importance in both VTE and ATE.

Swelling may not always be apparent, and objective measurement of the circumference of the

Table 2. Signs and symptoms in relation to the site of thrombosis and the suggested diagnostic imaging tests

Site of thrombosis	Sign(s) and symptom(s)	Suggested imaging	Detailed in
Limb (upper/lower) DVT	Pain, swelling, discoloration, collaterals, tenderness, increased temperature, impaired function of involved limb; may be asymptomatic	DUS[a], CTV/MRV[b], venography[c]	Chapter 14
Superior vena cava due to intrathoracic and jugular DVT	Neck/head pain and swelling, and/or with symptoms associated with upper limb DVT; may be asymptomatic	DUS (low sensitivity for intrathoracic)[a], CTV/MRV[b], venography (high sensitivity for intrathoracic)[c]	Chapter 14
Inferior vena cava, common iliac vein DVT	Back, buttock, and/or abdominal pain, ±symptoms associated with lower limb DVT; may be asymptomatic	DUS[a], CTV/MRV[b], venography[c]	Chapter 14
Right atrial thrombus	Bradycardia, tachyarrhythmia, new heart murmur, heart failure, respiratory distress; may be asymptomatic	Echocardiography	Chapter 14
Pulmonary embolism	Unexplained chest pain or shortness of breath with pleuritic chest pain, cough, hemoptysis, tachypnea, tachycardia, shock; may be asymptomatic	Spiral CT (CTPA)[a], V/Q scan[b], MRI[c], pulmonary angiography[c]	Chapter 14
Limb (upper/lower) arterial thrombosis	Pain, pallor, reduced temperature, absent pulses, or necrosis (late sign) of involved limb	DUS[a]	Chapter 15
Portal/hepatic/mesenteric/ -splenic vein thrombosis	Localized/diffuse abdominal pain, and/or hepatosplenomegaly; increased abdominal girth with or without ascites; may be asymptomatic	DUS[a], CTV/MRV[b]	Chapter 16
Renal vein thrombosis	Abdominal/flank pain, hematuria, oliguria, abdominal mass, thrombocytopenia	DUS[a]	Chapter 16
Central nervous system TE: Arterial ischemic stroke Sinus venous thrombosis	General neurologic symptoms: headache, altered level of consciousness, nausea, emesis, seizure (common in neonates), and/ or focal neurologic deficit	MRI/MRA MRV[a]/CTV[b]	Chapter 17

For details, see diagnostic imaging in the specific chapter. CT, computed tomography; CTPA, computed tomography pulmonary angiography; CTV, computed tomography venography; DVT, deep vein thrombosis; DUS, Doppler ultrasonography; MRA, magnetic resonance angiography; MRI, magnetic resonance imaging; MRV, magnetic resonance venography; TE, thromboembolism/thromboembolic event; V/Q scan, ventilation/perfusion scan. [a]Current practice. [b]Second choice (if [a] not available or nonconclusive). [c]Third choice.

affected and nonaffected limbs may help to quantify the degree of swelling. Standardized measurements of the affected limb can be done by measuring the limb circumference from a fixed distance of a bony landmark rather than measuring at the largest point of swelling, which may change during the course of a TE event. A number of specific clinical assessments used in adult patients may help in the assessment of older children suspected with lower limb TE. This includes calf pain induced either by dorsiflexion of the foot (Homan's sign), calf compression (May's sign), or sole pain induced by its compression (Payr's sign). The presence of superficial collateral vessels, skin induration, increased skin pigmentation, and ulcers are clinical signs of chronic venous stasis and PTS (see Chapter 14).

Malfunction of a CVC, such as difficulty with infusion, flushing, or getting blood return (a "blocked CVC"), or CVC-related infection may also suggest the presence of thrombosis.

A detailed neurological examination is required where there is suspicion of a cerebral TE (see Chapter 17).

Examination of the respiratory system may help to identify whether symptoms such as dyspnea and/or chest pain are possibly because of an infective condition or other causes other than those associated with a pulmonary embolism (PE) (see Chapter 14).

Diagnostic Imaging

The clinical suspicion of a TE should be followed by diagnostic imaging to confirm the presence of and extent of thrombosis. Knowledge of the different imaging techniques, their appropriate use and limitations, as well as an understanding of the normal vascular anatomy is important for the diagnosis of thrombosis in children.

Diagrams of the vascular anatomy for the upper and lower deep venous systems, major arteries, and umbilical circulation are presented in Figure 1. The cerebral venous sinus system and the cerebral arterial supply are further discussed in Chapter 17.

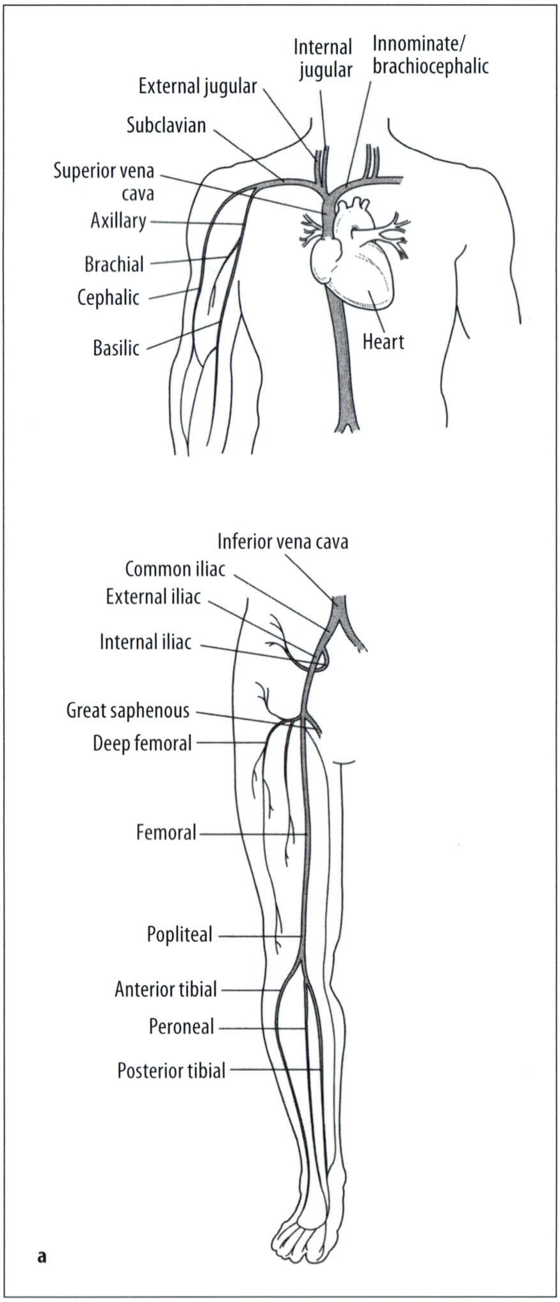

Fig. 1. a Anatomy of the upper and lower deep venous system. **b** Anatomy of major arteries. **c** Anatomy of the umbilical circulation. Reused with permission from Paul Monagle and Gabrielle deVeber [51].

(Figure continued on next pages.)

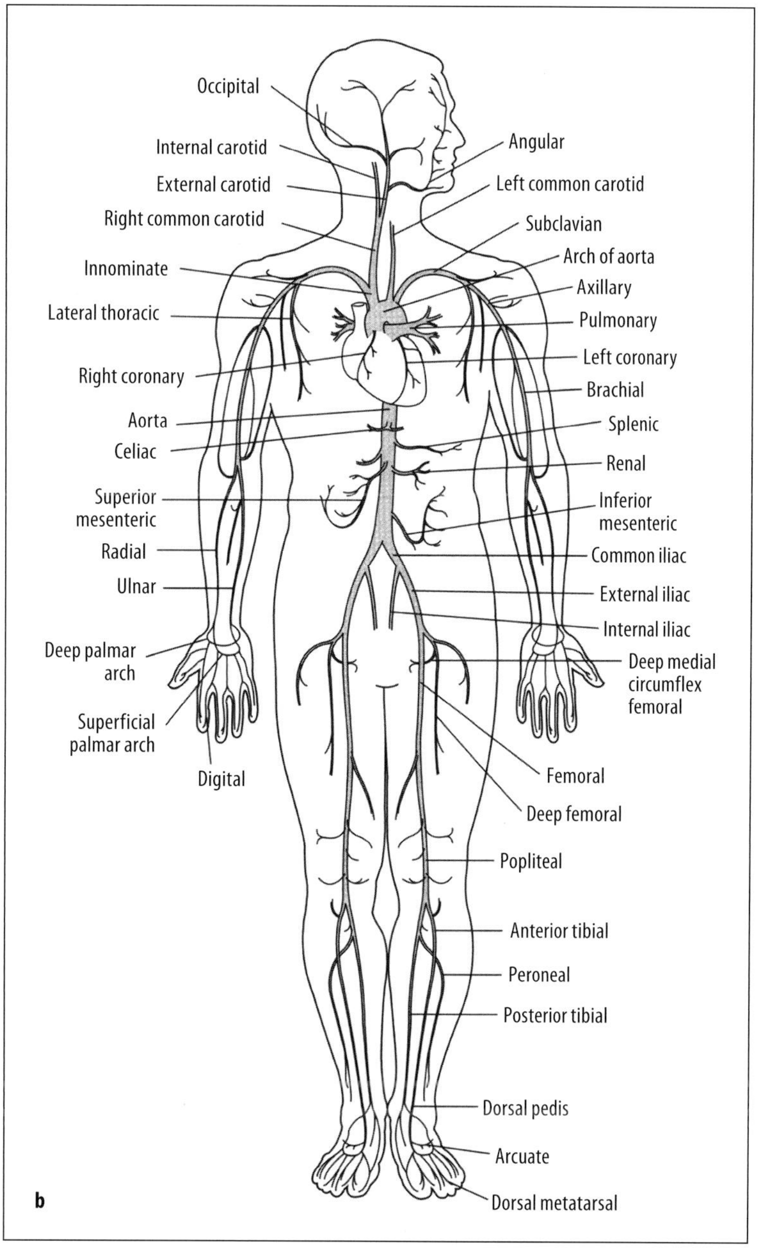

Fig. 1

(Figure continued on next page.)

Doppler Ultrasonography

Compression DUS is a noninvasive technique that is the preferred imaging option for the diagnosis of most thrombosis in children. In vessels with thrombosis, Doppler signals are absent, and the lumen cannot be compressed with direct pressure. Success of this technique is dependent on the experience of the examiner and on patient compliance. Its sensitivity in the assessment of the intrathoracic upper vessel system, including the proximal subclavian and innominate veins and the superior vena cava, is low because of the

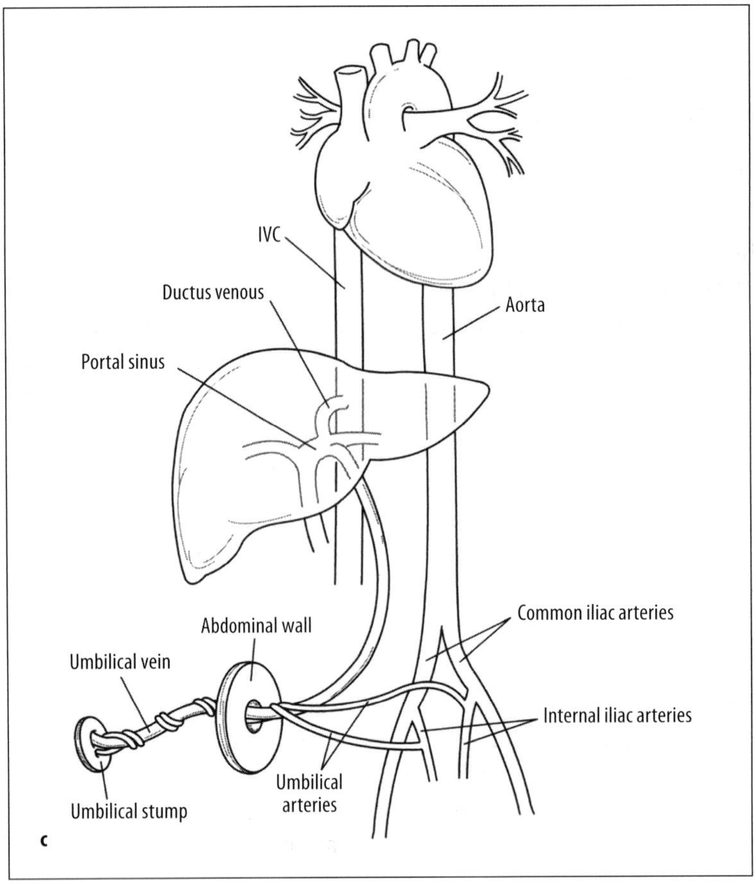

Fig. 1

inability to compress the vessels [1]. Similarly, the sensitivity of Doppler sonogram in diagnosis of thrombosis in the inferior vena cava is low. Other factors that may interfere with DUS imaging in children include small-diameter vessels, low pulse pressure, and the presence of a CVC that compromises the ability to clearly compress the veins. Other techniques such as computed tomography venography (CTV) or magnetic resonance venography (MRV) may be used in difficult cases. Echocardiography is a valuable noninvasive modality for the diagnosis of a thrombus occurring in the superior vena cava, heart, or to assess for right-sided heart strain in cases of PE.

Conventional Venography

Venography is a minimally invasive technique, where ionized dye is injected through a vein, thus enabling visualization of the vessels by X-ray. Except for the jugular veins, this technique enables the visualization of any portion of the venous system. Venography is considered the gold standard in the diagnosis of VTE in children; however, the need for good venous access, interventional radiologist, and anesthesia support, as well the exposure to contrast and ionizing radiation, makes this technique less suitable in children. In addition to a chest X-ray to visualize the line placement, a linogram (direct injection of contrast into the CVC of interest) and venography are occasionally used for the investigation of a malfunctioning CVC (see Chapter 14).

Computerized Tomography

X-ray-based computerized tomography (CT) with or without ionized contrast enables very rapid acquisition of images. Computerized tomography pulmonary angiography (CTPA), also termed spiral CT, is a noninvasive technique currently preferred in both pediatric and adult patients with clinically suspected PE (see Chapter 14). The most important disadvantages of CTPA are its exposure to ionizing radiation and the contraindication to using the contrast agent in children with impaired renal function.

Magnetic Resonance Imaging

Magnetic resonance imaging (MRI) with or without gadolinium-enhanced MRV or magnetic resonance arteriography (MRA) is the preferred imaging technique for assessing children presenting with stroke and has the advantage of not exposing children to radiation (see Chapter 17). Magnetic resonance venography may also have an important role for assessing thrombosis in the intrathoracic upper limb vessel system. Pulmonary contrast MRA should be considered as an alternative to CTPA for diagnosis of PE when ionized contrast injection or radiation is a significant consideration. Limitations of MRI in children include the need to remain immobile for extended periods of time, which typically warrants the use of sedation in younger children.

Ventilation/Perfusion Lung Scan

Ventilation/perfusion (V/Q) scan is a combination of scintigraphy with a radioisotope. In the ventilation phase, an aerosol form of a nuclide is inhaled, and in the perfusion phase, the nuclide is injected intravenously. A gamma camera acquires the images required to determine the ventilation/perfusion rate. The V/Q scan is interpreted according to criteria adapted from adults (classified as low, moderate, or high PE probability according to the documented mismatch in the ventilation and perfusion; see Chapter 14). A high-probability scan results in a peripheral basal perfusion defect with normal ventilation. However, this technique is not always available and requires a cooperative child (usually at least 5 years of age). Spiral CT has largely replaced V/Q scan in children with clinically suspected PE (see above).

Conventional Chest X-Ray

Conventional chest X-ray may help to identify or exclude alternative diagnoses, such as a pneumonia that occurs much more frequently than a PE, although identification of an infection does not preclude a concurrent PE. A chest X-ray should be performed to visualize the CVC position in cases with CVC dysfunction (see Chapter 14).

Laboratory Investigations

Laboratory Tests in the Acute Presentation

Specific diagnostic laboratory tests to confirm the presence of thrombosis are not available. Laboratory evaluation in the acute phase in a patient being assessed for TE may be helpful in assessing for other disorders or may be used to establish safety for a required treatment.

Complete Blood Count (Blood Collected into EDTA Anticoagulant)

A low platelet count may increase the risk of bleeding in patients who require antithrombotic therapy (see Chapter 20). Anemia and thrombocytopenia may suggest disseminated intravascular coagulation (DIC), especially in the presence of schistocytes, hypofibrinogenemia, and elevation of D-dimers.

Thrombocytopenia associated with hematuria (plus or minus a palpable flank mass) may suggest renal vein thrombosis (see Chapter 16). In addition, isolated thrombocytopenia in neonates is an important sign of CVC-associated thrombosis [10].

Prothrombin Time/International Normalized Ratio, Activated Partial Thromboplastin Time, Thrombin Time, Fibrinogen (Blood Collected into Citrate Anticoagulant)
Abnormal results may suggest coagulation factor deficiencies (see Chapter 4). Correction of factor deficiencies should be considered prior to initiation of antithrombotic therapy to minimize bleeding risks. A prolonged activated partial thromboplastin time (aPTT), if measured using an antiphospholipid-sensitive assay, may suggest the presence of antiphospholipid antibodies (APLAs) (see below). A shortened aPTT may reflect the presence of elevated factor VIII (FVIII) secondary to inflammatory disorders (see below). A prolonged prothrombin time (PT)/international normalized ratio (INR), aPTT, thrombin time, and/or a low fibrinogen level with thrombocytopenia may suggest DIC (see Chapter 11).

D-Dimer Test (Blood Collected into Citrate Anticoagulant)
D-dimers are degradation products of cross-linked fibrin that are formed during fibrinolysis (see Chapter 2). Although elevated D-dimer levels are associated with acute VTE, an elevated D-dimer level is often a nonspecific finding occurring in inflammation, sepsis, malignancy, or other proinflammatory states. In adults with low pretest probability of either deep vein thrombosis (DVT) or PE, normal D-dimer levels can be used to rule out a diagnosis. In contrast, a prospective study that recruited 296 children with or without objectively documented limb DVT (largely hospitalized patients) showed that D-dimer levels had poor discriminative and predictive ability for the diagnosis of limb DVT. Similarly, retrospective studies have also shown D-dimers to have high sensitivity but low specificity for the diagnosis of PE in children [11–14].

Elevated D-dimer plasma levels at diagnosis and after 3–6 months of treatment have been shown to be associated with persistent VTE, recurrent VTE, and/or development of PTS in a pediatric cohort [15].

Evaluation of Renal and Liver Function (Blood Collected into Heparin Anticoagulant)
Abnormal liver and/or renal function may lead to therapy adjustment in children with TE (see Chapter 20).

Laboratory Evaluation During Ongoing Anticoagulation
Effective and safe antithrombotic treatment requires appropriate monitoring (see Chapter 20).

Laboratory Thrombophilia

Thrombophilia refers to laboratory markers of hypercoagulability with an increased tendency to develop thrombosis. A number of inherited and acquired thrombophilias have been identified; however, the interpretation of thrombophilia test results in individual clinical scenarios may be difficult. Age-dependent normal laboratory values for many laboratory thrombophilia markers are presented in Appendix II. The inherited and acquired markers for thrombophilia are detailed below according to their mechanism of action. The impact of laboratory thrombophilia on acute systemic VTE, its recurrence, and stroke is presented in Table 3 [16–19].

Elevated Procoagulant Factors
Prothrombin (II) G20210A Variant (Blood Collected into EDTA Anticoagulant)
An elevated prothrombin (FII) level is caused by a point variant in the noncoding region of the prothrombin gene (nucleotide 20210 G to A) leading to augmented thrombin generation and potentially with an increased risk of thrombosis.

Elevated FVIII (Blood Collected into Citrate Anticoagulant)
There is limited evidence of the predictive role of persistently high levels of FVIII (>150 IU/dL) for VTE recurrence in children. In adults, evidence is conflicting; whereas some studies identified FVIII

Table 3. Prevalence and impact (expressed as pooled odds ratio) of laboratory thrombophilia in childhood thromboembolic events

Thrombophilia	Prevalence	First VTE odds ratio (95% CI)	Recurrent VTE odds ratio (95% CI)	First CSVT odds ratio (95% CI)	First AIS odds ratio (95% CI)
FV Leiden G1691A[a]	~1:20	3.8 (3–4.8)	0.6 (0.4–1.2)	2.7 (1.7–4.3)	3.7 (2.8–4.9)
Prothrombin G20210A[a]	~1:50	2.6 (1.6–4.4)	1.9 (1.0–3.5)	2.0 (0.9–4.1)	2.6 (1.7–4.1)
Protein C deficiency[a]	~1:200	7.7 (4.4–13.4)	2.4 (1.2–4.4)	6.3 (1.6–25.4)	11.0 (5.1–23.6)
Protein S deficiency[a]	~1:500	5.8 (3.0–11)	3.1 (1.5–6.5)	5.3 (1.5–18.2)	1.5 (0.3–6.9) (R)
Antithrombin deficiency[a]	~1:500–5,000	9.4 (3.3–26.7)	3.0 (1.4–6.3)	18.4 (3.3–104.3)	3.3 (0.7–15.5)
Lipoprotein(a)[a]	NA	4.5 (3.3–6.2)	0.8 (0.5–1.4)	NA	6.5 (4.5–9.6)
≥2 genetic traits[b]	NA	9.5 (4.9–18.4)	4.5 (2.9–6.9)	6.1 (0.9–43.1)	18.8 (6.5–54.1)
LAC/APLA	Variable	4.9 (2.2–10.9)	NA	NA	7.0 (3.7–13.1)
FVIII:C	NA	5.5 (2.0–15.1)	NA	NA	NA

Adapted from [16–19, 52–54]. AIS, arterial ischemic stroke; APLA, antiphospholipid antibodies; CI, confidence interval; CSVT, cerebral sinovenous thrombosis; FV, factor V; FVIII:C, factor VIII activity (>90th percentile); LAC, lupus anticoagulant; NA, not applicable; VTE, venous thromboembolism/thromboembolic event. [a]Heterozygote trait. [b]Including FV Leiden, prothrombin G20210A variant, lipoprotein(a) (>30 mg/dL), antithrombin deficiency, protein C, and/or protein S deficiency.

to be an independent predictor of TE recurrence, other studies found no evidence of effect [17, 20–22]. Given that plasma FVIII and von Willebrand factor levels may be increased during the acute phase response, we recommend that measurement of FVIII activity (FVIII:C) as a part of thrombophilia evaluation only be performed 3–6 months after VTE diagnosis and ideally following completion of anticoagulant therapy to minimize the impact of direct oral anticoagulants on FVIII:C. FVIII:C may be measured by one-stage clotting assay or chromogenic assay [23] (for normal values, see Appendix II).

Decreased Natural Inhibitors of Coagulation Factors

Deficiencies of natural inhibitors of coagulation, including protein C, protein S, and antithrombin, are uncommon but represent a potent thrombotic risk. Levels are age specific and may be influenced by secondary conditions affecting their production, consumption, or clearance. Deficiencies of these inhibitors are inherited in an autosomal dominant manner. All diagnostic laboratories processing pediatric samples for natural inhibitors of coagulation should use and interpret results according to age-, analyzer-, and reagent-specific reference ranges [24] (see Appendix II). It should be emphasized that a single laboratory test result below the 95% confidence limit for age is not enough to define an inherited state. The diagnosis of an inherited state should be based on the presence of compatible clinical phenotype, family history, and reproducible abnormal laboratory results.

Protein C and S Deficiency (Blood Collected into Citrate Anticoagulant)

Both proteins are vitamin K-dependent anticoagulant proteins, mainly synthesized in the liver. Activated protein C, together with protein S, thrombomodulin, and endothelial protein C receptor, forms a complex that inhibits activated factor V (FV) and activated FVIII (see Chapter 2).

Protein C deficiency is classified into two types: type I (most frequent) is characterized by both a low activity and antigen level (quantitative deficiency) and type II by a low activity but a normal antigen level (qualitative defect). The International Society on Thrombosis and Haemostasis recommends screening patients with protein C activity (using a chromogenic assay), since this will detect both type I (both protein C activity and antigen are decreased) and type IIa defects (abnormalities within the protein C activation or active sites). If persistently abnormal, protein C antigen levels can be measured using an enzyme-linked immunoassay (ELISA)-based test, to distinguish type IIa from type I defects, and a clot-based assay to rule out the rare type IIb defect (abnormalities with protein C substrate, surface, or cofactors binding to protein C) [25] (for normal values, see Appendix II). More than 400 putative variants in the protein C gene (*PROC*) have been described – type I deficiency is caused by both missense and null variants, which reduce protein synthesis or accelerate destruction, whereas type II deficiency is typically caused by missense variants affecting protein function [26].

Protein S, a cofactor for activated protein C, circulates in plasma in two states: a free active form and an inactive form bound to the complement component C4b-binding protein. Protein S deficiency is subdivided based on the amount of free and bound protein and its activity. Type I deficiency (quantitative) is characterized by reduced protein S activity, low free, and total protein S antigen. Type III, also a quantitative deficiency, is characterized by low free protein S antigen and activity but a normal total protein S antigen. Both types I and III are the most common defects. Type II deficiency (qualitative defect) is characterized by normal levels of free and total protein S antigen but reduced protein S activity [27].

Testing for protein S deficiency includes the measurement of free protein S antigen and, if abnormal, total protein S can be determined (both are measured using an ELISA-based test system; for normal values, see Appendix II). The distinction between type I and type III has no clinical implications. Functional protein S assays are difficult to perform and only rarely necessary as type II protein S deficiency is extremely rare. More than 200 putative variants in the protein S (*PROS1*) gene have been described. While the most common variants are missense, splice site, deletions, and nonsense variants have also been reported [28]. In a large cohort study, 69% of patients with protein C deficiency were found to have variants in the *PROC* gene. The pathogenic variant detection rate in the *PROS1* gene was 43% in patients with protein S deficiency [29].

Homozygous (or compound heterozygous) protein C or S cases generally present with neonatal purpura fulminans (separately addressed in this chapter) [6]. Acquired conditions with protein C and S deficiency reflect their increased consumption in sepsis- and nonsepsis-associated DIC, infections (typically varicella for protein S), or decreased production such as occurs in vitamin K deficiency, liver disorders, or medications (e.g., vitamin K antagonists [VKAs], oral contraceptives, L-asparaginase chemotherapy).

Antithrombin Deficiency (Blood Collected into Citrate Anticoagulant)

Antithrombin is a potent inhibitor of multiple coagulation factors, including activated FII and activated factor X (see Chapter 2). Antithrombin deficiency, a rare autosomal dominant thrombophilia, may be classified as type I (quantitative deficiency) or type II (qualitative defect). Subjects with type I antithrombin deficiency have low levels of antithrombin activity and antigen, whereas subjects with type II deficiency typically have low antithrombin activity, with a normal antigen level. The functional defect in type II variants involves either the heparin binding site (type IIHBS), the reactive site (type IIRS), or both (pleiotropic variants, type IIPE) [30]. While more prevalent in the general population, type II antithrombin deficiency, particularly type IIHBS, is thought to be less thrombogenic than type I deficiency [31]. Over 300 putative variants in the antithrombin (*SERPINC1*) gene have been described in adults and children with antithrombin deficiency. Carriers of null variants are predicted to have a significantly higher risk of VTE compared with carriers of missense variants [31].

Homozygous antithrombin deficiency is typically not compatible with life, with the exception of type IIHBS variants, where a severe thrombotic phenotype has been described with homozygosity [30]. Acquired antithrombin deficiency can occur in association with large protein losses (e.g., nephrotic syndrome), liver disease, sepsis, and treatment with L-asparaginase chemotherapy (see Chapter 14). Patients with antithrombin deficiency may be heparin resistant (see Chapter 20).

Resistance to Intrinsic Inhibitor of Coagulation

Activated Protein C Resistance (Blood Collected into Citrate Anticoagulant) – FV Leiden Variant (Blood Collected into EDTA)

A point variant in the FV gene (nucleotide 1691 A to G), also called the factor V Leiden (FVL) variant, is the most common genetic disorder associated with thrombosis in adults and children, with a carrier rate of 5% in the Caucasian population. The variant leads to a change in FV conferring resistance to inactivation by activated protein C. The presence of a heterozygous variant is associated with a low to mild risk of VTE and stroke in children [16, 18]. Patients with homozygous variants are at much greater risk of thrombosis compared with those with heterozygous variants. Acquired activated protein C resistance may occur in the setting of oral contraceptive use [7] or in association with high concentrations of coagulation FVIII.

Activation of Endothelial Cells

Lupus Anticoagulant (Blood Collected into Citrate Anticoagulant)

Lupus anticoagulant (LAC) detection consists of three sequential laboratory steps [32]: (1) demonstration of an abnormal phospholipid-dependent coagulation screening test (using diluted Russell viper venom test and/or a lupus-sensitive aPTT); (2) a mixing study to ensure that the abnormality of the screening test is due to the presence of a circulating inhibitor; (3) a confirmatory test, which incorporates the addition of exogenous phospholipids to prove that the abnormality is phospholipid dependent. Assessment for the presence of an LAC may be helpful prior to initiation of anticoagulation since anticoagulation may affect the interpretation of LAC screens [32].

Anticardiolipin Antibodies and Anti-β_2-Glycoprotein I Antibodies (Blood Collected into a Blood Tube without an Anticoagulant)

Both IgG and IgM anticardiolipin antibodies (ACLAs) and β_2-GPI antibodies are measured by immunoassay (ELISA) tests (for normal values, see Appendix II).

APLAs include LAC, ACLA, and anti-β_2-GPI. APLA may be transient in the setting of acute infection, inflammation, malignancy, and medications. APLA may also be transient in newborn infants with a positive maternal history for antiphospholipid syndrome (APS) but rarely cause neonatal TEs.

APS is defined by the presence of vascular thrombosis or pregnancy loss with the persistent (two tests performed 12 weeks apart) presence of APLA including LAC and/or ACLA and/or β_2-GPI antibodies [33]. In the pediatric population, similar criteria are suggested (excluding pregnancy as one of the clinical criteria), although never validated [34]. In contrast to the original Sapporo criteria, the Sydney criteria strongly advised that patients with APS be classified into those with positivity for one APLA (LAC only, ACLA only, or anti-β_2-GPI only) and those with >1 laboratory criterion present in any combination [33]. This was based on the concept that positivity for one APLA carries a lower risk of thrombosis or pregnancy complications compared with those with multiple (particularly triple) positivity. Two new antibodies, antiphosphatidylserine and prothrombin antibodies, are being investigated in

13

adults with thrombotic APS, and their role in children is unknown [35]. APS may occur either as a primary condition or in the setting of an underlying disease, usually systemic lupus erythematosus. Vascular thrombosis in the criteria for APS includes one or more clinical episodes of ATE, VTE, or small vessel thrombosis in any tissue or organ confirmed by imaging studies or histopathology (without significant vessel wall inflammation) [33]. VTE in APS is most commonly lower limb DVT and/or PE, but any part of the venous system may be involved, including portal, renal, mesenteric, and intracranial veins. The most frequent site of ATE in APS is in the cerebral vasculature resulting in transient ischemic attack (TIA)/AIS. Microvascular thrombosis in APS is least common but may manifest as the potentially lethal "catastrophic APS"; typically, multiorgan failure involving, but not confined to the lungs, brain, and kidneys [36]. Other abnormalities associated with APLA, known as noncriteria manifestations, include thrombocytopenia, hemolytic anemia, livedo reticularis, valvular heart disease (Libman-Sachs endocarditis), neurologic findings (cognitive deficits and white matter lesions), and renal dysfunction (thrombotic microangiopathy) [34].

Children presenting with unprovoked TE or in the setting of concomitant diagnosed or suspected autoimmune/rheumatologic disorders should be assessed for the presence of APLA. Testing should be repeated 12 weeks following an initial positive test. Children with persistent APLA (especially if positive for all three APLA) have a significant increased risk of recurrence, and prolonged (or long-term) anticoagulation may be considered [19, 37, 38]. Early recognition and aggressive initiation of anticoagulant therapy as well as other disease-directed therapies are critically important in the treatment of catastrophic APS [36]. For appropriate anticoagulants for this condition, see Chapter 20.

Homocysteine (Blood Collected into Heparin Anticoagulant)

Homocysteine is an amino acid that derives from dietary methionine. Elevated homocysteine may directly damage the endothelium conferring prothrombotic changes. No data are available on the significance of high homocysteine levels for the risk of VTE, ATE, and AIS and the efficacy of lowering homocysteine levels to prevent thrombotic recurrence in children. In adults, lowering the homocysteine levels was found to have no effect on recurrent events or risk for events.

Hyperhomocysteinemia may arise from dietary conditions such as vitamin deficiency, e.g., vitamin B6, vitamin B12, and folic acid, or increased dietary methionine intake, and has been linked to genetic defects, such as homocysteinuria, cobalamin C deficiency, or polymorphisms in the methylene tetrahydrafolate reductase (MTHFR) gene, such as MTHFR C677T variant. Even in homozygotes, there is only a mild elevation of the homocysteine level usually only in the presence of a subtherapeutic level of folic acid, thus MTHFR polymorphism independent of homocysteinemia does not increase the risk of TE and is no longer recommended as a part of a thrombophilia evaluation. Fasting homocysteine levels can be measured in the plasma by electrospray tandem mass spectrometry.

Increased Antifibrinolytic Activity

Elevated Lipoprotein(a) (Blood Collected into EDTA Anticoagulant)

Lipoprotein(a) [Lp(a)] is composed of a low-density lipid particle (LDL) and a polypeptide chain (apolipoprotein a). Lp(a) shares similar structural characteristics with plasminogen and tissue plasminogen activator and competes with plasminogen for its binding site to fibrin, leading to reduced fibrinolysis. Other thrombotic effects may be caused by the Lp(a)-induced secretion of plasminogen activator inhibitor and by inducing atherosclerosis because of its (high) LDL cholesterol content. The association between elevated LP(a) and the risk for VTE or ATE in children is not clear. Plasma Lp(a) levels can be measured by high-performance affinity liquid chromatography.

Impact of Thrombophilia in Childhood Thrombosis

The reported prevalence of laboratory thrombophilic risk factors in different studies in children with thrombosis varies (13%–79%) and mostly reflects differences in study design and differences in the clinically and demographic characteristics of the study populations [39]. Considering that TEs in children usually occur in the setting of one or more acquired clinical conditions, the presence of thrombophilia likely constitutes a risk factor rather than an isolated cause for TE complications. Systematic reviews, meta-analyses, or observational studies reported on the impact of thrombophilia specifically on the risk of developing primary VTE and its recurrence as well stroke in childhood, including CSVT and AIS (Table 3) [16–19, 40, 41]. These reviews, however, are limited by sample heterogeneity. The prevalence and impact of thrombophilia in noncerebral ATE are even less clear [4].

Who and When and What Should Be Tested

Given the heterogeneity of patient populations and the multifactorial pathogenesis of TEs in the pediatric population, it is difficult to present definitive recommendations regarding laboratory testing for the presence of a thrombophilic state. Diagnostic testing for thrombophilia in children should be discussed on an individual basis, at least for the symptomatic index patient. A tentative summary of circumstances in which testing for laboratory thrombophilia in children may be indicated is presented in Table 4.

Guidance for thrombophilia testing for children with VTE is largely based on expert opinion. In brief, diagnostic thrombophilia testing is recommended for neonates, children, and adolescents with first unprovoked and recurrent VTE. Unprovoked thrombosis and a family history of VTE may help to identify thrombophilia in children with VTE [41].

For the first episode of provoked VTE, it is suggested to discuss the utility of diagnostic thrombophilia testing with patients and parents. Thrombophilia testing is not suggested for neonates, children, or adolescents with asymptomatic or symptomatic CVC-related VTE.

The benefit of thrombophilia testing in neonates, children, and adolescents in the setting of ATE is less clear, and no current definitive guideline is available. For childhood-onset AIS, a systematic review and meta-analysis of previous observational studies suggest an association between the presence of the laboratory thrombophilia (inherited as well acquired) and the onset of AIS (Table 3) [16, 19]. However, there are insufficient data in the literature validating the utility of such testing, given the disparate setting in which AIS may occur. Additionally, the impact of thrombophilia on the risk of recurrent AIS is less clear. We do not recommend thrombophilia testing following perinatal AIS [42]. Noncerebral ATE mainly occurs as a complication of catheter placement (see Chapter 15). Thrombophilia testing is not suggested for neonates, children, and adolescents with asymptomatic or symptomatic catheter-related ATE [4]. For unprovoked (noncatheter-related) noncerebral ATE, only marginal data are available and do not enable a definitive recommendation [4].

Thrombophilia testing rarely influences the acute management of a patient with a TE, and the therapeutic treatment should be initiated independent of the laboratory thrombophilia results. Only in certain circumstances are selected laboratory thrombophilia tests required, e.g., neonates presenting with purpura fulminans. Decisions on extending anticoagulant therapy are individually based on the perceived risks of TE recurrence and anticoagulant-related bleeding. Whether long-term continuation of anticoagulant treatment or increased intensity should be considered after

Table 4. Laboratory thrombophilia testing in the pediatric population

Clinical scenario	Time/testing		Tests included	Rationale
***a** Proposal for laboratory thrombophilia testing in neonates, children and adolescents with VTEs and ATEs*				
Purpura fulminans or nonsepsis DIC	Acute	Recommended	Protein C and S, antithrombin	Deficiency of protein S, protein C, or antithrombin may warrant replacement therapy
Neonates/children/adolescents with unprovoked VTE	FU	Recommended	Thrombophilia workup	May help to determine the risk of recurrence and to identify homozygous or combined defect May allow screening of family members (if positive)
Children/adolescents with recurrent (noncatheter related) VTE	FU	Recommended	Thrombophilia workup	May help to determine the risk of recurrence and to identify homozygous or combined defect May allow screening of family members (if positive)
Children/adolescents with provoked (noncatheter related) VTE	FU	Suggest to discuss the utility with the patients/family	Thrombophilia workup	Insufficient data to recommend for or against
Neonates/children/adolescents with unprovoked, provoked (noncatheter related), or recurrent noncerebral ATE	FU	Suggest to discuss the utility with the patients/family	Thrombophilia workup	Insufficient data to recommend for or against
Neonates/children/adolescents with catheter-related VTE/ATE	FU	Not suggested		Does not influence treatment strategy
***b** Proposal for laboratory thrombophilia testing in children and adolescents without personal history of TE*				
Children/adolescents with family history of TE and known or unknown (not yet tested) thrombophilia trait	May be considered in selected patients: – to guide thromboprophylaxis in high-risk patient – concurrent exposure to other prothrombotic conditions (e.g., oral contraceptive, CVC insertion for acute lymphoblastic leukemia therapy, major surgery) – for research purposes		Proteins C and S, antithrombin; prothrombin gene and FV Leiden gene or test, according to known familial thrombophilia trait If familial trait is unknown, consider testing the index family member with TE first	Current data suggest that one or more positive test results increase the likelihood to experience a TE in life Testing needs to be discussed with the family for each individual situation
Children/adolescents without family history for TE and/or for thrombophilia trait in the setting of the presence or potential exposure to acquired prothrombotic condition(s)	Not recommended		–	No clinical trial demonstrating efficacy and risk/benefit of thromboprophylaxis No cost effectiveness

Acute, at the time of the event; FU, during follow-up; Thrombophilia workup, depending on clinician/center preferences and/or recommendations, may or may not include the following tests further addressed in the text: protein C activity, protein S-free antigen level, antithrombin activity, activated protein C resistance, FVIII activity, prothrombin gene variant, and FV Leiden gene variant analysis, lupus anticoagulant test, anticardiolipin IgM and IgG antibodies, β_2-GPI IgM and IgG antibodies, fasting homocysteine level, and Lp(a) plasma level. ATE, arterial thromboembolism/thromboembolic event; CVC, central venous catheter; DIC, disseminated intravascular coagulation; TE, thromboembolism/thromboembolic event; VTE, venous thromboembolism/thromboembolic event.

VTE in patients with a documented thrombophilia is still a matter of debate. In the current published pediatric VTE guidelines, it is recommended to manage children with VTE independent of the presence or absence of APLA or inherited thrombophilia [38]. In such cases, consultation with a reference thrombosis center is strongly recommended.

Laboratory testing for thrombophilia in the acute TE phase may be difficult and often impossible. In most cases, thrombophilia testing should be deferred for 3–6 months after the acute TE and after stopping the anticoagulant therapy. Testing of both parents should also be considered before concluding that an inherited deficiency of protein C, protein S, or antithrombin is present.

Thrombophilia test results in children with TE may provide an estimate of the risk of recurrence and assist in a decision regarding anticoagulant prophylaxis, such as in situations where a child will be exposed to one or more risk situations for recurrent thrombosis, e.g., major surgery, need of a CVC, oral contraceptive medication, and pregnancy. However, available evidence does not yet allow a definitive risk-based approach to be presented to patients and their families.

Comprehensive testing for laboratory thrombophilia in asymptomatic children on the basis of a positive family history for a TE remains controversial. Indeed, yet unknown inherited as well as environmental thrombotic risk factors may occur, and a normal thrombophilia workup may provide false reassurance. A prospective cohort study showed that the risk of VTE in relatives of pediatric index cases with VTE was markedly increased in relatives with protein C, protein S, or antithrombin deficiency. However, this was not the case for the more common thrombophilic traits, such as prothrombin (II) gene or FVL variants [9]. The European Prospective Cohort on Thrombophilia also showed that the risk of thrombosis in asymptomatic thrombophilia carriers was higher than for a control group; however, the risk did not exceed the 1%–3% annual risk of bleeding associated with long-term anticoagulation [40]. Therefore, screening for inherited thrombophilia in first-degree family members of pediatric VTE index cases with protein C, protein S, or antithrombin deficiency or combined inherited thrombophilia may be considered, particularly when considering exposing them to further thrombophilic risk factors such as oral contraception. If testing is considered, it seems rational to postpone testing of asymptomatic children until they are old enough to decide for themselves after weighing the pros and cons, given that the absolute incidence of VTE is very low in children with thrombophilia [41] (see Chapter 21). The use of prophylactic anticoagulation in children with positive thrombophilia trait in the presence of other TE risk factors remains controversial. It is recommended to counsel the family regarding the potential benefits and limitations prior to performing thrombophilia testing in children without a personal history of a TE only on the basis of a positive family history or the presence of a thrombophilic trait [39].

Testing of asymptomatic children or adolescents with a negative family history of thrombosis prior to surgery, oral contraceptive, or CVC insertion is not recommended. Depending on the specific treatment protocol used, there are some data to suggest that individual patient counseling may be considered for thrombophilia testing of children with acute lymphoblastic leukemia prior to CVC insertion [43] (see Chapter 14). However, there is yet no clear evidence for the safety and efficacy of primary prophylaxis with anticoagulation in this setting (see Chapter 20 for details on recent trials in this setting).

In general, it remains the responsibility of the involved physician to decide if, when and what tests are appropriate for the individual child, and in all cases, testing should involve detailed discussion with the patient and family.

Purpura Fulminans

Purpura fulminans is a rare life-threatening condition characterized by progressive hemorrhagic skin necrosis that occurs in the first days of life mostly because of congenital severe (homozygous or compound heterozygous) protein C and/or S deficiency. More commonly, purpura fulminans may occur secondary to consumption or decreased synthesis associated with acquired conditions such as infection (sepsis), hepatic dysfunction, or VKA therapy in older children and in adults [6]. Inherited neonatal purpura fulminans is estimated to occur in 1/250,000–1/4,000,000 births, and the presentation is that of DIC with a rapid (within hours) onset of small ecchymotic lesions, rapidly increasing in size with the formation of bullae leading to necrotic and gangrenous tissue. Neonates, and rarely, infants with severe genetic protein C deficiency may also present with large-vessel thrombosis such as renal vein thrombosis, DVT, or AIS. Evidence of prenatal thrombosis may be present and most commonly affects the eyes, the brain, and the renal veins.

The management of purpura fulminate should start by differentiating acquired versus inherited severe protein C/S deficiencies, as well as characterizing the degree of deficiency to tailor the mode and intensity of protein C/S replacement. Moreover, end organ damage including ocular, cutaneous, and vascular complications, need to be actively sought [44]. Anticoagulation may be started to prevent further skin necrosis. There may be a need for replacement of red blood cells, platelets, and factors lost because of both the procoagulable state and DIC (see Chapter 11). Early surgical debridement for areas that have become necrotic has been shown to decrease mortality. Neonates and children with purpura fulminans should be urgently tested for protein C and protein S deficiency followed closely with fresh frozen plasma transfusions (e.g., 10–15 mL/kg/dose every 8–12 h). Upon diagnostic confirmation, protein C concentrate can be added if severe (<0.01 IU/mL) or moderately severe (≥0.01–0.2 IU/mL) deficiencies are found (loading dose: intravenous 100–120 units/kg; followed by 50–100 units/kg/dose, every 6–8 h) [44]. Individuals with genetic severe protein C/protein S deficiency, who are promptly recognized, diagnosed, and appropriately supported, can survive to adulthood with a good quality of life. In cases suspected of congenital purpura fulminans, physicians should offer genetic testing for variants in the *PROC/PROS1* genes and genetic consultation.

Anatomical Thrombophilia

Certain anatomic conditions, though rare, may predispose to TEs and should be considered in patients with extensive, unprovoked, and recurrent thrombotic events. May-Thurner syndrome (e.g., iliac vein compression syndrome) is an anatomical thrombophilia that results from the obstruction of the left common iliac vein because of the compression from the overlying right common iliac artery. Patients are typically adolescents or young adults, more commonly females, who present with extensive proximal deep venous thrombosis of the left lower extremity. Additional risk factors such as estrogen exposure or inherited thrombophilia may be present. The diagnosis requires a high index of suspicion. CTV, MRV, and conventional venography have been used for diagnosis. A combination of pharmacomechanical thrombolysis, catheter-directed thrombolysis, angioplasty, stent placement, and anticoagulation can be considered in May-Thurner syndrome. Recurrent thrombosis and PTS are common [45].

Venous thoracic outlet syndrome (or Paget-Schroetter syndrome) refers to the extrinsic compression and impingement of the subclavian vein as it passes through the thoracic outlet, eventually resulting in upper extremity DVT. Thoracic outlet syndrome affects healthy and active adolescents, who typically give a history of repeated overhead activities. Diagnosis is suspected following the observation of the axillo-subclavian vein thrombosis on DUS and confirmed by dynamic ultrasound or venography. A combination of pharmacomechanical or catheter-directed thrombolysis in conjunction with angioplasty, anticoagulation, and decompressive rib resection may result in high rate of recanalization and excellent long-term outcomes [46].

For patients who do not undergo thrombolysis or surgery as treatment of the above anatomic thrombophilias, we would suggest following current guidelines for therapy of a spontaneous TE and consideration for longer-term treatment in the event of recurrence [38].

RAMs and Thromboprophylaxis

Thromboprophylaxis refers to measures taken to reduce the risk of TE. Successful thromboprophylaxis relies on the identification of children who are at significant risk for TEs and who therefore have the potential to benefit from preventative measures. Several recent initiatives have aimed at identifying such pediatric patient populations, although their aim has focused primarily on risk of VTE and not ATE.

Thromboprophylaxis in Hospitalized Pediatric Patients

RAMs to Prevent In-Hospital VTE

In adult medicine, the use of RAMs to identify patients requiring pharmacologic thromboprophylaxis is supported by the literature on both safety and efficacy [47]. Hence, most adult hospitals have standard algorithms for starting pharmacological prophylaxis in inpatients. Prospectively validated RAMs are not yet available in pediatrics. A recommendation to give thromboprophylaxis with pharmacological agents in children must be carefully balanced against the risk of bleeding and should be presented by informed members of the health care team to the subject (if old enough) or to the parents/guardians of young children using a shared decision model in which the risks, benefits, and alternatives to therapy are discussed in a nondirective manner. In cases where the responsible physician is not adequately informed/experienced in this area of pediatric medicine consultation with a reference thrombosis center is strongly recommended.

A recent meta-analysis of RAMs in pediatrics showed that admission to an intensive care unit, mechanical ventilation, the presence of a CVC, and prolonged length of hospital stay are risk factors for the development of hospital-acquired TE [48]. The CHAT consortium (children's hospital-acquired TE) is a multicenter initiative in the United States that collected data on cases of hospital-acquired VTE (HA-VTE) in children and controls matched by institution and year of admission. Logistic regression analysis was used to create a RAM that could predict which children would benefit from prophylactic anticoagulation. When evaluating children within 24 h of admission to hospital, the following risk factors were identified as independent predictors of risk of HA-VTE: age <1 year and 10–22 years, cancer, congenital heart disease, other high-risk conditions (autoimmune/inflammatory disease, blood-related disorder, protein losing state, total parenteral nutrition dependence, and thrombophilia/personal history of VTE), recent hospitalization, immobility, platelet count $>350 \times 10^9$/L, CVC, recent surgery, corticosteroid medication and mechanical ventilation. A prospective validation of the RAM derived from the CHAT database is underway that will hopefully help provide a validated RAM that can be utilized to decide on role of thromboprophylaxis in children [49, 50].

General Measures

Adequate hydration, early mobilization after surgery, and prompt removal of CVC and arterial catheters, when possible, are important to reduce the risk of TE in hospitalized children.

Mechanical Thromboprophylaxis

Graduated compression stockings may be used to prevent lower limb DVT in hospitalized children. Pneumatic calf compression devices may be used during surgery in children who are at risk of DVT.

Pharmacological Thromboprophylaxis

The risks and benefits of anticoagulant use will be discussed in Chapter 20. The usual agents for short-term thromboprophylaxis are the low-molecular-weight heparins (LMWHs) (see Table 5 for dosing). Monitoring is not usually required, but a trough anti-Xa activity level after 2–3 doses can be useful to rule out accumulation in children with significant renal impairment and in the very young, who might need higher dosages.

Long-term thromboprophylaxis may involve the use of a VKA. This is particularly the case for

Table 5. Prophylactic dosing of enoxaparin, tinzaparin, dalteparin, and nadroparin according to age

Type of LMWH	Prophylactic dose
Enoxaparin	
≤2 months of age	1.5 mg/kg SC once daily or 0.75 mg/kg SC twice daily
>2 months of age	1 mg/kg SC once daily or 0.5 mg/kg SC twice daily
Tinzaparin	
≤2 months of age	75 units/kg SC once daily
2–12 months of age	75 units/kg SC once daily
1–5 years	75 units/kg SC once daily
5–10 years	75 units/kg SC once daily
10–16 years	50 units/kg SC once daily
Dalteparin	
≤2 months of age	150 units/kg SC once daily
>2 months of age	100 units/kg SC once daily
Nadroparin	
≤2 months of age	150 units/kg SC once daily
2–24 months of age	120 units/kg SC once daily
2–12 years	100 units/kg SC once daily
12–18 years	85.5 units/kg SC once daily

LMWH, low-molecular-weight heparin; SC, subcutaneous.

the prevention of CVC-related thrombosis in children with an indwelling CVC for total parenteral nutrition. Some studies have supported the administration of warfarin, with an INR target range of 1.5–1.9 [38]. The potential use of direct oral anticoagulants as pharmacological thromboprophylaxis in children with cardiac disease will be discussed in Chapter 18 and in children with leukemia in Chapter 20.

Travel-Related TE

In children who have had a previous VTE and/or have significant risk factors, it is appropriate to offer advice regarding prevention of VTE for flights of >4–6 h duration and for long journeys using other modes of transport that involve immobility. This general advice includes adequate hydration and frequent mobilization in addition to early reporting of symptoms of VTE. The use of pharmacological thromboprophylaxis to prevent travel-related VTE is currently only recommended in high VTE risk adults, although the use of graduated compression stockings is listed as an alternative [47]. There is currently no evidence evaluating either practice in children.

Conclusion

TEs in childhood, even if rare, compared with adulthood, are increasingly diagnosed and recognized [5]. In most children, the TEs result from secondary complications of primary underlying diseases, such as infection, cancer, congenital heart disease, inflammatory conditions, or are related to therapeutic interventions such as CVC and/or arterial catheters. Idiopathic ("unprovoked") cases are rare. A detailed personal and family history and a careful physical examination are important steps to identify potential underlying conditions associated with an increased risk of thrombosis. Imaging studies and laboratory investigations are further determinants in the diagnostic approach to a child with thrombosis and will help in decisions about treatment options and counseling. RAMs are being identified to help recognize children at higher risk of TE for prevention of HA-VTE. The upcoming chapters (Chapters 14–18) are specifically dedicated to different aspects of TEs in children.

Acknowledgment

Our special thanks go to Dr. Mattia Rizzi and Dr. Chris Barnes who were the authors of this chapter/appendix in the first and second editions of this Handbook, which provided a valuable background for this updated chapter.

Conflict of Interest Statement

Christine Sabapathy declares to have no conflict of interest. Ali Amid reports consultancy fees paid to his Department of Hematology from Novo Nordisk Canada Inc, Octapharma AG, Roche Holding AG, and Shire Pharma Canada Inc. Riten Kumar has served on an Advisory Board for Bayer and has received research funding from Bioverativ. Laura Avila holds official copyrights for CAPTSure©. Heleen van Ommen reports consultancy fees paid to her academic department from Bayer BV, Boehringer Ingelheim, and Daiichi Sankyo, lecture honoraria paid to the Department from Boehringer Ingelheim, and an unrestricted grant paid to the Department from Octapharma, all outside the scope of the submitted work.

Author Contributions

Christine Sabapathy drafted the revised chapter, critically revised the chapter, and approved the final version. Ali Amid critically revised the chapter and approved the final version. Riten Kumar critically revised the chapter and approved the final version. Laura Avila critically revised the chapter and approved the final version. Heleen van Ommen drafted the revised chapter, critically revised the chapter, and approved the final version.

Abbreviations

ACLA	Anticardiolipin antibody
AIS	Arterial ischemic stroke
APLA	Antiphospholipid antibodies
APS	Antiphospholipid syndrome
aPTT	Activated partial thromboplastin time
ATE	Arterial thromboembolism/thromboembolic event
β_2-GPI	β_2-glycoprotein I
CT	Computed tomography
CTPA	Computed tomography pulmonary angiography
CTV	Computed tomography venography
CSVT	Cerebral sinovenous thrombosis
CVC	Central venous catheter
DIC	Disseminated intravascular coagulation
DUS	Doppler ultrasonography
DVT	Deep vein thrombosis
ELISA	Enzyme-linked immunosorbent assay
FII	Factor II (prothrombin)
FV	Factor V
FVIII	Factor VIII
FVL	Factor V Leiden
HA-VTE	Hospital-acquired venous thromboembolism
INR	International normalized ratio
LAC	Lupus anticoagulant
LMWH	Low-molecular-weight heparin
Lp(a)	Lipoprotein(a)
LDL	Low-density lipid
MRA	Magnetic resonance angiography
MRI	Magnetic resonance imaging
MRV	Magnetic resonance venography
MTHFR	Methylenetetrahydrofolate reductase
PE	Pulmonary embolism
PCR	Polymerase chain reaction
PT	Prothrombin time
PTS	Post-thrombotic syndrome
RAM	Risk assessment model
TE	Thromboembolism/thromboembolic event
VKA	Vitamin K antagonist
VTE	Venous thromboembolism/thromboembolic event
TIA	Transient ischemic attack
V/Q scan	Ventilation/perfusion scan

13

References

1 Macartney CA, Chan AK. Thrombosis in children. Semin Thromb Hemost. 2011; 37:763–1.
2 Yang JY, Chan AK. Neonatal systemic venous thrombosis. Thromb Res. 2010; 126:471–6.
3 Chalmers EA. Epidemiology of venous thromboembolism in neonates and children. Thromb Res. 2006;118:3–12.
4 Price VE, Chan AK. Arterial thrombosis in children. Expert Rev Cardiovasc Ther. 2008;6:419–28.
5 O'Brien SH, Stanek JR, Witmer CM, Raffini L. The continued rise of venous thromboembolism across US Children's Hospitals. Pediatrics. 2022;149: e2021054649.
6 Price VE, Ledingham DL, Krumpel A, Chan AK. Diagnosis and management of neonatal purpura fulminans. Semin Fetal Neonatal Med. 2011;16:318–22.
7 Trenor CC III, Chung RJ, Michelson AD, Neufeld EJ, Gordon CM, Laufer MR, et al. Hormonal contraception and thrombotic risk: a multidisciplinary approach. Pediatrics. 2011;127:347–57.
8 Bezemer ID, van der Meer FJ, Eikenboom JC, Rosendaal FR, Doggen CJ. The value of family history as a risk indicator for venous thrombosis. Arch Intern Med. 2009;169:610–5.
9 Holzhauer S, Goldenberg NA, Junker R, Heller C, Stoll M, Manner D, et al. Inherited thrombophilia in children with venous thromboembolism and the familial risk of thromboembolism: an observational study. Blood. 2012;120: 1510–5.
10 Sillers L, Van Slambrouck C, Lapping-Carr G. Neonatal thrombocytopenia: etiology and diagnosis. Pediatr Ann. 2015;44:e175–80.
11 Avila L, Amiri N, Pullenayegum E, Sealey VA, De R, Williams S, et al. Diagnostic value of D-dimers for limb deep vein thrombosis in children: a prospective study. Am J Hematol. 2021;96:954–60.
12 Biss TT, Brandao LR, Kahr WH, Chan AK, Williams S. Clinical probability score and D-dimer estimation lack utility in the diagnosis of childhood pulmonary embolism. J Thromb Haemost. 2009;7:1633–8.
13 Lee EY, Tse SKS, Zurakowski D, Johnson VM, Lee NJ, Tracy DA, et al. Children suspected of having pulmonary embolism: multidetector CT pulmonary angiography – thromboembolic risk factors and implications for appropriate use. Radiology. 2012;262:242–51.
14 Hennelly KE, Baskin MN, Monuteuax MC, Hudgins J, Kua E, Commeree A, et al. Detection of pulmonary embolism in high-risk children. J Pediatr. 2016;178: 214–8.
15 Goldenberg NA. Thrombophilia states and markers of coagulation activation in the prediction of pediatric venous thromboembolic outcomes: a comparative analysis with respect to adult evidence. Hematology Am Soc Hematol Educ Program. 2008;2008:236–44.
16 Kenet G, Lutkhoff LK, Albisetti M, Bernard T, Bonduel M, Brandao L, et al. Impact of thrombophilia on risk of arterial ischemic stroke or cerebral sinovenous thrombosis in neonates and children: a systematic review and meta-analysis of observational studies. Circulation. 2010;121:1838–47.
17 Kreuz W, Stoll M, Junker R, Heinecke A, Schobess R, Kurnik K, et al. Familial elevated factor VIII in children with symptomatic venous thrombosis and post-thrombotic syndrome: results of a multicenter study. Arterioscler Thromb Vasc Biol. 2006;26:1901–6.
18 Young G, Albisetti M, Bonduel M, Brandao L, Chan A, Friedrichs F, et al. Impact of inherited thrombophilia on venous thromboembolism in children: a systematic review and meta-analysis of observational studies. Circulation. 2008;118:1373–82.
19 Kenet G, Aronis S, Berkun Y, Bonduel M, Chan A, Goldenberg NA, et al. Impact of persistent antiphospholipid antibodies on risk of incident symptomatic thromboembolism in children: a systematic review and meta-analysis. Semin Thromb Hemost. 2011;37:802–9.
20 Jenkins PV, Rawley O, Smith OP, O'Donnell JS. Elevated factor VIII levels and risk of venous thrombosis. Br J Haematol. 2012;157:653–63.
21 Bosch A, Uleryk E, Avila L. Role of FVIII, IX and XI in venous thrombosis recurrence risk in adults and children: a systematic review. Res Pract Thromb Haemost. 2023;7:e100064.
22 Goldenberg NA, Knapp-Clevenger R, Manco-Johnson MJ; Mountain States Regional Thrombophilia Group. Elevated plasma factor VIII and D-dimer levels as predictors of poor outcomes of thrombosis in children. N Engl J Med. 2004;351(11):1081–8.
23 Scheres LJJ, Lijfering WM, Middeldorp S, Cheung YW, Barco S, Cannegieter SC, et al. Measurement of coagulation factors during rivaroxaban and apixaban treatment: results from two crossover trials. Res Pract Thromb Haemost. 2018;2:689–95.
24 Ignjatovic V, Kenet G, Monagle P. Developmental hemostasis: recommendations for laboratories reporting pediatric samples. J Thromb Haemost. 2012;10: 298–300.
25 Cooper PC, Pavlova A, Moore GW, Hickey KP, Marlar RA. Recommendations for clinical laboratory testing for protein C deficiency, for the subcommittee on plasma coagulation inhibitors of the ISTH. J Thromb Haemost. 2020;18: 271–7.
26 Reitsma PH, Bernardi F, Doig RG, Gandrille S, Greengard JS, Ireland H, et al. Protein C deficiency: a database of mutations, 1995 update. Thromb Haemost. 1995;73:876–89.
27 Marlar RA, Gausman JN, Tsuda H, Rollins-Raval MA, Brinkman HJM. Recommendations for clinical laboratory testing for protein S deficiency: communication from the SSC committee plasma coagulation inhibitors of the ISTH. J Thromb Haemost. 2021;19:68–74.
28 Alhenc-Gelas M, Plu-Bureau G, Horellou MH, Rauch A, Suchon P, for the GEHT Genetic Thrombophilia Group. PROS1 genotype phenotype relationships in a large cohort of adults with suspicion of inherited quantitative protein S deficiency. Thromb Haemost. 2016;115:570–9.
29 Caspers M, Pavlova A, Driesen J, Harbrecht U, Klamroth R, Kadar J, et al. Deficiencies of antithrombin, protein C and protein S – practical experience in genetic analysis of a large patient cohort. Thromb Haemost. 2012;108:247–57.

30 Luxembourg B, Pavlova A, Geisen C, Spannagl M, Bergmann F, Krause M, et al. Impact of the type of SERPINC1 mutation and subtype of antithrombin deficiency on the thrombotic phenotype in hereditary antithrombin deficiency. Thromb Haemost. 2014;111(02):249–57.
31 Kumar R, Bakeer N, Dawson J, Al-Mughairy A, Stanek J, Williams S, et al. Impact of SERPINC1 mutation on thrombotic phenotype in children with congenital antithrombin deficiency – first analysis of the International Society on Thrombosis and Haemostasis pediatric antithrombin deficiency database and biorepository. J Thromb Haemost. 2023;21:1248–57.
32 Pengo V, Tripodi A, Reber G, Rand JH, Ortel TL, Galli M, et al. Update of the guidelines for lupus anticoagulant detection. Subcommittee on Lupus Anticoagulant/Antiphospholipid Antibody of the Scientific and Standardisation Committee of the International Society on Thrombosis and Haemostasis. J Thromb Haemost. 2009;7:1737–40.
33 Miyakis S, Lockshin MD, Atsumi T, Branch DW, Brey RL, Cervera R, et al. International consensus statement on an update of the classification criteria for definite antiphospholipid syndrome (APS). J Thromb Haemost. 2006;4:295–306.
34 Aguiar CL, Soybilgic A, Avcin T, Myones BL. Pediatric antiphospholipid syndrome. Curr Rheumatol Rep. 2015;17: 27.
35 Vandevelde At, Chayoua W, de Laat B, Moore GW, Musial J, Zuily S, et al. Added value of antiphosphatidylserine/prothrombin antibodies in the workup of thrombotic antiphospholipid syndrome; Communication from the ISTH SSC Subcommittee on Lupus Anticoagulant/Antiphospholipid Antibodies. J Thromb Haemost. 2022;29(9):2136–50.
36 Berman H, Rodriguez-Pinto I, Cervera R, Gregory S, de Meis E, Rodrigues CEM, et al. Pediatric catastrophic antiphospholipid syndrome: descriptive analysis of 45 patients from the "CAPS Registry". Autoimmun Rev. 2014;13: 157–62.
37 Chalmers E, Ganesen V, Liesner R, Maroo S, Nokes T, Saunders D, et al. Guideline on the investigation, management and prevention of venous thrombosis in children. Br J Haematol. 2011;154:196–207.
38 Monagle P, Chan AK, Goldenberg NA, Ichord RN, Journeycake JM, Nowak-Gottl U, et al. Antithrombotic therapy in neonates and children: Antithrombotic Therapy and Prevention of Thrombosis, 9th ed: American College of Chest Physicians Evidence-Based Clinical Practice Guidelines. Chest. 2012;141:e737S–801S.
39 Raffini L, Thornburg C. Testing children for inherited thrombophilia: more questions than answers. Br J Haematol. 2009;147:277–88.
40 Nowak-Gottl U, Kurnik K, Manner D, Kenet G. Thrombophilia testing in neonates and infants with thrombosis. Semin Fetal Neonatal Med. 2011;16:345–8.
41 Klaassen IL, van Ommen CH, Middeldorp S. Manifestations and clinical impact of pediatric inherited thrombophilia. Blood. 2015;125:1073–7.
42 Curtis C, Mineyko A, Massicotte P, Leaker M, Jiang XY, Floer A, et al. Thrombophilia risk is not increased in children after perinatal stroke. Blood. 2017;129:2793–800.
43 Mitchell L, Lambers M, Flege S, Kenet G, Li-Thiao-Te V, Holzhauer S, et al. Validation of a predictive model for identifying an increased risk for thromboembolism in children with acute lymphoblastic leukemia: results of a multicenter cohort study. Blood. 2010;115: 4999–5004.
44 Minford A, Brandao LR, Othman M, Male C, Abdul-Kadir R, Monagle P, et al. Diagnosis and management of severe congenital protein C deficiency (SCPCD): communication from the SSC of the ISTH. J Thromb Haemost. 2022; 20:1735–43.
45 Avila L, Cullinan N, White M, Gaballah M, Cahill AM, Warad D, et al. Pediatric May-Thurner Syndrome-Systematic review and individual patient data meta-analysis. J Thromb Haemost. 2021;19: 1283–93.
46 Modi BP, Chewning R, Kumar R. Venous thoracic outlet syndrome and Paget-Schroetter syndrome. Sem Pediatr Surg. 2021;30(6):1–11.
47 Schünemann HJ, Cushman M, Burnett AE, Kahn SR, Beyer-Westendorf J, Spencer FA, et al. American Society of Hematology 2018 guidelines for management of venous thromboembolism: prophylaxis for hospitalized and nonhospitalized medical patients. Blood Adv. 2018;2:3198–225.
48 Mahajerin A, Branchford BR, Amankwah EK, Raffini L, Chalmers E, van Ommen CH, et al. Hospitalassociated venous thromboembolism in pediatrics: a systematic review and meta-analysis of risk factors and risk assessment models. Haematologica. 2015;100:1045–50.
49 Jaffray J, Mahajerin A, Branchford B, Nguyen ATH, Faustino EVS, Silvey M, et al. A new risk assessment model for hospital-acquired venous thromboembolism in critically ill children: a report from the Children's Hospital-Acquired Thrombosis Consortium. Pediatr Crit Care Med. 2022;23:e1–9.
50 Jaffray J, Branchford B, Goldenberg N, Malvar J, Croteau SE, Silvey M, et al. Development of a risk model for pediatric hospital-acquired thrombosis: a report from the CHAT Consortium. J Pediatr. 2021;228:252–9.
51 Monagle P. Andrew's Pediatric Thromboembolism and Stroke. Hamilton, ON: BC Decker Inc. 2014.
52 Goldenberg NA, Manco-Johnson MM. Protein C deficiency. Haemophilia. 2008;14:1214–21.
53 Ten Kate MK, Van Der Meer J. Protein S deficiency: a clinical perspective. Haemophilia. 2008;14:1222–8.
54 Patnaik MM, Moll S. Inherited antithrombin deficiency: a review. Haemophilia. 2008;14:1229–39.

Published online: December 5, 2024

Blanchette VS, Brandão LR, Carcao MD, Kumar R, Rand ML, Revel-Vilk S (eds): SickKids Handbook of Pediatric Thrombosis and Hemostasis, ed 3, rev. and ext. Basel, Karger, 2024, pp 256–274 (DOI: 10.1159/000538208)

Venous Thrombosis

Marie-Claude Pelland-Marcotte[a] Laura Avila[b] Michael Temple[c] Suzan Williams[b]

[a]Division of Pediatric Hematology-Oncology, Centre Hospitalier Universitaire de Québec, Québec City, QC, Canada; [b]Division of Paediatric Hematology-Oncology, The Hospital for Sick Children, Toronto, ON, Canada; [c]Interventional Radiology, St. Jude Children's Research Hospital, Memphis, TN, USA

Introduction

Venous thromboembolism (VTE) is a rare complication in pediatric medicine. There has, however, been an increase in the frequency of VTE in hospitalized children over the past 2 decades, likely because of a true increase in incidence and improvements in the detection of previously undiagnosed VTE. This is largely a result of advances in medical expertise and technology leading to an increase in the survival of children with previously fatal conditions and an increase in complications of complex conditions managed in tertiary care centers. The incidence of VTE in children was reported to be 5.3 cases per 10,000 hospital admissions in the 1990s, and more recently, 106 cases per 10,000 pediatric patients admitted to tertiary care hospitals [1–3]. The incidence follows a bimodal pattern with a peak occurring in infants <1 year and a second peak during adolescence [1, 4]. In contrast to VTE in adults, idiopathic VTE is rare, and 80–90% of VTE in children are associated with predisposing risk factors including the presence of a central venous catheter (CVC), the single most important risk factor, cardiovascular disease, nephrotic syndrome, surgery, infection, malignancy, inflammatory and autoimmune diseases, and vascular anatomic anomalies. Risk factors for hospital-associated deep venous thrombosis (DVT) include the aforementioned as well as the length of hospital stay and admission to the pediatric intensive care unit [5]. Analysis of risk factors associated with pediatric DVT has begun to inform pediatric risk assessment models [6]. VTE risk factors are discussed in Chapter 13.

Deep Vein Thrombosis

Clinical Presentation

The clinical presentation of DVT depends on the anatomical location of the thrombus (see Chapter 13). Symptoms of acute DVT in the upper and lower venous systems include localized pain, swelling, warmth, and discoloration of the overlying skin. Patients may present with complications of DVT, such as CVC occlusion, or with more severe manifestations, such as superior vena cava syndrome or pulmonary embolism (PE) (see below). Superior vena cava obstruction syndrome may present with swelling of the arms and face, dilated veins on the skin surface within the upper torso, skin discoloration, cough, chest pain, and/or hoarseness. Clinically unsuspected DVT may also be detected following surveillance imaging or investigations done for other conditions in the absence of DVT symptoms, often in association with the presence of a CVC [7] (see Catheter-Related Thrombosis section below). Chronic signs of DVT include the presence of collateral venous circulation (dilated blood vessels), chylothorax, chylopericardium, and post-thrombotic syndrome (PTS) [1].

Diagnosis

The approach to diagnosis of DVT in children includes recognition of the clinical presentation and radiological investigations. Venography is considered the reference standard for diagnosis of DVT, but in children, this is often not practical because of poor peripheral venous access and the concern for exposure to radiation. Doppler ultrasound has become the most common initial investigation. Advantages include that it is safe, painless, and portable. Compression ultrasound with Doppler is recommended to assess for DVT of the lower limb, peripheral upper limb, axillary, subclavian, and internal jugular veins [8]. The central intrathoracic venous system is contained within the bony thorax, making compression ultrasound with Doppler a less sensitive tool for diagnosis of DVT in this anatomical location. If central intrathoracic DVT is clinically suspected, venography, computed tomography venography (CTV), or magnetic resonance venography (MRV) should be used for the assessment of central veins. For clinically suspected lower limb DVT with a normal Doppler ultrasound, consider performing venography (if high index of suspicion) or repeating the compression ultrasound with Doppler after a week to assess for proximal progression of a calf vein thrombus. CTV or MRV should be considered in children with suspected proximal extension of femoral DVT, as there are limitations to compression ultrasound with Doppler in the evaluation of vessels located proximally to the iliac vessels, including the distal inferior vena cava (IVC). The diagnosis of PE will be discussed later in this chapter. Currently, there are no validated pediatric predictive scores to estimate the pretest probability of DVT, as those used in adults with suspected DVT. In contrast to adults with suspected DVT, D-dimers have a poor discriminative and predictive value for DVT in children, especially in the presence of comorbidities [9]. Thus, D-dimers should not be systematically used to assist in the diagnosis of DVT in children. More details regarding the diagnosis of VTE are available in Chapter 13.

Management

The aims of antithrombotic therapy in children with DVT are broadly similar to those for adults, that is, to reduce the risk of death because of thrombosis extension or embolization, reduce the incidence of recurrent thrombosis, reduce the incidence of PTS, and maintain vessel patency, where clinically relevant [8]. The majority of children with DVT can be managed with anticoagulation therapy alone; however, there are indications for thrombolysis, thrombectomy, and, in exceptional situations, the insertion of IVC filters (see below). Given the paucity of pediatric data, most of the recommendations detailed in this chapter are based on extrapolation from adult data and on expert opinion [8, 10, 11].

Anticoagulation

In children with a first symptomatic DVT, initial anticoagulation with heparinoids, including unfractionated heparin (UFH) or low-molecular-weight heparin (LMWH), is recommended for at least 5 days [10]. For ongoing therapy, LMWH, vitamin K antagonists (VKAs), or a direct oral anticoagulant (DOAC) is recommended. Rivaroxaban and dabigatran are the two DOACs approved by regulatory agencies (e.g., European Medicines Agency, Food and Drug Administration, Health Canada), as of 2022, for pediatric use in the acute VTE setting. The decision about which anticoagulant agent to use is dependent on the availability of each drug locally, the team's familiarity and expertise with their use, as well as patient preferences. Dosing and monitoring of antithrombotic therapy are detailed in Chapter 20. Since clinically unsuspected DVT appears to follow a more benign clinical course than symptomatic DVT [7], the decision to initiate anticoagulation or not in such cases should be individualized [11].

The duration of anticoagulation in children with DVT depends on whether the event was provoked or idiopathic [11]. However, there is no consensus on what constitutes a provoked DVT. While some risk factors are undoubtedly recognized as provoking factors, such as the presence of a CVC, surgery, or malignancy, whether DVT in the setting of oral contraceptives, physiologic disturbances such as severe dehydration, or obesity constitutes a provoked DVT remains debated. Children with idiopathic DVT should receive anticoagulation for 6–12 months, given these events have a higher risk of recurrence compared with provoked DVT [10, 11]. The decision to continue indefinite anticoagulation must be weighed against the risk of bleeding and the impact on the quality of life of the child and family because of restrictions on certain activities. In the case of recurrent idiopathic DVT, indefinite therapeutic or prophylactic anticoagulation is recommended based on extrapolation from adult data [10, 11]. The implication of inherited or acquired thrombophilia on long-term management of DVT is discussed in Chapter 13.

Children with provoked DVT in whom the risk factor has resolved are currently recommended to be treated with therapeutic anticoagulation for 6 weeks to 3 months. A recent pediatric randomized controlled trial has shown anticoagulation for 6 weeks to be noninferior to a 3-month duration for thrombotic recurrence and clinically relevant bleeding for clearly provoked DVT with no residual occlusive thrombi at the 6-week radiological re-evaluation. Whether a DVT was provoked was determined by the investigator, in the presence of provoking factors such as the presence of a CVC, infection, surgery, hospitalization, trauma, immobility, use of estrogen-containing contraceptives, or flare of an autoimmune or rheumatologic condition (although systemic lupus erythematosus was an exclusion criteria) [12]. Of note, this study excluded children with previous VTE, medical conditions putting the children at increased risk of recurrence (active malignancy, deficiencies of natural anticoagulants such as protein C, protein S, or antithrombin deficiencies, systemic lupus erythematosus) or high-risk thrombotic events (e.g., PE without DVT, more central PE, use or intent to use thrombolytic agents). If the risk factor for DVT is ongoing at the time of expected cessation of anticoagulation, such as asparaginase chemotherapy, active malignancy, or active nephrotic syndrome, anticoagulation should continue in either therapeutic doses or prophylactic doses until the risk factor has resolved. For DVT secondary to estrogen-containing contraceptives, it is not necessary to stop estrogen-containing contraceptives while the patient receives therapeutic anticoagulation. Afterward, the decision whether to continue estrogen-containing contraceptives or to transition toward an alternative progesterone only or nonhormonal form of contraception is individualized and based on patient preferences and indications for the estrogen-containing contraceptives (see Chapter 5). If the patient requires ongoing estrogen-containing therapy, ongoing anticoagulation (usually at a prophylactic dose) should be considered. For children and adolescents receiving pegylated-asparaginase, prophylactic or therapeutic anticoagulation should be administered until a minimum of 4 weeks after the last dose of asparaginase. In children with recurrent provoked DVT with an existing reversible risk factor, anticoagulation is recommended until the resolution of the precipitating factor and for a minimum of 3 months.

For children with vascular anatomic anomalies predisposing to DVT by venous extrinsic compression (e.g., thoracic outlet syndrome, May-Thurner syndrome), percutaneous or surgical intervention to correct the underlying anomaly may be needed in addition to anticoagulation [13]. For children with recurrent DVT secondary to such structural venous abnormalities, it is recommended to treat with indefinite anticoagulation unless successful percutaneous or surgical intervention addressing the anatomical abnormality has been performed [10, 11].

Complete or partial resolution of the DVT is expected in around 50% of children treated with anticoagulation and is more common in nonocclusive DVT. Progression of DVT on anticoagulation is rare. The presence of contributing factors such as noncompliance to antithrombotic medications, additional prothrombic risk factors, or drug malabsorption (e.g., subcutaneous edema for LMWH, gastrointestinal malabsorption for oral agents) should be sought. If progression occurs on VKA therapy despite an international normalized ratio (INR) within the therapeutic range of 2.0–3.0, UFH or LMWH should be started and subsequently switched back to VKA using a higher therapeutic range of INR of 3.0–4.0 [10]. If progression occurs on LMWH, increasing the dose of LMWH to a higher target anti-factor Xa level can be considered. If progression occurs on a DOAC, measurement of a DOAC-specific circulating level (i.e., anti-factor Xa for direct Xa inhibitors, diluted thrombin time for direct thrombin inhibitor, when locally available) might help determine whether the dosing was adequate. Alternative anticoagulation or additive antiplatelet therapy could be considered in the presence of clinically significant thrombotic progression despite therapeutic drug levels. Progression of an extensive lower limb DVT despite anticoagulation therapy may be an indication for thrombolysis or for the insertion of IVC filter (see below).

Thrombolysis

The indication for thrombolysis is a DVT-threatening organ or limb function in the absence of contraindications. Thrombolysis therapy may be administered systemically or locally via a catheter. Available data suggest that catheter-directed thrombolysis may achieve a higher response rate with a decreased rate of bleeding complications compared with systemic thrombolysis [14]. The use of pharmacomechanical or catheter-directed local thrombolysis depends on institutional experience, technical feasibility, and absence of contraindications [15]. The theoretical advantages of catheter-directed thrombolysis, i.e., the ability to deliver lower doses of a thrombolytic agent directly into the thrombus, may be mitigated by the increased risk of local vessel injury in children with small vessels. Local therapy may be used for catheter-related DVT when the catheter is already in situ. The benefit of using of pharmacomechanical or catheter-directed thrombolysis for DVT in an attempt to reduce the long-term complication of PTS remains unclear in children [8, 16]. It may be considered for patients with extensive symptomatic DVT, when there is a recent onset of symptoms, a perceived low risk of bleeding, and if local expertise is available. It may also be considered in patients with May-Thurner syndrome, as image-guided therapy such as local thrombolysis with or without angioplasty can improve vessel patency [17], which could potentially reduce the incidence of PTS. If thrombolysis is used, tissue plasminogen activator (tPA) rather than other thrombolytic agents is recommended [11]. Dosing, monitoring, and relative contraindications of thrombolysis therapy are detailed in Chapter 20.

Life-threatening DVT (e.g., in the immediate period after cardiac surgery) may warrant the consideration of thrombectomy, and this should be discussed with an experienced multidisciplinary pediatric team, including cardiothoracic surgeons, cardiologists, intensivists, and hematologists.

Importantly, children with DVT requiring initial therapy with thrombolysis and/or thrombectomy need ongoing anticoagulant therapy. The type and duration of anticoagulation should follow previous recommendations.

IVC Filter

IVC interruption with an IVC filter is used to prevent PE. Its use in children has been limited to case reports and few published series [18]. IVC filters should not be routinely used in children with VTE and should be reserved for cases in which absolute contraindications for anticoagulation exist or in children with refractory VTE at risk of embolization [11]. Data are limited regarding IVC filter placement in IVC <1 cm, age <2 years, weight <10 kg. Once the contraindication for anticoagulation is resolved, anticoagulation should be favored and the IVC filter removed.

Complications of filter placement include filter migration or fracture, extension of existing thrombus to the filter, risk of PE during manipulation of the filter at insertion, perforation of blood vessels, and perforation of adjacent structures as the child grows. In light of the increased long-term risk of lower limb DVT postinsertion of permanent IVC filters, retrievable devices are favored [19]. The retrievable IVC filter should be removed as soon as the contraindication to anticoagulation is resolved and the presence of thrombosis in the basket of the filter has been ruled out, ideally, before 2 weeks from its insertion. Previous reports on the range of successful filter removals in children have been as low as 54% to as high as almost 80%. While no absolute time limit can be established with regard to an effective filter retrieval, longer filter duration appears to negatively influence its retrievability [18]. The development of local quality control algorithms may improve filter removal in eligible patients [20].

Venous Stents

Angioplasty and venous stenting of the caval and iliofemoral veins are treatment modalities for eliminating (central) venous outflow obstructions and restoring venous flow to reduce post-thrombotic morbidity, and/or to relieve symptoms if PTS or chronic deep venous pathology have already developed, for DVT secondary to iliac vein compression syndrome and other etiologies [21]. The literature on stent outcomes in adults suggests approximately 90% primary patency at 12–18 months as well as objective and subjective clinical improvement [22–24]. In-stent thrombosis can reduce the effectiveness of venous interventions, and strategies to reduce the incidence of stent thrombosis are an important aspect of management. The risk of stent thrombosis is higher in the first 6 weeks after stent placement, although it may still occur later [25]. There is a decreased risk of in-stent thrombosis with increasing time spent within therapeutic range for anticoagulation [26]. There is significant heterogeneity in current clinical practice for postprocedural antithrombotic treatment after venous intervention, because of limited prospective randomized data, leading recommendations to be driven by consensus opinion and retrospective studies. Minimal antithrombotic therapy after venous interventions for thrombotic disease should adhere to the therapeutic anticoagulation guidelines for the underlying cause of thrombosis. Patients with higher periprocedural thrombotic risk based on patient and procedural factors may benefit from more intense antithrombotic therapy in the initial period after intervention, balancing risk of bleeding. In the setting of underlying thrombophilia, recurrent thrombosis, thrombosis without reversible risk factors, or cancer-associated thrombosis, extended therapeutic anticoagulation is warranted. Multidisciplinary management with interventional radiology, hematology, and/or vascular medicine involvement is recommended to determine the type and duration of anticoagulation therapy [27].

Enoxaparin or other LMWH is preferred for the first month after intervention. DOACs are acceptable anticoagulants for some patients, 1 month after the intervention, in the absence of specific contraindications to the agent being considered (e.g., end-stage renal disease). The benefit of adding single- or dual-agent antiplatelet therapy to anticoagulation regimens is unclear [27].

Catheter-Related Thrombosis

CVCs facilitate intravenous therapies in neonates, infants, and older children with difficult venous access. The mechanisms of CVC-related VTE include endothelial damage during catheter insertion, disruption of blood flow, infusion of prothrombotic agents, and thrombogenic catheter material. CVC-related VTE is well described in children with cancer, hemophilia, and other severe inherited bleeding disorders, cystic fibrosis, and children requiring total parenteral nutrition. The incidence of CVC-related VTE varies widely in the literature depending on whether clinically unsuspected VTE is included and the diagnostic modalities used. The highest frequency occurs in children <1 year of age, and this likely reflects the increased ratio of catheter-to-vessel size, as well as challenging venous access at this age. The most common location of CVC-related VTE is the upper venous system, as this is the site most commonly used for CVC placement in children. CVC-related VTE is associated with mortality (secondary to PE) and morbidity, including CVC infection, recurrence of VTE, venous hypertension secondary to chronic venous occlusion leading to either PTS or, very rarely, chylothorax/chylopericardium, and loss of venous access.

The occurrence of CVC-related VTE in neonates and children is associated with host- and catheter-related risk factors. Host-related risk factors include sepsis, low birth weight, and congenital heart disease. Catheter-related risk factors include CVC type, e.g., peripherally inserted central catheters (PICC) [28], previous CVC infections and/or occlusions, insertion technique, CVC location, duration of CVC insertion, type of therapy infused (e.g., total parenteral nutrition and hyperosmolar fluids), and concomitant therapies (e.g., corticosteroids).

Clinical Presentation

The most common signs of CVC-related DVT are edema, changes in skin color, temperature, or perfusion. A high index of suspicion is often required to investigate a child for CVC-related VTE as many of the signs of VTE can overlap with that of the underlying medical condition. CVC-related VTE commonly occurs in an intermittent and subacute manner, when periods of partial or complete vessel occlusion are accompanied by optimal or suboptimal parallel development of increasing venous collateral drainage, ultimately leading to a complete absence of symptoms. Therefore, repeated mechanical occlusion and CVC-related infection may be the first sign of VTE. Neonates with CVC or umbilical vein catheter (UVC)-related VTE may present with thrombocytopenia. Specific symptoms of superior vena cava occlusion include swelling of the head and neck, conjunctival edema, plethora, and pleural effusion. Occlusion of the IVC may present with lower extremity edema. There may be visible collateral vessels on the chest and/or abdominal wall. Right atrial thrombosis related to CVC may present with loss of CVC patency, respiratory distress, and/or arrhythmia. Asymptomatic right atrial thrombosis may be an incidental finding on echocardiography.

Diagnosis

Depending on the location of the catheter, various radiological techniques may be used to evaluate for the presence of VTE (see "Deep Vein Thrombosis" and "Diagnosis"). Contrast dye study through the line (linogram) may aid in the diagnosis of catheter occlusion because of a fibrin sheath at the tip of CVC but is inadequate to diagnose or exclude CVC-related VTE [8]. Doppler ultrasound, conventional venography, CTV, or MRV may be required to exclude large-vessel thrombosis. Echocardiography can be used to detect right atrial thrombus. Blood flow problems, particularly soon after CVC placement, may be secondary to a catheter kink, malposition of the catheter tip, or a constricting suture. This may be diagnosed on a chest X-ray.

Management

If the CVC is no longer necessary or is not functioning, the catheter should be removed to eliminate the source of the thrombus. It is recommended to delay CVC removal until after a few days of anticoagulation, whenever possible because of the anecdotal reports of PE following CVC removal. However, a recent study reported the risk of PE following CVC removal to be lower than previously shown [29]. Thereafter, anticoagulation should be continued for a total duration of between 6 weeks and 3 months [11]. If the CVC remains in place afterward, a prophylactic regimen of anticoagulation should be considered until the CVC is removed. If recurrent VTE occurs while on prophylaxis, consider increasing the anticoagulation dose to a therapeutic dose until the CVC is removed and for a minimum of 3 months following the VTE. For neonates with CVC- or UVC-related VTE, refer to the section "Venous Thrombosis in Neonates."

For children with right atrial thrombosis related to CVC, risk stratification based on thrombus size and mobility is suggested [30]. Removal of the CVC is advised, when possible, with or without anticoagulation depending on the individual risk factors [11]. For patients with high-risk features on echocardiography, such as atrial thrombus with a size approximating that of the pulmonary valve of the patient in any dimension, mobile, pedunculated, or snake-shaped thrombus, anticoagulation with appropriately timed CVC removal is recommended [30]. Surgical thrombectomy or thrombolysis should be considered based on individualized risk-benefit assessment. Dosing and monitoring of anticoagulation and thrombolysis therapy are detailed in Chapter 20.

Prophylaxis

A summary of the evidence published in a recent Cochrane systematic review showed low certainty that the use of primary prophylactic anticoagulation prevents CVC-related VTE [31]. This conclusion was due to the low number of studies addressing this question and their heterogeneity. The exception to this is in the case of long-term total parenteral nutrition administration, where prophylaxis with VKA is recommended to maintain a target INR of 1.5–1.9 [10].

Thrombotic recurrences are seen in approximately a third of children with a previous CVC-related VTE requiring a new CVC [32]. Most of these events are diagnosed within 2 weeks after the insertion of the new CVC (median time 11 days, 25th–75th percentile, 4–44 days). Therefore, secondary thromboprophylaxis should be considered on a case-by-case basis, notably informed by the risk of bleeding. The presence of thrombophilia did not predict CVC-related DVT recurrence, and thrombophilia testing is not recommended following a first episode of CVC-related VTE [33].

There has been much debate as to the clinical significance of clinically unsuspected (asymptomatic) catheter-related VTE. Surveillance for asymptomatic VTE in children who have a CVC in place is currently not recommended.

Table 1. Initial management of blocked central venous catheter

Chemical-related blockage	Blood-related blockage
Indications	
Infusion running then sudden unexplained occlusion	Blood sampling Blood administration Blood backup in infusion
Initial action	
1. Attempt to aspirate 2. Flush with 0.9% NaCl 3. Follow hydrochloric acid local instillation guidelines (Table 2)	1. Attempt to aspirate 2. Flush with 0.9% NaCl 3. Follow guidelines for tPA local instillation (Table 2) If unsuccessful clearing, a second attempt may be indicated If able to flush the catheter but unable to get blood return, proceed to diagnostic workup, if clinically indicated
4. If no blood return, follow guidelines for tPA local instillation (Table 2) If able to flush the catheter but no blood return, proceed to diagnostic workup if clinically indicated 5. If unable to flush the catheter, proceed to diagnostic workup, if clinically indicated	4. If unable to flush the catheter, proceed to diagnostic workup, if clinically indicated

See text for the recommended diagnostic workup. Adapted from SickKids formulary. tPA, tissue plasminogen activator.

Occlusion

Occlusion of a CVC may occur because of fibrin sheaths, intraluminal thrombus, VTE around the CVC, mechanical problems, or chemical precipitation. Catheter occlusion is associated with an increased risk of CVC-related infection and leads to increased need for CVC replacement. Flushing with normal saline, UFH, or intermittent urokinase is recommended to prevent CVC occlusion [10]. The current available data do not recommend one option over others. For blocked CVCs, tPA or intermittent urokinase should be instilled in the catheter for 30 min, to be repeated once if the catheter remains occluded. See Tables 1 and 2 for suggested guidelines for the management of blocked CVCs.

If a CVC remains blocked following two doses of local thrombolytic therapy, radiological imaging to rule out a CVC-related thrombosis is recommended. A chest X-ray is suggested to visualize the CVC position. A contrast linogram is recommended to determine potential occlusion at the tip of the CVC, presence of retrograde flow, and potential leak. Doppler ultrasound, conventional venography, CTV, or contrast-enhanced MRV may be required to exclude large vessel VTE. Echocardiography can be used to detect right atrial thrombus.

Pulmonary Embolism

PE, although uncommon, is an increasingly recognized complication in children and can be a significant cause of morbidity and mortality. The incidence of PE in population-based studies has been age specific and sex specific, varying from no reported cases to several per 100,000 [1, 34]. Two specific patterns of PE are recognized in children: classic thromboembolic PE and in situ pulmo-

Table 2. Guidelines for local installation for blocked central venous catheter

Type of catheter	Chemical occlusion hydrochloric acid 0.1 M	Blood-related occlusion	
		Body weight	Alteplase (tPA)
Single lumen (e.g., Hickman, Cook Roko, PICC)	2 mL	>10 kg	1 mg/mL; use amount required to fill volume of line to maximum; 2 mL = 2 mg
		≤10 kg	1 mg diluted to 2 mL; 1 mL = 0.5 mg
Double lumen (e.g., Hickman, Cook, PICC, Quinton)	2 mL per lumen	>10 kg	1 mg/mL; use amount required to fill volume of line to maximum; 2 mL = 2 mg per lumen; treat one lumen at a time; second lumen may not need to be treated if catheter cleared
		≤10 kg	1 mg diluted to 2 mL per lumen; 1 mL = 0.5 mg
Subcutaneous ports (e.g., Port-A-Cath, PASport)	3 mL	>10 kg	2 mg diluted with normal saline to 3 mL; 1 mL = 0.65 mg per lumen; if double lumen port, treat one lumen at a time; second lumen may not need to be treated if port cleared
		≤10 kg	1.5 mg diluted with normal saline to 3 mL; 1 mL = 0.5 mg
Hemodialysis catheters[a]			
Small quinton	1 mL	>10 kg	See guidelines above for single-lumen catheter
Large quinton	1.5 mL	≤10 kg	0.75 mg diluted to 1.5 mL

After a minimum of 2 h instillation of each drug, withdraw drug; if possible, flush the catheter with normal saline; attempt to aspirate blood. Adapted from SickKids formulary. PICC, peripherally inserted central catheter; tPA, tissue plasminogen activator. [a]For non-nephrology patients, use double lumen guidelines.

nary artery thrombosis, which is often because of local causes, such as congenital heart disease, pulmonary artery anomalies, or lung transplantation [35]. Risk factors for classic thromboembolic PE include the presence of a CVC, the use of estrogen-containing contraceptives, surgery and immobility, cancer, vascular malformations with slow blood flow (e.g., capillary lymphatic venous malformation or Klippel-Trenaunay syndrome, diffuse and/or multifocal pure venous malformation), nephrotic syndrome, long-term total parenteral nutrition, systemic lupus erythematosus, ventriculoatrial shunts, and congenital and/or acquired thrombotic tendencies [34, 36]. About half of children with PE have evidence of acute DVT in the extremities. High-risk (massive) PE is defined as acute PE causing cardiopulmonary arrest, sustained hypotension or normotension with signs or symptoms of shock, whereas intermediate risk (submassive) PE is an acute PE with evidence of right ventricular strain, myocardial necrosis or both, in the absence of hypotension or compensated shock [37]. The diagnosis of PE in children requires an increased level of clinical suspicion to enable timely recognition and appropriate therapy.

Clinical Presentation

Clinical signs of PE are nonspecific in children and may be masked by underlying conditions. Shortness of breath, pleuritic pain, dyspnea, unexplained and persistent tachycardia are possible findings, but it may be difficult to differentiate the overlapping signs of PE in a critically ill child. Moreover, even in children who develop PE and who are not critically ill, the classical signs of PE may be absent, making the diagnosis even more challenging [38]. Rarely, PE can present with hypoxemia, hemoptysis, syncope, shock, or cardiac arrest. In adults, clinical prediction scores are used to identify those in whom PE can be ruled out by a negative D-dimer without further investigation. Currently, there are no data to support the use of these scores in children [39]. Children with PE were as likely as children without PE to have a D-dimer value within the normal range.

Diagnosis

The diagnosis of PE requires confirmatory diagnostic radiographic imaging. Ventilation/perfusion (V/Q) scanning was historically the first-line investigation for children with suspected PE and may still be appropriate for use in young women to avoid breast irradiation. V/Q scanning is not possible in very young children (generally less than 5–6 years) because of the inability of very young children to cooperate with testing requirements. The V/Q scan in children and adolescents is usually interpreted according to criteria adapted from adults, being classified as low, moderate, or high PE probability for Prospective investigation of PE – diagnosis (PIOPED) and normal, near normal, abnormal not consistent with PE and abnormal consistent with PE for Prospective investigation study of acute PE – diagnosis (PISAPED).

Computed tomography pulmonary angiography (CTPA) is being used increasingly in children, although there are no published studies on sensitivity or specificity. Currently, CTPA has become the noninvasive first-line imaging study in both pediatric and adult patients with clinically suspected PE, as it also provides information on the differential diagnosis for the patients' symptomatology and can detect right ventricular strain. With young and uncooperative children, the risk of sedation or anesthetic to facilitate the investigation must be weighed against the benefit of identifying the PE. CTPA is contraindicated in patients with known or suspected allergy to contrast media, patients with renal failure, and requires precautions in patients who are pregnant or on metformin. Magnetic resonance pulmonary angiography (MRPA) is an alternative to conventional pulmonary angiography in patients with suspected PE in whom CTPA is contraindicated. The experience with MRPA in children is limited.

Conventional catheter pulmonary angiography has been considered the "gold-standard" diagnostic test in both adults and children. Pulmonary angiography is expensive, invasive, and requires expertise and sedation in children. Thus, it may not be readily available. Pulmonary angiography may be considered when less invasive diagnostic tests are indeterminate and clinical suspicion is high.

In a child with a suspected PE, findings on echocardiography, and extremity imaging (ultrasound, venogram, CTV, and MRV) can add relevant information for management. Echocardiography may help identify signs of right ventricular strain, such as tricuspid regurgitation, septal flattening, and right ventricle flattening or reduced function. Echocardiography can also be preferred to diagnose PE in neonates, when the need for contrast, sedation, and vessel size limit the utility of other diagnostic tests. In children with symptomatic acute PE, cardiac troponin levels may help detect myocardial necrosis.

Management

Treatment should be instituted promptly upon confirmation of the presence of PE. Initiation of therapy may also be considered in selected unstable patients with a high clinical suspicion while awaiting diagnostic confirmation. In adults, predictive mortality risk stratification assessment takes into account clinical features at presentation, comorbidities, presence or absence of a concomitant

DVT, electrocardiography, imaging findings (i.e., echocardiographic and/or CTPA), and biomarkers (i.e., troponin, brain natriuretic peptide). Conversely, no prognostic risk stratification strategies have been developed for children diagnosed with PE, and the adult-based prognostic clinical indices had moderate discrimination and thus, limited clinical usefulness in children [40].

As the clinical presentation of acute PE can be highly variable ranging from asymptomatic, nonspecific, or mild symptomatology to severe hypoxemia, right ventricular failure, shock, and even death, the treatment of pediatric patients should be guided by the risks associated with the individual clinical condition of the patient.

Anticoagulation is considered the main treatment in the majority of patients with PE. The choice of the initial and subsequent anticoagulant and guidelines for duration of anticoagulant therapy are similar to those of extremity DVT (see the section above).

In patients with high-risk PE, more aggressive therapy is warranted. Thrombolysis should be considered (see Chapter 20). Embolectomy performed percutaneously (using catheters) or surgically should be considered when systemic thrombolysis is contraindicated or unsuccessful. The choice of embolectomy technique depends on patient-related factors, availability of resources, and expertise at the local institution. For intermediate-risk PE, thrombolysis or other reperfusion therapies are not routinely indicated [11] but can be considered on a case-by-case basis by a multidisciplinary team, based on the patient's overall clinical condition, cardiac impairment, anticipated bleeding risk, and available local expertise [37].

Chronic Thromboembolic Pulmonary Hypertension

Chronic thromboembolic pulmonary hypertension (CTEPH) is a potential long-term complication of acute PE or recurrent PE with considerable morbidity and mortality, reported to affect approximately less than 5% of children with PE [41, 42]. CTEPH is defined as mean pulmonary artery pressure >25 mm Hg that persists for 6 months after PE diagnosis. Exercise intolerance, fatigue, and dyspnea are the most commonly reported symptoms of CTEPH, followed by chest discomfort, syncope, hemoptysis, light-headedness, or peripheral leg edema. In the majority of patients, echocardiography, which detects the presence of elevated pulmonary artery pressure, provides the first indication of CTEPH. Diagnosis is based on findings on CTPA or V/Q scan and confirmed with right heart catheterization and pulmonary angiography [42]. Pulmonary thromboendarterectomy surgery is well tolerated with improved functional status. Pulmonary vasodilators may contribute to increased survival in inoperable disease [41]. Due to high risk of recurrent thrombosis, adherence to long-term anticoagulation is important.

Venous Thrombosis in Neonates

Neonates are at highest risk of developing VTE among the childhood age group. Risk factors include the use of intravascular catheters in small-caliber and umbilical vessels, sepsis, inflammation, hypotension, and hypoxia [43, 44]. Renal vein thrombosis is the most common type of non-catheter-related VTE in neonates, being associated with gestational diabetes (see Chapter 16). Purpura fulminans, because of homozygous or compound heterozygous states of protein C or protein S deficiency, is an acute life-threatening syndrome requiring specific management (see Chapter 13).

The current guidelines for the management of neonatal VTE suggest considering treatment options based on site, extent, clinical consequences of the thrombosis, and the risk of bleeding associated with the use of anticoagulation therapy or thrombolytic therapy [11]. The potential risk of hemorrhage vs. the benefit of anticoagulation or thrombolysis needs to be carefully considered in the neonate. The risk of bleeding is associated with gestational age, birth weight, and comorbidities, such as lung disease, necrotizing enterocolitis, sepsis, and the presence of intraventricular hemorrhage. The incidence of recurrent VTE, PTS, and other more specific complications of neonatal VTE, e.g., portal hypertension after UVC-related thrombosis, is unknown both in treated and untreated neonates. Thus, in neonates, management options include supportive care only, anticoagulant therapy, thrombolytic therapy, or surgery.

For neonatal VTE, initial anticoagulation or supportive care with radiologic monitoring for extension of thrombosis is recommended. If extension of the thrombus occurs, anticoagulation should be strongly considered. Initial anticoagulation may be with LMWH alone or UFH followed by LMWH or a DOAC (when adequate formulations are available) for a total of 6 weeks to 3 months depending on the presence of risk factors and VTE resolution [11]. Premature or low birth weight neonates, as well as neonates in whom oral feedings had not been established, were not eligible for the currently published DOAC trials. Additional prospective phase IV studies are ongoing to address some of these limitations, evaluating the efficacy and safety of DOACs in young-aged children. Until further data are available, UFH or LMWH should be preferred for these patients. For catheter-related VTE in neonates, removal of the catheter is suggested after a few days of therapeutic anticoagulation, although a recent study reported lower than expected rates of PE following CVC removal [29]. If thrombolysis is required, tPA rather than other thrombolytic agents and plasminogen (frozen plasma) administration prior to or during therapy is recommended. Dosing and monitoring of anticoagulation and thrombolysis therapy in neonates are detailed in Chapter 20.

Venous Thrombosis in Cancer Patients

The etiology of VTE in childhood cancer is multifactorial. The risk factors include increased thrombin generation related to disease (e.g., leukemia), age (highest risk during adolescence), the use of CVC, chemotherapy including asparaginase, corticosteroids, and anthracyclines, the use of total parenteral nutrition, and infection [45]. Non-CVC-related VTE complications in children with cancer include: (1) cerebral sinovenous thrombosis (CSVT) in children with acute lymphoblastic leukemia, mostly during the induction phase of their chemotherapy; (2) DVT adjacent to tumor site (e.g., soft tissue or bone tissue origin); and (3) vascular bed invasion of the IVC from tumors of renal or hepatic origin. According to the current recommendations, the management of VTE in children with cancer should follow the general recommendations for management of VTE in children [11]. LMWH is the preferred anticoagulant in children with cancer because of the ease of maintaining the anticoagulation therapy around the usual frequent procedures, although adult experience and subgroup analysis from the pediatric EINSTEIN-Jr trial suggest that DOACs might be an adequate option for patients with cancer [46, 47].

As the presence of cancer presents a unique challenge in terms of balancing risk vs. benefit, the decision to initiate anticoagulation should be made on an individual basis. For example, there are no evidence-based guidelines for anticoagulation in patients with VTE who develop chemotherapy-induced thrombocytopenia. Most experts recommend a platelet count of greater than 50×10^9/L for full-dose anticoagulation and of greater than 30×10^9/L for prophylactic dose anticoagulation. In the presence of thrombocytopenia, whether to hold or reduce anticoagulation doses or to use platelet transfusions to maintain a platelet count at a higher level in order to give full-dose anticoagulation should be decided on an individual basis (see Chapter 20). For planned in-

14

trathecal chemotherapy, omission of anticoagulation for at least 24 h is suggested. For asparaginase-associated thrombotic complications, it is suggested that after a VTE, asparaginase can be restarted, after reimaging demonstrates thrombus stabilization or improvement, with closely monitored anticoagulation [48]. Following VTE treatment, thromboprophylaxis is usually continued up to 4 weeks after the last dose of pegylated-asparaginase, given its longer half-life compared with native asparaginase formulations.

The role of thromboprophylaxis is not yet established in children with cancer. A randomized controlled trial suggested that thromboprophylaxis with LMWH might be efficacious and safe to reduce VTE in children with acute lymphoblastic leukemia [49, 50] and two randomized controlled trials are underway in this high-risk population [51, 52]. Until further research is available, thromboprophylaxis can be considered in high-risk situations, such as children with important vascular compression by tumor, children with a history of a previous thrombosis, or in the presence of a positive family history of thrombosis (see Chapter 13).

Post-Thrombotic Syndrome

PTS is a syndrome of chronic venous insufficiency following DVT. The pathophysiology of PTS is thought to involve venous hypertension as a result of venous valvular reflux, thrombotic venous occlusion, or other causes of impaired venous return [53]. In a systematic review of the literature, the overall weighted mean frequency of PTS following upper extremity DVT or lower extremity DVT in children was 26% (95% CI: 23–28%) among a total of nearly 1,000 patients studied [54]. Younger patients, children with CVC-related thrombosis, and the presence of complete resolution of the index thrombotic event may indicate a lower risk of developing PTS in the pediatric population [55].

Clinical Presentation

The most common symptoms of PTS in children are pain, easily tired limb, poor endurance, heaviness, and swelling in the affected limb [56]. PTS symptoms may be persistent or intermittent, may be aggravated by physical activity and improve with resting, leg elevation, or supine position. The most common sign of PTS is edema in the affected limb. In the upper extremity, there may be dilation of the superficial veins of the upper arm and chest wall and dependent cyanosis of the arm. Clinical findings, such as skin induration, skin inflammation, and skin pigmentation, are unusual in children. In severe cases, venous leg ulcers may occur, which can be precipitated by minor trauma. These are generally chronic, painful, and slow to heal.

Diagnosis

PTS is a clinical diagnosis based on the development of characteristic symptoms and signs in a patient with prior DVT. In some patients, it may take up to 6 months for resolution of the initial pain or swelling; therefore, the diagnosis of PTS should be deferred until after the acute DVT phase.

There are three clinical tools for diagnosis of PTS in children, the modified Villalta Scale [57], the Manco-Johnson instrument [58], and the index for the Clinical Assessment of PTS in Children (CAPTSure©) [59] (Table 3). In the modified Villalta Scale, two symptoms and nine signs of PTS are graded on a scale of 0–1 or 0–2, depending on the clinical finding, with an automatic score of 9 given for ulceration. Scores for symptoms and signs are added to provide a final numerical score that is categorized as mild (1–3 points), moderate (4–8 points), or severe PTS (≥9 points). The Manco-Johnson instrument includes the assessment of four signs of PTS as well as pain at rest, pain-limiting activities of daily living, and pain-limiting aerobic activities. Pain is assessed with the use of the Wong-Baker faces pain scale. The finding of ≥1 sign or symptom in-

Table 3. Components of standardized outcome measures for PTS employed in pediatric studies

Outcomes measures and components	Scoring
Modified Villalta scale	
Symptoms[a]	
Pain or abnormal use	1
Swelling	1
Signs	
Increased limb circumference[b]	1
Change in skin color	1
Pitting edema	1
Venous collaterals on skin	1
Pigmentation of skin	1
Tenderness on palpations of deep veins	1
Varicosities	1 moderate, 2 severe
Head swelling	1 moderate, 2 severe
Ulceration	9
Mild PTS	1–3
Moderate PTS	4–8
Severe PTS	≥9
Manco-Johnson instrument	
Signs	
Edema[c]	1
Dilated superficial collateral veins	1
Venous stasis dermatitis	1
Venous stasis ulcers	1
Symptoms	
Chronic lower-extremity pain	
Limiting aerobic activities	0–5
Limiting activities of daily living	0–5
At rest	0–5
Any PTS present	≥1
Physically and functionally significant PTS	Symptoms ≥1
CAPTSure©[d]	
Upper extremity subindex	
Pain intensity	0 none, 8 mild, 15 moderate, 24 severe
Endurance, compared to other limb	0 same, 9 slightly worse, 16 worse
Swelling	0 never, 5 rarely, 13 often
Heaviness	0 never, 6 rarely, 13 often
Visible veins (collateral circulation)	0 no, 5 mild, 13 moderate/severe
Paresthesia, tingling	0 never, 5 rarely, 12 often
Arm circumference difference	0 0–1 cm, 5 1.1–2 cm, and 9 >2 cm
Lower extremity subindex	
Pain intensity	0 none, 7 mild, 15 moderate, 25 severe
Venous ulcers	Present: 21
Endurance, compared to other limb	0 same, 7 slightly worse, 13 worse
Swelling	0 never, 4 rarely, 10 often
Paresthesia (tingling)	0 never, 4 rarely, 9 often
Tightness, heaviness, tired limb	0 never, 3 rarely, 8 often
Redness, purple, or blotchy skin	0 never, 3 rarely, 7 often
Limb circumference difference	0 0–1 cm, 4 1.1–2 cm, and 7 >2 cm
Any PTS present	>10
Moderate to severe PTS	>30

PTS, post-thrombotic syndrome. [a]Reported by patient, parent, caregiver, or proxy. [b]>3% compared with contralateral side. [c]>1 cm increase in circumference in the affected extremity compared with the contralateral extremity. [d]Interested individuals may contact pts.research@sickkids.ca for potential licensing of the tool at their institutions.

dicates the presence of any PTS, and the presence of pain indicates clinically significant PTS [54, 60]. CAPTSure© was developed with the participation of an international panel of pediatric thrombosis experts and a group of pediatric patients, who proposed the signs and symptoms to be included to diagnose and rate the severity of pediatric PTS. The elicited signs and symptoms were tested in children at risk for PTS [61], and the obtained results were used to guide pediatric thrombosis experts and select the final items through a Delphi process [59]. The scoring system is based on the relative importance of the included signs and symptoms, according to health care providers, patients, and parents [59]. The tool has proven validity and reliability [62]. The final score ranges between 0 and 100 points, with higher scoring indicating higher PTS severity; a score of 0–10 points indicates no PTS, a score of 11–30 points indicates mild PTS, and a score of ≥31 points indicates moderate to severe PTS [63]. Training videos were developed for the administration of the Manco-Johnson instrument (at the Kids-DOTT clinical trial website) [64] and for CAPTSure© [65].

In a patient with previously documented DVT with symptoms and signs compatible with PTS, no further investigations are needed. In a patient with clinical manifestations compatible with PTS with no prior history of DVT, a Doppler ultrasound can be useful to detect a previously undiagnosed DVT. Excluding a recurrent thrombotic event is warranted in the setting of acute worsening of PTS symptoms. An unequivocal change in the extent of thrombosis on the current ultrasound compared with the previous is indicative of new ipsilateral DVT.

Management

Despite limited evidence, graduated compression garments and intermittent compression are used to manage PTS in adults [66]. In children, the use of low-pressure compression garments (15–20 mm Hg) for 8–12 h per day, 3 or more days per week, was associated with lower PTS severity at follow-up [67]. Although adherence to therapy can be low, it can be enhanced through education and specialized care [68].

Venous ulcers are rare in children but can be quite debilitating; multidisciplinary care may be required. The cornerstone of venous ulcer treatment in adults is compression therapy. Other relevant measures in adults include ulcer cleansing and debridement, management of cellulitis and infection, and topical dressings [69]. Wound care expertise should be utilized.

Prevention

Given the limited treatment options and impact on health-related quality of life and health care costs, prevention of PTS has been the focus of research in adults for many years. Nevertheless, the role of elastic compression stockings after DVT and of pharmacomechanical and catheter-directed thrombolysis to prevent PTS in adults remains uncertain [70]. No prevention studies have been performed on children. In children and adults, compression garments could be used to reduce edema or pain after acute DVT.

Conclusion

Although VTE is increasingly recognized in children, most data related to diagnosis and management are extrapolated from studies conducted in adults. For older children, this extrapolation may be acceptable in some circumstances. However, differences in the hemostatic systems of neonates, infants, and younger children compared with adults may limit the generalization of recommendations for adults with VTE, to children. Until further studies are available, it is suggested to follow the American Society of Hematology guidelines for the management of children with acute symptomatic VTE [11], with anticoagulation being the cornerstone of therapy. The clinical significance and management of clinically unsuspected (asymptomatic) VTE in children is still debated. Similarly, while awareness of pediatric PTS is increasing, pediatric guidelines for prevention and management of PTS are lacking.

Acknowledgments

The authors express their gratitude to Drs. Victoria E. Price and Leonardo R. Brandão, who wrote previous versions of this chapter, and their appreciation for the thoughtful comments provided by the reviewers and the editors who reviewed this chapter for the third edition of the "SickKids Handbook of Pediatric Thrombosis and Hemostasis."

Conflict of Interest Statement

Dr. Laura Avila holds official copyrights for CAPT-Sure©. Drs. Marie-Claude Pelland-Marcotte, Michael Temple, and Suzan Williams have no conflicts of interest to declare.

Author Contributions

Marie-Claude Pelland-Marcotte prepared the first version of this manuscript. Laura Avila provided critical reviews of drafts and approved the final submitted versions. Michael Temple provided critical reviews of drafts and approved the final submitted versions. Suzan Williams provided critical reviews of drafts and approved the final submitted versions.

Abbreviations

ALL	Acute lymphoblastic leukemia
CSVT	Cerebral sinovenous thrombosis
CTEPH	Chronic thromboembolic pulmonary hypertension
CTPA	Computed tomography pulmonary angiography
CTV	Computed tomography venography
CVC	Central venous catheter
DOAC	Direct oral anticoagulant
DVT	Deep vein thrombosis
INR	International normalized ratio
IVC	Inferior vena cava
LMWH	Low-molecular-weight heparin
MRPA	Magnetic resonance pulmonary angiography
MRV	Magnetic resonance venography
PE	Pulmonary embolism
PICC	Peripherally inserted central catheter
PIOPED	Prospective investigation of pulmonary embolism – diagnosis
PISAPED	Prospective investigation study of acute pulmonary embolism – diagnosis
PTS	Post-thrombotic syndrome
tPA	Tissue plasminogen activator
UFH	Unfractionated heparin
UVC	Umbilical vein catheter
VKA	Vitamin K antagonist
VTE	Venous thromboembolism/thromboembolic event
V/Q scan	Ventilation/perfusion scan

14

References

1 Andrew M, David M, Adams M, Ali K, Anderson R, Barnard D, et al. Venous thromboembolic complications (VTE) in children: first analyses of the Canadian Registry of VTE. Blood. 1994;83(5):1251–7.

2 van Ommen C, Peters M. Venous thromboembolic disease in childhood. Semin Thromb Hemost. 2003;29:391–404.

3 O'Brien SH, Stanek JR, Witmer CM, Raffini L. The continued rise of venous thromboembolism across US children's hospitals. Pediatrics. 2022;149(3):e2021054649.

4 Tuckuviene R, Christensen AL, Helgestad J, Johnsen SP, Kristensen SR. Pediatric venous and arterial noncerebral thromboembolism in Denmark: a nationwide population-based study. J Pediatr. 2011;159(4):663–9.

5 Mahajerin A, Branchford BR, Amankwah EK, Raffini L, Chalmers E, van Ommen CH, et al. Hospital-associated venous thromboembolism in pediatrics: a systematic review and meta-analysis of risk factors and risk-assessment models. Haematologica. 2015;100(8):1045–50.

6 Kerlin BA, Stephens JA, Hogan MJ, Smoyer WE, O'Brien SH. Development of a pediatric-specific clinical probability tool for diagnosis of venous thromboembolism: a feasibility study. Pediatr Res. 2015;77(3):463–71.

7 Sharathkumar AA, Biss T, Kulkarni K, Ahuja S, Regan M, Male C, et al. Epidemiology and outcomes of clinically unsuspected venous thromboembolism in children: a systematic review. J Thromb Haemost. 2020;18(5):1100–12.

8 Chalmers E, Ganesen V, Liesner R, Maroo S, Nokes T, Saunders D, et al. Guideline on the investigation, management and prevention of venous thrombosis in children. Br J Haematol. 2011;154(2):196–207.
9 Avila L, Amiri N, Pullenayegum E, Sealey VA, De R, Williams S, et al. Diagnostic value of D-dimers for limb deep vein thrombosis in children: a prospective study. Am J Hematol. 2021;96(8):954–60.
10 Monagle P, Chan AKC, Goldenberg NA, Ichord RN, Journeycake JM, Nowak-Gottl U, et al. Antithrombotic therapy in neonates and children: Antithrombotic Therapy and Prevention of Thrombosis, 9th ed: American College of Chest Physicians Evidence-Based Clinical Practice Guidelines. Chest. 2012;141(2 suppl):e737S-801S.
11 Monagle P, Cuello CA, Augustine C, Bonduel M, Brandão LR, Capman T, et al. American Society of Hematology 2018 Guidelines for management of venous thromboembolism: treatment of pediatric venous thromboembolism. Blood Adv. 2018;2(22):3292–316.
12 Goldenberg NA, Kittelson JM, Abshire TC, Bonaca M, Casella JF, Dale RA, et al. Effect of anticoagulant therapy for 6 weeks vs 3 months on recurrence and bleeding events in patients younger than 21 years of age with provoked venous thromboembolism: the kids-DOTT randomized clinical trial. JAMA. 2022;327(2):129–37.
13 Arthur LG, Teich S, Hogan M, Caniano DA, Smead W. Pediatric thoracic outlet syndrome: a disorder with serious vascular complications. J Pediatr Surg. 2008;43(6):1089–94.
14 Albisetti, M. Thrombolytic therapy in children. Thromb Res. 2006;118(1):95–105.
15 Kukreja K, Vaidya S. Venous interventions in children. Tech Vasc Interv Radiol. 2011;14(1):16–21.
16 Goldenberg NA, Branchford B, Wang M, Ray Jr C, Durham JD, Manco-Johnson MJ. Percutaneous mechanical and pharmacomechanical thrombolysis for occlusive deep vein thrombosis of the proximal limb in adolescent subjects: findings from an institution-based prospective inception cohort study of pediatric venous thromboembolism. J Vasc Interv Radiol. 2011;22(2):121–32.
17 Avila L, Cullinan N, White M, Gaballah M, Cahill AM, Warad D, et al. Pediatric May-Thurner syndrome—systematic review and individual patient data meta-analysis. J Thromb Haemost. 2021;19(5):1283–93.
18 Kukreja KU, Gollamudi J, Patel MN, Johnson ND, Racadio JM. Inferior vena cava filters in children: our experience and suggested guidelines. J Pediatr Hematol/Oncol. 2011;33(5):334–8.
19 Group PS. Eight-year follow-up of patients with permanent vena cava filters in the prevention of pulmonary embolism: the PREPIC (Prevention du Risque d'Embolie Pulmonaire par Interruption Cave) randomized study. Circulation. 2005;112(3):416–22.
20 Sutphin PD, Reis SP, McKune A, Ravanzo M, Kalva SP, Pillai AK. Improving inferior vena cava filter retrieval rates with the define, measure, analyze, improve, control methodology. J Vasc Interv Radiol. 2015;26(4):491–8.
21 O'Sullivan GJ, Semba CP, Bittner CA, Kee ST, Razavi MK, Sze DY, et al. Endovascular management of iliac vein compression (May-Thurner) syndrome. J Vasc Interv Radiol. 2000;11(7):823–36.
22 Mabud TS, Cohn DM, Arendt VA, Jeon G-S, An X, Fu J, et al. Lower extremity venous stent placement: a large retrospective single-center analysis. J Vasc Interv Radiol. 2020;31(2):251–9.
23 Eijgenraam P, ten Cate H, Arina J. Venous stenting after deep venous thrombosis and antithrombotic therapy: a systematic review. Vasc Med Rev. 2014;2(3):88–97.
24 Taha MA, Busuttil A, Bootun R, Davies AH. A systematic review on the use of deep venous stenting for acute venous thrombosis of the lower limb. Phlebology. 2019;34(2):115–27.
25 Gwozdz A, Saha P, Silickas J, Kahn T, Jones L, Stephenson L, et al. Early duplex surveillance following deep venous stenting for the treatment of post-thrombotic syndrome can predict patients at greatest risk for re-intervention. Eur J Vasc Endovasc Surg. 2018;56(6):e27.
26 Notten P, van Laanen JH, Eijgenraam P, de Wolf MA, Kurstjens RL, Ten Cate H, et al. Quality of anticoagulant therapy and the incidence of in-stent thrombosis after venous stenting. Res Pract Thromb Haemost. 2020;4(4):594–603.
27 Kishore S, Khaja MS, Thornburg B, Sharma AM, Knuttinen M-G, Shamoun F, et al. Antithrombotic therapy after venous interventions: AJR expert panel narrative review. Am J Roentgenol. 2022;219(2):175–187.
28 Jaffray J, Witmer C, O'Brien SH, Diaz R, Ji L, Krava E, et al. Peripherally inserted central catheters lead to a high risk of venous thromboembolism in children. Blood. 2020;135(3):220–6.
29 Jaffray J, Kreuziger LB, Branchford B, Wee CP, Faustino EVS, Zakai NA, et al. Symptomatic pulmonary embolus after catheter removal in children with catheter related thrombosis: a report from the CHAT consortium. J Thromb Haemost. 2022;20(1):133–7.
30 Yang JY, Williams S, Brandão LR, Chan AK. Neonatal and childhood right atrial thrombosis: recognition and a risk-stratified treatment approach. Blood Coagul Fibrinolysis. 2010;21(4):301–7.
31 Pelland-Marcotte M-C, Amiri N, Avila ML, Brandão LR. Low molecular weight heparin for prevention of central venous catheter-related thrombosis in children. Cochrane Database Syst Rev. 2020(6):CD005982.
32 Avila ML, Amiri N, Stanojevic S, Vu TT, Barron K, Krol P, et al. Can thrombophilia predict recurrent catheter-related deep vein thrombosis in children? Blood. 2018;131(24):2712–9.
33 O'Brien SH, Badawy SM, Rotz SJ, Shah MD, Makarski J, Bercovitz RS, et al. The ASH-ASPHO choosing wisely campaign: 5 hematologic tests and treatments to question. Blood Adv. 2022;6(2):679–85.
34 Biss TT, Brandao LR, Kahr WH, Chan AK, Williams S. Clinical features and outcome of pulmonary embolism in children. Br J Haematol. 2008;142(5):808–18.
35 Rajpurkar M, Biss T, Amankwah EK, Martinez D, Williams S, Van Ommen CH, et al. Pulmonary embolism and in situ pulmonary artery thrombosis in paediatrics. A systematic review. Thromb Haemost. 2017;117(6):1199–207.
36 Lee EY, Tse SK, Zurakowski D, Johnson VM, Lee NJ, Tracy DA, et al. Children suspected of having pulmonary embolism: multidetector CT pulmonary angiography—thromboembolic risk factors and implications for appropriate use. Radiology. 2012;262(1):242–51.

37 Ross C, Kumar R, Pelland-Marcotte M-C, Mehta S, Kleinman ME, Thiagarajan RR, et al. Acute management of high- and intermediate-risk pulmonary embolism in children: a review. Chest. 2022;161(3):791–802.
38 Brandão LR, Labarque V, Diab Y, Williams S, Manson DE. Pulmonary embolism in children. Semin Thromb Hemost. 2011;37(7):772–85.
39 Biss TT, Brandao LR, Kahr WH, Chan AK, Williams S. Clinical probability score and D-dimer estimation lack utility in the diagnosis of childhood pulmonary embolism. J Thromb Haemost. 2009;7(10):1633–8.
40 Pelland-Marcotte M-C, Tucker C, Klaassen A, Avila ML, Amid A, Amiri N, et al. Outcomes and risk factors of massive and submassive pulmonary embolism in children: a retrospective cohort study. Lancet Haematol. 2019;6(3):e144–53.
41 Madani MM, Wittine LM, Auger WR, Fedullo PF, Kerr KM, Kim NH, et al. Chronic thromboembolic pulmonary hypertension in pediatric patients. J Thorac Cardiovasc Surg. 2011;141(3): 624–30.
42 Piazza G, Goldhaber SZ. Chronic thromboembolic pulmonary hypertension. N Engl J Med. 2011;364(4):351–60.
43 Revel-Vilk S, Ergaz Z. Diagnosis and management of central-line-associated thrombosis in newborns and infants. Semin Fetal Neonatal Med. 2011;16(6): 340–4.
44 Yang JY, Chan AK. Neonatal systemic venous thrombosis. Thromb Res. 2010; 126(6):471–6.
45 Athale UH, Chan AK. Thromboembolic complications in pediatric hematologic malignancies. Semin Thromb Hemost. 2007;33(4):416–26.
46 Lyman GH, Carrier M, Ay C, Di Nisio M, Hicks LK, Khorana AA, et al. American Society of Hematology 2021 guidelines for management of venous thromboembolism: prevention and treatment in patients with cancer. Blood Adv. 2021; 5(4):927–74.
47 Palumbo JS, Lensing AWA, Brandão LR, Hooimeijer HL, Kenet G, van Ommen H, et al. Anticoagulation in pediatric cancer–associated venous thromboembolism: a subgroup analysis of EINSTEIN-Jr. Blood Adv. 2022;6(22): 5821–8.
48 Grace RF, Dahlberg SE, Neuberg D, Sallan SE, Connors JM, Neufeld EJ, et al. The frequency and management of asparaginase-related thrombosis in paediatric and adult patients with acute lymphoblastic leukaemia treated on Dana-Farber Cancer Institute consortium protocols. Br J Haematol. 2011; 152(4):452–9.
49 Greiner J, Schrappe M, Claviez A, Zimmermann M, Niemeyer C, Kolb R, et al. THROMBOTECT-a randomized study comparing low molecular weight heparin, antithrombin and unfractionated heparin for thromboprophylaxis during induction therapy of acute lymphoblastic leukemia in children and adolescents. Haematologica. 2109;104(4):756–65.
50 Pelland-Marcotte M-C, Tole S, Pechlivanoglou P, Brandão LR. Effectiveness and safety of primary thromboprophylaxis in children with cancer: a systematic review of the literature and network meta-analysis. Thromb Haemost. 2019; 119(12):2034–42.
51 O'Brien SH, Li D, Mitchell LG, Hess T, Zee P, Yee DL, et al. PREVAPIX-ALL: apixaban compared to standard of care for prevention of venous thrombosis in paediatric acute lymphoblastic leukaemia (ALL)-rationale and design. Thromb Haemost. 2019;119(5):844–53.
52 Klaassen IL, Lauw MN, van de Wetering MD, Biemond BJ, Middeldorp S, Abbink FC, et al. TropicALL study: thromboprophylaxis in children treated for acute lymphoblastic leukemia with low-molecular-weight heparin—a multicenter randomized controlled trial. BMC Pediatr.. 2017;17(1):122.
53 Kahn SR. The post-thrombotic syndrome. Hematology Am Soc Hematol Educ Program. 2016;2016(1):413–8.
54 Goldenberg NA, Donadini MP, Kahn SR, Crowther M, Kenet G, Nowak-Göttl U, et al. Post-thrombotic syndrome in children: a systematic review of frequency of occurrence, validity of outcome measures, and prognostic factors. Haematologica. 2010;95(11):1952–9.
55 Engel ER, Nguyen ATH, Amankwah EK, Albisetti M, Brandão LR, Goldenberg NA, et al. Predictors of postthrombotic syndrome in pediatric thrombosis: a systematic review and meta-analysis of the literature. J Thromb Haemost. 2020;18(10):2601–12.
56 Avila ML, Stinson J, Lumia C, Williams S, Montoya MI, Feldman BM, et al. Characteristics of pain, other symptoms and function in pediatric post-thrombotic syndrome. Res Pract Thromb Haemost. 2018;2(2):334–8.
57 Kuhle S, Koloshuk B, Marzinotto V, Bauman M, Massicotte P, Andrew M, et al. A cross-sectional study evaluating post-thrombotic syndrome in children. Thromb Res. 2003;111(4–5):227–33.
58 Manco-Johnson M, Knapp-Clevenger R, Miller B, Hays T. Post-thrombotic syndrome (PTS) in children: validation of a new pediatric outcome instrument and results in a comprehensive cohort of children with extremity deep vein thrombosis (DVT). Blood. 2003; 102(11):553.
59 Avila M, Brandão L, Williams S, Montoya M, Stinson J, Kiss A, et al. Development of CAPTSure™ – a new index for the assessment of pediatric postthrombotic syndrome. J Thromb Haemost. 2016;14(12):2376–85.
60 Smith J, Thornhill D, Goldenberg NA, Brandão L, Knapp-Clevenger R, Warren BB, et al. Validation of outcome instruments for pediatric postthrombotic syndrome: introducing the Peds-VEINES-QOL, a new health-related quality of life instrument. Thromb Haemost. 2021; 121(10):1367–75.
61 Avila M, Brandao L, Williams S, Ward L, Montoya M, Stinson J, et al. Pediatric post-thrombotic syndrome in children: toward the development of a new diagnostic and evaluative measurement tool. Thromb Res. 2016;144:184–91.
62 Avila ML, Feldman BM, Pullenayegum E, Lumia C, Montoya MI, Vincelli J, et al. Post-thrombotic syndrome in children: measurement properties of CAPT-Sure, a new diagnostic tool. Res Pract Thromb Haemost. 2019;3(4):652–7.
63 Avila L, Amiri N, De R, Vincelli J, Pullenayegum E, Williams S, et al. Characteristics of upper- and lower-extremity deep vein thrombosis and predictors of postthrombotic syndrome in children. Blood Adv. 2021;5(19):3737–47.
64 MJI Educational Video. PTS Assessment training video. Available from: www.allkids.org/academics/research/multicenter-studies/kids-dott
65 Avila L, Brandao LR, Vincelli J. CAPTSure instructional video. Available from: https://www.sickkids.ca/en/care-services/clinical-departments/thrombosis-program/.

14

66 Kahn SR, Comerota AJ, Cushman M, Evans NS, Ginsberg JS, Goldenberg NA, et al. The postthrombotic syndrome: evidence-based prevention, diagnosis, and treatment strategies—a scientific statement from the American Heart Association. Circulation. 2014;130(18): 1636–61.
67 Avila L, Amiri N, De R, Vincelli J, Pullenayegum E, Brandão LR. Compression garments for the management of pediatric post-thrombotic syndrome: a prospective longitudinal study. J Thromb Haemost. 2021;19(12):3073–9.
68 Montoya MI, Avila ML, Vincelli J, Williams S, Brandão LR. Understanding the barriers in compliance to elastic compression garments in the treatment of pediatric post-thrombotic syndrome: a qualitative study. Thromb Res. 2016; 144:113–5.
69 O'Donnell TF, Passman MA, Marston WA, Ennis WJ, Dalsing M, Kistner RL, et al. Management of venous leg ulcers: clinical practice guidelines of the Society for Vascular Surgery® and the American Venous Forum. J Vasc Surg. 2014; 60(2):3S-59S.
70 Makedonov I, Kahn SR, Galanaud J-P. Prevention and management of the post-thrombotic syndrome. J Clin Med. 2020;9(4):923.

Published online: December 5, 2024

Blanchette VS, Brandão LR, Carcao MD, Kumar R, Rand ML, Revel-Vilk S (eds): SickKids Handbook of Pediatric Thrombosis and Hemostasis, ed 3, rev. and ext. Basel, Karger, 2024, pp 275–287 (DOI: 10.1159/000538207)

Arterial Thrombosis

Mattia Rizzi[a, b] Anthony K.C. Chan[c] Alessandra Bosch[d, e] Manuela Albisetti[e, f]

[a]Pediatric Hematology/Oncology Service, Pediatric Institute of Southern Switzerland, Bellinzona, Switzerland; [b]Pediatric Hematology/Oncology Unit, Department "Woman-Mother-Child", Lausanne University Hospital and University of Lausanne, Lausanne, Switzerland; [c]Division of Pediatric Hematology/Oncology, Department of Pediatrics, McMaster Children's Hospital, McMaster University, Hamilton, ON, Canada; [d]Division of Hematology/Oncology, The Hospital for Sick Children, Toronto, ON, Canada; [e]Division of Hematology, University Children's Hospital Zurich, Zurich, Switzerland; [f]Children's Research Center, University Children's Hospital Zurich, University of Zurich (UZH), Zurich, Switzerland

Introduction

Arterial thromboembolism/thromboembolic events (ATEs) in children are less common than venous thromboembolic events [1]. In a Danish nationwide pediatric population study, the incidence of ATE and venous thromboembolic event was 0.29 and 2.09 per 100,000 person-years, respectively [2]. Analysis of an Australian prospective single-center pediatric tertiary hospital showed that the incidence of pediatric ATE was 8.5 per 10,000 hospital admissions [3]. Outside the central nervous system, most ATEs develop secondary to catheterization including extremity indwelling arterial catheters (EICs), umbilical artery catheters (UACs), or cardiac catheterization (CC) [3, 4]. Catheter-related ATEs generally occur in neonates and infants with severe underlying medical conditions, particularly cardiac diseases. Noncatheter-related ATEs are much less frequent than catheter-related ATEs and usually occur in rare disorders affecting the vascular system.

This chapter will focus mainly on ATE occurring in the limb arteries and/or abdominal aorta, and mostly secondary to CC. In addition, noncatheter-related ATE in the context of Takayasu's arteritis and Alagille syndrome will be reported.

Extremity Catheter-Related Arterial Thrombosis

Arterial catheters can be placed either peripherally or centrally. EICs are inserted peripherally to monitor blood pressure and oxygen saturation and facilitate frequent blood sampling in critically ill children. In infants and older children, the preferred site is the radial artery. Alternative EIC-insertion sites include the ulnar, brachial, axillary, dorsalis pedis, and tibialis posterior arteries (vascular anatomy is described in Chapter 13, Fig. 1b). If a peripheral arterial access is not possible, cannulation of the more central femoral or iliac arteries is chosen.

In addition, femoral artery cannulation occurs during CC for the diagnosis and treatment of children with congenital heart disease (CHD) or

Table 1. Risk factors for catheter-related arterial thrombosis

	For EIC[a]	For CC	For UAC
Patient related			
Younger age (e.g., newborn)	X	X	X[b]
Low body weight	X	X	
Congenital heart disease	X	X	
Poor perfusion (i.e., severe sepsis, shock)	X		
Catheter related			
Longer duration of insertion/CC procedure	X	[X]	
Longer length	X		
Larger diameter of the catheter for a given weight	X	(X)	[X]
Repeated catheter manipulation/puncture attempts	X	(X)	
Nonheparin-bonded arterial catheter	X		[X]
Proximal placement of UAC	n/a	n/a	X
Side-hole UAC	n/a	n/a	X
Treatment related			
Infusion of hyperosmolar solutions	X		X

CC, cardiac catheterization; EIC, extremity indwelling arterial catheter; n/a, not applicable; UAC, umbilical arterial catheter; (X), trend toward increased risk; [X], controversial data. [a]Particularly for femoral location. [b]Prematurity.

acquired heart disease (see Chapter 18). Femoral artery cannulation can also be required for children undergoing extracorporeal membrane oxygenation (see Chapter 19) or in those who require cerebral angiography (see Chapter 17).

Increased thrombotic potential of the damaged vessel wall by a catheter, thrombogenic catheter materials, and/or disruption of blood flow in the vessel are factors that may lead to thrombotic complications [3–7].

The overall reported cumulative incidence of catheter-related ATE in children was 21% [4]. The incidence rates differed consistently among studies and types of catheters and varied depending on whether diagnosis of ATE was based on routinely performed imaging (including both symptomatic and asymptomatic catheter-related ATE) or on imaging performed because of the presence of clinical signs and/or symptoms (symptomatic catheter-related ATE) [4].

The reported incidence of EIC-related ATE ranged from 3.4 to 63% [4, 6]. The relative incidence of EIC-related ATE according to insertion site was 13% for femoral location, 9% in the brachial location, and 4% in the umbilical location in a single-center study [6]. Younger age (mainly newborns) and/or the presence of CHD were significantly associated with increased risk for femoral catheter-related ATE [4, 6]. In contrast, placement of the arterial catheter into the radial artery was found to be safe and not associated with increased risk of ATE in children of all ages [4, 6]. Additional reported risk factors for catheter-related ATE include longer duration of insertion, longer length and larger diameter of the catheter, conditions associated with poor perfusion such as severe sepsis or shock, low body weight (BW), and cyanotic CHD [1, 4, 6] (Table 1).

The pooled incidence of CC-related ATE reported in prospective studies was 11% (95% CI: 3–21) [4, 5]. The relative incidence of CC-related ATE reported in a single-center study was 32% in infants and 2% in older children [5]. When considering only patients aged ≤4 weeks, the relative incidence of CC-related ATE was 57% [5]. Younger age and low BW were significantly associated

Table 2. Classification of arterial thrombotic events

Mild	Moderate	Severe
• Early signs of threatened limb without risk for an irreversible limb/organ dysfunction (i.e., no evidence for moderate or severe state)	• Capillary return >8 s for >24 h • Absent oxygen saturation pulse • Dampened Doppler wave • Tight tissue compartments	• Complete limb ischemia • Pregangrenous changes • Paralyzed limb >24 h • Doppler/angiogram obstruction with no distal flow >24 h • Failure of reperfusion after 4 h of UFH ± thrombolysis

UFH, unfractionated heparin.

with increased risk of CC-related ATE [5]. Additional reported risk factors for CC-related ATE include balloon dilation, larger sheath size for a given weight, and repeated catheter manipulation [5] (Table 1).

Clinical Presentation

The clinical presentation of ATE varies according to the anatomical location and degree of occlusion of the artery involved. Children have a spectrum of symptoms ranging from asymptomatic to signs of a severely threatened limb or severe organ dysfunction. Signs of threatened limb include absence of palpable pulses, difference in blood pressure of over 10 mm Hg between limbs, decreased skin temperature, skin discoloration (pale or cyanosed), and prolonged capillary refill time. Classification of ATE may be based on the clinical signs and the risk for the related limb or organ (Table 2).

Diagnosis

Diagnosis of catheter-related ATE can be made clinically or objectively. Objective tests for suspected ATE can be performed at the bedside including hand-held Doppler examination for absent pulses, a difference in blood pressure of >10 mm Hg between two limbs (using appropriate age-related cuff size and segmental plethysmography [pulse volume recording]).

Doppler ultrasound (DUS) examination can confirm the clinical diagnosis of ATE [4]. Although the gold standard for diagnosis of ATE is contrast angiography, it is rarely performed in this setting because of its invasiveness.

Health care providers should be aware that catheterization of an artery can result in arterial spasm. The clinical signs and Doppler findings can be similar to ATE; however, arterial spasm usually resolves approximately 6 h after catheterization.

Management

Only limited information is available, and current guidelines for the treatment of ATE are based on weak evidence. If arterial occlusion is suspected, the catheter should be removed immediately [8]. If blood flow cannot be restored and ATE is diagnosed, anticoagulation should be strongly considered with or without thrombolysis or surgical thrombectomy, depending on the urgency to restore patency of the vessels [8]. Heparin is an efficient treatment modality for pediatric non-life/organ-threatening ATE [9].

An algorithm for the acute management of catheter-related ATE is presented in Figure 1. The algorithm is based on expert opinion as minimal evidence exists regarding the management of ATE in children. The potential risk of hemorrhage vs. the benefit of therapy, available local expertise, surgical accessibility, and the predicted

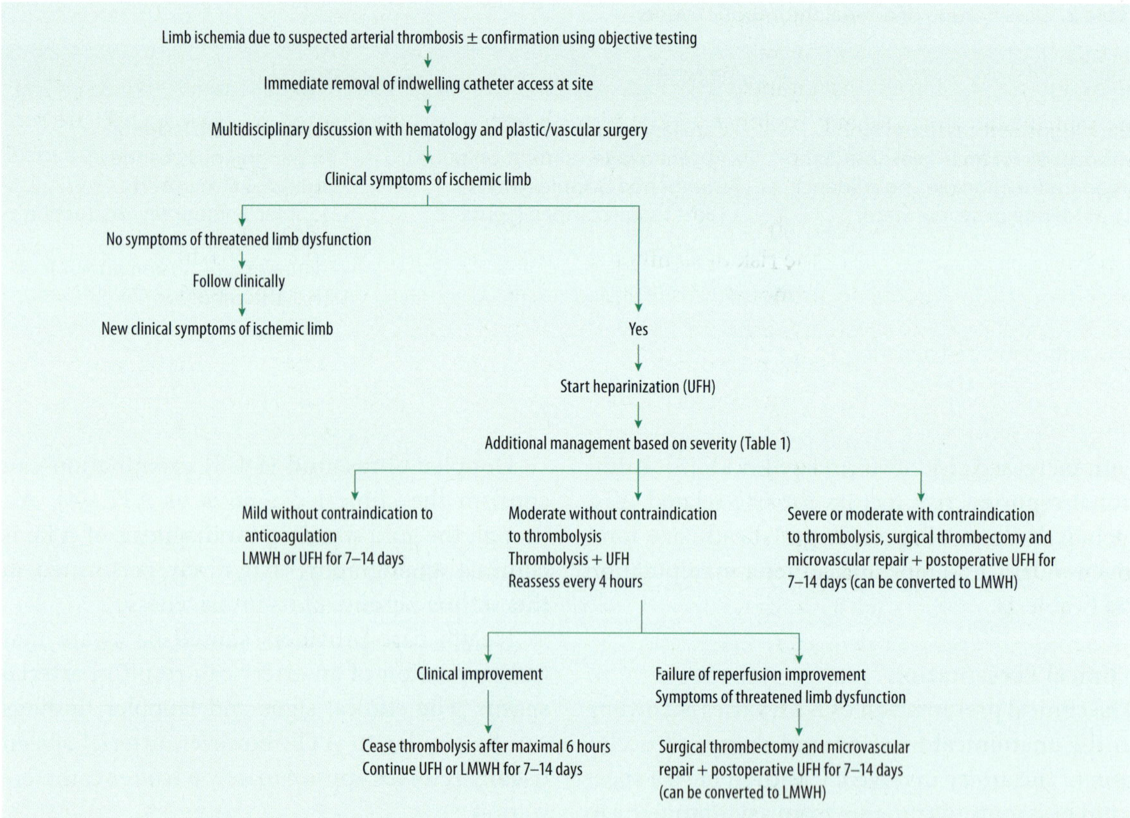

Fig. 1. Acute management of catheter-related arterial thrombosis. For additional therapy after 7–14 days, refer to text. Dosing and monitoring details for UFH, LMWH, and thrombolytic therapy are outlined in Chapter 20. LMWH, low-molecular-weight heparin; UFH, unfractionated heparin.

time course need to be carefully considered in all cases, especially in neonates and severely ill children who are more prone to hemorrhagic complications. In general, a higher risk of losing a limb or essential organ function will inform a recommendation to use a management strategy with higher risks. A multidisciplinary discussion is often required, involving the pediatric hematologist, vascular surgeon, plastic surgeon, interventional radiologist, and neonatologist/pediatrician.

For ATE following CC, therapeutic unfractionated heparin (UFH) should be commenced as an intravenous continuous infusion (see Chapter 20). No UFH bolus should be administered if <4 h have passed since the last dose of UFH given immediately after CC [8]. Low-molecular-weight heparin (LMWH) may be a valuable alternative to UFH and can be used per algorithm (Fig. 1). However, initial therapy with UFH is preferred over LMWH in patients who require more invasive procedures such as surgical thrombectomy or thrombolysis, because of higher bleeding risks associated with these procedures and the full reversibility properties of UFH, in contrast to the partial reversibility properties of LMWH (see Chapter 20).

In case of vasospasm, vasodilators, such as topical nitroglycerine, have been utilized as a therapeutic option either alone or as adjunctive therapy in the management of neonatal peripheral ischemia because of arterial cannulation or venous cannulation, with variable success [10]. However, in premature neonates, topical nitroglycerin should be used with caution because of the risk of significant drug absorption leading to pronounced systemic effects complicated by severe hypotension [10].

A follow-up DUS is usually performed after 7–14 days of therapy. In the case of persistent complete or partial occlusion of the vessel, options include stopping anticoagulation, switching to antiplatelet therapy, i.e., acetylsalicylic acid (ASA), or continuing anticoagulation therapy up to 3 months. The continuation of antithrombotic therapy beyond the first 7–14 days is based on single-center experiences [9, 11, 12]. Currently, no evidence is available to recommend one of these therapeutic options over the other. A case-by-case decision considering the safety and efficacy of each option in the context of the patient is recommended. Dosing and monitoring details for anticoagulation, antiplatelet, and thrombolytic therapy are outlined in detail in Chapter 20. The role of thrombophilia testing in children with ATE is discussed in Chapter 13. There is too little evidence and experience to inform the use of direct oral anticoagulants in this situation.

Prevention

UFH is frequently used to maintain the patency of peripheral arterial catheters. Continuous infusion of UFH in a concentration of 0.5 U/mL of 0.45% NaCl at a rate of 0.11 mL/h for a BW of <1,800 g and of 1 U/mL of 0.45% NaCl at a rate of 0.1–1 mL/h for a BW of >1,800 g is recommended for neonates and children to decrease the incidence of catheter occlusion and prolong the patency of peripheral artery catheters [8]. Intermittent flushes with UFH do not prevent the loss of catheter patency and do not prevent arterial thrombosis.

Considering the current evidence for CC, a bolus dose of at least 50 U/kg UFH is suggested immediately after arterial puncture. For prolonged procedures, further doses of UFH are recommended [8]. In a randomized-controlled study comparing high-dose UFH (100 U/kg bolus followed by age-based continuous infusion) vs. low-dose UFH (50 U/kg bolus) during CC in children, no association was observed between laboratory markers of UFH in plasma and clinical outcome [13]. In addition, a Cochrane review was unable to determine the effects of low-dose (<100 U/kg) vs. high-dose (≥100 U/kg) UFH for the prevention of vascular thrombosis during CC in children [14].

The use of nitroglycerin with various routes of administration and doses was shown to prevent radial artery spasm and occlusion during transradial catheterization in children and adults [15, 16].

UAC-Related Arterial Thrombosis

UACs are primarily used in newborns for monitoring of arterial blood pressure or blood gases and blood sampling. They may be used to give fluids, medications, and nutrition, if no vascular access is available.

The pooled incidence of UAC-related ATE encompassing prospective and retrospective studies was 20% (95% CI: 10–33) [4].

Host-related risk factors for UAC-related ATE include underlying conditions of patients, such as prematurity, respiratory distress syndrome, asphyxia, infection, persistent ductus arteriosus, meconium aspiration, and CHD [4]. Conversely, inherited prothrombotic genetic variants do not appear to increase the risk of UAC-associated ATE [17].

In addition to patient characteristics, there are catheter-related risk factors for UAC-related ATE. For example, longer duration of UAC was found to be associated with an increased risk of

ATE. The adjusted odds ratio for developing ATE for each additional day of using the UAC was 1.2 (95% CI: 1.1–1.3) [17]. Thus, it is strongly recommended to limit the use of UAC to as short period as possible. Several other UAC-related risk factors for ATE have been identified (Table 1). As more proximal placement of the UAC (defined as a position between T_6 and T_{10}) was associated with a lower incidence of clinical vascular complications, this positioning is preferred [8]. End-hole catheters were associated with a significantly decreased risk of aortic thrombosis compared with side-hole catheters. Infusion of hyperosmolar solutions was associated with higher risk of ATE. The size and the material (polyvinyl chloride, polyurethane, or Teflon) of the catheters as well as the type of infused solution have been associated with an increased risk of UAC-related ATE. However, one study comparing two different types of UACs, heparin-bonded polyurethane catheter vs. polyvinyl chloride catheter, did not identify a difference in their thrombogenicity [4].

Clinical Presentation

Systematic ultrasound screening identified UAC-related ATE in 17–32.3%, occurring several days after the UAC was removed [4, 17]. However, only a minority of cases (1–3%) were symptomatic.

The clinical presentation of UAC-related ATE varies according to the anatomical location, including isolated aortic thrombosis or other arteries such as renal artery (unilateral/bilateral), mesenteric arteries, iliac arteries, and/or spinal arteries, as well as the degree of occlusion of the artery involved. In a systematic review, UAC-related ATE was located in the aorta in 90% (95% CI: 72–100) of cases, whereas other locations reported in few studies were the lower extremity arterial system in 66% (95% CI: 6–100) of cases, or thrombosis extending from the aorta to the lower extremity arteries or the renal artery in 43% (95% CI: 31–56) and 22% (95% CI: 3–48) of cases, respectively. The clinical spectrum of UAC-related ATE may range from asymptomatic to a threatened limb or severe organ dysfunction, including [4]:

- acute limb ischemia (nonpalpable lower limb pulses, decreased temperature, and/or skin discoloration of the lower limbs or feet, prolonged capillary refill time, difference in blood pressure of over 10 mm Hg)
- systemic arterial hypertension. The onset of hypertension and narrowing of the pulse pressure may be early signs of UAC-related aortic thrombosis
- congestive heart failure, such as poor feeding
- renal dysfunction with oliguria and/or hematuria
- mesenteric ischemia with necrotizing enterocolitis
- paraplegia presents classically with loss of lower limb motor function and bladder retention if the spinal artery of Adamkiewicz is involved
- other reported clinical findings include evidence of irritability, thrombocytopenia, and/or catheter dysfunction

Classification of aortic thrombosis may be based on the clinical signs and the risk for the related limb or organ (Table 3).

Diagnosis

DUS is the diagnostic test of choice because it is noninvasive and can be performed at the bedside; however, its validity in the diagnosis of UAC-related ATE has not been established [4]. Additional investigations include echocardiography, CC, computed tomography angiography (CTA), magnetic resonance angiography (MRA), and contrast angiography.

Management

Similar to extremity catheter-related ATE, the management of UAC-related ATE is largely dependent on the clinical scenario and the further requirement of the catheter. If possible, the UAC should be removed. The indication for anticoagulation depends on the extent of thrombosis. If there is no contraindication to anticoagulation therapy, UFH or LMWH is suggested for a duration of at least 7–14 days similar to previously reported management of other catheter-related ATE. Nonetheless, there are insufficient data to recommend an optimal treatment modality and/or duration. Duration of antithrombotic therapy may be guided by the clinical (±persistent risk factor) and repeat imaging (complete resolution vs. persistent partial/complete occlusion). Dosing and monitoring details for UFH, LMWH, and thrombolytic therapy in neonates are outlined in Chapter 20.

Cranial ultrasound is recommended before a decision to treat a newborn with anticoagulation or thrombolytic therapy is made [18]. The potential risk of hemorrhage vs. the benefit of anticoagulation needs to be carefully considered in the neonate, particularly in the presence of recent intracranial hemorrhage (ICH) and prematurity. The optimal time to commence anticoagulation in the setting of ICH or other major bleeding events is not clear, and it largely depends on the risk of thrombosis progression and/or recurrence. A reported pooled rate of minor or major treatment-related bleeding in a systematic review was below 0.1% [4]. Serial head ultrasound imaging may be useful in guiding the use of anticoagulation treatment in this setting. If the ATE is potentially life-, organ-, or limb-threatening, thrombolytic or surgical therapy should be considered.

The recommended management of radiographically detected asymptomatic UAC-related ATE is less clear. If the UAC is no longer required, the catheter should be removed. As spontaneous resolution is reported in most cases, close clinical follow-up and administration of anticoagulation therapy only for symptomatic cases seems to be a reasonable option. Similar management should be applied in asymptomatic UAC-related ATE that is radiographically detected after the catheter has been removed.

There are no consistent data to make a firm recommendation for thrombophilia screening for neonates with UAC-related ATE [18, 19]. In general, thrombophilia testing is not suggested in this scenario (see Chapter 13).

The management of renal artery thrombosis and/or mesenteric arterial thrombosis is reported in Chapter 16.

Prevention

Continuous infusion of low-dose UFH (for BW ≤1,800 g: 0.5 U/mL of 0.45% NaCl at a rate of 0.11 mL/h, and for BW >1,800 g: 1 U/mL of 0.45% NaCl; total UFH dose of 25–200 U/kg/day) is recommended to maintain patency of UAC [8]. This dose does not prevent ATE [8].

15

Aortic Thrombosis

Most cases of aortic thrombosis are located in the abdominal aorta and occur in the newborn secondary to UAC (see above).

Spontaneous cases of aortic thrombosis and occurrence beyond the neonatal period are extremely rare. Aortic thrombosis can involve the thoracic aorta as well.

Clinical Presentation

The presentation of aortic thrombosis may vary depending on the location and the extent of the thrombus (Table 3) from being asymptomatic to signs and symptoms of a threatened limb or severe organ dysfunction as detailed above (paragraph UAC-related ATE).

Thoracic aortic thrombosis can present with signs mimicking coarctation, such as poor peripheral perfusion, impaired left ventricular function, and diminished femoral pulses.

Diagnosis

Noninvasive ultrasound studies are usually performed to diagnose aortic thrombosis. However, false-negative ultrasound results have been reported in infants. Additional investigations include echocardiography, CC, CTA, MRA, and contrast angiography.

Table 3. Clinical classification and therapeutic options of aortic thrombosis

	Mild	Moderate	Severe
Signs and symptoms	Decreased femoral pulses Inability to withdraw blood Hypertension	Mild signs *plus* Absent femoral pulses Peripheral ischemia Congestive heart failure	Mild and moderate signs *plus* Severe limb-threatening ischemia Renal failure Visceral involvement Acidosis Sepsis
Therapeutic options	Anticoagulation (UFH or LMWH)	Thrombolysis + UFH If contraindication to thrombolysis, consider surgical thrombectomy followed by postoperative UFH/LMWH	Surgical thrombectomy *plus* postoperative UFH/LMWH

LMWH, low-molecular-weight heparin; UFH, unfractionated heparin. Modified from Nagel et al. [18].

Management

The classification of neonatal aortic thrombosis according to minor, moderate, and major degree of thrombosis was developed in 1992 and can be used to provide a standardized description of thrombosis and for management decisions [18, 20] (Table 3).

Similar to other ATE, the therapeutic options include anticoagulation (LMWH or UFH), thrombolytic therapy, and/or surgical thrombectomy. Therapeutic decisions may be based on the above-mentioned clinical classification (Table 3). A child with aortic thrombosis should be followed closely as severity could increase with time requiring a change in management. The therapeutic recommendations are based on expert opinion, as minimal evidence exists on the management of aortic thrombosis in children. The potential risk of hemorrhage vs. the benefit of therapy, i.e., thrombolysis and anticoagulation, the local expertise, surgical accessibility, and predicted time course need to be carefully considered in all cases, especially in neonates and severely ill children who are more prone to hemorrhagic complications. The optimal duration of anticoagulation therapy for persistent complete or partial aortic thrombosis is not known, and duration of antithrombotic therapy may be guided by the clinical presentation (± persistent risk factor/underlying disease) and repeat imaging (complete resolution vs. persistent partial/complete occlusion). Dosing and monitoring details for anticoagulation and thrombolytic therapy are outlined in detail in Chapter 20.

Arterial Stents – Noncardiac, Non-Central Nervous System

Endovascular arterial stents are used in children for the management of a variety of noncardiac vascular disorders, such as branch pulmonary artery stenosis, coarctation of the aorta, traumatic arterial injuries, arterial dissection, renovascular disease, antiphospholipid syndrome, and hepatic stenosis. The small vessel size in young children increases the risk of thrombosis. There are no studies assessing the role of anticoagulation or antiplatelet therapy to prevent stent occlusion in children. However, for children having endovascular stents inserted, administration of UFH at the time of insertion is suggested [8]. The dose of UFH is not specified in the recommendation; however, the common practice is to give a bolus dose of UFH 100 U/kg as a bolus. A common practice is to then continue with ASA therapy (1–5 mg/kg per dose) for 3–6 months.

Renal Artery Stents

Percutaneous transluminal renal angioplasty, with or without stenting, is a valuable treatment option in pediatric renal artery stenosis. This method is usually undertaken from a femoral arterial approach, with either a long vascular sheath or a guiding catheter. Angioplasty equipment designed for use in adult coronary arteries is ideal for the renal arteries of children and, in particular, in segmental arteries. Intra-arterial UFH (100 U/kg) is given before percutaneous transluminal renal angioplasty [21]. To further minimize the risk of immediate thrombotic complications, LMWH (age-appropriate prophylactic dose) or UFH (at 10 U/kg/h) for 12–24 h can be given after the procedure [21]. Moreover, to promote renal function protection after the acute period of stent insertion, antiplatelet therapy seems to play an important role in the prevention of distal embolization in adult patients. For children, ASA (1–5 mg/kg/dose once daily) is usually prescribed for 3–6 months postrenal artery stent insertion [21].

Noncatheter-Related Arterial Thrombotic Events

Spontaneous or noncatheter-related ATE are rare in children of all ages but more so in neonates and have a high risk of morbidity and mortality [3, 22].

Reported cases of noncatheter ATE have been associated with congenital diseases, including Alagille syndrome (discussed below), primary hyperlipidemia, or hyperhomocysteinemia, or can develop secondary to trauma, circumferential burns of the limbs, or peripheral arterial embolization. In addition, noncatheter-related ATE may develop secondarily to inflammatory vascular diseases, such as Kawasaki's disease (see Chapter 18), Takayasu's arteritis (discussed below), or organ transplantation (see Chapter 16), and may affect specific organ sites, such as liver, kidney, heart, and the central nervous system.

The clinical presentation and management of renal artery thrombosis and hepatic ATE are discussed in Chapter 16. Central nervous system (including spinal cord ischemia) and cardiac-related ATE are discussed in Chapters 17 and 18, respectively. Here, we will specifically address arterial complications related to Takayasu's arteritis, Alagille syndrome, and the midaortic syndrome.

Takayasu's Arteritis

Takayasu's arteritis is a rare large vessel vasculitis, which affects the aorta and major aortic branches. The incidence increases with increasing age. In children, the mean age at onset is 12 years (0.63/100,000) [23]. A higher incidence rate is observed in adult females and in Asian populations.

Takayasu's arteritis presents with local and systemic inflammation, and disease flares with nonspecific symptoms including fever and malaise [24]. Granulomatous inflammation of the arterial wall can result in segmental arterial stenosis, thrombus formation, occlusion, aneurysms, or dissection. In children, the aorta is most commonly inflamed (arch, thoracic, and abdominal) leading to mid aortic syndrome or by carotid, subclavian, renal, and splanchnic artery involvement. End-organ ischemia of the affected arterial territories depends on the location and extent of arterial wall inflammation.

Treatment of this inflammatory disease includes immunosuppressive agents, such as corticosteroids, TNF-alpha-, IL-6-, or JAK inhibitors, and the treatment of midaortic syndrome as outlined below [23].

15

Alagille Syndrome

Alagille syndrome is a rare autosomal dominant genetic disorder of variable penetrance, with pathogenic variants in the *JAG1* or *NOTCH2* genes and an estimated incidence of 1/30,000 births [25]. The gene variants cause abnormal development of intrahepatic bile ducts (chronic cholestasis), and the syndrome can involve the heart (peripheral pulmonary artery stenosis), eyes (posterior embryotoxon, retinopathy), kidneys (dysplastic kidney), skeleton (butterfly vertebrae), and be associated with characteristic facies [26]. In addition, the variants cause defective angiogenesis and subsequent arterial anomalies, including structural abnormalities, aneurysms, aortic coarctation, and stenosis [26–29].

Arterial anomalies can involve the aorta, renal, celiac, mesenterial, subclavian, and cerebral arteries. Midaortic syndrome may be caused by stenosis of the abdominal aorta and its visceral branches – as described below [29, 30].

Some individuals develop Moyamoya syndrome, with progressive stenosis up to occlusion of the carotid artery, with complications including stroke and ICH (see Chapter 17) [26, 27]. Therapy focuses on medical and surgical management of the liver and heart disease, and if necessary, of the midaortic syndrome (see below) and/or Moyamoya syndrome (see Chapter 17) [28].

Midaortic Syndrome

Midaortic syndrome is caused by diffuse or segmental narrowing of the abdominal or distal descending aorta and can involve arterial visceral branches and/or renal arteries [30]. Midaortic syndrome is most often idiopathic but can also be seen in Takayasu's arteritis or Alagille syndrome and other congenital syndromes [23, 29, 31]. It can present as severe hypertension with headaches (in case of renal artery involvement), blood pressure discrepancies between extremities, associated decreased peripheral pulses or even claudication of extremities, bruits over large arteries, abdominal claudication, and failure to thrive. Diagnosis is made with vascular imaging such as contrast angiography, CTA, MRA, or DUS.

Renal hypertension is treated with medical therapy, whereas stenosis with associated clinical symptoms can be treated with endovascular interventions (stent or balloon angioplasty) or revascularization procedures (renal angioplasty, kidney auto transplant, arterial bypass surgery, or the TESLA (tissue expander stimulated lengthening of arteries) or MAGIC (mesenteric artery growth improves circulation) procedures) [30]. Treatment of aortic and arterial thrombosis is previously outlined in this chapter and in Chapter 20.

Complications of Arterial Thrombosis

Like adults, children may develop acute complications or chronic complications after an ATE. Reperfusion syndrome and limb and organ necrosis are significant acute complications of ATE. Chronic complications of ATE depend on the anatomical location of the thrombus, and may manifest as hypertension, renal function impairment, leg length discrepancies, muscle wasting, claudication, chronic pain, paraplegia and loss of arterial access.

Acute Reperfusion Injury

Reperfusion injury occurs when blood supply returns to the tissue after a period of ischemia and results in inflammation and oxidative damage. Acute ischemia-reperfusion injury of the limbs is characterized by edema, compartment syndrome, and neuromuscular dysfunction. Metabolic consequences of reperfusion injury can be variable, ranging from transient symptoms in the limb to systemic inflammation with multiple organ dysfunction [32]. Inflammatory mediators of the reperfusion injury can result in acute lung injury and rhabdomyolysis-induced acute renal failure. Consultation with vascular surgery/plastic surgery is recommended for the comanagement of reperfusion injury, particularly in instances when a vascular injury is present [33]. Prompt fasciotomy is necessary for reducing compartment pressure and limiting the degree of rhabdomyolysis. Treatment of rhabdomyolysis should focus on preventing life-threatening complications from hyperkalemia and preserving renal function. In adults, the use of hypertonic mannitol infusion has been suggested to decrease the need for fasciotomy and minimize neuromuscular dysfunction, but no data exist for pediatric patients. Reconstructive vascular procedures include primary vessel repair (lateral and/or mouth-to-mouth anastomoses), interposition grafts, bypasses, patches, or endovascular techniques. The ideal postrepair anticoagulant regimen is unknown (anticoagulant vs. antiplatelet) and, in general, thrombotic complications postsurgical repair occur in up to 5% of patients, usually within the initial 4 weeks [33].

Long-Term Complications and Peripheral Arterial Insufficiency

Studies on children with CHD complicated by femoral and/or iliac ATE secondary to indwelling arterial catheter or CC have reported a high percentage of persistent occlusion [9, 34]. The prevalence of persistent occlusion was significantly increased in children with CC-related ATE (44–48%) compared with children with indwelling arterial catheter-related ATE (12–14%). The occluded artery increased the risk for leg growth retardation [34]. The loss of arterial access in patients with complex CHD requiring repeated CCs is also a problem [34].

Children with peripheral ATE should be followed regularly for measurement of the extremity length and circumference, and for measurement of the systolic blood pressure in both extremities (ankle-brachial index [ABI]; see below). Some clinicians will follow with DUS imaging 3 and 6 months following the acute event. Subsequently, if imaging findings are stable, only clinical observation is continued. The clinical value and therapeutic consequence for follow-up DUS in peripheral ATE are not clear. However, routine DUS can objectively confirm clinical signs of no or partial resolution of the thrombus and can provide information on the flow in the collaterals.

The ABI is the first-line test for diagnosis of peripheral arterial insufficiency. The ABI is the ratio of the blood pressure in the ankle to the blood pressure in the arm (brachial); an index lower than 0.9 is diagnostic for peripheral arterial insufficiency. Values below 0.8 indicate moderate disease and below 0.5 imply severe arterial insufficiency [34]. If the ABI is abnormal, the next steps for diagnosis are DUS examination, CTA, MRA, and/or contrast angiography study.

Treatment of children with peripheral arterial insufficiency includes the elimination of other risk factors for arterial insufficiency, e.g., smoking, hypertension, hypercholesterolemia, and instructions for regular exercise. No evidence supports the use of medical therapy for children with peripheral arterial insufficiency. If symptoms persist, consultation with a vascular surgeon is recommended for possible balloon angioplasty, stenting, or bypass surgery.

For UAC-related ATE, the reported pooled rate of complete thrombus resolution was 75% (95% CI: 48–96) and 31% (95% CI: 17–47) for partial resolution [4]. The long-term morbidity of UAC-related ATE remains uncertain. Reported complications included chronic arterial hypertension and amputation [4].

Conclusion

Catheter-related ATEs are serious iatrogenic complications seen mainly in the neonatal and pediatric intensive care units and following CCs. Noncatheter-related ATEs are very rare in children of all ages. Treatment strategies for ATE in children for all ages and causes (catheter and noncatheter related) may vary widely depending on the clinical situation and can impact short-term and long-term outcomes. Data from pediatric cohorts suggest that early recognition and more aggressive therapeutic approaches, i.e., initiation of anticoagulation therapy in most patients and in severe cases that do not respond to medical antithrombotic therapy, the usage of interventional therapies (such as thrombolytic therapy and/or endovascular or surgical thrombectomy) may result in improved short-term and long-term outcomes [3, 22, 34].

Acknowledgments

Our special thanks go to Dr. M. Patricia Massicotte and Dr. Shoshana Revel-Vilk (who were the authors of this chapter in the first and second editions of this Handbook), which provided a valuable background for this updated chapter. We dedicate this chapter to the memory of Dr. M. Patricia Massicotte who passed away in 2020.

Conflict of Interest Statement

Mattia Rizzi declares no potential conflicts of interest related to this work. Anthony K.C. Chan declares no potential conflicts of interest related to this work. Alessandra Bosch received research grants from Rudolf-Marx Research Grant of the German Society for Thrombosis and Haemostasis Research e.g., (GTH) and from the Clinical Medicine Plus Scholarship of the Prof. Dr. Max Cloetta Foundation. Manuela Albisetti declares no potential conflicts of interest related to this work.

Author Contributions

Mattia Rizzi drafted the chapter, critically revised the chapter, and approved the final version. Anthony K.C. Chan critically revised the chapter and approved the final version. Alessandra Bosch drafted the chapter, critically revised the chapter, and approved the final version. Manuela Albisetti drafted the chapter, critically revised the chapter, and approved the final version.

Abbreviations

ABI	Ankle-brachial index
ASA	Acetylsalicylic acid
ATE	Arterial thromboembolism/thromboembolic event
BW	Body weight
CC	Cardiac catheterization
CTA	Computed tomography angiography
DUS	Doppler ultrasound
EIC	Extremity indwelling arterial catheter
ICH	Intracranial hemorrhage
LMWH	Low-molecular-weight heparin
MRA	Magnetic resonance angiography
UAC	Umbilical artery catheter
UFH	Unfractionated heparin

References

1 Price VE, Chan AK. Arterial thrombosis in children. Expert Rev Cardiovasc Ther. 2008;6:419–28.
2 Tuckuviene R, Christensen AL, Helgestad J, Johnsen SP, Kristensen SR. Pediatric venous and arterial noncerebral thromboembolism in Denmark: a nationwide population-based study. J Pediatr. 2011;159:663–9.
3 Monagle P, Newall F, Barnes C, Savoia H, Campbell J, Wallace T, et al. Arterial thromboembolic disease: a single-centre case series study. J Paediatr Child Health. 2008;44:28–32.
4 Rizzi M, Goldenberg N, Bonduel M, Revel-Vilk S, Amankwah E, Albisetti M. Catheter-related arterial thrombosis in neonates and children: a systematic review. Thromb Haemost. 2018;118:1058–66.
5 Brotschi B, Hug MI, Kretschmar O, Rizzi M, Albisetti M. Incidence and predictors of cardiac catheterisation-related arterial thrombosis in children. Heart. 2015;101:948–53.
6 Brotschi B, Hug MI, Latal B, Neuhaus D, Buerki C, Kroiss S, et al. Incidence and predictors of indwelling arterial catheter-related thrombosis in children. J Thromb Haemost. 2011;9:1157–62.
7 Rizzi M, Albisetti M. Treatment of arterial thrombosis in children: methods and mechanisms. Thromb Res. 2018;169:113–9.
8 Monagle P, Chan AKC, Goldenberg NA, Ichord RN, Journeycake JM, Nowak-Göttl U, et al. Antithrombotic therapy in neonates and children: Antithrombotic Therapy and Prevention of Thrombosis, 9th ed: American College of Chest Physicians Evidence-Based Clinical Practice Guidelines. Chest. 2012;141(2 suppl):e737S–801S.

9 Crameri O, Brotschi B, Achini F, Rizzi M, Albisetti M. Treatment of catheter-related arterial thrombosis in children: a 15-year single-center experience. J Pediatr. 2021;239:182–6.
10 Mosalli R, Khayyat W, Al Qarni S, Al Matrafi A, El Baz M, Paes B. Topical nitroglycerin in newborns with ischemic injuries: a systematic review. Saudi Pharm J. 2021;29:764–74.
11 Cohen CT, Anderson V, Desai SB, Arunachalam A, Ahmed M, Diaz R. Patient characteristics and treatment outcomes of symptomatic catheter-related arterial thrombosis in infants: a retrospective cohort study. J Pediatr. 2021; 231:215–22.
12 Glatz AC, Keashen R, Chang J, Balsama LA, Dori Y, Gillespie MJ, et al. Outcomes using a clinical practice pathway for the management of pulse loss following pediatric cardiac catheterization. Catheter Cardiovasc Interv. 2015;85:111–7.
13 Hanslik A, Kitzmuller E, Tran US, Thom K, Karapetian H, Prutsch N, et al. Monitoring unfractionated heparin in children: a parallel-cohort randomized controlled trial comparing 2 dose protocols. Blood. 2015;126:2091–7.
14 Avila ML, Shah PS, Brandao LR. Different unfractionated heparin doses for preventing arterial thrombosis in children undergoing cardiac catheterization. Cochrane Database Syst Rev. 2020; 2:CD010196.
15 Abdelazeem B, Abuelazm MT, Swed S, Gamal M, Atef M, Al-Zeftawy MA, et al. The efficacy of nitroglycerin to prevent radial artery spasm and occlusion during and after transradial catheterization: a systematic review and meta-analysis of randomized controlled trials. Clin Cardiol. 2022;45:1171–83.
16 Jang YE, Ji SH, Kim EH, Lee JH, Kim HS, Mossad EB, et al. Subcutaneous nitroglycerin for radial arterial catheterization in pediatric patients: a randomized controlled trial. Anesthesiology. 2020; 133:53–63.
17 Revel-Vilk S, Ergaz Z. Diagnosis and management of central-line-associated thrombosis in newborns and infants. Semin Fetal Neonatal Med. 2011;16: 340–4.
18 Nagel K, Tuckuviene R, Paes B, Chan AK. Neonatal aortic thrombosis: a comprehensive review. Klin Padiatr. 2010; 222:134–9.
19 Raffini L. Thrombophilia in children: who to test, how, when, and why? Hematology Am Soc Hematol Educ Program. 2008:228–35.
20 Colburn MD, Gelabert HA, Quinones-Baldrich W. Neonatal aortic thrombosis. Surgery. 1992;11:21–8.
21 Tullus K, Roebuck DJ. Renovascular hypertension in small children – is it Takayasu arteritis or fibromuscular dysplasia? J Am Soc Hypertens. 2018;12: 506–8.
22 Rashish G, Paes BA, Nagel K, Chan AK, Thomas S; Thrombosis and Hemostasis in Newborns (THiN) Group. Spontaneous neonatal arterial thromboembolism: infants at risk, diagnosis, treatment, and outcomes. Blood Coagul Fibrinolysis. 2013;24:787–97.
23 Aeschlimann FA, Yeung RSM, Laxer RM. An update on childhood-onset Takayasu arteritis. Front Pediatr. 2022; 10:872313.
24 Aeschlimann FA, Twilt M, Yeung RSM. Childhood-onset Takayasu arteritis. Eur J Rheumatol. 2020;7(suppl1):S58–66.
25 Habash N, Ibrahim SH. The Global Alagille Alliance study: redefining the natural history of Alagille syndrome. Hepatology. 2023;77:347–9.
26 Turnpenny PD, Ellard S. Alagille syndrome: pathogenesis, diagnosis and management. Eur J Hum Genet. 2012; 20:251–7.
27 Kamath BM, Spinner NB, Emerick KM, Chudley AE, Booth C, Piccoli DA, et al. Vascular anomalies in Alagille syndrome: a significant cause of morbidity and mortality. Circulation. 2004;109: 1354–8.
28 Kohaut J, Pommier R, Guerin F, Pariente D, Jacquemin E, Martelli H, et al. Abdominal arterial anomalies in children with Alagille syndrome: surgical aspects and outcomes of liver transplantation. J Pediatr Gastroenterol Nutr. 2017;64:888–91.
29 Salem JE, Bruguiere E, Iserin L, Guiochon-Mantel A, Plouin PF. Hypertension and aortorenal disease in Alagille syndrome. J Hypertens. 2012;30:1300–6.
30 Lazea C, Al-Khzouz C, Sufana C, Miclea D, Asavoaie C, Filimon I, et al. Diagnosis and management of genetic causes of middle aortic syndrome in children: a comprehensive literature review. Ther Clin Risk Manag. 2022;18:233–48.
31 Delis KT, Gloviczki P. Middle aortic syndrome: from presentation to contemporary open surgical and endovascular treatment. Perspect Vasc Surg Endovasc Ther. 2005;17(3):187–203.
32 Eliason JL, Wakefield TW. Metabolic consequences of acute limb ischemia and their clinical implications. Semin Vasc Surg. 2009;22:29–33.
33 Wahlgren CM, Kragsterman B. Management and outcome of pediatric vascular injuries. J Trauma Acute Care Surg. 2015;79:563–7.
34 Rizzi M, Kroiss S, Kretschmar O, Forster I, Brotschi B, Albisetti M. Long-term outcome of catheter-related arterial thrombosis in infants with congenital heart disease. J Pediatr. 2016;170:181–7.

15

Chapter 16

Published online: December 5, 2024

Blanchette VS, Brandão LR, Carcao MD, Kumar R, Rand ML, Revel-Vilk S (eds): SickKids Handbook of Pediatric Thrombosis and Hemostasis, ed 3, rev. and ext. Basel, Karger, 2024, pp 288–306 (DOI: 10.1159/000538205)

Thromboembolic Events at Specific Organ Sites

Veerle Labarque[a] Noa Mandel-Shorer[b] Jeremy Robertson[c] Suzan Williams[d]

[a]Department of Pediatric Hematology-Oncology, University Hospitals Leuven, Leuven, Belgium; [b]Department of Pediatric Hematology-Oncology, Ruth Rappaport Children's Hospital, Rambam Health Care Campus, Haifa, Israel; [c]Haematology & Haemophilia Service, Queensland Children's Hospital, South Brisbane, QLD, Australia; [d]Division of Hematology/Oncology, The Hospital for Sick Children, Toronto, ON, Canada

Introduction

Thromboembolic events (TEs), occurring with and without underlying risk factors, most frequently involve the deep venous, peripheral arterial, and central nervous systems. Although rare, TEs may occur in the renal and hepatic veins and arteries as well as other abdominal vessels such as portal, splenic, and mesenteric veins or mesenteric arteries. These TEs may be associated with significant morbidity and mortality, posing a challenge for the caregiver.

In this chapter, we describe TEs in the kidney, liver, splanchnic system, and retinal vessels with focus on clinical presentation, diagnosis, and management. Because of the rarity of such events in children, most of the information related to management summarized herein is based on expert opinion and extrapolation from adult literature.

Kidney-Related TEs

Renal Vein Thrombosis

Renal vein thrombosis (RVT) is uncommon but is predominantly a disease of children, primarily affecting newborns [1]. RVT accounts for 16–20% of all TEs in newborns and is the most prevalent noncatheter-related cause of TEs outside the central nervous system during the neonatal period [1]. Almost 80% of all RVT presents within the first month of life, one-third of which are diagnosed in the first week. Some cases develop in utero and are detected prenatally [1]. Males are more commonly affected than females (2:1 ratio). In approximately 70% of the cases, neonatal RVT is unilateral, with left-sided predominance. Extension of the thrombus into the inferior vena cava (IVC) occurs in 40% of patients. Coexisting risk factors, other than the presence of a central venous catheter (CVC), such as perinatal asphyxia, maternal diabetes, dehydration, infection, and cyanotic congenital heart disease, are found in up to 80% of the affected neonates [1] (Table 1). A

Table 1. Predisposing conditions for neonatal and childhood renal vein thrombosis

Neonates
Umbilical venous catheter
Perinatal asphyxia
Infant of a diabetic mother
Dehydration, shock
Infection
Prematurity
Cyanotic congenital heart disease
Older children
Dehydration, shock
Acute blood loss
Nephrotic syndrome
Renal transplantation
Consumptive coagulopathy
Angiographic studies
Corticosteroids

predisposing condition and/or prothrombotic state may also be present in children (Table 1).

Clinical Presentation

Neonates may be asymptomatic, but most have at least one of the three cardinal RVT signs at presentation: hematuria (56%); thrombocytopenia (48%); and palpable flank mass (45%) [1]. Of note, the entire classic triad occurs in less than a quarter of cases. Other possible presenting symptoms include vomiting, pallor, metabolic acidosis with electrolyte abnormalities, proteinuria, renal impairment, disseminated intravascular coagulation, and shock.

Diagnosis

Accurate and prompt diagnosis requires a high level of clinical suspicion. The diagnosis can be suspected on the basis of hematuria and renal masses in the presence of predisposing factors and can be confirmed on imaging.

Because of its wide availability, practicality, sensitivity, and lack of adverse effects, Doppler ultrasonography has gained popularity over renal venography and has become the first-line investigation of choice [1]. Findings vary according to the time of onset, severity, extent of the thrombus, and development of collateral circulation. Gray-scale ultrasound demonstrates globular enlargement of the kidney, increased echogenicity, and attenuation or loss of corticomedullary differentiation, whereas color Doppler ultrasound (DUS) detects high arterial resistance or absent flow in the renal veins. However, the performance to detect a thrombus is poor. Alternatively, computed tomography (CT) angiography and magnetic resonance venography display an almost 100% sensitivity to detect a thrombus in the renal veins and may therefore be required in case of unclear initial imaging on ultrasonography. Details regarding the role of a prothrombotic work-up are outlined in Chapter 13.

Management

During the acute phase, a collaborative approach amongst subspecialists (neonatologists, radiologists, pediatric hematologists, and pediatric nephrologists) is essential. All children with RVT need urgent treatment of concurrent shock, sepsis, cyanosis, and electrolyte imbalances. In severe cases, renal replacement therapy (e.g., peritoneal dialysis/hemodialysis/continuous renal replacement therapy) may be needed.

Regarding the role of anticoagulation, a review of retrospective case series reported no difference in renal outcomes irrespective of whether the infant received no anticoagulation, unfractionated heparin (UFH), or low-molecular-weight heparin (LMWH), as approximately 75% of affected kidneys become atrophic regardless of treatment [2]. However, prospective controlled trials are needed to generate evidence-based recommendations on anticoagulation treatment of RVT. The potential risk of thrombus extension without anticoagulation must be balanced against the bleeding risk imposed by using anticoagulation.

The current American Society of Hematology guidelines [3] suggest anticoagulation in neonates with RVT because of potential long-term beneficial effect of reducing hypertension and/or renal damage. Possible benefit of anticoagulation may be more pertinent with high thrombus burden, such as with bilateral involvement or with thrombus extension into the IVC. Nevertheless, treatment decisions should also take into account the potential bleeding risk associated with anticoagulation, as it varies with severity of disease, age, gestational age, and degree of thrombocytopenia. Similarly, the degree of residual renal function may help on the decision-making process. The presence or absence of thrombophilia is not relevant for determining initial therapy. In case of an in situ umbilical venous catheter, it remains unclear whether the catheter should be removed at diagnosis, in association with supportive therapy and radiologic monitoring, and whether anticoagulation should be withheld until extension occurs, or initiated prior to catheter removal.

For the management of neonates with unilateral RVT with or without extension into the IVC, starting anticoagulation is suggested, unless there is a contraindication (e.g., severe intraventricular hemorrhage). In life-threatening (i.e., bilateral) cases of RVT, initial thrombolysis followed by anticoagulation rather than anticoagulation alone is suggested. If there is a strong suspicion of bilateral fetal RVT, delivery should be considered and postnatal treatment will not be different from the management of noncatheter-related neonatal RVT. As LMWH may accumulate in the presence of renal impairment, it is preferable to start therapy with UFH in those patients or to reduce the dose of LMWH and adjust it according to the anti-Xa level monitoring. Particularly in younger patients, the efficacy and safety of direct oral anticoagulants (DOACs) is less studied, as the pediatric trials published to date included a minimal number of neonates, infants, and toddlers. Duration of anticoagulation treatment may be guided by radiological imaging to determine status of thrombosis, assessed risk, and benefit of continued anticoagulation. Longer duration of anticoagulation may be considered in the setting of thrombus progression, presence of proximal extension of the thrombosis, and bilateral RVT with IVC or atrial involvement. Dosing and monitoring details for anticoagulation and thrombolytic therapy in neonates are outlined in Chapter 20.

There are no evidence-based recommendations for treatment of RVT in non-neonates (i.e., infants and children older than 1 month of age at the time of presentation). Of note, particularly in older pediatric patients, non-neonatal RVT may occur in the setting of nephrotic syndrome or with systemic lupus erythematosus complicated by systemic lupus erythematosus-related proteinuria. Similar to treating adults with RVT, the main goal of therapy should be the preservation of renal parenchyma and prevention of embolic events. Therefore, we suggest prompt initiation of anticoagulation with UFH or LMWH in the absence of contraindications. In older patients, pending the renal clearance being affected by either the acute RVT or any potential underlying renal disease, DOACs less prone to renal accumulation (e.g., apixaban) may be considered. If a child presents with an acute onset of symptoms, thrombolysis followed by anticoagulation should be considered. Although nephrectomy may eventually be required to control resulting hypertension, surgery has limited utility in the acute treatment of RVT [1]. Dosing and monitoring details for anticoagulation and thrombolytic therapy in children are outlined in Chapter 20.

Outcome

Although mortality rates are low, morbidity is considerable. In almost half of the neonates, RVT is associated with adrenal hemorrhage [2]. Other acute complications of RVT include paradoxical arterial ischemic stroke, pulmonary embolism (PE), and cerebral sinovenous thrombosis [1]. Long-term outcomes depend on severity and laterality of kidney involvement and may vary from normal renal function to end-stage renal disease. Atrophy of the affected kidney occurs in 75% of cases. Approximately 20% of children develop hypertension on long-term follow-up, and 3% of children develop end-stage renal disease requiring renal replacement therapy (e.g., hemodialysis/peritoneal dialysis and even renal transplantation). Overall, children with a history of RVT have a 15.5-fold risk of hypertension, chronic kidney disease, or all-cause mortality. Hence, they warrant long-term close follow-up of growth, blood pressure, renal function, and urinalysis and should be followed regularly by a nephrologist. Renal DUS should be performed at regular intervals to monitor the sizes of, and blood flow to, the affected kidney(s) [1].

Renal Artery Thrombosis

Renal artery thrombosis (RAT) is extremely rare in children, with a paucity of informative literature available to aid clinical decisions. It is most commonly reported following renal transplantation but may also occur after blunt abdominal trauma. Rarely, it has been identified in inflammatory vascular conditions, including Takayasu's arteritis, Behcet's disease, or Alagille syndrome (Chapter 15). Traumatic RAT is usually unilateral, the left side is involved more often, almost never occurs as an isolated event, and indicates major associated injuries. Rare cases can occur in the neonatal period; however, neonatal RAT is less common than RVT but strongly associated with umbilical catheters and patent ductus arteriosus.

Clinical Presentation

The clinical symptoms of acute RAT include steady, aching flank pain, abdominal pain, fever, nausea, vomiting, and hematuria. Acute renal failure may develop. The presentation of chronic progressive thrombosis is often silent, causing refractory hypertension and leading to chronic kidney disease.

History of a kidney transplant or trauma to the back or abdomen may be helpful.

Diagnosis

Renal ultrasound findings can be minimal unless Doppler imaging is used. In the absence of renal failure, contrast-enhanced CT scan is the modality of choice for diagnosis, for prediction of the level of occlusion and follow-up of RAT. Angiography is equally useful for predicting the blockage and can be relied upon if segmental obstruction to the blood flow is present. Unlike CT scan, angiography will not be helpful to delineate the extent of associated injuries but can be helpful to discern between RAT and renal artery stenosis. Magnetic resonance imaging (MRI), magnetic resonance angiography, and unenhanced magnetic resonance angiography techniques constitute promising alternatives for the evaluation of vascular complications following renal transplantation and renal artery stenosis [4].

Management

RAT must be diagnosed and treated as soon as possible to avoid progressive and permanent loss of renal function. The optimal treatment for RAT is uncertain, given the absence of comparative studies. Conservative treatment with anticoagulation is reserved for unilateral cases [5]. For bilateral RAT and RAT in a solitary kidney, revascularization is usually indicated [5]. It can be performed either surgically or more preferably by less invasive percutaneous techniques. Local thrombolysis or thrombectomy with minimally invasive percutaneous endovascular therapy for acute occlusions of the main renal artery or significant branch can be considered.

Prevention

In the setting of renal transplantation, a systematic review has suggested that prophylactic antithrombotic management could reduce the risk of renal vessel thrombosis. However, because of the nonexperimental design of the studies included and data heterogeneity, the authors could not make strong recommendations in favor or against the use of prophylaxis in these patients [6].

Hemodialysis-Related Thrombosis

CVCs and arteriovenous fistulae are frequently used to gain vascular access for hemodialysis in children, both of which are associated with thrombotic complications. Immediate failure of the vascular access is caused by technical problems, whereas late dysfunction usually results from an intraluminal thrombus or a thrombus at the tip of the catheter. CVC-related TEs may occur in the right atrium, on the vessel wall, or may completely occlude the vessel causing a deep vein thrombosis (DVT). In addition, formation of a fibrin sheath that can elongate and cover the intake and outflow holes of the catheter may lead to catheter dysfunction or catheter-related infection, shortening the survival of the CVC. Factors that increase the risk of CVC-related TEs include larger catheters relative to the size of the vessel and the fluid shifts occurring during intermittent dialysis. Alternatively to CVCs, renal failure patients may rely on arteriovenous fistulas to undergo dialysis treatment. A thrombus in an arteriovenous fistula mainly develops as a consequence of venous stasis produced by stenotic lesions. Excessive vessel compression after needle withdrawal to avoid bleeding and dialysis-related hypotensive episodes are contributors to thrombus formation, and major inherited (e.g., protein C/S and antithrombin deficiencies) or acquired (e.g., antiphospholipid syndrome) prothrombotic risk factors may also play a role on increasing the risk.

Clinical Presentation

A CVC-related TE in the setting of hemodialysis may present solely as catheter malfunction but may also lead to right atrial thrombosis and/or DVT. The clinical presentation of these TEs is detailed in Chapter 14. An intraluminal thrombus results in a blocked catheter (i.e., the catheter is unable to deliver the required blood flow).

Thrombosis of an arteriovenous fistula can present with the absence of a thrill (vibration), discontinuous bruit, or edema distal to the fistula. Occasionally, thrombosis of the arteriovenous fistula may only be noted during the dialysis session because of difficulties with cannulation, aspiration of thrombi, inability to achieve the target dialysis blood flow, or prolonged bleeding from the needle puncture sites.

Diagnosis

CVC-related TE in the setting of hemodialysis is diagnosed with a similar approach as described for a CVC-related DVT and/or blocked CVC (see Chapter 14). In case of an arteriovenous fistula, close monitoring (presence of a thrill, growth of the fistula, surveillance using noninvasive DUS), and collaboration with a vascular surgeon is important for early diagnosis of complications, prolonged patency, and fewer TEs. Abnormalities on physical examination of the arteriovenous fistula or problems during the dialysis session should prompt a fistulogram to diagnose a stenosis and/or thrombosis of the fistula.

Management

Management of a blocked CVC used for hemodialysis is similar to the management of a blocked CVC in nonhemodialysis patients (see Chapter 14). Similarly, management of DVT related to a CVC used for hemodialysis is similar to the management of DVT related to CVC in nonhemodialysis patients. The dose of LMWH should be reduced upfront in renal insufficiency, as elimination happens primarily via the kidney. Close monitoring of the anti-Xa level is important, as accumulation may occur (see Chapter 20). In addition, there are no evidence-based guidelines to suggest whether LMWH should be administered prior to or after the hemodialysis session. As predicting long-term drug elimination may be challenging in the setting of hemodialysis, we suggest administration of LMWH after the dialysis session. In terms of preferable DOACs in patients with reduced renal clearance, although studies investigating apixaban (Eliquis) in adult patients on dialysis are promising, the use of DOACs has not been approved in this setting. Moreover, there are no pediatric data available yet.

Stenosis of an arteriovenous fistula may be managed by percutaneous transluminal angioplasty and stent placement. However, once thrombosis has occurred, urgent surgical revision is the standard treatment. Today, percutaneous endovascular correction of the thrombosed arteriovenous fistula has become a valid alternative option and includes purely mechanical thrombectomy or pharmacomechanical thrombolysis using tissue plasminogen activator (tPA).

Prevention

Many approaches to prevent CVC dysfunction have been proposed and are mainly based on the use of anticoagulant or thrombolytic CVC locks. The use of tPA (1 mg/mL) has been shown to be more effective than high-dose heparin (5,000 U/mL) in reducing intraluminal thrombus formation between hemodialysis sessions. However, the benefit of tPA as a routine CVC lock requires further studies.

Vitamin K antagonist (VKA) or LMWH have been used between hemodialysis sessions to prevent TEs of the arteriovenous fistula or the CVC used for hemodialysis [7]. In a small cohort, it has been shown that a prophylactic dose of enoxaparin (Clexane) of 0.5 mg/kg/day was effective in preventing TEs in the majority of patients (anti-factor Xa levels: peak 0.25–0.5 U/mL); in patients at high risk for TEs, dosing at 1 mg/kg/day may be necessary (anti-factor Xa level: peak 0.5–1 U/mL) [8].

During hemodialysis, anticoagulation with LMWH or UFH is recommended to prevent thrombosis within the artificial circuit, independent of the type of vascular access used [7]. Nevertheless, clinical practice varies from dosing according to body weight to empirical dosing, even in children. Most authors recommend calculating the appropriate dose based on body weight (e.g., enoxaparin [Clexane]: 0.5–1 mg/kg/day; UFH: a loading dose of 50 U/kg, followed by a maintenance infusion at 25 U/kg/h or a loading dose of 50 U/kg followed by a second bolus of 25 U/kg halfway through the dialysis session) [9], and adjustments can be based on clinical signs and/or laboratory monitoring (i.e., activated clotting time or activated partial thromboplastin time; see Chapter 20). The most frequently used nonheparin anticoagulant is citrate (hypertonic sodium citrate or 3% acid citrate dextrose). As the half-life of citrate is minutes, this anticoagulant option offers the potential to anticoagulate the circuit but not the patient. The activated clotting time test can be used to monitor the anticoagulant effect of citrate, whereas calcium levels should be monitored to detect hypocalcemia.

Finally, in addition to a systemic pharmacological treatment, local interventions including unique catheter designs, advanced coating technologies, and new surgical techniques may be beneficial in preventing thrombosis of CVCs for hemodialysis or arteriovenous fistula, but discussing these is beyond the scope of this handbook.

Nephrotic Syndrome-Associated Thrombosis

Thrombotic complications are not rare in children with nephrotic syndrome. The overall incidence is about 3% but may increase to 10% or even 25% in children with congenital nephrotic syndrome or membranous nephropathy, respectively [10]. The incidence seems higher at the time of first presentation of nephrotic syndrome, but TEs were also reported at relapses. The most important risk factors for nephrotic syndrome-associated TE are age (<1 year; ≥12 years) and severity of proteinuria [11].

The pathophysiology of nephrotic syndrome-associated TEs is thought to be multifactorial including a genetic predisposition as well as acquired thrombophilia, hyperlipidemia, diuretics, and hemoconcentration [10]. Acquired thrombophilia occurs as a result of increased procoagulant activity (i.e., increased production of fibrinogen, factor V, and factor VIII by the liver), increased platelet activation and aggregability, reduced natural anticoagulant activity (i.e., urinary loss of antithrombin, protein S), and reduced fibrinolysis [10].

Both venous and arterial TEs have been described. The majority of the events (76.3%) are a lower limb DVT [11], followed by TEs in the IVC, and they are most frequently associated with the presence of CVC. PE has been found in up to 28% of children, whereas RVT, a well-known complication in adults with nephrotic syndrome, occurs less commonly in children, except for infants with congenital nephrotic syndrome. Involvement of cerebral vessels has also been reported and has probably been underdiagnosed in the past. Peripheral artery thrombosis is usually secondary to arterial punctures or arterial catheters.

Clinical Presentation

Symptoms of TEs in children with nephrotic syndrome are the same as those of children without nephrotic syndrome and are described in the relevant chapters (Chapters 14 [DVT or PE], 15 [arterial TE], and 17 [arterial and venous strokes]). TEs in children with nephrotic syndrome may also be subclinical [11].

Diagnosis

Diagnostic measures in children with nephrotic syndrome do not differ from the methods used in children without nephrotic syndrome and are described in Chapters 14, 15, and 17. Special consideration should be paid in the setting of decreased renal function, as iodinated contrast, as well as gadolinium, should be used with caution.

Management

The initial treatment of TEs in children with nephrotic syndrome is similar to children without nephrotic syndrome as discussed in the relevant chapters (Chapters 14, 15, and 17). It is recommended to continue anticoagulation therapy until the nephrotic syndrome is no longer active. As antithrombin levels may be low, LMWH treatment is preferred. In children who do not rapidly go into remission, VKA may be a useful alternative. The use of DOACs is emerging in adults with nephrotic syndrome, but the efficacy and safety in pediatric patients requires further evaluation. In addition to anticoagulation and/or thrombolysis or thrombectomy, it is crucial to simultaneously control the activity of the nephrotic syndrome. Close collaboration with a pediatric nephrologist is important for the management of these patients.

Prevention

Several nonpharmacologic strategies to limit the likelihood of a TE in childhood nephrotic syndrome may be considered, including regular ambulation, adequate hydration, avoidance of CVCs whenever possible, and the use of graduated compression stockings for bedridden children. The appropriateness of prophylactic anticoagulation in all patients with nephrotic syndrome continues to be highly debated. Current guidelines recommend prophylactic anticoagulation at times of active nephrotic syndrome recurrence for children with a previous history of a venous TE [7] or for children with congenital nephrotic syndrome who are at increased thrombotic risk (i.e., acute illness, dehydration, presence of a CVC, thrombocytosis), but clinical trials establishing benefits and risks of prophylactic anticoagulation in childhood nephrotic syndrome are lacking. Interval re-evaluation of long-term prophylaxis in children with congenital nephrotic syndrome is suggested. What to do in children with a previous catheter-related TE, who have no CVC at the time of nephrotic syndrome recurrence also remains an unanswered question.

According to the current practice at The Hospital for Sick Children (SickKids), all children with a history of nephrotic syndrome-associated TE are started on prophylactic anticoagulation as soon as recurrent prominent proteinuria (albumin-to-creatinine ratio: 30–300 mg/g) occurs. As children with severe congenital nephrotic syndrome are at high risk for TE, they receive anticoagulation to target therapeutic levels, at times of active disease even in the absence of a previous TE. Of note, achieving adequate thromboprophylaxis in congenital nephrotic syndrome can be challenging and requires close drug monitoring. For congenital nephrotic syndrome patients in critically ill conditions complicated by a thrombotic event, given that heparinoids rely on circulating antithrombin levels to reach their therapeutic effect that will likely be reduced, the use of direct thrombin inhibitors (i.e., bivalirudin) or the concomitant infusion of antithrombin concentrate may be considered (see Chapter 20).

Liver-Related TEs

Portal Vein Thrombosis

Portal vein thrombosis (PVT) is a major cause of extrahepatic portal hypertension and an important cause of variceal bleeding in children. Although the thrombosis might date back to the newborn period (i.e., related to the use of umbilical catheter), presentation may occur later. PVT is also a well-known vascular complication of liver transplantation in children, associated with the difficult reconstitution of the portal vein, especially in living donor transplantation. Intra-abdominal sepsis, umbilical venous catheterization in the newborn period, prothrombotic abnormalities, and cirrhosis are the most frequent risk factors in nontransplanted children. Other possible risk factors include splenectomy and sickle cell anemia. An underlying etiology is not identified in approximately 50% of children with PVT [12].

Clinical Presentation

PVT in children is usually diagnosed as part of the investigation for splenomegaly, upper gastrointestinal bleeding (from esophageal varices), or peripheral (pan)cytopenia (because of increased destruction of blood cells resulting from hypersplenism). In neonates, thrombocytopenia may be seen at the time of diagnosis, but this is usually secondary to other concomitant conditions [12]. In children, mild elevation of alanine aminotransferase may be seen, but liver function is usually normal. Transient ascites can occur in acute PVT, but in chronic PVT, ascites is rarely seen even in the presence of significant portal hypertension, unless the PVT is a complication of already-established cirrhosis.

Diagnosis

Abdominal ultrasound with color Doppler remains the imaging modality of choice to diagnose PVT. In acute PVT, findings may be limited to the loss of flow in the portal vein, evidence of progressive splenomegaly and, occasionally, ascites. However, the accuracy of DUS depends on technical factors such as the skills of the sonographer, patient cooperation, and the presence of abdominal gas and anatomic variations, which may preclude the visualization of the portal vein and its collaterals. Typical findings in chronic PVT include loss of visualization of the main portal vein for at least part of its length, associated cavernous transformation around the portal vein at the porta hepatis, splenomegaly, and the presence of portosystemic collaterals, e.g., at the splenic hilum or around the stomach and esophagus. Other investigations (such as CT scan, MRI, and angiography) may also identify PVT, with MRI performing at least as well or better than CT [12]. However, those modalities have limited utility because of their disadvantages, including the use of ionizing radiation, need for sedation, accessibility, and/or invasiveness.

Management

Currently, there is little evidence for a net benefit from anticoagulation in patients with PVT. However, if the PVT is identified in the acute phase (within approximately 2–4 weeks of its likely occurrence for neonatal PVT, or while the underlying condition associated with a hypercoagulable state is still present for non-neonatal PVT), the

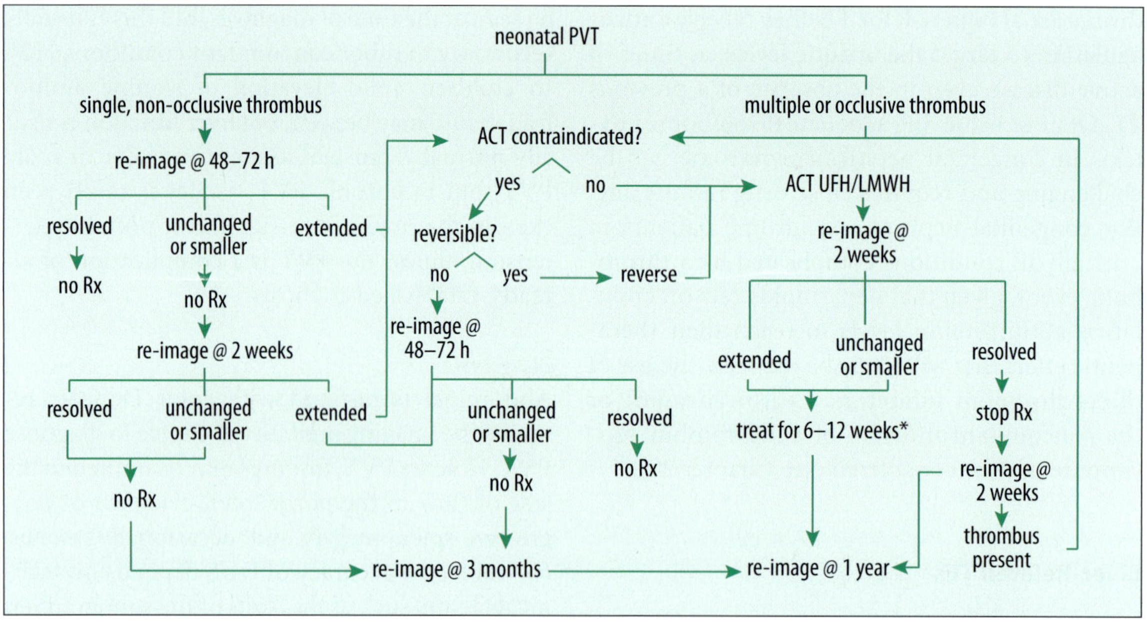

Fig. 1. Proposed algorithm for the management of neonatal portal vein thrombosis. ACT, anticoagulant therapy; LMWH, low-molecular-weight heparin; PVT, portal vein thrombosis; Rx, treatment; UFH, unfractionated heparin. Adapted and updated from Williams and Chan [12]. *Re-image after 6 weeks. Discontinuation of therapy can be considered if thrombus is non-occlusive but should be continued for an additional 6 weeks if thrombus remains occlusive. Figure created with BioRender.com.

available evidence favors anticoagulation for occlusive, idiopathic, and post-liver transplantation PVT [3]. Thrombolysis should be approached with caution and may be considered in non-neonates, with acute progressive PVT and signs of mesenteric ischemia [13]. The choice of therapy will also depend on thrombus location (main portal vein vs. left or right portal venous branch), patient age, and comorbidities. Separate algorithms for the management in neonates (shown in Fig. 1) and older children (shown in Fig. 2) are proposed, but these are not the only potential strategies. Importantly, thrombocytopenia, coagulopathy, and renal dysfunction should be ruled out prior to the start of anticoagulation. In neonates, removal of an umbilical venous catheter should be strongly considered.

Most often, PVT in children is diagnosed long after its original occurrence, with evidence of complete occlusion and well-established cavernous transformation and portal hypertension. In these circumstances, anticoagulation is not indicated. Management of chronic PVT is focused on the complications of portal hypertension (e.g., esophageal varices, hypersplenism) and portosystemic shunting (e.g., minimal hepatic encephalopathy and hepatopulmonary syndrome). Involvement of a pediatric hepatologist, pediatric interventional radiologist, and pediatric surgeon (preferably involving colleagues with liver transplant expertise) is important when planning appropriate care. The advent of a surgical procedure to create a conduit from mesenteric vein to left portal vein ("meso-Rex bypass") has enabled restitution of portal venous flow and resolution of complications of portal hypertension and portosystemic shunting for many affected children [14]. However, this is associated with a substantial risk of thrombosis and need for reintervention. A side-to-side splenorenal shunt is a less in-

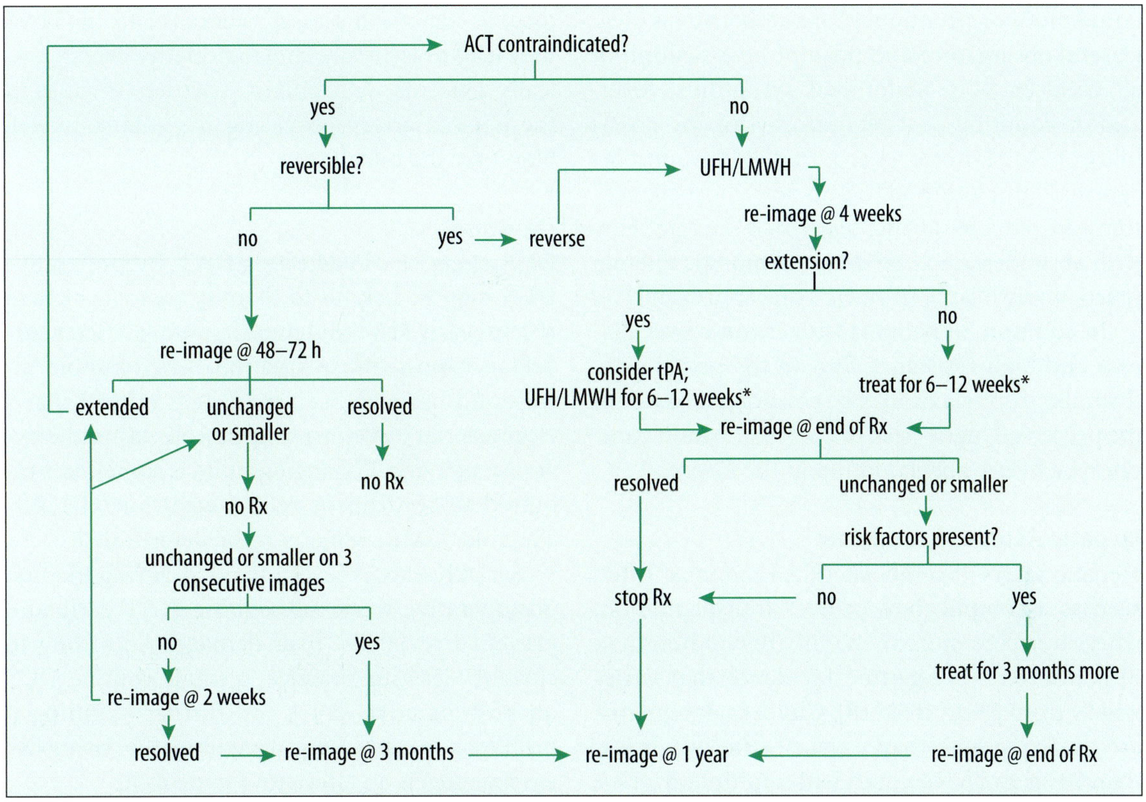

Fig. 2. Proposed algorithm for the management of non-neonatal portal vein thrombosis. ACT, anticoagulant therapy; LMWH, low-molecular-weight heparin; Rx, treatment; tPA, tissue plasminogen activator; UFH, unfractionated heparin. *Re-image after 6 weeks. Discontinuation of therapy can be considered (except for cancer, antiphospholipid syndrome, severe thrombophilia) if thrombus is non-occlusive but should be continued for an additional 6 weeks if thrombus remains occlusive. Figure created with BioRender.com.

vasive alternative and may be associated with fewer complications. There are no (high-quality) randomized trials available to advise on primary prophylaxis of esophageal variceal bleeding.

The optimal management of PVT in children with cirrhosis and portal hypertension is also unclear. It is desirable to prevent progression to complete occlusion because this may adversely affect the options for surgical treatment including transplantation. However, because of the potential risk of fatal variceal bleeding, many physicians are reluctant to offer anticoagulation. Nevertheless, the 9th Antithrombotic Chest Guidelines recommend treatment in symptomatic adults with PVT, irrespective of the presence or the absence of underlying liver disease [15]. Anticoagulation with LMWH may be preferred over VKA in patients with liver dysfunction and thrombocytopenia.

Prevention

The need for primary thromboprophylaxis in children undergoing splenectomy is still under debate. Currently, it is suggested that thromboprophylaxis (acetylsalicylic acid [ASA] or LMWH) should not be used routinely in children undergoing splenectomy. Thromboprophylaxis could be considered for those with a particularly large spleen or pronounced thrombocytosis [16]. Careful observation and prompt investigation of all children with abdominal symptoms, fever, and/or vomiting postsplenectomy for the possibility of PVT is however required. For prompt diagnosis, completing a DUS on day 7 postsplenectomy in patients at increased risk, i.e., patients with an underlying hereditary hemolytic anemia (particularly if large spleen), is one approach [17].

In addition, in patients with chronic liver disease and high resistance flow in the portal vein, thromboprophylaxis may be considered based on the perceived higher risk of PVT that would complicate a liver transplantation in the future.

Hepatic Artery Thrombosis

Hepatic artery thrombosis (HAT) is most often seen as a complication of liver transplantation, where it occurs more frequently in children than in adults, with a reported incidence that varies widely from 5% to 20% [18]. Children at high risk are those younger than 3 years, who weigh less than 10 kg and have a graft with multiple arteries, or a hepatic artery diameter <2 mm. Surgical risk factors include an abnormal arterial anatomy in the graft requiring reconstruction and a delay in arterial reperfusion, whereas microscope assisted anastomosis and split, reduced, or living-donor grafts might reduce the risk of HAT.

Clinical Presentation

HAT can present early (<1 month post-transplantation) or late (>1 month post-transplantation). While early HAT is associated with an aggressive course, a high rate of allograft loss, and increased patient mortality, late HAT may follow a more indolent course.

In children, early HAT may present with fulminant hepatic necrosis and graft failure, sepsis, liver abscesses, or worsening of graft function and is reason for urgent early retransplantation. Late HAT, on the other hand, may be asymptomatic or have a milder clinical course. Acute presentations include fever, right upper quadrant pain, jaundice, or hepatic abscesses, whereas chronic HAT may lead to ischemic cholangiopathy, which typically presents with biliary strictures because of the hepatic artery providing the sole source of blood for the bile ducts.

Diagnosis

DUS is sensitive in detecting HAT. Intraoperative DUS may be helpful to identify patients at high risk for early HAT and thus deserving stricter surveillance post-transplantation. Microbubble ultrasound has also been used. It is critical that a clear arterial waveform is seen well within the liver parenchyma. CT angiography is sometimes required to confirm or refute suspicion of HAT. The role of MRI remains to be determined.

Serial testing is recommended during the first postoperative week to diagnose HAT early and prevent irreversible liver damage. According to current SickKids practice, a single routine DUS on postoperative day 1 and further scanning if problems are noted (e.g., coagulopathy, rising liver enzymes) is an alternative approach.

Management

Early HAT is an indication for immediate return to the operating room to attempt surgical reconstruction of the arterial anastomosis, when occurring within 7 days post-transplantation. Surgical revascularization has been associated with improved graft salvage: a 20-year graft survival rate of almost 80% was reported in children who had undergone successful revascularization compared with 24% when revascularization was not attempted or failed [19]. Outside the immediate postoperative period (>3 days postoperatively), nonsurgical interventions such as transcatheter arterial thrombolysis, balloon angioplasty, or intraluminal stenting are emerging as a less invasive alternative to open surgery. Anticoagulant therapy alone is not effective. Repeat liver transplantation is the appropriate therapeutic choice in the setting of unsuccessful revascularization, acute hepatic decompensation, or chronic problems

Table 2. European Bone Marrow Transplant (EBMT) diagnostic criteria for hepatic sinusoidal obstruction syndrome in children

No limitation for time of onset of sinusoidal obstruction syndrome The presence of two or more of the following criteria (after exclusion of other potential diagnoses): • unexplained consumptive and transfusion-refractory thrombocytopenia • otherwise unexplained weight gain on 3 consecutive days despite the use of diuretics or a weight gain 45% above baseline value • hepatomegaly above baseline value, best if assessed by imaging • ascites above baseline value, best if assessed by imaging • rising bilirubin from an individual baseline value on 3 consecutive days or bilirubin ≥2 mg/dL within 72 h

Adapted from Corbacioglu et al. [20].

16

with ischemic cholangiopathy with cholestasis, progressive fibrosis, and recurrent biliary sepsis.

The management of late HAT is not based on revascularization and goes beyond the scope of this handbook.

Prevention

The risks and benefits of prophylactic LMWH and antiplatelet drugs are unproven. Published data suggest that prophylactic antiplatelet drugs, such as ASA, might prevent late HAT, but the role in the prevention of early HAT is more controversial. The current liver transplantation protocols at SickKids include prophylaxis with intravenous administration of UFH and dipyridamole, replaced by oral ASA as soon as enteral feeds are tolerated.

Sinusoidal Obstruction Syndrome

Sinusoidal obstruction syndrome (SOS), also termed hepatic veno-occlusive disease, is a serious complication of hematopoietic stem cell transplantation (HSCT). In children, SOS has also been described as occurring postirradiation or after the administration of certain chemotherapeutic agents outside the setting of HSCT (i.e., Wilm's tumor). In addition, the risk of SOS is influenced by patient-related factors, e.g., underlying disease and genetic predisposition, which may play a more important role in children than in adults. SOS is most likely because of sinusoidal endothelial cell damage, loss of sinusoidal integrity, and consequent obstruction of the hepatic sinusoids [20].

Clinical Presentation

SOS usually peaks around day +12 after HSCT, but late-onset SOS seems to be more frequent in children than in adults. Clinical symptoms include hepatomegaly, ascites, and weight gain. Importantly, up to one-third of children suffer anicteric SOS.

Diagnosis

The diagnosis of SOS remains primarily a clinical diagnosis, and in children, this diagnosis should be based on the revised European Group for Blood and Marrow Transplant (EBMT) diagnostic criteria for SOS in children (Table 2) [20]. Once SOS is suspected, ultrasonography is most helpful in accurately assessing the liver size and presence of ascites compared with a baseline evaluation. No other ultrasonography finding (i.e., reversal of flow in the portal vein, a hepatic artery resistance index greater than 0.75, and marked thickening of the gallbladder wall) is useful for early diagnosis of SOS. Although transjugular liver biopsy and hepatic sinusoidal pressure gradient measurements may have value for diagnosing SOS in adults, these investigations are not recommended in children, because of the absence of data.

Following the diagnosis, assessment of the severity of SOS is required to identify patients in need of pre-emptive treatment. The EBMT recently proposed new criteria for severity grading of SOS in children, distinguishing mild, moderate, severe, and very severe SOS [20]. Children with (very) severe SOS develop multiorgan failure, including renal failure, confusion or disorientation, bleeding, and cardiopulmonary failure, and have a very high mortality rate.

Management
Symptomatic measures should be initiated first to treat established SOS and will likely suffice for mild and moderate SOS. These measures include fluid restriction, diuretics, and albumin (in case of hypoalbuminemia) to achieve baseline weight and restore euvolemia. Hepatotoxic or nephrotoxic medications should be avoided. Platelet and red cell transfusions and correction of coagulopathy using fresh frozen plasma may also be necessary. Early specific measures are indicated in all children with severe or progressive disease and consist of defibrotide (Defitelio) at a dose of 6.25 mg/kg/dose in a 2-h infusion, given intravenously every 6 h for 21 days or until resolution of multiorgan failure and/or signs of SOS, whichever comes later [21]. Although defibrotide has a relatively mild anticoagulant activity, it should be used cautiously in patients with high bleeding risk, and it is contraindicated in patients receiving systemic thrombolysis or systemic anticoagulation and in children with clinically significant uncontrolled bleeding. If therapeutic anticoagulation were to be initiated to treat a DVT occurring while on defibrotide, there would be concern regarding increased bleeding risk. Therefore, the risk and benefit of administering both anticoagulation and defibrotide concomitantly would need to be carefully considered. During therapy, if possible, platelet count should be kept $\geq 30 \times 10^9$/L.

Prevention
The mainstay of the management of SOS however consists of prevention and supportive care. Whenever possible, HSCT should be delayed if acute hepatitis exists, or a reduced-intensity conditioning regimen should be considered. Also, the use of treosulfan compared with busulfan was associated with a reduced incidence of SOS. Besides, fluid overload should be avoided in all children undergoing HSCT. Studies on pharmacological prevention are most convincing for the use of ursodeoxycholic acid (Ursochol), a synthetic bile acid (10 mg/kg/dose, 3 times per day), which is currently recommended in the prevention of SOS for children at risk. More conflicting data or limited experience exist regarding the prophylactic use of low-dose UFH, LMWH, or *N*-acetylcysteine. A 2015 Cochrane systematic review concluded that there is still insufficient evidence for the prophylactic use of defibrotide [22], but in 2022, the European Medicines Agency strongly advised against the use of defibrotide for the prophylaxis of SOS, based on the premature closure of a phase 3 randomized clinical trial comparing defibrotide vs. best supportive care for the prevention of SOS in both adult and pediatric patients because of futility.

Budd-Chiari Syndrome
Budd-Chiari syndrome (BCS) is caused by obstruction of the hepatic venous outflow anywhere between the small branch hepatic veins to the suprahepatic IVC and right atrium [23]. BCS is rare in children, most frequently reported in the Indian subcontinent and is usually associated with congenital or acquired webs of the hepatic venous outflow tract, an underlying malignancy or myeloproliferative neoplasm, inflammatory processes, or inherited or acquired thrombophilia [23]. In adults, approximately half of the patients with primary BCS have a *JAK2*-V617F-associated myeloproliferative neoplasm. Other genes include the *JAK2* exon 12, *MPL*, or *CALR*. Their percentage is unclear in children. Thrombosis in children with a myeloproliferative neoplasm may present as BCS.

Clinical Presentation
The acute symptoms of BCS clinically resemble those of the SOS: hepatic dysfunction associated with abdominal pain, jaundice, ascites, and hepatosplenomegaly. The presentation may be fulminant or acute but is mostly chronic in children. The slower onset form can be painless and may progress silently to cirrhosis, presenting ultimately with manifestations of portal hypertension or liver failure.

Diagnosis
DUS is the most useful diagnostic test to screen for the presence of BCS. In cases in whom the results are negative or nondiagnostic but there is a strong clinical suspicion, venography of the hepatic veins should be performed. CT or MRI are generally not as sensitive but may provide useful complementary information in challenging cases. Genetic testing for a *JAK2*^{V617F}, *JAK2* exon 12, *MPL*, or *CALR* variants may be performed in children to rule out suspected underlying myeloproliferative disorder. For further laboratory thrombophilia screening, refer to Chapter 13.

Management
There are no guidelines available for the management of pediatric BCS. However, the common approaches used in adults have been extrapolated for use in children [24]. Historically, a step-by-step strategy was utilized for the management of BCS. The first-line treatment consisted of medical therapy including anticoagulation, treatment of the underlying disease, and symptomatic therapy of complications of portal hypertension (ascites, varices, and encephalopathy). Angioplasty with or without local thrombolysis and stenting was performed in patients with short-length stenosis who did not respond to medical therapy and transjugular intrahepatic portosystemic shunt, or surgical portosystemic shunt was indicated when medical therapy failed, and angioplasty and stenting were not possible or not successful. Liver transplantation was considered the last step if all the above therapies failed, in children with fulminant liver failure or in those with decompensated end-stage cirrhosis at presentation or during follow-up. However, currently, this strategy is debated as patients initially receiving medical treatment alone have a high failure rate [25], and thus, valuable time to salvage the functioning liver may be lost. Hence, early use of radiological intervention is now recommended. Transjugular intrahepatic portosystemic shunts, angioplasty, and stenting have all been shown to be effective and safe in children [26]. The choice usually depends on the available experience. Liver transplantation remains a salvage treatment. In patients with myeloproliferative neoplasms, a combination of anticoagulation and cytoreduction may lower the risk of recurrence.

Mesenteric Vascular Thrombosis

Thrombosis into the mesenteric vein and/or artery primarily occurs in adults and is a highly lethal condition. Although extremely rare, this entity may also be encountered in childhood, but only case reports and small case series of children with mesenteric vascular thrombosis (MVT) have been published. Idiopathic MVT or primary MVT has been described in otherwise healthy children, but MVT occurs more frequently in association with a broad spectrum of predisposing conditions (systemic vasculitis, abdominal infection, inflammatory bowel disease, and paroxysmal nocturnal hemoglobinuria) [27]. If none of these conditions are found, the patient should be investigated for the presence of a *JAK2* (V617F or exon 12) and secondly a *CALR* variant. Inherited or acquired prothrombotic risk factors may be present concomitantly.

Clinical Presentation

The onset of an MVT is characterized by acute abdominal pain in the vast majority of patients. Other common symptoms include diarrhea, nausea, vomiting, and lower gastrointestinal bleeding [27]. Acute thrombosis of either the mesenteric vein or artery result in bowel infarction, but a chronic presentation of thrombosis in the mesenteric vein with protracted symptoms of recurrent abdominal pain and growth failure has also been described.

Diagnosis

Diagnosis by ultrasonography is often limited by overlying bowel gas. A magnetic resonance venography is the most reliable diagnostic tool, but a CT scan with and without oral and intravenous contrast is usually considered the initial screening study because of its lower cost and widespread availability. The CT scan can show signs of infarcted or ischemic bowel, and it may be diagnostic for venous thrombosis. In cases of arterial thrombosis, selective angiography is more specific [27].

Management

There are no evidence-based guidelines for the treatment of MVT in children. Therapeutic options are extrapolated from studies in adults, but high-quality evidence is limited even in this population. Immediate surgical exploration to evaluate bowel viability and anticoagulation are the mainstay of the management of acute MVT in adults and should be carried out without delay. However, the optimal long-term approach is still unclear [28]. Balancing the benefit of anticoagulation with the risk of bleeding is challenging, but the mortality rate from MVT is significantly higher than the mortality rate from bleeding in these patients. Based on these results, experts recommend anticoagulation in symptomatic patients for at least 3 months, unless evidence of active bleeding or a very high risk of bleeding. The need for prolonged or indefinite anticoagulation must be evaluated on an individual basis but should be considered in patients at risk for recurrence (e.g., patients with a myeloproliferative neoplasm) and with a low or moderate risk of bleeding. The use of anticoagulation in asymptomatic patients remains a matter of debate. In cases of arterial thrombosis or when it is important to rapidly resolve the venous thrombosis (e.g., when infarction of the bowel is imminent), thrombolysis may also be considered and has been reported successful [28].

Splenic Vein Thrombosis

Splenic vein thrombosis (SpVT) is extremely rare. It usually accompanies a PVT or MVT, but isolated SpVT has also been reported. Isolated SpVT in children has been described as a complication of umbilical vein catheterization, postsplenectomy, as well as post liver transplantation. Pancreatic pathologies represent the most common risk factors in adults [29].

Clinical Presentation

Many patients with isolated SpVT remain asymptomatic. The most frequent presenting symptom is gastrointestinal bleeding because of gastric or gastroesophageal varices. Splenomegaly is usually present and may be accompanied by thrombocytopenia.

Diagnosis

Despite limited accuracy, DUS is noninvasive and should therefore be the initial test. Sensitivity is improved if the sonographer is asked to specifically look for this entity. A venous phase angiography is the reference standard confirmatory test. However, the diagnosis of SpVT may be challenging, even with angiography, and SpVT should be considered in patients with gastrointestinal bleeding and unexplained splenomegaly but normal liver function [29].

Management

Endoscopic management of gastric or esophageal varices may be sufficient. Splenectomy is the management of choice for children with recurrent variceal hemorrhage or problematic hypersplenism. The role for splenectomy in asymptomatic patients remains controversial. Splenic arterial embolization has also been reported in the management of SpVT, provoking splenic necrosis with the need for control of significant symptoms including pain and fever in the week or so thereafter, achieving loss of the spleen without the need for surgery. On the other hand, anticoagulant therapy has not been described in management of isolated SpVT. Moreover, caution is highly recommended in case of associated necrohemorrhagic pancreatitis.

Prevention
Children following splenic arterial embolization and splenectomy are at increased risk of life-threatening infections because of encapsulated bacteria. According to local guidelines, pneumococcal (13-valent [conjugated] and 23-valent [polysaccharide]), *Haemophilus influenzae* (type B), meningococcal (against serotypes A, C, Y, and W135, in addition to the serogroup B meningococcal vaccine), and influenza vaccines should be considered, as well as prophylactic antibiotics, with oral penicillin being the drug of choice in areas with low rates of penicillin-resistant pneumococcus. The ideal timing of vaccination is 2 weeks prior or 2 weeks post the procedure. For guidelines on primary thromboprophylaxis in children undergoing splenectomy, refer to section on PVT.

Retinal Vein Occlusion

Retinal vein occlusion (RVO) is common in middle-aged and older adults and highly associated with cardiovascular comorbidities. In younger patients, other risk factors, such as inflammation, vasospasm, compression, and thrombophilia, have also been described [30]. However, RVO is extremely rare in children and reported only in a few case reports. In neonates, RVO has been described in association with cyanotic heart disease causing an elevated hematocrit.

Clinical Presentation
RVO usually presents with visual loss, but symptoms may be more subtle. Visual field abnormalities may be present but are commonly asymptomatic.

Diagnosis
The diagnosis of RVO is made based on a funduscopic examination, demonstrating dilated tortuous retinal veins with hemorrhages and/or cotton wool spots. The presence of macular edema should be confirmed by optical coherence tomography, and fluorescein angiography facilitates the visualization of peripheral capillary nonperfusion and macular ischemia, and the detection of subtle neovascularization [30].

Management
The current management of RVO is based on data from studies directed at the consequences, i.e., the macular edema and neovascularization, rather than re-establishing normal circulation [30]. In adults, several attempts to resolve the vein occlusion have not proven beneficial because of complications of the intervention performed. More recently, a single intravitreal injection of 1.25 mg bevacizumab (Avastin) provides promising results in a few reported cases, both in adults and children [31, 32]. Additionally, in patients with recent onset of symptoms, no local risk factors (i.e., glaucoma), and no contraindications, LMWH is suggested for a period of 1–3 months. Therapeutic doses for 10–15 days should be followed by half therapeutic doses for up to 3 months [33].

Long-Term Complications

Post-thrombotic syndrome (PTS) is a well-known long-term complication of DVT (see Chapter 14). However, the assessment and study of incidence and risk factors for PTS in children with TEs in specific organs is limited by the absence of assessment tools. The 3 existing scales measuring severity of PTS in children cannot be applied to non-extremity TEs. Recommendations for the assessment of outcomes of neonates and children with RVT and PVT were published [34]. For children with BCS, it was recommended that long-term follow-up should be done by a subspecialist with a specific expertise in liver diseases. Recommendations about outcomes of other rare site TEs, such as mesenteric veins, could not be made owing to lack of information. The management of acquired coagulopathy secondary to liver disease is discussed in Chapter 11.

Conclusion

Apart from the well-known TEs in the deep venous, peripheral arterial, and central nervous system, children may also develop thromboses in specific organs. Most of these events occur in specific circumstances but need to be recognized early as they are usually associated with high rates of morbidity and mortality. General principles of TE management apply in most cases, but specific management approaches may be necessary, incorporating involvement of the relevant multidisciplinary experts. As very few guidelines are available, further studies are required to improve care for affected children.

Acknowledgments

Our special thanks go to Anthony K.C. Chan who was coauthor of this chapter in the first and second editions of this Handbook, which provided a valuable background for this updated chapter.

Conflict of Interest Statement

Veerle Labarque reports receiving speaker and/or consultancy fees from Bayer, Novartis, Novo-Nordisk, Octapharma, Roche, Sobi, and Takeda and has received financial support for travel, accommodations, and expenses from Jazz Pharmaceuticals, Roche, and Sobi. She is recipient of a research grant from CSL Behring. Noa Mandel-Shorer, Jeremy Robertson, and Suzan Williams have no conflicts of interest to declare.

Author Contributions

Veerle Labarque designed, drafted, revised, and approved the final version of chapter. Veerle Labarque, Noa Mandel-Shorer, Jeremy Robertson, and Suzan Williams discussed the content of the chapter. Noa Mandel-Shorer, Jeremy Robertson, and Suzan Williams contributed substantially to the design of the chapter, revised the chapter, and approved the final version. Veerle Labarque, Noa Mandel-Shorer, Jeremy Robertson, and Suzan Williams agree to be accountable for all aspects of the work.

Abbreviations

Anti-Xa	Anti-factor Xa
ASA	Acetylsalicylic acid
BCS	Budd-Chiari syndrome
CT	Computed tomography
CVC	Central venous catheter
DOAC	Direct oral anticoagulant
DUS	Doppler ultrasound
DVT	Deep vein thrombosis
EBMT	European Group for Blood & Marrow Transplantation
HAT	Hepatic artery thrombosis
HSCT	Hematopoietic stem cell transplantation
IVC	Inferior vena cava
LMWH	Low-molecular-weight heparin
MRI	Magnetic resonance imaging
MVT	Mesenteric vascular thrombosis
PE	Pulmonary embolism
PTS	Post-thrombotic syndrome
PVT	Portal vein thrombosis
RAT	Renal artery thrombosis
RVO	Retinal vein occlusion
RVT	Renal vein thrombosis
SOS	Sinusoidal obstruction syndrome
SpVT	Splenic vein thrombosis
TE	Thromboembolism/thromboembolic event
tPA	Tissue plasminogen activator
UFH	Unfractionated heparin
VKA	Vitamin K antagonist

References

1 Brandão LR, Simpson EA, Lau KK. Neonatal renal vein thrombosis. Semin Fetal Neonatal Med. 2011;16(6):323–8.

2 Lau KK, Stoffman JM, Williams S, McCusker P, Brandao L, Patel S, et al. Neonatal renal vein thrombosis: review of the English-language literature between 1992 and 2006. Pediatrics. 2007;120(5):e1278–84.

3 Monagle P, Cuello CA, Augustine C, Bonduel M, Brandão LR, Capman T, et al. American Society of Hematology 2018 Guidelines for management of venous thromboembolism: treatment of pediatric venous thromboembolism. Blood Adv. 2018;2(22):3292–316.

4 Chavhan GB, Babyn PS, John P, Yoo SJ, Rigsby CK. Pediatric body MR angiography: principles, techniques, and current status in body imaging. Am J Roentgenol. 2015;205(1):173–84.

5 Singh O, Gupta SS, Sharma D, Lahoti BK, Mathur RK. Isolated renal artery thrombosis because of blunt trauma abdomen: report of a case with review of the literature. Urol Int. 2011;86(2):233–8.

6 Bapistella S, Zirngibl M, Buder K, Toulany N, Laube GF, Weitz M. Prophylactic antithrombotic management in adult and pediatric kidney transplantation: a systematic review and metaanalysis. Pediatr Transplant. 2021;25(4):e14021.

7 Monagle P, Chan AKC, Goldenberg NA, Ichord RN, Journeycake JM, Nowak-Göttl U, et al. Antithrombotic therapy in neonates and children: Antithrombotic Therapy and Prevention of Thrombosis, 9th ed: American College of Chest Physicians Evidence-Based Clinical Practice Guidelines. Chest. 2012;141(2 suppl):e737S–801S.

8 Sharathkumar A, Hirschl R, Pipe S, Crandell C, Adams B, Lin JJ. Primary thromboprophylaxis with heparins for arteriovenous fistula failure in pediatric patients. J Vasc Access. 2007;8(4):235–44.

9 Davenport A. Alternatives to standard unfractionated heparin for pediatric hemodialysis treatments. Pediatr Nephrol. 2012;27(10):1869–79.

10 Kerlin BA, Ayoob R, Smoyer WE. Epidemiology and pathophysiology of nephrotic syndrome associated thromboembolic disease. Clin J Am Soc Nephrol. 2012;7(3):513–20.

11 Kerlin BA, Blatt NB, Fuh B, Zhao S, Lehman A, Blanchong C, et al. Epidemiology and risk factors for thromboembolic complications of childhood nephrotic syndrome: a Midwest Pediatric Nephrology Consortium (MWPNC) study. J Pediatr. 2009;155(1):105–10.

12 Williams S, Chan AKC. Neonatal portal vein thrombosis: diagnosis and management. Semin Fetal Neonatal Med. 2011;16(6):329–39.

13 Hall TC, Garcea G, Metcalfe M, Bilku D, Dennison AR. Management of acute non-cirrhotic and non-malignant portal vein thrombosis: a systematic review. World J Surg. 2011;35(11):2510–20.

14 Shneider BL, Bosch J, de Franchis R, Emre SH, Groszmann RJ, Ling SC, et al. Portal hypertension in children: expert pediatric opinion on the report of the Baveno v Consensus Workshop on Methodology of Diagnosis and Therapy in Portal Hypertension. Pediatr Transplant. 2012;16(5):426–37.

15 Kearon C, Akl EA, Comerota AJ, Prandoni P, Bounameaux H, Goldhaber SZ, et al. Antithrombotic therapy for VTE disease: Antithrombotic Therapy and Prevention of Thrombosis, 9th ed: American College of Chest Physicians Evidence-Based Clinical Practice Guidelines. Chest. 2012;141(2 suppl):e419S–96S.

16 Stringer MD, Lucas N. Thrombocytosis and portal vein thrombosis after splenectomy for paediatric haemolytic disorders: how should they be managed? J Paediatr Child Health. 2018;54(11):1184–8.

17 Iolascon A, Andolfo I, Barcellini W, Corcione F, Garçon L, de Franceschi L, et al. Recommendations regarding splenectomy in hereditary hemolytic anemias. Haematologica. 2017;102(8):1304–13.

18 Sevmis S, Karakayali H, Tutar NU, Boyvat F, Ozcay F, Torgay A, et al. Management of early hepatic arterial thrombosis after pediatric living-donor liver transplantation. Transplant Proc. 2011;43(2):605–8.

19 Ackermann O, Branchereau S, Franchi-Abella S, Pariente D, Chevret L, Debray D, et al. The longterm outcome of hepatic artery thrombosis after liver transplantation in children: role of urgent revascularization. Am J Transplant. 2012;12(6):1496–503.

20 Corbacioglu S, Carreras E, Ansari M, Balduzzi A, Cesaro S, Dalle JH, et al. Diagnosis and severity criteria for sinusoidal obstruction syndrome/veno-occlusive disease in pediatric patients: a new classification from the European society for blood and marrow transplantation. Bone Marrow Transplant. 2018;53(2):138–45.

21 Bajwa RPS, Mahadeo KM, Taragin BH, Dvorak CC, McArthur J, Jeyapalan A, et al. Consensus report by pediatric acute lung injury and sepsis investigators and pediatric blood and marrow transplantation consortium joint working committees: supportive care guidelines for management of veno-occlusive disease in children and adolescents, part 1:focus on investigations, prophylaxis, and specific treatment. Biol Blood Marrow Transplant. 2017;23(11):1817–25.

22 Cheuk DKL, Chiang AKS, Ha SY, Chan GCF. Interventions for prophylaxis of hepatic venoocclusive disease in people undergoing haematopoietic stem cell transplantation. Cochrane Database Syst Rev. 2015;2015(5):CD009311.

23 Cauchi JA, Oliff S, Baumann U, Mirza D, Kelly DA, Hewitson J, et al. The Budd-Chiari syndrome in children: the spectrum of management. J Pediatr Surg. 2006;41(11):1919–23.

24 DeLeve LD, Valla DC, Garcia-Tsao G, American Association for the Study Liver Diseases. Vascular disorders of the liver. Hepatology. 2009 May;49(5):1729–64.

25 Sharma VK, Ranade PR, Marar S, Nabi F, Nagral A. Long-term clinical outcome of Budd-Chiari syndrome in children after radiological intervention. Eur J Gastroenterol Hepatol. 2016;28(5):567–75.

26 Redkar R, Bangar A, Hathiramani V, Raj V, Swathi C. Pediatric Budd-Chiari syndrome: a case series. Indian Pediatr. 2018;55(10):871–3.

27 Oğuzkurt P, Senocak ME, Ciftci AO, Tanyel FC, Büyükpamukçu N. Mesenteric vascular occlusion resulting in intestinal necrosis in children. J Pediatr Surg. 2000;35(8):1161–4.

28 Mancuso A. An update on the management of Budd-Chiari syndrome: the issues of timing and choice of treatment. Eur J Gastroenterol Hepatol. 2015;27(3):200–3.

29 Köklü S, Köksal A, Yolcu OF, Bayram G, Sakaoğullari Z, Arda K, et al. Isolated splenic vein thrombosis: an unusual cause and review of the literature. Can J Gastroenterol. 2004;18(3):173–4.
30 Ip M, Hendrick A. Retinal vein occlusion review. Asia Pac J Ophthalmol. 2018;7(1):40–5.
31 Pidro A, Pidro A, Nadarevic-Vodencarevic A, Halilbasic M, Lepara O, Nisic F. Short term and long term results after intravitreal bevacizumab therapy for macular oedema in branch retinal vein occlusion. Romanian J Ophthalmol. 2022;66(1):22–6.
32 Zheng L, Gillies M, Martin FJ. Central retinal vein occlusion in an otherwise healthy child treated successfully with a single injection of bevacizumab. J AAPOS. 2015;19:473–4.
33 Abbattista M, Capecchi M, Martinelli I. Treatment of unusual thrombotic manifestations. Blood. 2020;135(5):326–34.
34 Rajpurkar M, Sharathkumar A, Williams S, Lau K, Ling SC, Chan AKC, et al. Recommendations for the assessment of non-extremity venous thromboembolism outcomes: communication from the SSC of the ISTH. J Thromb Haemost. 2015;13(3):477–80.

Published online: December 5, 2024

Blanchette VS, Brandão LR, Carcao MD, Kumar R, Rand ML, Revel-Vilk S (eds): SickKids Handbook of Pediatric Thrombosis and Hemostasis, ed 3, rev. and ext. Basel, Karger, 2024, pp 307–335 (DOI: 10.1159/000538198)

Stroke

Elizabeth Pulcine[a] Andrea Andrade[b] Adriana Carolina Vargas Nino[a]
Suzan Williams[c] Rebecca N. Ichord[d] Nomazulu Dlamini[a]

[a]Division of Neurology, Department of Paediatrics, The Hospital for Sick Children, University of Toronto, Toronto, ON, Canada; [b]Department of Paediatrics, Schulich School of Medicine and Dentistry, Western University, London, ON, Canada; [c]Department of Paediatrics, Division of Haematology/Oncology, The Hospital for Sick Children, University of Toronto, Toronto, ON, Canada; [d]Department of Neurology & Pediatrics, Perelman School of Medicine, University of Pennsylvania, Philadelphia, PA, USA

Introduction

Cerebrovascular diseases involving thrombosis or thromboembolism in children are well-recognized entities and can be divided in two main categories: arterial ischemic stroke (AIS) and cerebral sinovenous thrombosis (CSVT). Both conditions can affect all ages from newborns to adolescents. Early recognition allows prompt initiation of treatment that may prevent thrombus propagation, infarct expansion, stroke recurrence, and life-threatening complications, thereby improving survival and long-term functional outcome. Multidisciplinary collaboration of varied disciplines including pediatric stroke/neurology, interventional neuroradiology, thrombosis/hematology, intensive care physicians, and neurosurgery are required in the care of pediatric stroke patients.

Arterial Ischemic Stroke

AIS is an acute neurologic syndrome manifesting with focal cerebral, spinal, or retinal deficits because of infarction conforming to an arterial territory on neuroimaging. This may be caused by thromboembolic occlusion or critical focal hypoperfusion in the involved artery. Thromboembolic occlusion affects large-, medium-, or sometimes small-vessel territories, whereas critical hypoperfusion more commonly affects those areas of the brain located in the border zones between two different arterial territories. These border zone infarcts, also referred to as watershed infarcts, most commonly affect the border zone between the anterior cerebral artery (ACA) and the middle cerebral artery (MCA) and within the internal MCA watershed zone, in the setting of intracranial carotid steno-occlusive disease or global hypoperfusion (shown in Fig. 1).

The incidence of pediatric AIS in North America has been estimated to be 2.4/100,000/year [1].

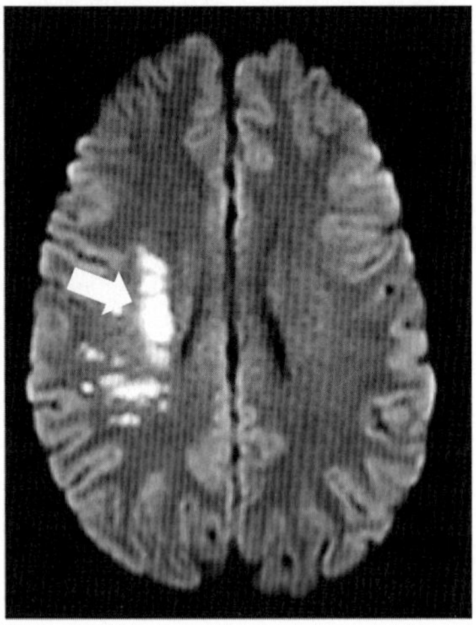

Fig. 1. Axial MRI of the brain. Diffusion-weighted sequence showing a right watershed distribution (ACA/MCA) ischemic infarct. 11-year-old boy with no identifiable risk factors for stroke.

There is a male predominance [2]. Neonates comprise 25% of pediatric patients with AIS, with an estimated prevalence of 1 per 3,500 live term births [1, 2]. AIS in the perinatal period is now estimated to be as frequent as large vessel AIS in adults with an incidence 17 times higher than during childhood [3]. The reported incidence rates of pediatric AIS have increased in part due to an increasing awareness of the condition and to improved imaging techniques [4]. AIS is one of the top 10 causes of death in the pediatric population. Approximately 10–50% of children with initial AIS occurring after the newborn period experience recurrent AIS or transient ischemic attacks (TIAs). Increased recurrence rates generally reflect children with underlying arteriopathy or congenital heart disease (CHD) not receiving antithrombotic therapy [5, 6].

Perinatal AIS may result from combinations of maternal, intrapartum, and neonatal factors [7]. Most infants beyond the newborn period and children with AIS have a medical condition that predisposes them to AIS [8]. Congenital or acquired heart disease and sickle cell disease (SCD) are common causes of AIS in children. Heart disease is responsible for 20–25% of AIS in children [8]. Additional acute or chronic systemic risk factors include common childhood illnesses, such as infection, dehydration, iron deficiency anemia, prothrombotic disorders, or other chronic diseases. Individual children often have multiple converging risk factors for AIS. No stroke etiology is found in up to a third of neonates and approximately 10% of older infants and children, even after extensive diagnostic investigations [9].

Clinical Presentation

The clinical presentation varies among age groups. In the newborn period (0–28 days), the most common clinical presentation is acute encephalopathy with altered mental status (lethargy, obtundation, and coma) and focal seizures typically with onset beyond 12 h after delivery [3]. Less common presentations in this age group are unexplained irritability and hemiparesis [9]. AIS in the asymptomatic neonate may be incidentally detected on imaging done for other reasons.

A separate category of perinatal AIS termed presumed perinatal AIS is recognized in children who present in the 4- to 12-month age period with an emerging hemiparesis or early hand dominance. These children have imaging findings of a remote vaso-occlusive pattern of AIS, presumed to have occurred in utero or silently in the early neonatal period [9]. The relevant information in the history and physical examination of neonates and older children with suspected AIS are described in Table 1 [10, 11].

Diagnosis

The gold-standard test to confirm a clinical diagnosis of AIS in the acute setting is magnetic resonance imaging (MRI)/magnetic resonance angiography (MRA) of the brain and the vessels of the head and neck. The most useful MRI/MRA sequences in the stroke imaging protocol include diffusion weighted images (DWI) and apparent diffusion coefficient (ADC), which are essential

Fig. 2

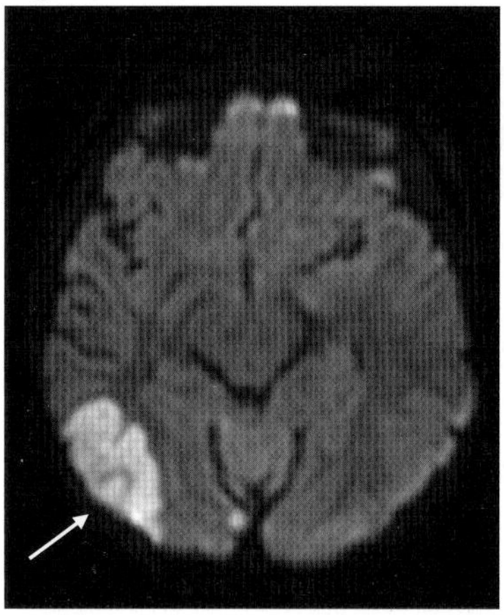

Fig. 3

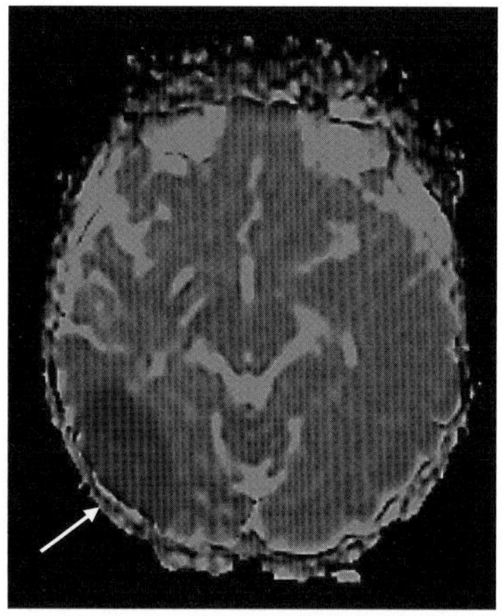

Fig. 2. MRI of the brain in an axial view using a diffusion-weighted sequence. The arrow demonstrates an area of restricted diffusion involving the inferior branch of the right MCA, indicative of an acute ischemic infarct.

Fig. 3. MRI of the brain in an axial view using apparent diffusion coefficient sequence of the same patient. The arrow shows the counterpamap sequence with hypointense signal in the same vascular territory.

Table 1. Relevant history and physical exam in suspected arterial ischemic stroke by age group

Neonates	
Clinical presentation	Acute focal motor seizures after the first 12 h of life
Past medical history	Maternal thrombosis, gestational/obstetric disorders
Physical exam	Gaze preference, asymmetric limb tone and movements, subtle seizures Heart murmur suggests possible congenital heart disease
Older infant or child	
Clinical presentation	Acute focal neurological deficit, usually abrupt onset, can be self-resolving (hemiparesis, hemisensory deficit, visual field deficit, aphasia, facial weakness, other cranial nerve deficits, and unilateral ataxia)
Past medical history	Recent head or neck trauma, head or neck irradiation, migraine headaches, varicella infection or vaccination (in the past 12 months), use of oral contraceptives, use of illicit drugs such as cocaine or amphetamines
Family history	Hyperlipidemia, migraines, thrombotic events (age <55 years with stroke, myocardial infarction, deep venous thrombosis, maternal recurrent fetal loss)
Physical examination	Carotid/head bruits, skin lesions of neurocutaneous disease (NF-1, PHACE syndrome, Sturge-Weber syndrome), cardiac murmur If febrile search for physical stigmata of infectious endocarditis Baseline neurological exam should very clearly define severity of deficits

NF-1, neurofibromatosis, type 1; PHACE, Posterior fossa, Hemangioma, Arterial lesions, Cardiac abnormalities, Eye abnormalities.

for the detection of acute brain infarction. Briefly, DWI and ADC are techniques based on measuring the random motion of water molecules through tissues. Changes in the integrity of the tissue and the cells in the area being scanned (i.e., ischemic area in contrast to a well-perfused one) generate different image signals that allow neuroradiological evaluation for the presence of cytotoxic edema because of acute ischemic injury (shown in Fig. 2, 3). Unenhanced computerized tomography (CT) scans are frequently normal up to 12 h after symptom onset in childhood AIS. In

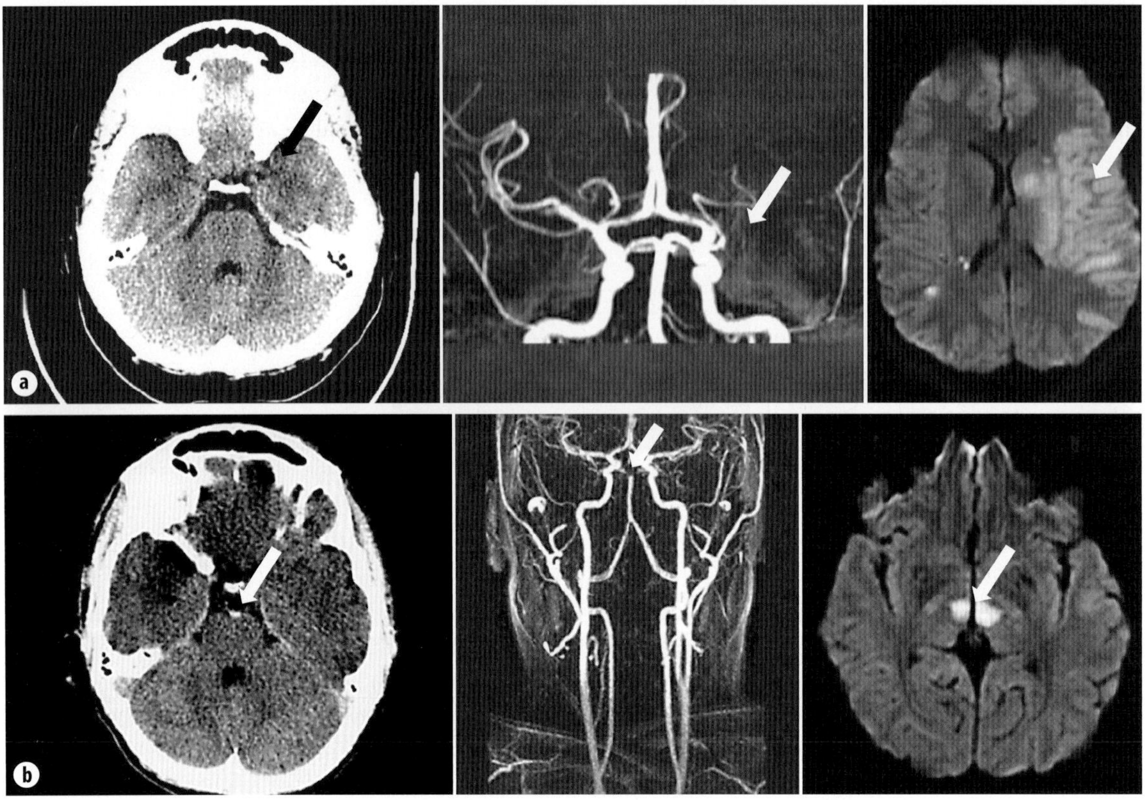

Fig. 4. a From left to right: Sequence of imaging of a 13-year-old girl that presented to the ER with acute right hemiparesis. Noncontrast CT on axial view, with a left "hyperdense" MCA sign, representing an acute thrombus occluding the artery (arrow). Time-of-flight MRA showing absent flow in the location of left MCA, confirming the acute occlusion (arrow). DWI on axial view, showing an area of restricted diffusion over the left MCA territory, representing an acute AIS (arrow). **b** From left to right: Sequence of imaging of a 14-year-old boy with an acute onset of difficulty walking and "seizure-like" activity, followed by acute loss of consciousness and collapse. Noncontrast CT on axial view with a "hyperdense" basilar artery (arrow), representing an acute thrombus occluding the artery. MRA with gadolinium, showing a filling defect at the top of the basilar (arrow), confirming the acute occlusion. Diffuse-weighted imaging on axial view, showing bilateral areas of restricted diffusion over the medial thalami (arrow) representing an AIS of the basilar-posterior circulation territories (arrow).

patients with larger infarcts involving complete large vessel territories, or in those whose symptoms started in the prior 24 h, unenhanced CT may show large areas of hypodensity, involving specific vascular territories. Sometimes the only radiological evidence in a noncontrast CT is a hyperdense sign within the artery where an occlusive thrombus is located (shown in Fig. 4a). This hyperdensity is most commonly found in the MCA and is referred to as the "hyperdense MCA sign" and/or the "dot sign" (shown in Fig. 4a) [12]. Although, it is mainly described in adults with MCA stroke, it can also be found within other large vessels, such as the basilar artery (shown in Fig. 4b). It is important to remember that stroke is a vascular disease and therefore requires vascular imaging. The importance of MRA or computed tomography angiography (CTA), as a part of the initial screen, is to evaluate the integrity of the cervical, vertebrobasilar, and intracranial circulation. Additionally, the presence of a filling defect on CTA or contrast-enhanced MRA in a major artery may be indicative of the presence of a thrombus and requires further investigation. Both thrombotic occlusions and arteriopathies (i.e., focal cerebral arteriopathy [FCA], moyamoya disease, vasculitis, and dissection) are detectable by MRA or CTA.

Initial blood work before starting therapy should include an activated partial thromboplastin time (aPTT), prothrombin time (PT)/international normalized ratio (INR), fibrinogen, and a complete blood count. Results of screening coagulation parameters and platelet count are assessed to establish the safety of antithrombotic treatment for acute AIS. It is reasonable and common practice to obtain a complete profile of studies for hypercoagulable states in all cases of confirmed acute AIS, regardless of a known risk factor such as heart disease or arterial dissection, given that pediatric stroke is often multifactorial.

As initial treatment considerations are not related to laboratory markers of a hypercoagulable state, blood tests can be sent after starting therapy and might include, as follows: (a) natural anticoagulants; protein C and antithrombin activity, protein S-free antigen; procoagulant factors (genetic tests) – factor V Leiden, prothrombin gene variant (plasma-based test) – factor VIII; miscellaneous; homocysteine, antiphospholipid antibodies including lupus anticoagulant, anticardiolipin (IgM/IgG), and anti-β2 glycoprotein antibodies (IgM/IgG), and lipoprotein(a) (see Chapter 13 and Appendix II). Acutely, the antiphospholipid antibody panel should be considered before anticoagulation is initiated. Subsequently, especially in neonates or in patients with less than 10 kg, the remainder of the laboratory investigation, starting with the natural anticoagulants, can be obtained within 4–6 weeks and the remainder, any time up to 3–6 months from the initial event.

The stroke work up should include a transthoracic echocardiogram to evaluate for a cardiac source of thrombus. These include formation of a thrombus in a dyskinetic ventricle because of cardiac arrhythmia, thrombus formation, or vegetation on an abnormal heart valve or paradoxical embolism from a venous thrombus in the presence of an intracardiac right-to-left shunt because of congenital structural heart defects. It is also reasonable to consider a transesophageal echocardiogram for evaluation of cardioaortic source if neuroimaging and history are suggestive of cardioembolic stroke or in the investigation of cryptogenic stroke.

Further testing should be considered on a case-by-case basis and may include cerebral angiogram, vasculitis work-up (erythrocyte sedimentation rate, C3 and C4, rheumatoid factor, antinuclear antibody, and C-reactive protein), cerebrospinal fluid analysis looking for evidence of vasculitis or infection, and other blood testing (varicella titers, vitamin B12, and metabolic work up, formal eye examination, and sickle cell testing) [10, 11].

In neonates and children whose initial symptom is a focal seizure, and in those whose level of consciousness is compromised, or neurological exam is obscured by pharmacological paralysis, continuous electroencephalography (EEG) monitoring is warranted to evaluate and treat for subclinical seizures [11].

Management

The acute management of suspected AIS entails optimizing cerebral perfusion pressure and oxygenation while considering reperfusion therapies and antithrombotic therapy (antiplatelet or anticoagulant) to prevent stroke recurrence. Monitoring for secondary complications including seizures and malignant cerebral edema is important. It should be noted that none of these therapies have been evaluated in clinical trials in children, and therefore, they are established from consensus-based expert opinion and extrapolated from adult stroke literature [10, 13].

Neuroprotective Measures

Neuroprotective measures aim to protect neurons by reducing cerebral metabolic demands and ensuring adequate perfusion. This is to prevent recruitment of the ischemic core into the penumbra, minimize the final volume of the infarct, and avoid secondary complications such as malignant cerebral edema. Neuroprotective measures include:

- aggressive treatment to prevent and reverse fever
- anticonvulsant medication to treat seizures
- maintenance of normoglycemia
- avoidance of relative hypotension
- maintenance of normovolemia.

Antithrombotic Therapy

Antithrombotic therapy aims to reduce the risk of recurrent thrombotic occlusion of cerebral arteries in children with AIS and in neonates with cardioembolic AIS.

For children (non-neonates) with AIS, consensus guidelines recommend antithrombotic therapy in the absence of significant intracranial hemorrhage (ICH) to treat and prevent thromboembolic complications, all of which are used off label. Antithrombotic therapy can be divided into three main groups: antiplatelet (cyclooxygenase [COX] inhibitor-1 class: acetylsalicylic acid [ASA]; P2Y12-receptor blocker class: clopidogrel), anticoagulants (heparinoids: unfractionated heparin [UFH], low-molecular-weight heparin [LMWH]; vitamin K antagonists (VKAs): warfarin, acenocumarol, and phenprocoumon), and fibrinolytic agents: (tissue plasminogen activator [tPA]). In terms of new antiplatelet agents, there is little pediatric experience with the new P2Y12 compounds named ticagrelor, cangrelor, and prasugrel. Similarly, there is no pediatric literature on the fibrinolytic agent tenecteplase (TNKase®), and therefore, they will not be included. Conversely, the limited reports on the use of new direct oral anticoagulants (DOACs) for children with CSVT (e.g., rivaroxaban) will be covered.

Five international consensus-based guidelines exist that address the use of antiplatelet, anticoagulant, and fibrinolytic therapy in children with AIS: The American Heart Association/American Stroke Association [10, 14]; The American College of Chest Physicians [13]; The American Heart Association Scientific Statement on Prevention and Treatment of Thrombosis in Pediatric CHD [15]; The Royal College of Paediatrics and Child Health and Stroke Association [16]; and The Australian Clinical Consensus Guidelines [17]. In general, the available guidelines recommend anticoagulation for secondary stroke prevention if there is confirmed dissection or cardioembolic source. The duration of treatment largely depends on the underlying condition and individual risk factors and varies widely across institutions and experts. If the above etiologies are ruled out, the recurrence risk is deemed to be lower, and antiplatelet therapy with ASA or clopidogrel is then reasonable for secondary stroke prevention. At The Hospital for Sick Children, it is common to continue daily ASA prophylaxis therapy for a minimum of 2 years. For children with recurrent AIS while on ASA therapy, it is reasonable to change to clopidogrel therapy or to anticoagulant therapy [13]. For children with AIS secondary to a cardioembolic cause, anticoagulation with LMWH or VKA is recommended for at least 3 months followed by step-down to antiplatelet therapy [13, 15]. For management of children with AIS secondary to dissection, see below. Dosing and monitoring of UFH, LMWH, VKA, ASA, and clopidogrel therapy are detailed in Chapter 20.

Antithrombotic therapy in children with AIS is considered relatively safe with an estimated 4% risk of symptomatic ICH [18]. If there is hemorrhagic conversion, systolic hypertension, or other bleeding risk factors are present, antithrombotic therapy in patients with AIS may be neither safe nor feasible. In patients with large territorial infarctions (e.g., >2/3 of the MCA territory), postponing initiation of antithrombotic therapy beyond 48–72 h after stroke onset can be considered in hopes of minimizing the risk of hemorrhagic conversion and other systemic bleeding complications. However, the risk-benefit ratio must be weighed in each case and management approach individualized. Early (i.e., 12–24 h, depending on clinical situation) follow-up neuroimaging (CT or MRI) is reasonable and may lead to temporary discontinuation or cessation of antithrombotic therapy if hemorrhagic conversion or systemic bleeding complications arise [10, 13, 19].

Pediatric AIS: Special Considerations

AIS in the Neonatal Period

The mortality rate following AIS in newborns is less than 10%. Neurologic deficits are detected in about two-thirds of survivors by young childhood age as children often grow into their deficits. Lesions that involve the motor cortex, internal capsule, and basal ganglia together are associated with increased motor disability compared with lesions limited to the cortex or the basal ganglia alone. Epilepsy is common in children after neonatal stroke with estimates of incidence approaching up to 15% by age 2 years. The diagnostic investigations in neonatal stroke include MRI/MRA of the brain and continuous EEG monitoring if there is a suspicion of subclinical seizures. The importance of inherited thrombophilia in the pathophysiology and long-term outcomes of perinatal stroke is not yet known. Therefore, currently, there is no evidence to support routine extensive thrombophilia screening in this setting outside the research protocols [7]. In contrast to older infants and children, fewer than 5% of newborns with AIS have recurrent systemic or cerebral thrombosis. Thus, for neonates with noncardiogenic AIS, the use of antithrombotic therapy is not recommended [13]. For neonates with a first cardioembolic AIS, anticoagulation should be considered with either UFH or LMWH for 3–6 months, followed by ASA if the cardiac defect has not been fully repaired, given a high risk of recurrent AIS [13, 20]. For neonates with recurrent AIS, anticoagulation therapy or ASA therapy for an indefinite time may be considered. Dosing and monitoring of UFH, LMWH, VKA, and ASA therapy in neonates are detailed in Chapter 20.

Cardioembolic AIS

The incidence of cardioembolic AIS in neonates and children with cardiac disease is reported to be as high as 1 in 757 [21] and affects up to 8% of children with CHD preoperatively. Cardioembolic stroke can arise via different pathophysiological mechanisms, including formation of a mural thrombus in a dyskinetic ventricle, thrombus formation, or vegetation on an abnormal heart valve, arrhythmia resulting in pooling of blood and nonlaminar flow or paradoxical embolism of a venous thrombus in right-to-left shunting because of congenital structural heart defects [10, 14, 15, 22]. Children with CHD are at high risk of developing thrombosis, and the risk can vary over the life span [22]. Cardiac surgery itself poses a significant thromboembolic risk in addition to a risk of global hypoxic-ischemic injury. During surgical repair, the use of cardiopulmonary bypass temporarily exposes the patient's blood to plastic tubing and other thrombogenic materials in the artificial circulatory system [23]. This results in activation and aggregation of platelets and the fibrin-forming coagulation system with subsequent thrombus formation within the tubing or circuitry of the machine. A retrospective study from The Hospital for Sick Children examined 5,526 children with CHD who underwent cardiac surgery from 1992 to 2001 and found that the incidence of ischemic stroke (28 with AIS and 2 with CSVT) was 5.4 per 1,000 children from 1992 to 2001 [24]. Risk factors associated with procedural stroke included older age at the time of the surgery, longer duration of cardio-

17

pulmonary bypass, reoperation, and number of days hospitalized after the operation [24]. The authors hypothesized that children who require reoperation likely have more severe underlying cardiac disease placing them at higher risk for procedure-related complications [24]. It remains unknown which individual patient characteristics further alter the risk of AIS in the procedural period, for instance, congenital or acquired resistance to antithrombotic therapy. In infants and young children, normal developmental changes in the hemostatic system may also contribute to this risk.

For recommended thromboprophylaxis of AIS in children with congenital and acquired heart disease, including patients placed on extracorporeal life support, see Chapters 18 and 19.

AIS because of Arterial Dissection

Cervicocephalic arterial dissection (CCAD) is an under-recognized cause of AIS in pediatric patients, accounting for 6.4–9.1% of cases described recently in two large pediatric prospective cohorts [25, 26]. There are two types of CCAD in children, extracranial and intracranial dissection. These entities have different risk factors and management and are described further below.

Pathophysiology

Two different mechanisms are proposed in the formation of an intramural hematoma within the vessel wall layers, which can result in AIS. The first is that the tear in the intima leads to the accumulation of blood between the vessel wall layers exposing the endothelial basement membrane and the extracellular matrix proteins to blood products, resulting in platelet adhesion and aggregation and local thrombus formation [27]. Once a thrombus has formed, ischemia occurs from vessel occlusion at the site of the dissection or from artery-to-artery embolization downstream [28]. The second proposed mechanism is the mechanical obstruction of the lumen by the expanding intramural hematoma as the result of a primary bleed in the vessel wall [29]. In addition, a pseudoaneurysmal dilatation of the vessel can occur in the context of an intramural hematoma located within the tunica media and the adventitia [29]. Subsequently, AIS can occur either immediately after formation of the intramural hematoma or up to several months later because of delayed artery-to-artery embolization from the downstream dissected vessel or from an associated pseudoaneurysm thrombus.

Extracranial Dissection

Extracranial dissection accounts for up to 5–25% of childhood AIS and is often preceded by trauma. Typically, extracranial dissection affecting the anterior circulation, especially the distal segment of the internal carotid artery, presents with focal neurological symptoms such as hemiparesis and aphasia. Posterior circulation dissection, affecting the vertebral arteries, is more challenging to diagnose, presenting with nonspecific symptoms, such as vertigo, ataxia, nausea and vomiting, and/or decreased level of consciousness. For more, please see the section on Posterior Circulation AIS below. Clues to the diagnosis include recent history of trauma and/or cranial nerve abnormalities. CCAD can occur spontaneously or after blunt or penetrating trauma or high velocity head flexion, extension, or rotation with stretch injury of the arterial wall. When children present with spontaneous CCAD, it is important to investigate for an underlying genetic predisposition of the affected artery, such as collagen defects associated with Ehlers-Danlos syndrome (EDS) type IV, vascular EDS that weakens the artery wall, making the child more prone to dissection. For more information on clinical and genetic testing for the diagnosis of EDS, see Appendix IV.

Treatment of Extracranial Arterial Dissection

Therapy for CCAD aims to prevent stroke until the dissection site has healed or recanalized. Treatment of AIS secondary to extracranial dissection with anticoagulation therapy is an acceptable and widely used approach [10, 30]. Treatment with ASA alone, or other antiplatelet agent, is also reasonable, as there are no data from clinical trials in children evaluating the effectiveness of anticoagulation compared with antiplatelet therapy. The results of the Cervical Artery Dissection in Stroke Study, the largest randomized clinical trial to date in adults evaluating the use of antiplatelet agents vs. anticoagulation, did not report significant differences in terms of recurrent AIS, angiographic recanalization on MRA/CTA at 3 months, risk of intracranial bleed, or mortality [31]. If the patient requires an invasive procedure such as a cerebral angiogram, it is reasonable to start treatment with UFH, which can be more easily held for a procedure and restarted. Duration of treatment with LMWH or VKA typically is guided by clinical and radiologic status at regularly scheduled follow-up intervals. It is common practice for children with extracranial CCAD to receive LMWH for a minimum of 3 months, followed by transition to ASA, which is continued for a minimum of 2 years after AIS. This duration of treatment is based on the concern for risk of recurrence from pseudoaneurysm or other vascular abnormalities at the site of the dissection [4]. The risk of recurrent AIS in children with CCAD is highest in the 12 months after the initial stroke with an estimated recurrence risk of 19% in the first year [32].

Intracranial Dissection
Intracranial arterial dissection also referred to as FCA dissection type (FCA-d) is considered an extremely rare occurrence in children. There are few cases reported in the literature, and the majority of these have been confirmed postmortem at the time of autopsy [33]. The most common presentation is headache, followed by focal neurological deficit. The arteries affected are the distal segment of the internal carotid artery and the proximal segments of the MCA and ACA. In case of suspected intracranial dissection, the differentiation from inflammatory FCA is challenging [33]. Features that distinguish intracranial dissection from inflammatory FCA (or transient cerebral arteriopathy) include the findings on angiography of double lumen and intimal flap in the artery [33]. On wall imaging MRI, the presence of a wall hematoma is highly suggestive of intracranial dissection.

Treatment of Intracranial Arterial Dissection
As in cases of extracranial CCAD, it is common practice to treat with some form of antithrombotic therapy for a minimum of 2 years after sentinel AIS. Some authors suggest that children with an intracranial dissection should avoid anticoagulation because of an increased risk of subarachnoid hemorrhage (SAH). However, the treatment among these patients is controversial because the concern for increased risk of ICH is only based on anecdotal and sporadic cases [4]. In the study by Metso et al. [34], which aimed to assess the safety of anticoagulation in adult patients with intracranial dissection, those without SAH at presentation underwent anticoagulation with intravenous (IV) UFH or LMWH and were then switched to warfarin to complete 3 months of anticoagulation with no subsequent SAH cases identified [34].

AIS in the Setting of Infections
The most common viral infection associated with AIS in unvaccinated children is *Varicella zoster* virus [5]. There is evidence that varicella can infect the walls of the arteries of the circle of Willis, particularly the terminal internal carotid artery, the proximal MCA, and the ACA, which are innervated by branches of the trigeminal nerve. Spread of varicella along the "trigeminovascular" nerve pathways following reactivation of the latent virus in the trigeminal ganglion has been documented. Viral invasion of the implicated arterial segments results in an inflammatory response. Other infectious agents implicated in cerebral arteriopathies include parvovirus B19, cytomegalovirus, *Mycoplasma pneumoniae*, *Borrelia burdgoferi*, enterovirus, and *Helicobacter*

pylori. The clinical presentation of FCA inflammatory type (FCA-i), also known as transient cerebral arteriopathy, is acute hemiparesis and/or aphasia caused by infarction, most commonly of the basal ganglia and internal capsule. These findings are associated with unifocal stenosis/occlusion of the proximal MCA, sometimes extending to the bifurcation of the internal carotid artery [35]. FCA-i is characterized by a monophasic course of stenosis lasting 3–6 months associated with basal ganglia infarction. Following the initial 3–6 months, the vascular stenosis typically stabilizes or improves. However, recurrence may occur within this initial course or beyond. Treatment includes ASA or anticoagulation (based on the degree of vascular involvement or stenosis) for a minimum of 3–6 months. The total duration of treatment is based on the vascular findings, and longer duration is warranted when persistent stenosis is found. Some experts advise a 3- to 5-day pulse of IV methylprednisolone followed by an oral prednisone taper [36], particularly when there is severe progression of the initial stenosis. However, the use of steroids is controversial [37] and is now the subject of two clinical trials, namely the High-Dose Steroids in Children with Stroke (PASTA) and the Focal Cerebral Arteriopathy Steroid (FOCAS) trials.

AIS can occur as a direct complication of central nervous system bacterial infection, particularly pneumococcal and tuberculosis meningitis [38]. The extensive involvement of the basal cisterns in tuberculosis meningitis may induce an exudative encasement of the circle of Willis, causing arteritis, stenosis, and vasospasm. This may progress to full arterial occlusion resulting in AIS that can be recurrent and multifocal involving both the anterior and posterior circulation with small, medium, and large artery involvement. Exudative encasement with thrombosis can also affect the arteries and veins coursing over the convexity of the hemispheres resulting in subsurface infarction. The use of antithrombotic therapy in conjunction with antibiotic and in some instances steroid therapy has been reported with minimal risk for hemorrhagic conversion in children with stroke in the setting of aggressive bacterial or tuberculous meningitis. Recent data from our own center suggest considerable safety and efficacy of anticoagulation therapy in reducing the risk of recurrent brain infarction, in a carefully selected subgroup of children with tuberculosis-related meningitis [38]. Nevertheless, further studies are required to replicate these findings. In recent times, AIS has been found to be a complication of the severe acute respiratory syndrome coronavirus-2 (SARS-CoV-2) infection in neonates and children, although this is much less frequent compared with adults [39]. When considered the primary stroke risk factor for AIS, SARS-CoV-2 is thought to cause AIS because of an inflammatory arteriopathy [39].

Posterior Circulation AIS

Posterior circulation (vertebrobasilar system) AIS accounts for 20–30% of pediatric AIS cases. Clinical diagnosis is more challenging than anterior circulation AIS because of the nonspecific and diffuse neurological manifestations, like vertigo, hearing loss, cranial nerve palsies, quadriplegia, ataxia, and encephalopathy in varying combinations resulting in delayed diagnosis. In addition, visual field deficits because of occipital infarction can be subtle and not reported by patients. Vertebral artery dissection is an important but under-recognized cause. AIS involving the brainstem and cerebellum are particularly at risk of upward cerebellar and downward tonsillar herniation as well as obstructive hydrocephalus and brainstem compression because of limited space for expansion of the infarcted tissue resulting in life-threatening consequences if not detected early.

An anatomical cause of posterior circulation stroke, known as Bowhunter's syndrome (BHS), presents with vertebrobasilar insufficiency provoked by dynamic impingement and mechanical obstruction to blood flow in the vertebral arteries because of normal and physiological head rotation [40]. BHS must be suspected in the case of ectasia or dilatation affecting the V3 segment of a vertebral artery, which could be unilateral or bilateral. It is hypothesized that BHS represents an abnormal response of a susceptible vertebral artery to the normal mechanical impact of the bony structures in its proximity [14]. Patients with BHS often have posterior circulation stroke with recurrence despite therapeutic anticoagulation and antiplatelet therapy. In certain cases, a surgical approach can be considered [14]. In a small case series of 11 children with BHS followed for a mean duration of 33.3 months, Braga et al. [41] reported that the use of vertebral artery decompression or first and second cervical vertebrae (C1–C2) fusion is linked to a reduction of stroke recurrence.

The role for dual antiplatelet and anticoagulant therapy in this setting may be warranted since there is a higher risk of recurrence compared with anterior circulation strokes [42]. Increased recognition of posterior circulation AIS related to small vessel disease is an important consideration given the association with hemorrhagic stroke risk [43]. The outcome from posterior circulation stroke in children including basilar artery occlusion is more favorable compared with adults with brainstem infarction [44].

Moyamoya Disease

Moyamoya disease is characterized by progressive stenosis of the distal internal carotid arteries with formation of secondary collateral vessels distal to the stenosis. Other cranial arteries may be affected as well. When moyamoya occurs in isolation, it is classified as moyamoya disease, while patients with recognized genetic or acquired risk factors have moyamoya syndrome. The clinical conditions commonly associated with moyamoya syndrome include cranial radiotherapy, neurofibromatosis type I, SCD, and trisomy 21 [4]. Genetic consulting is recommended in relevant cases. Moyamoya disease is most commonly seen in children of Asian descent but has also been described in other ethnicities. The incidence of moyamoya disease is highest in countries in East Asia, such as Japan and Korea. In Japan, the annual prevalence and incidence have been estimated to be 3.16–10.5 and 0.35–0.94 per 100,000, respectively. Conversely, the annual incidence in the USA and Europe has been reported to be about 10% of that in Japan [4].

Moyamoya disease has a bimodal age distribution of clinical presentation, with one peak in the first decade and a second peak in adults 30–40 years of age. Affected family members can be identified in 6–20% of cases, and an autosomal dominant inheritance with variable expression has been proposed. A major founder susceptibility gene for familial moyamoya has been identified at p. R4810K on the *RNF213* gene [45]. Moyamoya disease is genetically heterogeneous and has been linked to 3p24.2-26, 17q25, and other genetic loci. An expanded phenotype associated with *RNF213* variants is now recognized [46]. The most common clinical features in patients with moyamoya disease and/or syndrome include recurrent TIAs or AIS, cognitive decline (approximately 50% of children, especially in those who developed the disease prior the age of 4 years), headaches, and seizures (20–30%). However, there appear to be distinct clinical phenotypes, which are associated with a variable profile of ischemic risk [47]. The diagnosis can usually be confirmed with noninvasive vascular imaging (i.e., 3 Tesla MRI/MRA) (shown in Fig. 5). Evaluation with a cerebral angiogram is needed for surgical planning. Measurement of cerebral perfusion with gadolinium-contrast or arterial spin labeling techniques and assessment of blood flow reserve with acetazolamide challenge may contribute to the evaluation and follow-up of individuals with moyamoya disease. Transcranial Doppler (TCD) is sometimes used to evaluate and follow-up children with moyamoya because of SCD [10].

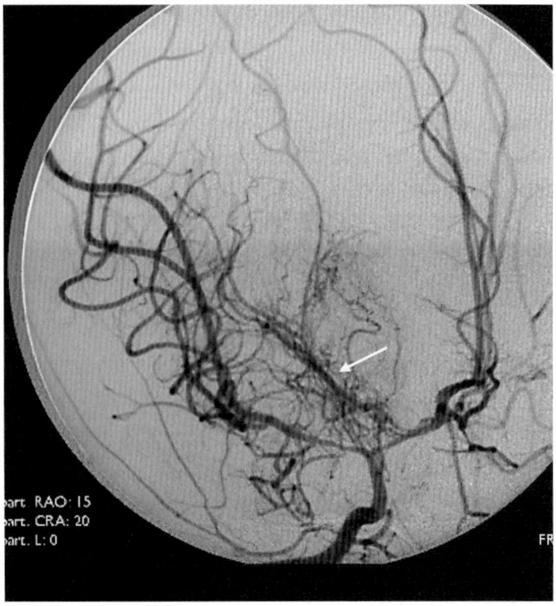

Fig. 5. Conventional cerebral angiography on a coronal view of a child with moyamoya disease. The arrow shows the collateral moyamoya vessels arising from the lenticulostriate branches of the stenosed proximal right MCA.

Children should be referred to neurosurgery centers experienced in the management of moyamoya. Various surgical revascularization techniques are used for moyamoya disease, including direct bypass procedures and indirect encephaloduroarteriosynangiosis (EDAS). Direct bypass procedures are typically used in selected older children where the superficial temporal artery is sutured to the MCA. EDAS procedure implants an extracranial artery intracranially resulting in the growth of new collateral branches into the underperfused cerebral territories over time. Two large long-term follow-up studies have indicated that surgical treatment of moyamoya is reasonably safe (4% risk of stroke within 30 days of surgery per hemisphere) and effective (96% probability of remaining stroke free over a 5-year follow-up period) [10].

Antiplatelet therapy may be useful in preventing moyamoya-related AIS both for primary and secondary stroke prevention [10]. Anticoagulants are rarely recommended because of the perceived risk of hemorrhagic stroke, which increases with age and is more commonly seen in adult moyamoya patients.

Children with moyamoya disease/syndrome are at additional risk of ischemic symptoms during the perioperative period. Hyperventilation related to crying can lower the partial pressure of carbon dioxide and induce ischemia secondary to cerebral vasoconstriction. Adequate intraoperative blood pressure maintenance, postoperative pain control, and procedures to reduce the discomfort and anxiety related to dressing changes and suture removal may reduce the risk of ischemic symptoms and shorten the hospitalization [10].

Sickle Cell Disease

Cerebral ischemic injury is common among children with SCD, where clinically overt AIS may occur in up to 11% of children not receiving primary prevention therapy by age 20 years, with the peak age of onset between 2–5 years [48]. The pathophysiology is complex and multifactorial, involving sickling in the microcirculation, abnormal cerebral autoregulation, anemia-related thrombophilia, and large vessel progressive stenosis. The postulated mechanism for large vessel intracranial disease is proliferation of vascular intima, leading to progressive stenosis of intracranial portions of the internal carotid, middle, and ACA arteries. Silent cerebral infarcts, defined as small foci of T2 hyperintensity with no history or physical findings of focal neurologic deficit, are the most common neurologic injury in SCD [48]. Unlike overt AIS located in the cortex and deep white matter, silent cerebral infarcts are typically in the deep white matter in the frontal, parietal, and temporal lobes. Silent cerebral infarcts are recognized as a cause of school problems and neurocognitive deficits. After abnormal TCD velocities, the presence of silent cerebral infarcts is the greatest risk factor for overt AIS in patients with SCD [48].

The use of antithrombotic therapy in primary and secondary AIS prevention in patients with SCD is controversial, because of the complex pathophysiology of stroke in SCD, and the perceived increased risk of hemorrhage in patients with moyamoya-type vasculopathy.

The basic principle for SCD stroke treatment is to improve tissue-level oxygen delivery to the brain. In addition to the general neuroprotective measures for AIS, supportive measures include oxygen and red blood cell (RBC) transfusion. Exchange RBC transfusion is generally the preferred option. Because of the time involved in arranging an exchange transfusion, and associated risks of fluctuating blood pressure, if the initial hemoglobin is less than 100 g/L, a simple RBC transfusion may be considered while arranging an exchange transfusion [48]. In addition to oxygen and RBC transfusion, a septic work-up should be completed, and empiric antibiotics should be administered in the setting of fever.

Following the initial exchange transfusion, a long-term chronic transfusion program is generally recommended after the first AIS in SCD, given the high recurrence rates. Fifty percent will have a second stroke within 2 years. However, transfusion therapy is not completely effective; approximately 20% of children experience second overt AIS despite transfusion therapy [49]. The transfusion interval and volumes are tailored to the transfusion targets of a hemoglobin S less than 30% and avoiding hyperviscosity; tailoring target hematocrit to incorporate patient's baseline hematocrit and pretransfusion hemoglobin S percentage. An example of a chronic transfusion program would be transfusion intervals of 3–4 weeks with volume of 15 mL/kg. At the earliest opportunity, optimally prior to the first transfusion, all SCD patients should have extended antigenic phenotyping: ABO, Rh (C, D, E), Kell, Duffy, Kidd, and MNS blood groups (see Appendix III). Prophylactic red cell antigen matching for Rh and Kell reduces alloimmunization rates, and additional matching for Kidd, Duffy, and S minimizes the risk of alloimmunization with transfusion even further. Despite the complications of chronic RBC transfusion program, a practical alternative has not been yet identified [50]. Long-term chronic RBC transfusion program is also recommended to prevent AIS in children with SCD identified at high risk for stroke [48]. TCD velocities are tested on an annual basis from age 2 to 16 years in children with SCD. Children with abnormal TCD velocities, defined as greater than 200 cm/s in the large cerebral vessels, have a 40% stroke risk within 3 years, which can be reduced by chronic RBC transfusion. Regular transfusions decrease the incidence and recurrence of cerebral infarction from 14% to 6% in children with prior silent infarction [51]. In a recent trial, TCD with transfusions changing to hydroxyurea (TWiTCH), hydroxyurea therapy was shown to be noninferior to RBC transfusion for primary stroke prevention in children with SCD [52]. Curative treatment by hematopoietic stem cell transplantation with an HLA-matched sibling donor may offer secondary stroke prevention. Gene therapy may be a future option.

Genetics in AIS

Inherited disorders that lead to vascular disease in children and adults have been recognized, and specific clinical and radiologic phenotypes have been identified. In a recent study from the United Kingdom, single gene pathogenic variants were identified in 1.5% of individuals of European origin with lacunar strokes [53]. Thus, investigating for these single gene variants in this patient population appears to be worthwhile. The main clinical and radiologic features of the most common monogenic vascular syndromes are depicted in Table 2 [54].

Thrombolysis in Hyperacute AIS

In adults, IV tPA at 0.9 mg/kg (maximum dose of 90 mg) significantly improves clinical outcome when given within 4.5 h of AIS onset, despite a 6.4% risk of ICH [55]. In the absence of contrain-

Table 2. Monogenetic disorders associated with childhood ischemic and hemorrhagic stroke

Condition	Gene variant	Clinical features	Radiologic features
Aicardi-Goutières	*RNASEH2A, 2B, 2C* *SAMHD1* *TEX1*	Newborns or infants with impaired development, irritability, and arthropathy	Basal ganglia calcification Leukoencephalopathy Moyamoya vasculopathy
ADAMTS13 Thrombotic microangiopathy	*ADAMTS13*	Arterial ischemic stroke in children because of increased high-molecular-weight multimers: von Willebrand factor	Ischemic stroke and intracranial hemorrhage
Fabry disease	*Alpha-GAL-A*	Multisystemic (cardiac, renal) X-linked lysosomal storage disease Acroparesthesia Small vessel ischemia, especially in the posterior circulation	Basilar artery dolichoectasia T2-hyperintensities in the white matter of the frontal and parietal lobes T1-weighted images demonstrate high signal in the deep gray matter especially the pulvinar (characteristic)
Large vessel vasculopathies	*ACTA2*	Early onset coronary and thoracic disease Arterial ischemic stroke	White matter disease Abnormal internal carotid arterial morphology with dilation and straightening of the carotid, vertebral, anterior, middle, and posterior cerebral arteries Territorial infarcts
Alagille syndrome	*JAG1*	Multisystemic involvement Abnormal vertebrae	Intracranial stenosis Cerebral aneurysms
Moyamoya disease	*RNF213*	Progressive childhood arteriopathy Transient ischemic attacks with hyperventilation Can involve other vascular beds including renal and cardiac	Progressive noninflammatory nonatherosclerotic bilateral occlusive disease of the terminal internal carotid and proximal middle and anterior cerebral arteries with formation of basal collaterals
Deficiency of Adenosine Deaminase 2 (DADA2)	*CECR1*	Recurrent fevers Tendril-like skin discolorations Enlarged liver and spleen Recurrent stroke-like episodes Immune system abnormalities	Small-vessel vasculitis with lacunar infarcts
Ehlers-Danlos syndrome type IV (vascular Ehlers-Danlos syndrome)	*COL3A1*	Easy bruising Thin skin with visible veins Characteristic facial features At risk of arterial, gastrointestinal, and uterine rupture	Recurrent spontaneous dissection in the cervical or vertebrobasilar circulation Cerebral aneurysms
COL4A1-related disorders	*COL4A1*	Perinatal arterial ischemic and/or hemorrhagic stroke Retinal arterial tortuosity, retinal hemorrhages, cataracts Cardiac arrhythmias Renal cysts, proteinuria, hematuria Elevated creatine kinase	Porencephaly White matter changes Cerebral or cerebellar hemorrhage Cerebral aneurysms Microhemorrhage

dications, it is the standard of care in acute AIS across all stroke etiologies in adults. Observational studies report the use of IV tPA in pediatric patients, but safety and efficacy have not been established in pediatric AIS [56]. Children increasingly reach tertiary centers within the time window required for tPA administration. Data on safety and dosing in children are needed to guide therapy because physiologically immature fibrinolytic and coagulation systems are different than those in adults [13] (Appendix II). As per the American Heart Association guidelines, tPA is not recommended for AIS in children outside of study settings [10, 14]; however, in adolescents, no consensus against its use has been established.

At The Hospital for Sick Children, in the absence of any contraindications, IV tPA can be administered to a child over 2 years of age within 4.5 h of symptom onset with a persistent focal neurological deficit (Pediatric National Institutes of Health Stroke Scale [PedNIHSS] score >4) and confirmed arterial occlusion on MRA/CTA in consultation with thrombosis and pediatric stroke teams. The dose used for children who are 12 years and younger is 0.75 mg/kg (maximum dose of 75 mg) and for children older than 12 years is 0.9 mg/kg (maximum dose of 90 mg) with an initial 10% of the full calculated dose administered as a bolus over 5 min and the remainder 90% of the full dose as an infusion over 1 h.

In the adult stroke literature, a recent open-label, parallel-group, randomized-controlled trial has shown that IV tenecteplase as a 0.25 mg/kg single bolus dose (maximum dose of 25 mg) is noninferior in recanalization of large vessel occlusion when compared with IV tPA at 0.9 mg/kg (maximum dose of 90 mg) given as an initial 10% bolus over 5 min and 90% as infusion over 1 h [57]. Therefore, tenecteplase is now routinely considered as an alternative to alteplase within 4.5 h of acute stroke symptom onset in adult stroke patients who meet standard criteria for thrombolysis. There is no pediatric stroke literature on the fibrinolytic agent tenecteplase, and its efficacy, safety, and potential uses in pediatric stroke are therefore not known.

Hyperacute Code Stroke Response and Multidisciplinary Stroke Teams

Adult stroke experts have developed networks and interdisciplinary teams that aim to facilitate hyperacute stroke care across large geographic areas [58]. Across the USA and Canada, designated stroke centers have been established and accredited. Although pediatric stroke is one of the top 10 causes of morbidity and mortality, there are challenges in developing similar models of care because of numerous barriers. For one, the mimics for pediatric stroke are vast and more frequently encountered in the emergency department. In addition, lack of awareness regarding pediatric stroke amongst primary care providers leads to delay in diagnosis [59] precluding the use of hyperacute therapies [58]. Selecting the optimal type of neuroimaging modality to diagnose childhood AIS in a timely fashion while excluding stroke mimics also poses a barrier given that MRI is often preferred; however, not all pediatric emergency rooms have 24-h MRI availability. The only prospective treatment trial of IV tPA to date in children, the Thrombolysis in Pediatric Stroke [60] trial, was closed because of lack of enrollment. However, it allowed for the establishment of pediatric stroke treatment centers and hyperacute intrahospital guidelines (one example shown in Fig. 6) [61]. Prospective studies to evaluate the effectiveness of multidisciplinary stroke teams and guidelines will be beneficial to expand this model of care.

Endovascular Therapy

In adults, mechanical thrombectomy with stent retrievers is now recommended as the standard of care in AIS caused by a proximal large vessel occlusion in the anterior circulation [62, 63]. In comparison, mechanical thrombectomy is rarely used in children with a recently reported rate of 10% from a Swiss cohort [64]. This is primarily because

1. CLINICAL PRESENTATION WITH SUDDEN ONSET OF:

B is for **B**alance: sudden trouble with balance or coordination?
E is for **E**yes: sudden blurred or double vision or sudden loss of vision in one or both eyes?

F is for **F**ace: does one side of the face droop or feels numb? Ask your child to smile
A is for **A**rm: is one arm weak or numb? Ask your child to raise both arms. Does one arm drift downward?
S is for **S**peech: is speech slurred or is your child unable to speak or hard to understand? Ask your child to repeat a simple sentence like „the sky is blue." Is the sentence repeated correctly?
T is for **T**ime: call 911 if your child shows one or more of these symptoms, even if the symptoms go away, call 911 and get them to the hospital immediately

↓

2. HIGH LEVEL OF CLINICAL SUSPICION OF STROKE
STROKE ALERT CRITERIA ARE MET (if 'yes' to any of the questions listed above)

Multi-D team discussion including Neurology, Neuroradiology, Anesthesia, Hematology +/– Neurosurgery in selected circumstances
Initiate neuroprotective measures
Confirm time last seen well
Keep NPO and determine timing of last meal
Confirm accurate body weight
Insert PIV and order STAT labs
CBC, PT/INR, aPTT, fibrinogen, blood type & screen, electrolytes, glucose and creatinine
Call referral hospital centralized triage system for all possible acute strokes, even if stable
Look for stroke risk factors → chronic systemic disease, trauma, infection, congenital heart disease, toxicology

↓

3. TRANSFER DECISION
Is urgent CT/CTA or MRI/MRA and general anesthesia available?

YES ↓ → 4.

NO → **TRANSFER FOR FULL DIAGNOSTIC MRI/MRA ASAP <24 HOURS** ↓ → 4.

4. RADIOLOGICAL ASSESSMENT

Urgent neuroimaging using standardized protocol
Non-contrast head CT to rule out hemorrhage
If cooperative, no braces, and access to MRI → obtain STAT MRI/MRA within 1 hour
If MRI not possible and transfer not feasible/swift → obtain CT/CTA within 1 hour
Vascular imaging of head +/– neck from aortic arch to vertex → especially with history of trauma
Do not be afraid to order a CTA (except in sickle cell disease or with renal impairment)

↓

STROKE CONFIRMED

a

6

(Figure continued on next page.)

STROKE CONFIRMED (transfer to PICU for both hyperacute/immediate post-treatment care)

↓

5. INTERVENTIONAL DECISIONS

Assess eligibility for IV-tPA, endovascular intervention +/– antithrombotic therapy, and neurointerventional consult:
IV-tPA criteria: ***is the child ≥ 2 years old AND within 4.5 hours of symptom onset with a thrombus seen on vascular imaging with MRA/ CTA?***

OR

Endovascular criteria: ***is the child ≥ 2 years old AND within 24 hours of symptom onset with a large vessel occlusion seen on vascular imaging with MRA/CTA?***

AND

Assess for urgent neurosurgical consult:
Is there neuroimaging confirmed intracranial hemorrhage, malignant middle cerebral arterial infarction, posterior circulation infarction, and/or clinical signs of raised intracranial pressure?

↓

6. MANAGEMENT DECISIONS

Intensive neurological surveillance (≥48 hours), continuous EEG monitoring, intensive blood pressure monitoring, stabilize modifiable risk factors, neuroprotective measures (see below)

AND

Assess eligibility for secondary stroke prevention management (anticoagulation, antiplatelet therapy, other measures; see text for details)

↓

7. INITIAL INVESTIGATIONS TO LOOK FOR ETIOLOGY („triple P")

Pump – echocardiography
Plasma – standardized prothrombotic work-up
Pipes – vascular imaging

Acute Stroke Neuroprotective Care

- **NPO**, head of bed flat (if tolerated and no signs of increased ICP)
- **Normotension:** Target SBP 50–95%ile f or age to maintain cerebral perfusion pressure. Tx hypotension (< 50%ile for age): NS, inotropes Tx hypertension (> 33%ile for age): labetalol: lower by ~25% over 24 hours
- **Normovolemia:** maintenance NS, bolus PRN
- **Normothermia:** Treat >37°C with antipyretics +/– cooling
- **Normoglycemia:** No IV glucose unless hypoglycemic, target: 5–10 mmol/L
- **Seizure control:** ASAP with any suspected seizure activity. Consider EEG

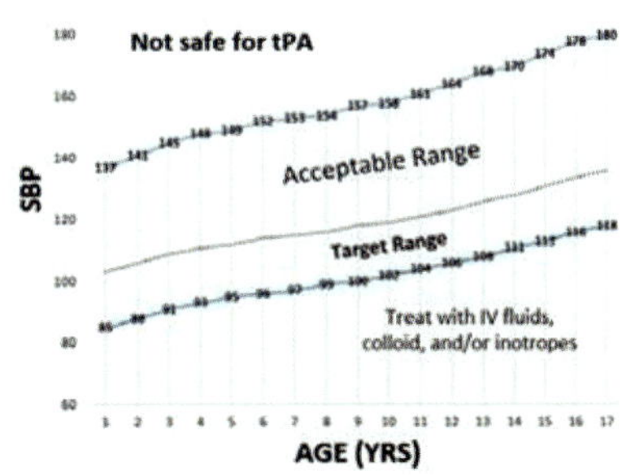

b

6

(For legend see next page.)

of delays in diagnosis and uncertainty regarding clinically efficacy and safety, chief among them being fatal bleeding complications. It is not known whether thrombectomy has the same increased or decreased rate of hemorrhagic complications in children as compared with that of adults [64]. To address this question, a recent systematic review [65] identified 110 children who underwent mechanical thrombectomy. Their results showed that 90% of children had a good long-term neurological outcome (modified Rankin Scale [mRS] 0–2) and 87% had successful angiographic recanalization, two died and only one had symptomatic ICH [65]. However, the lack of a control group is an important limitation to this study, especially given the known high rate of good outcome (mRS 0–2) in children with stroke not treated with embolectomy. Data regarding PedNIHSS severity vs. outcome in pediatric stroke are awaited to resolve the question of natural pediatric outcomes following severe initial stroke and ascertain a target group that will be most likely to benefit.

Fig. 6. a The Hospital for Sick Children pathway of care for confirmed or suspected hyperacute pediatric arterial ischemic stroke (AIS) at an outside centre. **b** A simplified SickKids hyperacute AIS algorithm. See text for further details. This clinical care guideline is meant as a guide for the health care provider, does not establish a standard of care, and is not a substitute for medical judgment, which should be applied based upon the individual circumstances and clinical condition of the patient. Reproduced with permission from the Children's Stroke Program at The Hospital for Sick Children. aPTT, activated partial thromboplastin time; ASAP, as soon as possible; C, Celsius; CBC, complete blood count; CT/CTA, computerized tomography/angiography; EEG, electroencephalogram; ICP, intra-cranial pressure; IV, intravenous; IV-tPA, intravenous tissue plasminogen activator; mmol/L, millimoles per liter; MRI/MRA, magnetic resonance imaging/angiography; Multi-D, multidisciplinary; NPO, no diet/liquid intake by mouth; NS, normal saline; PICU, pediatric intensive care unit; PIV, peripheral intravenous line; PRN, as needed; PT/INR, prothrombin time/international normalized ratio; SBP, systolic blood pressure; STAT, short turnaround time; Tx, treatment; %ile, percentile; YRS, years.

One of the limiting factors of using mechanical thrombectomy in children is the uncertainty as to the youngest age where an adult-sized device can be used safely for retrieval of the thrombus. A recent study showed that around 94% of 5-year-old children have developed the adult artery caliber in the circle of Willis [66]. Until safety data and optimal selection criteria of children who would benefit the most from mechanical thrombectomy are known, it should be only considered in carefully selected cases, in consultation with a vascular neurologist and an interventional radiologist with expertise in the management of pediatric stroke.

Complications of AIS

Malignant MCA Infarction

Malignant MCA (MMCA) infarction presents with anterior circulation focal neurological deficits, followed by decreased level of consciousness culminating in transtentorial herniation and death. It is more frequent in adolescents and young adults who have limited skull compliance and physiological brain atrophy that can compensate for the mass effect secondary to progressive cerebral edema in the setting of ischemia. In adults, MMCA infarction occurs in 10–20% of large (>50% territory) MCA-AIS with a high mortality rate (80%). Decompressive hemicraniectomy can be lifesaving [67]. In pediatric MCA-AIS, the frequency of MMCA infarction varies from 1.3 to 12.5% [68]. In a cohort of 66 children, 12 (18%) developed malignant cerebral edema [68]. In this study, authors found that prolonged seizures, longer than 5 min in duration in the first 24 h, and a high initial PedNIHSS score (≥8), are independent predictors for MMCA [68]. Therefore, it is imperative to closely monitor for clinical and subclinical seizures using continuous EEG monitoring and aggressively implement neuroprotective measures in children presenting with acute AIS during their first 24–48 h.

The use of anticoagulation in a large territory AIS during the first 72 h is controversial, and there are no specific guidelines. Adult stroke specialists advocate holding anticoagulation in such cases because of a higher risk of hemorrhagic conversion; however, in children, this risk seems to be lower. The decision should be made on a case-by-case basis and must include a multidisciplinary team including a pediatric neurologist, hematologist, neurosurgeon, and intensive care physicians balancing the risk of bleeding versus the risk of reinfarction. Additionally, in patients that may require decompressive hemicraniectomy, if anticoagulation is considered, UFH may be the best option given the ability to rapidly reverse its effect and its short half-life [67].

Hemorrhagic Transformation

Hemorrhagic transformation of acute AIS may occur spontaneously, as a complication of anticoagulation or secondary to systemic factors like hypertension. This complication has been widely studied in the adult population. A commonly used classification system was developed for the European Cooperative Acute Stroke Study (ECASS), which divides hemorrhagic transformation into four subtypes [69, 70]: "H0 – no hemorrhage detected; HI1 – scattered heterogenous petechiae along the margins of the infarct; HI2 – more confluent petechia; PH1 – small parenchymal hemorrhage with less than 30% of infarcted area with no to mild mass effect; and PH2 – large parenchymal hemorrhage with greater than 30% infarcted area with significant mass effect or hemorrhage remote from the stroke location" [70]. In adults, ECASS grade HI1, HI2, and PH1 within the first 36 h of stroke onset were not associated with a higher risk of neurological morbidity or mortality when compared with patients without hemorrhagic transformation [69, 70]. PH2, however, was associated with a significantly increased risk of early and 3-month mortality as well as acute neurological deterioration [70]. Childhood AIS studies have been adopting this classification [18, 71, 72]. An important MRI mimic of HI1 in young children and infants is "cortical laminar necrosis" or mineralization of the cortical ribbon, which can develop rapidly (days to a few weeks) in this age group. In a single center prospective cohort, hemorrhagic transformation was observed in 19 of 63 (30%; 95% CI, 19–43%) childhood AIS cases [71]. Most cases (96%) were asymptomatic with an isolated radiological finding consisting of HI1, i.e., tiny asymptomatic petechiae [71]. Antithrombotic therapy and hypertension were not associated with hemorrhagic transformation [71]. The risk for hemorrhagic transformation was higher in children treated with combined antiplatelet and anticoagulant therapies [71]. In a child with hemorrhagic transformation of AIS, a multidisciplinary discussion can be beneficial in deciding the risks vs. benefit ratio of continuing versus withholding antithrombotic therapy. An extended discussion with parents/guardians about the risks and benefits of antithrombotic therapy is important.

Long-Term Outcomes

Long-term outcomes of pediatric stroke include not only sensorimotor deficits such as hemiparesis and cerebral palsy but also expressive and receptive language impairments, visual filed deficits, cognitive impairment, mental health disorders, and epilepsy [73]. The full impact of AIS in a child may not be known for years as the child grows and matures and reaches various developmental stages. In other words, children with AIS often "grow into their deficits" [73, 74]. There may be ongoing and emerging needs throughout growth and development. Therefore, children who have experienced a stroke require long-term monitoring and follow-up throughout maturation to ensure optimal achievement of developmental, functional, and psychosocial potentials [73, 74].

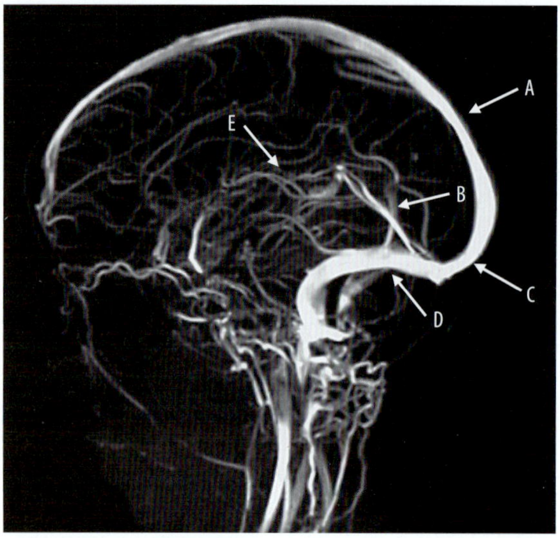

Fig. 7. Sagittal MRV demonstrating normal cerebral venous anatomy: (A) superior sagittal sinus; (B) straight sinus; (C) torcula; (D) left transverse sinus; (E) internal cerebral veins.

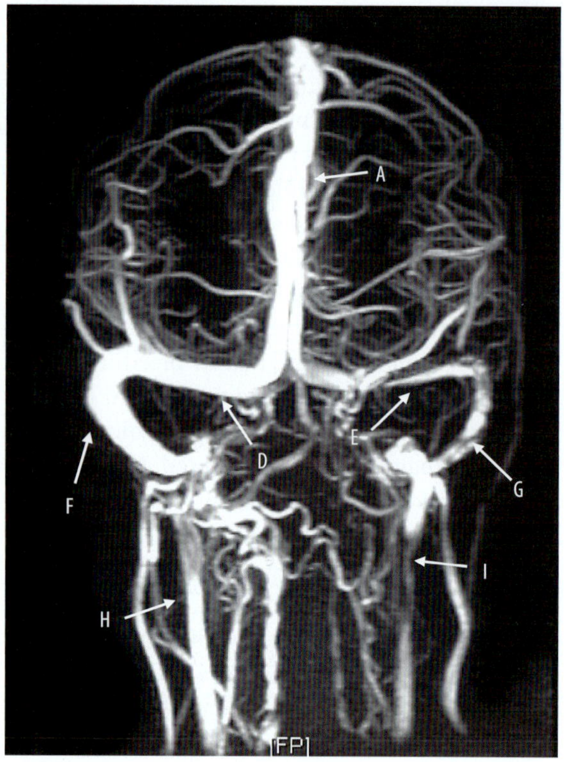

Fig. 8. Coronal MRV demonstrating normal cerebral venous anatomy: (A) superior sagittal sinus; (D) right transverse sinus; (E) left transverse sinus (nondominant); (F) right sigmoid sinus; (G) left sigmoid sinus; (H) right internal jugular vein; (I) left internal jugular vein.

Cerebral Sinovenous Thrombosis

CSVT, with or without infarction, occurs when a thrombus develops in the veins of the brain or venous sinuses and obstructs venous outflow [75, 76]. The incidence of CSVT is approximately 0.4–0.7 per 100,000 children per year. Around 40% of cases occur during the neonatal period, giving an incidence in newborns of 1–12 per 100,000 per year [75, 76].

Venous sinuses and veins are located within the subarachnoid space. Arachnoid villi project into the venous sinuses of the dura and are concentrated in the superior sagittal sinus, serving an important role in the absorption and drainage of cerebrospinal fluids [75]. The cerebral venous system is divided into two major networks of veins and sinuses (shown in Fig. 7, 8). The superficial system includes (a) the superficial cortical veins; (b) the superior sagittal vein; (c) the confluence of the sinuses; (d) the transverse sinuses; (e) the sigmoid sinuses; and (f) the internal jugular veins. The deep system is formed by (1) the basal veins that are responsible for the drainage from the basal ganglia and, in preterm newborns, the germinal matrix; (2) the galenic system that is composed of the two internal cerebral veins and the vein of Galen; (3) the straight sinus; (4) the basal vein of Rosenthal; and (5) the torcula. Normal anatomic variations in the cerebral venous anatomy exist, the most common of which is hypoplasia or the absence of a major dural sinus, usually the left or less commonly, the right transverse sinus (86%). A retrospective case-control analysis showed that the presence of anatomical variations does not predispose children to the development of CSVT, and these variations appear

Table 3. Relevant history and physical examination findings in suspected cerebral sinus venous thrombosis (CSVT) by age group

Neonates	
Clinical presentation	Acute seizures after the first 12 h of life, hydrocephalus, altered mental status
Past medical history	*Maternal factors:* chorioamniotis, gestational diabetes, and maternal hypertension *Perinatal factors:* meconium aspiration, hypoxic-ischemic encephalopathy, polycythemia, and neonatal infection
Physical exam	Increased head circumference, hypotonia. Focal motor deficit
Older infant or child	
Clinical presentation	Headache, vision problems (blurred vision, double vision), less frequent seizures, and focal deficits
Past medical history	*Acute Illness:* head and neck infection (otitis media, mastoiditis), dehydration, trauma, central nervous system tumors, recent intracranial surgery, and anemia (iron deficiency) *Chronic conditions:* congenital heart disease, nephrotic syndrome, systemic lupus erythematosus, and malignancy *Drugs:* L-asparaginase, oral contraceptives, steroids, epoetin-alpha, adenoviral vector-based vaccine for COVID-19[a] (i.e., ChAdOx1 CoV-19 [AstraZeneca], Ad26.COV2.S [Janssen; Johnson & Johnson])
Family history	Thrombotic events (age <55 years with stroke, myocardial infarction, deep venous thrombosis, and maternal recurrent fetal loss)
Physical examination	*General exam:* signs of ear infection or trauma, nausea, and vomiting *Neurological exam:* papilledema, pupil asymmetries, ocular palsies (especially cranial nerve VI), facial sensory deficits, hemiparesis, hemisensory deficit, and psychiatric symptoms

[a]Causative of vaccine-induced immune thrombotic thrombocytopenia, rarely complicated by CSVT. Of note, children have not received adenoviral-based immunization for COVID-19.

17

equally in children with CSVT and in healthy controls [77].

The two main mechanisms implicated in the physiopathology of CSVT are venous congestion and parenchymal ischemic lesions. Thrombosis within the cerebral venous system results in outflow obstruction, venous congestion, and a consequent increase in capillary hydrostatic pressure, driving fluid into the interstitial space and producing edema and ultimately infarction [78]. In most cases, infarction is hemorrhagic. In term and preterm newborns, there is an association between intraventricular hemorrhage and CSVT. Positioning of the neonate has a major influence on venous outflow. Neck flexion and compression of the superior sagittal sinus by the occipital bone in supine lying patients have been implicated in venous stasis and thrombosis, and further study of these associations is ongoing [78].

Clinical Presentation

CSVT in children is usually multifactorial, with a predisposing comorbid condition identified in up to 95% of children (Table 3). The clinical picture of children with CSVT can be nonspecific and subtle. Progressive headache, altered level of consciousness, focal deficits, and seizures (focal or generalized) are the most common presenting symptoms as reported in a multicenter cohort of 170 children [79]. Less commonly, cranial nerve abnormalities and papilledema are also found. The most common risk factors include chronic

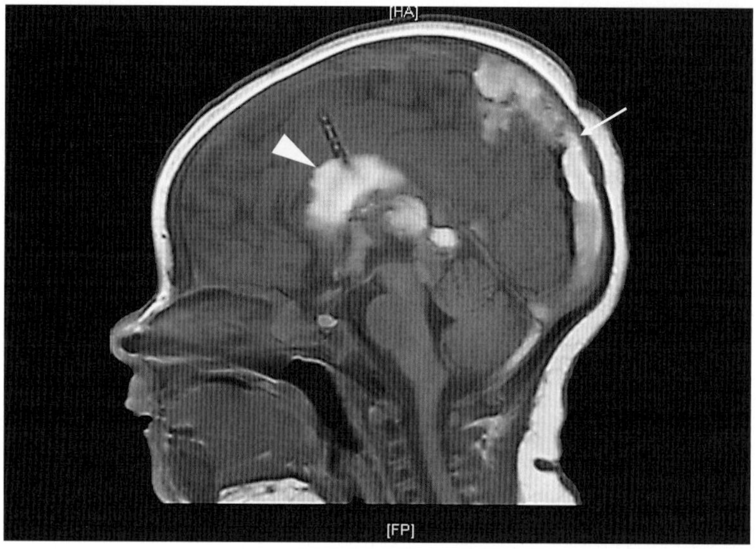

Fig. 9. Sagittal MRV with contrast of a neonate with extensive CSVT involving the superior sagittal sinus (arrow) and associated intraventricular hemorrhage (arrowhead) because of involvements of the internal cerebral veins.

disease (such as malignancies) in 50% followed by head and neck disorders in 41% (Table 3). In the same cohort, a prothrombotic state was found in 20%, whereas other hematological abnormalities such as severe iron deficiency were found in 19% [79].

Diagnosis

Contrast-enhanced venous imaging with magnetic resonance venography (MRV) with gadolinium or computed tomography venography (CTV) are the methods of choice for the accurate diagnosis of CSVT (shown in Fig. 9). The diagnosis is established by demonstrating a lack of flow or filling defect in the cerebral veins. Although not reliable to rule out CSVT, unenhanced CT scans may occasionally detect CSVT as hyperintensity in the expected locations of the superficial deep sinuses. However, these findings are not specific and may have a similar appearance in cases of generalized hemoconcentration as is common in neonates. The addition of contrast may show a filling defect, referred to as the "empty delta sign" in the posterior part of the sagittal sinus. While simple CT scan with contrast misses the diagnosis of CSVT in up to 40% of patients, dedicated CTV confirms the diagnosis reliably. Diffusion and perfusion MRI may play a role in detecting venous congestion in CSVT and in the differentiation of cytotoxic and vasogenic edema but does not reliably differentiate venous from arterial infarction. Time-of-flight MRV can present false-positive findings suggesting CSVT including flow gaps in the venous sinuses. The superficial venous system is more frequently involved than the deep system, and the most common sites of CSVT are the transverse, superior sagittal, sigmoid, and straight sinuses. Between one- and two-thirds of children with CSVT may have parenchymal brain lesions such as venous infarction and hemorrhage.

Management

Anticoagulation is the mainstay treatment for children with CSVT, based on the current adult recommendations. Other risk factors, such as hypertension, comorbid bleeding diathesis, or other risks of bleeding, such as head trauma or recent surgery, may impact the decision to treat with anticoagulation [80]. If anticoagulation is started, follow-up imaging within 2–5 days may be needed if the patient worsens or fails to improve clinically to assess for hemorrhage or thrombus propagation. In a recent multicenter cohort study evaluating the treatment practices among 10 countries in children diagnosed with CSVT, the antithrombotic therapy of choice varied according to the region, with LMWH being the most used anticoagulant agent across North America [79]. A study evaluating the efficacy and safety of rivaroxaban, a new oral direct factor X inhibitor, randomized 114 children (aged 0–18 years) diagnosed with CSVT in comparison to standard-of-care anticoagulation (rivaroxaban [73 patients] vs. standard anticoagulation [41]) [81]. In both arms, anticoagulation had a low risk of CSVT propagation/recurrence and clinically relevant bleeding [81]. In terms of intervention, it may be reasonable to consider endovascular thrombolysis only in rare cases of catastrophic and life-threatening thrombosis failing to respond to systemic anticoagulation [82].

Additional supportive interventions are commonly needed. These include correcting fluid and electrolyte disturbances, treating infection especially of the head and neck, optimizing hemoglobin and platelet count, and monitoring and treating seizures. In cases where an associated provoking condition exists, it is important to optimize treatment of the comorbid disease such as exchange transfusion in SCD, mastoidectomy and abscess drainage for mastoiditis, and immune modulation for autoimmune-mediated thrombophilia (e.g., Bechet's, inflammatory bowel disease). In cases with persistent intracranial hypertension, acetazolamide to reduce cerebrospinal fluid production may be helpful.

CSVT in the Neonatal Period

Over 90% of newborns will survive their CSVT. In the Canadian Registry, the outcomes at a mean of 1.6 year follow-up were normal in 59%, neurological deficits in 22% including seizures, and recurrent thrombosis in 8%. However, studies applying standardized outcome measures found unfavorable outcomes (death or neurological deficit) in 37 of 63 (59%) of children with neonatal CSVT [83]. The presence of venous infarction was associated with worse outcome [78].

For neonates with CSVT that have no evidence of ICH or large parenchymal infarct, it is reasonable to treat with anticoagulation using LMWH, or UFH followed by LMWH, for 6 weeks to 3 months [13, 80]. In neonates, the experience with DOACs is limited, and ongoing studies will, hopefully, clarify their efficacy and safety in younger patients. For neonates who have CSVT with radiological evidence of significant ICH or large ischemic infarct, it is reasonable to hold anticoagulation, to repeat neuroimaging early (2–5 days) with CT/CTV or MRI/MRV and start anticoagulation if progression of the thrombus is observed [13, 79]. Dosing and monitoring of UFH and LMWH therapy in neonates are detailed in Chapter 20. In a single-center retrospective study of CSVT in preterm infants, more than one-quarter were asymptomatic at the time of diagnosis [84]. Anticoagulation in this small cohort appeared to be safe [84]. However, larger studies of preterm infants are needed.

CSVT in Older Infants and Children

About 90% of older children with CSVT survive the acute thrombosis event. In the Canadian Registry, the outcome was evaluated in 82 older infants and children at a mean interval from thrombosis to the last follow-up visit of 1.6 (range of 0.05–5.2) years [83]. There were 42 (51%) with a normal outcome, 32 (39%) with neurological deficits, and 8 (10%) deaths because of CSVT [83]. Standardized outcome studies demonstrate unfavorable outcome (death or neurological deficit) in 25 of 68 (37%) [83]. In a multicenter study, the mortality as a result of CSVT was 4% [79]. Mortality and neurological deficits were related to altered mental status as an initial symptom and no anticoagulation therapy [79].

For children with CSVT without significant ICH, anticoagulation initially with UFH or LMWH, and subsequently with LMWH, VKA, or

DOAC for a minimum of 3 months is recommended [13]. In children who still experience occlusion of CSVT or ongoing symptoms after 3 months of therapy, it is reasonable to treat a further 3 months [13]. Recently, a prospective trial enrolled 417 children (aged 0–21 years) after 6 weeks of anticoagulation if their thrombus burden at that point was only partially occlusive [85]. Patients were randomized to receive either 6 weeks or 3 months of anticoagulation for their provoked venous thrombotic event (excluding cancer, acquired/inherited major thrombophilia, or unprovoked events) [85]. The study included 59 children with CSVT (length of therapy: 6 weeks [25 patients] vs. 3 months [34]) [85]. The results revealed noninferiority of the patients treated on the 6-week arm, and practitioners may consider a similar approach for patients diagnosed with low-risk CSVT [85]. For children with CSVT with associated significant hemorrhagic parenchymal venous infarction, an extended discussion with the parents/guardians about the risks and benefits of anticoagulation is necessary. In cases of extensive and rapidly progressive thrombosis and infarction, the risk of mortality without anticoagulation is high, and anticoagulation may be the only life-saving treatment available. In less severe cases of CSVT with ICH, it may be reasonable to repeat radiologic monitoring of the thrombosis at 3–5 days and consider anticoagulation if thrombus extension is noted at that time, and if the ICH is stable or resolving [13]. Dosing and monitoring of UFH, LMWH, DOAC, and VKA therapy in children are detailed in Chapter 20.

In children with severe progressive CSVT that is unresponsive to a trial of therapeutic anticoagulation, other alternatives could include thrombolysis or surgical decompression [13]. Surgical or endovascular thrombectomy has been used in gravely ill patients, including children, usually in coma and with extensive thrombosis of superficial and deep venous structures and no response to anticoagulation [13]. In children with a history of CSVT who are at risk of recurrence, such as nephrotic syndrome or asparaginase chemotherapy, prophylactic anticoagulation may be considered when the patient is exposed to the inciting agent (e.g., asparaginase) or has an exacerbation of the underlying provoking disease condition [13].

Complications of CSVT

The most common acute complications of CSVT include new ICH or worsening of pre-existing ICH, intracranial venous hypertension, CSVT propagation, and rarely, hydrocephalus. ICH occurs in up to 30–40% children with CSVT at diagnosis. Anticoagulation-related hemorrhage is rare (6%) and in most cases nonfatal, does not worsen outcome, and does not require surgical intervention [80]. Intracranial venous hypertension is seen in most children with CSVT but may not require specific measures for its control once anticoagulation therapy is initiated. However, persistent severe cases may need mannitol, acetazolamide, or neurosurgical intervention. Chronic gradual visual loss because of optic nerve compression can result from persistent raised intracranial pressure, and visual field monitoring is advisable in some cases. CSVT propagation is usually seen in untreated CSVT cases and may be associated with additional brain injury [80]. Hence, in untreated cases, radiological monitoring of CSVT is important, and in cases of propagation, anticoagulation therapy should be strongly considered. Although communicating hydrocephalus because of decreased function cerebrospinal fluid absorption by the affected arachnoid granulations is common, obstructive hydrocephalus is rarely seen in children with CSVT and is associated with a poor outcome [80]. It is more frequent in children with CSVT of the deep cerebral venous system causing hemorrhagic infarction of the thalami resulting in swelling and compression of cerebrospinal fluid pathways and intraventricular hemorrhage. Coma as a presenting feature is often seen in these children.

Transient Ischemic Attack

Transient ischemic attack (TIA) is defined as a transient episode of neurological dysfunction caused by a focal brain, spinal cord, or retinal ischemia without evidence of infarction on neuroimaging. TIAs are frequent in the adult population and are usually associated with atherosclerotic disease. In children, TIAs are poorly understood, and the exact incidence has not been described. TIA should be suspected in children with transient neurological deficits, in the context of risk factors for AIS, for example, in children with a known vasculopathy such as moyamoya disease/syndrome, SCD, arterial dissection, and CHD [10].

Clinical Presentation

TIAs can present as any focal neurological deficit depending on the vascular territory that is affected (hemiparesis, hemisensory deficit, visual deficits, aphasia, and cerebellar symptoms). The main feature is that these deficits resolve before 24 h and that they are associated with the absence of radiological evidence of acute ischemia (restricted diffusion on MRI in the affected vascular territory) [10].

In the clinical setting, it is important to be cautious and recognize other neurological disorders that may mimic TIAs, like postictal neurological deficits (Todd's paralysis) in the setting of epileptic seizures and hemiplegic or complicated migraine, particularly in patients with a positive family history. The attacks related to demyelinating disorders such as multiple sclerosis may also be confused with TIAs, since these can present as a transient focal neurological deficit; however, they generally present with a more gradual symptom onset.

Diagnosis

The diagnosis of TIA can be made on a clinical basis, after excluding other common causes of acute neurological deficit in children (see the above section); and when the acute focal neurological deficit happens in the context of a stroke or an existing stroke risk factor (cardiac, prothrombotic, or vascular conditions). However, MRI to rule out ischemic infarction with rapid resolution of clinical signs is necessary.

Management

There is a lack of data regarding TIAs among the pediatric population, and none of the current available guidelines in pediatric stroke specifically cover this issue. It is nonetheless reasonable to follow adult guidelines in evaluating children with a high clinical suspicion of TIA, where other causes of transient neurological deficits have been ruled out. This would typically start with MRI/MRA of the brain, MRA of the neck, echocardiogram, and a complete prothrombotic work up. For patients with TIAs, in the setting of any given risk factor for AIS, treatment with antiplatelet therapy may be considered. In patients who are already on ASA, and present with further TIAs, the underlying etiology informs the decision whether to switch to clopidogrel or to start LMWH or VKA. For example, in patients with dissection and prior AIS who continue having TIAs while treated with ASA, switching to anticoagulation with LMWH or VKAs is reasonable. In patients with moyamoya and stroke who continue having TIAs while treated with ASA, switching to clopidogrel is preferred, and in appropriately selected cases, neurosurgical intervention with indirect bypass, because of the increased risk for ICH in this specific population. Dosing and monitoring of UFH, LMWH, VKA, ASA, and clopidogrel therapy are detailed in Chapter 20. Further long-term studies of pediatric patients with TIAs are warranted since there are currently insufficient data to support guidelines for treatment and prevention.

Conclusion

Pediatric cerebrovascular diseases are well-recognized entities and result mainly from cardiac, hematological, and vascular disorders. The accurate and prompt diagnosis and treatment of these conditions can help to prevent death and neurological sequelae that interfere with the child's development and quality of life.

Acknowledgment

The authors express their gratitude to Dr. Gabrielle deVeber, former director of the Children's Stroke Program at The Hospital for Sick Children between 1998 and 2018, who wrote previous versions of this chapter, and their appreciation for the thoughtful comments provided by the editors who reviewed this chapter for the third edition of the "SickKids Handbook of Pediatric Thrombosis and Hemostasis."

Conflict of Interest Statement

The authors have no conflicts of interest to declare.

Author Contributions

Elizabeth Pulcine contributed to the drafting, revision, addition of important intellectual content, and final approval of the version of the manuscript. Andrea Andrade contributed to the drafting, revision, addition of important intellectual content, and final approval of the version of the manuscript. Adriana Carolina Vargas Nino contributed to the addition of important intellectual content and final approval of the version of the manuscript. Suzan Williams contributed to the revision, addition of important intellectual content, and final approval of the version of the manuscript. Rebecca N. Ichord contributed to the revision, addition of important intellectual content, and final approval of the version of the manuscript. Nomazulu Dlamini contributed to the revision, addition of important intellectual content, and final approval of the version of the manuscript.

Abbreviations

ACA	Anterior cerebral artery
ADC	Apparent diffusion coefficient
AIS	Arterial ischemic stroke
aPTT	Activated partial thromboplastin time
ASA	Acetylsalicylic acid
BHS	Bowhunter's syndrome
CHD	Congenital heart disease
COX	Cyclooxygenase
CSVT	Cerebral sinovenous thrombosis
CT	Computed tomography
CTA	Computed tomography angiography
CTV	Computed tomography venography
DOAC	Direct oral anticoagulant
DWI	Diffusion weighted images
EDAS	Encephaloduroarteriosynangiosis
EDS	Ehlers-Danlos syndrome
EEG	Electroencephalography
FCA	Focal cerebral arteriopathy
ICH	Intracranial hemorrhage
INR	International normalized ratio
IV	Intravenous
LMWH	Low-molecular-weight heparin
MCA	Middle cerebral artery
MMCA	Malignant MCA
MRA	Magnetic resonance angiography
MRI	Magnetic resonance imaging
MRV	Magnetic resonance venography
PedNIHSS	Pediatric National Institutes of Health Stroke Scale
PT	Prothrombin time
RBC	Red blood cell
SAH	Subarachnoid hemorrhage
SARS-CoV-2	Severe acute respiratory syndrome coronavirus-2
SCD	Sickle cell disease
TCD	Transcranial Doppler
TIA	Transient ischemic attack
tPA	Tissue plasminogen activator
UFH	Unfractionated heparin
VKA	Vitamin K antagonist

References

1 Agrawal N, Johnston SC, Wu YW, Sidney S, Fullerton HJ. Imaging data reveal a higher pediatric stroke incidence than prior US estimates. Stroke. 2009;40(11):3415–21.

2 Golomb MR, Fullerton HJ, Nowak-Gottl U, Deveber G, International Pediatric Stroke Study Group. Male predominance in childhood ischemic stroke: findings from the international pediatric stroke study. Stroke. 2009;40(1):52–7.

3 Lehman LL, Rivkin MJ. Perinatal arterial ischemic stroke: presentation, risk factors, evaluation, and outcome. Pediatr Neurol. 2014;51(6):760–8.

4 deVeber G, Roach ES, Riela AR, Wiznitzer M. Stroke in children: recognition, treatment, and future directions. Semin Pediatr Neurol. 2000;7(4):309–17.

5 Amlie-Lefond C, Bernard TJ, Sebire G, Friedman NR, Heyer GL, Lerner NB, et al. Predictors of cerebral arteriopathy in children with arterial ischemic stroke: results of the International Pediatric Stroke Study. Circulation. 2009;119 (10):1417–23.

6 Bigi S, Fischer U, Wehrli E, Mattle HP, Boltshauser E, Burki S, et al. Acute ischemic stroke in children versus young adults. Ann Neurol. 2011;70(2):245–54.

7 O'Brien SH. Perinatal thrombosis: implications for mothers and neonates. Hematology Am Soc Hematol Educ Program. 2015;2015:48–52.

8 Mackay MT, Wiznitzer M, Benedict SL, Lee KJ, Deveber GA, Ganesan V, et al. Arterial ischemic stroke risk factors: the International Pediatric Stroke Study. Ann Neurol. 2011;69(1):130–40.

9 Kirton A, deVeber G. Advances in perinatal ischemic stroke. Pediatr Neurol. 2009;40(3):205–14.

10 Roach ES, Golomb MR, Adams R, Biller J, Daniels S, Deveber G, et al. Management of stroke in infants and children: a scientific statement from a Special Writing Group of the American Heart Association Stroke Council and the Council on Cardiovascular Disease in the Young. Stroke. 2008;39(9):2644–91.

11 Bowers KJ, Deveber GA, Ferriero DM, Roach ES, Vexler ZS, Maria BL. Cerebrovascular disease in children: recent advances in diagnosis and management. J Child Neurol. 2011;26(9):1074–100.

12 Ernst M, Romero JM, Buhk JH, Kemmling A, Fiehler J, Groth M. Sensitivity of visual and quantitative detection of middle cerebral artery occlusion on non-contrast-enhanced computed tomography. Neuroradiology. 2014;56 (12):1063–8.

13 Monagle P, Chan AKC, Goldenberg NA, Ichord RN, Journeycake JM, Nowak-Gottl U, et al. Antithrombotic therapy in neonates and children: Antithrombotic Therapy and Prevention of Thrombosis, 9th ed: American College of Chest Physicians Evidence-Based Clinical Practice Guidelines. Chest. 2012;141(2 suppl): e737S-801S.

14 Ferriero DM, Fullerton HJ, Bernard TJ, Billinghurst L, Daniels SR, DeBaun MR, et al. Management of stroke in neonates and children: a scientific statement from the American Heart Association/American Stroke Association. Stroke. 2019; 50(3):e51–96.

15 Giglia TM, Massicotte MP, Tweddell JS, Barst RJ, Bauman M, Erickson CC, et al. Prevention and treatment of thrombosis in pediatric and congenital heart disease: a scientific statement from the American Heart Association. Circulation. 2013;128(24):2622–703.

16 Kmietowicz Z. Guidelines aim to help identify and treat stroke in children. BMJ. 2017;357:j2521.

17 Medley TL, Miteff C, Andrews I, Ware T, Cheung M, Monagle P, et al. Australian Clinical Consensus Guideline: the diagnosis and acute management of childhood stroke. Int J Stroke. 2019; 14(1):94–106.

18 Schechter T, Kirton A, Laughlin S, Pontigon AM, Finkelstein Y, MacGregor D, et al. Safety of anticoagulants in children with arterial ischemic stroke. Blood. 2012; 119(4):949–56.

19 DeVeber G. In pursuit of evidence-based treatments for paediatric stroke: the UK and Chest guidelines. Lancet Neurol. 2005;4(7):432–6.

20 Rodan L, McCrindle BW, Manlhiot C, MacGregor DL, Askalan R, Moharir M, et al. Stroke recurrence in children with congenital heart disease. Ann Neurol. 2012;72(1):103–11.

21 Hoffman JL, Mack GK, Minich LL, Benedict SL, Heywood M, Stoddard GJ, et al. Failure to impact prevalence of arterial ischemic stroke in pediatric cardiac patients over three decades. Congenit Heart Dis. 2011;6(3):211–8.

22 Sinclair AJ, Fox CK, Ichord RN, Almond CS, Bernard TJ, Beslow LA, et al. Stroke in children with cardiac disease: report from the International Pediatric Stroke Study Group Symposium. Pediatr Neurol. 2015;52(1):5–15.

23 Silvey M, Brandao LR. Risk factors, prophylaxis, and treatment of venous thromboembolism in congenital heart disease patients. Front Pediatr. 2017; 5:146.

24 Domi T, Edgell DS, McCrindle BW, Williams WG, Chan AK, MacGregor DL, et al. Frequency, predictors, and neurologic outcomes of vaso-occlusive strokes associated with cardiac surgery in children. Pediatrics. 2008;122(6):1292–8.

25 deVeber GA, Kirton A, Booth FA, Yager JY, Wirrell EC, Wood E, et al. Epidemiology and outcomes of arterial ischemic stroke in children: the Canadian Pediatric Ischemic Stroke Registry. Pediatr Neurol. 2017;69:58–70.

26 Rafay MF, Shapiro KA, Surmava AM, deVeber GA, Kirton A, Fullerton HJ, et al. Spectrum of cerebral arteriopathies in children with arterial ischemic stroke. Neurology. 2020;94(23):e2479–90.

27 Bergmeier W, Hynes RO. Extracellular matrix proteins in hemostasis and thrombosis. Cold Spring Harb Perspect Biol. 2012;4(2):a005132.

28 Kennedy F, Lanfranconi S, Hicks C, Reid J, Gompertz P, Price C, et al. Antiplatelets vs anticoagulation for dissection: CADISS nonrandomized arm and meta-analysis. Neurology. 2012;79(7):686–9.

29 Schievink WI. Spontaneous dissection of the carotid and vertebral arteries. N Engl J Med. 2001;344(12):898–906.

30 Nash M, Rafay MF. Craniocervical arterial dissection in children: pathophysiology and management. Pediatr Neurol. 2019;95:9–18.

31 Markus HS, Levi C, King A, Madigan J, Norris J, Cervical Artery Dissection in Stroke Study I. Antiplatelet therapy vs anticoagulation therapy in cervical artery dissection: the cervical artery dissection in stroke study (CADISS) randomized clinical trial final results. JAMA Neurol. 2019;76(6):657–64.

32 Fullerton HJ, Wintermark M, Hills NK, Dowling MM, Tan M, Rafay MF, et al. Risk of recurrent arterial ischemic stroke in childhood: a prospective international study. Stroke. 2016;47(1):53–9.

33 Dlamini N, Freeman JL, Mackay MT, Hawkins C, Shroff M, Fullerton HJ, et al. Intracranial dissection mimicking transient cerebral arteriopathy in childhood arterial ischemic stroke. J Child Neurol. 2011;26(9):1203–6.

34 Metso TM, Metso AJ, Helenius J, Haapaniemi E, Salonen O, Porras M, et al. Prognosis and safety of anticoagulation in intracranial artery dissections in adults. Stroke. 2007;38(6):1837–42.

35 Sebire G. Transient cerebral arteriopathy in childhood. Lancet. 2006;368(9529):8–10.

36 Andrade A, Yau I, Moharir M. Current concepts in pediatric stroke. Indian J Pediatr. 2015;82(2):179–88.

37 Steinlin M, Bigi S, Stojanovski B, Gajera J, Regenyi M, El-Koussy M, et al. Focal cerebral arteriopathy: do steroids improve outcome? Stroke. 2017;48(9): 2375–82.
38 Boelman C, Shroff M, Yau I, Bjornson B, Richrdson S, deVeber G, et al. Antithrombotic therapy for secondary stroke prevention in bacterial meningitis in children. J Pediatr. 2014;165(4):799–806.
39 Beslow LA, Linds AB, Fox CK, Kossorotoff M, Zuniga Zambrano YC, Hernandez-Chavez M, et al. Pediatric ischemic stroke: an infrequent complication of SARS-CoV-2. Ann Neurol. 2021;89(4): 657–65.
40 Qashqari H, Bhathal I, Pulcine E, Muthusami P, Moharir M, MacGregor D, et al. Bow hunter syndrome: a rare yet important etiology of posterior circulation stroke. J Clin Neurosci. 2020;78:418–9.
41 Braga BP, Sillero R, Pereira RM, Urgun K, Swift DM, Rollins NK, et al. Dynamic compression in vertebral artery dissection in children: apropos of a new protocol. Childs Nerv Syst. 2021;37(4):1285–93.
42 Mackay MT, Prabhu SP, Coleman L. Childhood posterior circulation arterial ischemic stroke. Stroke. 2010;41(10): 2201–9.
43 Caorsi R, Penco F, Grossi A, Insalaco A, Omenetti A, Alessio M, et al. ADA2 deficiency (DADA2) as an unrecognised cause of early onset polyarteritis nodosa and stroke: a multicentre national study. Ann Rheum Dis. 2017;76(10):1648–56.
44 Goeggel Simonetti B, Rafay MF, Chung M, Lo WD, Beslow LA, Billinghurst LL, et al. Comparative study of posterior and anterior circulation stroke in childhood: Results from the International Pediatric Stroke Study. Neurology. 2020;94(4):e337–44.
45 Liu W, Morito D, Takashima S, Mineharu Y, Kobayashi H, Hitomi T, et al. Identification of RNF213 as a susceptibility gene for moyamoya disease and its possible role in vascular development. PLoS One. 2011;6(7):e22542.
46 Bang OY, Chung JW, Kim DH, Won HH, Yeon JY, Ki CS, et al. Moyamoya disease and spectrums of RNF213 vasculopathy. Transl Stroke Res. 2020; 11(4):580–9.
47 Kaseka ML, Slim M, Muthusami P, Dirks PB, Westmacott R, Kassner A, et al. Distinct clinical and radiographic phenotypes in pediatric patients with moyamoya. Pediatr Neurol. 2021;120: 18–26.
48 Brousse V, Kossorotoff M, de Montalembert M. How I manage cerebral vasculopathy in children with sickle cell disease. Br J Haematol. 2015;170(5): 615–25.
49 Hulbert ML, McKinstry RC, Lacey JL, Moran CJ, Panepinto JA, Thompson AA, et al. Silent cerebral infarcts occur despite regular blood transfusion therapy after first strokes in children with sickle cell disease. Blood. 2011;117(3):772–9.
50 Ware RE, Helms RW, Investigators SW. Stroke With Transfusions Changing to Hydroxyurea (SWiTCH). Blood. 2012; 119(17):3925–32.
51 DeBaun MR, Gordon M, McKinstry RC, Noetzel MJ, White DA, Sarnaik SA, et al. Controlled trial of transfusions for silent cerebral infarcts in sickle cell anemia. N Engl J Med. 2014;371(8):699–710.
52 Ware RE, Davis BR, Schultz WH, Brown RC, Aygun B, Sarnaik S, et al. Hydroxycarbamide versus chronic transfusion for maintenance of transcranial doppler flow velocities in children with sickle cell anaemia-TCD With Transfusions Changing to Hydroxyurea (TWiTCH): a multicentre, open-label, phase 3, non-inferiority trial. Lancet. 2016; 387(10019):661–70.
53 Tan RYY, Traylor M, Megy K, Duarte D, Deevi SVV, Shamardina O, et al. How common are single gene mutations as a cause for lacunar stroke? A targeted gene panel study. Neurology. 2019; 93(22):e2007–20.
54 Doig D, Davagnanam I, Taranath A, Zlatareva D, Alwis A, Siddiqui A, et al. Monogenetic stroke syndromes in children and young adults. AJR Am J Roentgenol. 2020;215(3):695–705.
55 Emberson J, Lees KR, Lyden P, Blackwell L, Albers G, Bluhmki E, et al. Effect of treatment delay, age, and stroke severity on the effects of intravenous thrombolysis with alteplase for acute ischaemic stroke: a meta-analysis of individual patient data from randomised trials. Lancet. 2014;384(9958): 1929–35.
56 Bernson-Leung ME, Rivkin MJ. Stroke in neonates and children. Pediatr Rev. 2016;37(11):463–77.
57 Menon BK, Buck BH, Singh N, Deschaintre Y, Almekhlafi MA, Coutts SB, et al. Intravenous tenecteplase compared with alteplase for acute ischaemic stroke in Canada (AcT): a pragmatic, multicentre, open-label, registry-linked, randomised, controlled, non-inferiority trial. Lancet. 2022;400(10347):161–9.
58 Rivkin MJ, Bernard TJ, Dowling MM, Amlie-Lefond C. Guidelines for urgent management of stroke in children. Pediatr Neurol. 2016;56:8–17.
59 Rafay MF, Pontigon AM, Chiang J, Adams M, Jarvis DA, Silver F, et al. Delay to diagnosis in acute pediatric arterial ischemic stroke. Stroke. 2009;40(1):58–64.
60 Rivkin MJ, deVeber G, Ichord RN, Kirton A, Chan AK, Hovinga CA, et al. Thrombolysis in pediatric stroke study. Stroke. 2015;46(3):880–5.
61 Bernard TJ, Friedman NR, Stence NV, Jones W, Ichord R, Amlie-Lefond C, et al. Preparing for a "pediatric stroke alert". Pediatr Neurol. 2016;56:18–24.
62 Casaubon LK, Boulanger JM, Blacquiere D, Boucher S, Brown K, Goddard T, et al. Canadian stroke best practice recommendations: hyperacute stroke care guidelines, update 2015. Int J Stroke. 2015;10(6):924–40.
63 Goyal M, Menon BK, van Zwam WH, Dippel DW, Mitchell PJ, Demchuk AM, et al. Endovascular thrombectomy after large-vessel ischaemic stroke: a meta-analysis of individual patient data from five randomised trials. Lancet. 2016; 387(10029):1723–31.
64 Bigi S, Dulcey A, Gralla J, Bernasconi C, Melliger A, Datta AN, et al. Feasibility, safety, and outcome of recanalization treatment in childhood stroke. Ann Neurol. 2018;83(6):1125–32.
65 Bhatia K, Kortman H, Blair C, Parker G, Brunacci D, Ang T, et al. Mechanical thrombectomy in pediatric stroke: systematic review, individual patient data meta-analysis, and case series. J Neurosurg Pediatr. 2019;24(5):558–71.
66 Wu C, Honarmand AR, Schnell S, Kuhn R, Schoeneman SE, Ansari SA, et al. Age-related changes of normal cerebral and cardiac blood flow in children and adults aged 7 months to 61 years. J Am Heart Assoc. 2016;5(1):e002657.

67 Shah S, Murthy SB, Whitehead WE, Jea A, Nassif LM. Decompressive hemicraniectomy in pediatric patients with malignant middle cerebral artery infarction: case series and review of the literature. World Neurosurg. 2013;80(1–2):126–33.
68 Andrade A, Bigi S, Laughlin S, Parthasarathy S, Sinclair A, Dirks P, et al. Association between prolonged seizures and malignant middle cerebral artery infarction in children with acute ischemic stroke. Pediatr Neurol. 2016;64:44–51.
69 Beghi E, Boglium G, Cosso P, Fiorelli G, Lorini C, Mandelli M, et al. Stroke and alcohol intake in a hospital population. A case-control study. Stroke. 1995;26(9):1691–6.
70 Fiorelli M, Bastianello S, von Kummer R, del Zoppo GJ, Larrue V, Lesaffre E, et al. Hemorrhagic transformation within 36 hours of a cerebral infarct: relationships with early clinical deterioration and 3-month outcome in the European Cooperative Acute Stroke Study I (ECASS I) cohort. Stroke. 1999;30(11):2280–4.
71 Beslow LA, Smith SE, Vossough A, Licht DJ, Kasner SE, Favilla CG, et al. Hemorrhagic transformation of childhood arterial ischemic stroke. Stroke. 2011;42(4):941–6.
72 Pulcine E, Seed M, Brandao LR, Slim M, Palasamudram S, Shroff M, et al. Hemorrhagic transformation and stroke recurrence in children with cardiac disease receiving antithrombotic therapy for secondary stroke prevention. J Thromb Haemost. 2021;19(10):2428–39.
73 Dunbar M, Kirton A. Perinatal stroke: mechanisms, management, and outcomes of early cerebrovascular brain injury. Lancet Child Adolesc Health. 2018;2(9):666–76.
74 Teasell R, Salbach NM, Foley N, Mountain A, Cameron JI, Jong A, et al. Canadian stroke best practice recommendations: rehabilitation, recovery, and community participation following stroke. Part one—Rehabilitation and Recovery Following Stroke; 6th Edition Update 2019. Int J Stroke. 2020;15(7):763–88.
75 Ichord R. Cerebral sinovenous thrombosis. Front Pediatr. 2017;5:163.
76 Wasay M, Dai AI, Ansari M, Shaikh Z, Roach ES. Cerebral venous sinus thrombosis in children: a multicenter cohort from the United States. J Child Neurol. 2008;23(1):26–31.
77 Kouzmitcheva E, Andrade A, Muthusami P, Shroff M, MacGregor DL, deVeber G, et al. Anatomical venous variants in children with cerebral sinovenous thrombosis. Stroke. 2019;50(1):178–180.
78 Kersbergen KJ, Groenendaal F, Benders MJ, de Vries LS. Neonatal cerebral sinovenous thrombosis: neuroimaging and long-term follow-up. J Child Neurol. 2011;26(9):1111–20.
79 Ichord RN, Benedict SL, Chan AK, Kirkham FJ, Nowak-Gottl U, International Paediatric Stroke Study G. Paediatric cerebral sinovenous thrombosis: findings of the International Paediatric Stroke Study. Arch Dis Child. 2015;100(2):174–9.
80 Moharir MD, Shroff M, Stephens D, Pontigon AM, Chan A, MacGregor D, et al. Anticoagulants in pediatric cerebral sinovenous thrombosis: a safety and outcome study. Ann Neurol. 2010;67(5):590–9.
81 Connor P, Sanchez van Kammen M, Lensing AWA, Chalmers E, Kallay K, Hege K, et al. Safety and efficacy of rivaroxaban in pediatric cerebral venous thrombosis (EINSTEIN-Jr CVT). Blood Adv. 2020;4(24):6250–8.
82 Dlamini N, Billinghurst L, Kirkham FJ. Cerebral venous sinus (sinovenous) thrombosis in children. Neurosurg Clin N Am. 2010;21(3):511–27.
83 Moharir MD, Shroff M, Pontigon AM, Askalan R, Yau I, Macgregor D, et al. A prospective outcome study of neonatal cerebral sinovenous thrombosis. J Child Neurol. 2011;26(9):1137–44.
84 Christensen R, Krishnan P, deVeber G, Dlamini N, MacGregor D, Pulcine E, et al. Cerebral venous sinus thrombosis in preterm infants. Stroke. 2022;53(7):2241–8.
85 Goldenberg NA, Kittelson JM, Abshire TC, Bonaca M, Casella JF, Dale RA, et al. Effect of anticoagulant therapy for 6 weeks vs 3 months on recurrence and bleeding events in patients younger than 21 years of age with provoked venous thromboembolism: the Kids-DOTT randomized clinical trial. JAMA. 2022;327(2):129–37.

Chapter 18

Published online: December 5, 2024

Blanchette VS, Brandão LR, Carcao MD, Kumar R, Rand ML, Revel-Vilk S (eds): SickKids Handbook of Pediatric Thrombosis and Hemostasis, ed 3, rev. and ext. Basel, Karger, 2024, pp 336–358 (DOI: 10.1159/000538194)

Bleeding and Thrombotic Complications in the Setting of Cardiac Disease

Christina J. VanderPluym[a] Brian McCrindle[b] Leonardo R. Brandão[c]

[a]Heart Center, Boston Children's Hospital, Harvard School of Medicine, Boston, MA, USA; [b]Division of Cardiology, The Hospital for Sick Children, University of Toronto, Toronto, ON, Canada; [c]Division of Hematology, The Hospital for Sick Children, University of Toronto, Toronto, ON, Canada

Introduction

Pediatric cardiac disease represents a major health burden affecting a large group of children in tertiary pediatric centers. For example, congenital heart disease (CHD) is 60 times more prevalent than pediatric cancer, constituting the leading cause of death in the first year of life [1]. CHD affects about 1% of live births and accounts for the majority of cardiac pathology in children. In the United States, more than 35,000 neonates are born with CHD annually, and by the age of 5 years, approximately 80% of these children will undergo one or more cardiac surgical interventions. Besides mortality, disease- and treatment-related complications in children with CHD include hemorrhagic and/or thrombotic events (TEs). The increased frequency of these complications is attributed to advances in medical and surgical care of this patient population with increased utilization of invasive cardiovascular procedures, indwelling vascular devices (i.e., catheters, stents, transvenous pacemakers, septal occluders, mechanical and bioprosthetic heart valves), and intensive antithrombotic therapies, as well as to increased awareness and recognition.

CHD can be broadly classified, depending on the underlying lesion, into acyanotic and cyanotic [1]. Common CHDs and their estimated distribution include acyanotic CHD: ventricular septal defect (VSD) 20%, patent ductus arteriosus (PDA) 10%, coarctation of the aorta 10%, critical aortic stenosis 5%, atrial septal defect 5%, interrupted aortic arch 1%, and cyanotic CHD: tetralogy of Fallot 10%, transposition of the great arteries 5%, tricuspid atresia 1%, pulmonary stenosis 1%, Ebstein anomaly 1%, and hypoplastic left heart syndrome 1%. A notable differentiating feature of cyanotic CHD is the mixing of venous and arterial circulation, either intracardiac or extracardiac, resulting in systemic desaturation and placing these children at risk of paradoxical emboli from venous to arterial circulations. In addition to these, there is a myriad of different constellations of congenital lesions in combination, such as with right atrial isomerism.

Acquired heart disease is less common than CHD in children but encompasses a number of disorders with significant morbidity and mortality. Important pediatric acquired heart disorders where bleeding and/or TE complications are also clinically relevant include Kawasaki disease, infective endocarditis (IE), and cardiomyopathies. In some populations, rheumatic heart disease remains a major problem. More recently, the coronavirus disease 2019 (COVID-19) pandemic has revealed a new type of acquired heart disease with variable organ involvement termed either pediatric inflammatory multisystem syndrome temporarily associated with COVID-19 (PIMS-TS) by the Royal College of Paediatrics and Child Health and by the World Health Organization or multisystem inflammatory syndrome in children (MIS-C) by the Centers for Disease Control and Prevention [2–4]. This condition is a delayed hyperinflammatory syndrome temporally related to SARS-CoV-2 infection, with variable cardiac manifestation of ventricular dysfunction (myocarditis), coronary artery (CA) dilation, and/or conduction abnormalities.

Given the high burden of bleeding and TE complications in children with heart disease, there has been a surge in the development of specific antithrombosis recommendations for this highly heterogeneous population. As such, there are evidence-based graded statements on primary or secondary anticoagulation for children undergoing cardiac catheterization, single-ventricle physiology, Kawasaki disease with CA involvement, mechanical valves (MVs) or stents, cardiomyopathy, and management of intracardiac thrombosis or cardioembolic arterial ischemic strokes (AISs) [5]. Additionally, the American Heart Association has also issued a scientific statement identifying high-risk groups for TE complications among children with cardiac disease (e.g., shunt-dependent single ventricles, Fontan circulation, Kawasaki disease with coronary arteriopathy, and myocarditis), expanding the recommendation portfolio published in the last guideline with a combined evidence-based and consensual approach to grading their recommendations [6]. The emergence of COVID-19-associated illnesses in children has spurred research from basic science to trials, resulting in evidence-based recommendations and guidance statements for prophylactic antithrombotic regimens in this evolving population [7–9].

Despite this growing body of literature, strong evidence-based recommendations addressing hemostatic/TE disorders in children with cardiac disease are only starting to appear, and the current published guidelines continue to be largely derived from small pediatric studies, single-center experiences, and extrapolations from adult trials. Hence, current clinical practices may vary significantly according to provider preference, local policies, and clinical needs. With the significantly decreased mortality in children with CHD, more emphasis is being placed toward prevention and optimal management of complications, including bleeding and TE in this population. Given that in the USA alone around 1.3 million newborns diagnosed with CHD survive to adulthood, it became imperative for referral centers to develop their own anticoagulation/hemostasis protocols to optimize the care of children with these conditions.

In this chapter, an up-to-date overview of important hemostatic and TE issues in children with cardiac disease, including the practices reflective of our local institutional protocols, is presented, with particular emphasis on a practical diagnostic approach and therapeutic management.

Bleeding

Children with cardiac disease are unique in that they are at higher risk not only of thrombosis but also of bleeding because of several intrinsic and extrinsic risk factors. In addition to the inherent risk of bleeding related to cardiovascular surgery and catheterization, CHD in itself has been associated with several acquired hemostatic abnormalities, including thrombocytopenia, platelet dysfunction, decreased coagulation proteins (e.g., acquired von Willebrand syndrome [AVWS]), low-grade disseminated intravascular coagulation, and primary hyperfibrinolysis. AVWS, characterized by loss of high-molecular-weight multimers of von Willebrand factor (VWF) because of enhanced shear stress, is associated with high-velocity turbulent flow such as in patients with restrictive septal defects, stenotic or regurgitant valves, and narrowed shunts or conduit (see Chapter 11). In addition, children with progressive heart failure/dysfunction may also develop different degrees of acquired coagulopathy because of infradiaphragmatic venous hypertension leading to congestive hepatopathy [10]. Moreover, certain syndromic forms of CHD can be associated with specific hemostatic defects, such as chromosome 22q11.2 microdeletion syndrome (DiGeorge/velocardiofacial syndrome) and Jacobsen syndrome (see Chapter 6). Similarly, Noonan syndrome can also be associated with thrombocytopenia, platelet dysfunction, and multiple coagulation factor deficiencies, most commonly factor XI deficiency [11].

Risk factors for perioperative bleeding include cyanotic CHD, young age (neonates and infants are at increased risk for hemodilution), congestive hepatopathy, use of cardiopulmonary bypass (CPB), deep hypothermic circulatory arrest, complex surgical procedures with extensive dissections and multiple sternotomies. Longer storage duration of transfused packed red blood cells (RBCs) was identified as a risk factor for bleeding in children undergoing high-risk cardiac surgeries [12]. Last, higher intensity, combination regimens, and extended or even indefinite length of antithrombotic therapies are more often being utilized in children with cardiac disease, further increasing the bleeding risk.

End-organ dysfunction, namely renal and hepatic, places children at higher risk of anticoagulation-related bleeding because of impaired drug metabolism and/or clearance, consequently resulting in supratherapeutic drug levels. Additionally, platelet activation and thrombin generation may also be impaired because of ensuing renal and hepatic dysfunction, leading to an ineffective hemostatic response that contributes to an excessive bleeding tendency associated with antiplatelet/anticoagulant therapy.

Clinical Presentation and Diagnosis

Bleeding can be classified with respect to severity into *major bleeding* (fatal, symptomatic involving a critical area such as intracranial or retroperitoneal, causing a fall in hemoglobin ≥2 g/dL over 24 h), *clinically relevant nonmajor* (overt bleeding for which a blood product is administered and which is not directly attributable to the child underlying medical condition, bleeding that requires medical or surgical intervention to restore hemostasis, other than in an operating suite), or *minor bleeding* (other than the above) [13]. Bleeding complications in children with cardiac disease are usually provoked in the setting of an invasive procedure, such as cardiac surgery, cardiac catheterization, or extracardiac invasive procedures. This type of bleeding presents in the form of persistent intraoperative oozing from the surgical field and/or excessive postoperative bleeding. The most common causes of bleeding immediately after CPB include inability to achieve surgical hemostasis, platelet abnormalities, hypofibrinogenemia, inadequate reversal of heparin with protamine, and combinations of these factors [14]. Interestingly, AVWS, detected in half of the children with cardiac anatomy, resolves completely after surgical or interventional procedures [15, 16]. Prolonged use of intravenous phosphodiesterase-3-inhibitors such as milrinone has been shown to result in platelet inhibition and may contribute to increased surgical bleeding [16].

Spontaneous (unprovoked) bleeding is generally less common, but all children should have a thorough history assessed for bleeding and/or family history of bleeding events/disorders to ascertain for inherited bleeding conditions, preferably using a standardized validated bleeding questionnaire (see Appendix I) [17]. For children with CHD undergoing any invasive procedure, a minimum preoperative hemostatic screening, including complete blood count, prothrombin time (PT)/international normalized ratio (INR), activated partial thromboplastin time (aPTT), thrombin time, and fibrinogen, may be considered. Further laboratory investigations may be indicated if there is a history of bleeding or abnormal results on screening tests (see Chapter 4). Testing children at risk for AVWS should be considered (see Chapter 11), particularly when the pediatric bleeding score is abnormal (see Appendix I) and/or if the cardiac lesion is associated with a high-flow cardiac defect. In AVWS associated with cardiovascular disorders, the ristocetin cofactor activity (VWF:RCo) or collagen binding (VWF:CB) activity to VWF:antigen ratio is often, but not always, reduced [18]. Decreased high-molecular-weight von Willebrand factor multimers and prolongation of the platelet function analyzer-100® (PFA-100®) closure times are diagnostic and considered the main risk factor associated with bleeding.

When performing coagulation testing on children with CHD, it is important to remember that cyanotic CHD is often associated with secondary polycythemia, which, if present, will reduce the amount of plasma in a given volume of whole blood. Coagulation laboratory results (INR/PT, aPTT) in children with high hematocrit (>55%) may be falsely prolonged [19]. Therefore, when the hematocrit exceeds 55%, the reduced plasma volume requires a decrease in the volume of citrate anticoagulant used to maintain the recommended ratio of 9:1 using the following formula: $C = 1.85 \times 10^{-3} \times (100 - HCT) \times V$, where C = mL of 3.2% sodium citrate anticoagulant, HCT = hematocrit of the patient in %, and V = mL of whole blood in tube.

A common cause of bleeding events in children with cardiac disease is the use of antiplatelet and/or anticoagulation for treatment or prevention of thrombosis. Bleeding events, such as epistaxis, mucosal bleeding, and heavy menstrual bleeding (see Chapter 5), can significantly affect quality of life and should be addressed with supportive measures. Having dedicated teams that monitor and manage antithrombotic agents for children with cardiac disease may help reduce the risk of bleeding and TEs [20, 21].

Management

Treatment of bleeding in children with cardiac disease is best guided by clinical assessment of the child's hemodynamic status, assessment of severity of bleeding, and results of the hemostasis laboratory analyses. An important challenge is that anticoagulation is indispensable in preventing thrombus formation during or after cardiac procedures with high TE risk. Hence, an individualized case-by-case assessment should be performed based on the risk and gravity of TE complication (based on local and overall prevalence) vs. the severity of the bleeding event. At The Hospital for Sick Children (SickKids) cardiac conditions/procedures considered high risk for TE include mechanical artificial valves, most cardiovascular stents, systemic to pulmonary artery shunts, post-Fontan procedure, preheart and postheart transplantation, Kawasaki disease with significant CA involvement, mechanical circulatory support, and history of previous TEs.

In general, minor bleeding events require only symptomatic management with no or minimal adjustment of antithrombotic therapy, whereas major bleeding will often require interruption or reversal of antithrombotic therapy and/or hemostatic interventions (as detailed below). Reversal of anticoagulation should follow the protocols detailed in Chapter 20 and in Appendix III.

Empirical management based solely on clinical assessment is often employed for early postoperative bleeding since delaying treatment while awaiting diagnostic information may not be appropriate in many cases. Alternatively, targeted

18

hemostatic interventions guided by clinical algorithms based on clinical and thromboelastography parameters may be associated with decreased transfusions with equivalent or less bleeding in cardiac surgery [22]; however, this approach requires further validation in the pediatric population.

Transfusion of blood products is used for children with thrombocytopenia, platelet dysfunction, coagulopathies, low plasma fibrinogen levels, and AVWS. Suggested doses of platelet, frozen plasma (FP)/fresh frozen plasma (FFP), and cryoprecipitate are detailed in Appendix III. Treatment of AVWS is discussed in Chapter 11. RBC transfusion is recommended to keep the hematocrit between 28% and 30% for noncyanotic CHD and 35–40% for cyanotic CHD or children with low cardiac output, as evidenced by impaired perfusion and low mixed venous saturation [23].

The use of desmopressin (DDAVP) may be considered for platelet dysfunction (see Chapters 6 and 7).

Antifibrinolytic agents are routinely used to decrease bleeding and transfusions in children undergoing cardiac surgery involving CPB. Tranexamic acid has been shown to reduce the need for blood product transfusions across multiple studies [24].

The off-label use of recombinant activated factor VII (rFVIIa) may be considered for severe bleeding refractory to other therapies. The suggested initial dosing is 20–45 µg/kg, which can be escalated to 90 µg/kg every 4 h until bleeding is controlled; if no response, discontinue after maximum 3 doses. Importantly, the use of rFVIIa is associated with an increased risk of thrombosis [25]. Similarly, the off-label use of prothrombin complex concentrates (PCC) for the treatment of life-threatening bleeding refractory to conventional therapy after cardiac surgery has been described as rescue therapy. In adults, the suggested initial dosing is 20 IU/kg, leading to a 7- and 5-fold reduction of plasma and platelet transfusion, respectively, and an estimated 4% risk of thrombosis [26]. Very little pediatric literature is available relevant to bleeding post-CPB in children. The suggested initial dosing is based on the INR prior to PCC administration and on child's weight (i.e., INR <3: <10 kg – 250 IU factor IX [FIX], 10–25 kg – 500 IU FIX, and 25–50 kg – 750 IU FIX; INR >3: <10 kg – 500 IU FIX, 10–25 kg – 750 IU FIX, and 25–50 kg – 1,000 IU FIX) [27].

Thromboprophylaxis

The modern management of pediatric cardiac disease often requires complex surgical and/or transcatheter interventional procedures, which can involve creation of extracardiac conduits and shunts, placement of intravascular and/or intracardiac stents and devices, or MVs that can alter the blood flow shear stress, disrupt the endothelium, and activate the coagulation system, increasing the risk for TEs. Given this burden of artificial material interfacing the endothelium and blood surface and altered rheology, primary thromboprophylaxis is often indicated to prevent the formation of pathological thrombosis. TE is an important complication in children with cardiac disease and often necessitates continued thromboprophylaxis beyond the initial treatment of the TE if the underlying cardiac risk factor has not been corrected (secondary thromboprophylaxis). Primary and secondary thromboprophylaxis regimens in pediatric cardiac disease at SickKids are detailed in Table 1. Important cardiac settings in which thromboprophylaxis is often required are discussed below.

Cardiac Baffles, Conduits, Shunts, and Stents

Baffles, conduits, and shunts used in pediatric cardiovascular surgery can be classified by the type of material used (biologic or synthetic) as well as by the location of the connections made (intra-atrial, venoatrial, intraventricular, ventric-

Table 1. Thromboprophylaxis for pediatric cardiac disease/procedures[a]

Procedure/condition	Thromboprophylaxis
Cardiac catheterization via an artery	UFH bolus dose (100 U/kg) and further doses (50 U/kg) in prolonged procedures (≥2 h)
Intravascular/intracardiac stents	
PDA stent	ASA and clopidogrel for 3 months
mBTS stent	Add ASA to LMWH (until the next palliative surgical intervention occurs)
Systemic venous system (includes pulmonary arteries in single-ventricle patients)	LMWH for 3 months and ASA indefinitely
Pulmonary vein stent	LMWH for 3 months and ASA indefinitely
Pulmonary artery stent <5 mm	ASA indefinitely
ASD stent	LMWH and ASA until stent removal
RVOT and coarctation of the aorta stent	None
Coronary artery stents	Periprocedural UFH, ASA ± clopidogrel ± GPIIb/IIIa antagonist[b] followed by ASA and clopidogrel for ≥1 month for bare metal stents and ≥6 months for drug-eluting stents followed by indefinite ASA. Indefinite ASA and clopidogrel may be continued in high-risk patients
Staged surgery for single ventricle physiology	
MBTS (Norwood procedure)	Intraoperative UFH followed by therapeutic LMWH until Glenn procedure (Note: no anticoagulation is given after Sano modification or hybrid procedure)
SCPC (Glenn procedure)	None for single shunt, therapeutic LMWH, or VKA (target INR 2–3) for patients with bilateral shunts until the time of Fontan completion
Fontan procedure	DOAC or VKA (target INR 2.0–3.0) for at least 6 months or until fenestration closure and ASA after VKA stopped. Consider DOAC or VKA if any additional risk factors (arrhythmia, AVVR, dysfunction, h/o thrombosis, and PLE)
Prosthetic heart valves	
Mechanical prosthetic heart valves	VKA (target 2–3 for AVR, 2.5–3.5 for MVR) and ASA for all mechanical, except the On-X® aortic valve (target 1.5–2.0) with ASA
Bioprosthetic heart valves	VKA (target 1–3) for 3–6 months and then lifelong ASA
Acquired cardiac disease	
Cardiomyopathy	Therapeutic LMWH, DOAC, and VKA (target INR 2.0–3.0) for all patients with dilated cardiomyopathy and LV ejection fraction <20% or cardiomyopathy with qualitatively severely reduced function/severe arrhythmia, left ventricular noncompaction, arrhythmogenic right ventricle, restrictive cardiomyopathy, and history of TE
Kawasaki disease	See Figure 2

AVR, aortic valve replacement; ASA, acetylsalicylic acid; DOAC, direct oral anticoagulant; GP, glycoprotein; INR, international normalized ratio; LMWH, low-molecular-weight heparin; mBTS, modified Blalock-Taussig shunt; MVR, mitral valve replacement; PDA, patent ductus arteriosus; PLE, protein-losing enteropathy; ROVT, right ventricular outflow tract; SCPC, superior cavopulmonary connection; TE, thromboembolism/thromboembolic event; UFH, unfractionated heparin; VKA, vitamin K antagonist. [a]Data from [2, 3] and current practice at The Hospital for Sick Children, Toronto, Canada. [b]Eptifibatide is the preferred GPIIb/IIIa inhibitor.

uloarterial, or total cavopulmonary anastomosis/Fontan). The type of material used primarily depends on the indication for and anatomic placement of the conduit or shunt. Polytetrafluoroethylene (PTFE, or Gore-Tex®) grafts are primarily used for systemic to pulmonary artery shunts and in the creation of some Fontan connections between the inferior vena cava (IVC) and the pulmonary artery. The Contegra® bioprosthetic valved conduit is a glutaraldehyde-preserved valve-containing bovine jugular vein graft (Contegra®; Medtronic Inc., MN, USA) that has been used for reconstruction of a dysfunctional right ventricular outflow tract such as in children with pulmonary atresia and has also been used to construct the extracardiac Fontan connection. Surgically created conduits and shunts are an integral part of the three-stage palliative surgical approach to a heterogeneous group of complex CHD characterized by single-ventricle physiology (Fig. 1).

Percutaneously placed stents are increasingly used in pediatric cardiac disease to manage congenital obstructive lesions in the pulmonary circulations or systemic circulations (e.g., tetralogy of Fallot, native/recurrent coarctation of the aorta, pulmonary artery, and vein stenoses), as well as acquired obstructive lesions (Fontan pathway obstruction) [28]. Balloon-expandable stents, which can be redilated later, are preferred over self-expandable stents [29], given their ability to "grow" with the child.

Published guidelines for thromboprophylaxis for endovascular stents recommend unfractionated heparin (UFH) perioperatively but do not provide additional guidance because of the lack of data [30]. Thromboprophylaxis regimens used for cardiac catheterization via an artery, stents, and cardiovascular shunts at SickKids are detailed in Table 1.

Prosthetic Valves

Infants and children with valvular heart disease whose innate valves cannot be surgically repaired require valve replacement surgery. The three main types of prosthetic valves utilized in children are bioprosthetic valves (BVs; surgical and transcatheter), pulmonary autograft (Ross procedure), and MVs. While the risk of TE is lower with BVs, their durability is poor as compared with MV, with valve leaflet thickening and degradation. Hence, in most centers, BVs are reserved for right-sided valve replacement or when there is a contraindication to anticoagulation. Transcatheter BV such as the Sapien™ 3 valve (Edwards Lifesciences Corp., Irvine, CA, USA) for the aortic/mitral position and Melody™ valve (Medtronic Inc., MN, USA) for mitral/pulmonary position have gained more traction in the pediatric and adult CHD population. These bovine valves are placed within an expandable stent for transcatheter placement. Optimal thromboprophylaxis for this indication and population is not well established, with variable recommendations ranging from lifelong monotherapy with acetylsalicylic acid (ASA) to limited or lifelong vitamin K antagonist (VKA) or direct oral anticoagulants (DOACs) [31].

MVs have exceptional durability and, as such, are preferred for most children. MVs, however, are thrombogenic, necessitating lifelong anticoagulation. The three most commonly used MV designs are the caged ball (Starr-Edwards), the tilting disc (Bjork-Shiley, Medtronic-Hall), and the bileaflet (St. Jude) [32]. TE complications of MVs and recommendations for thromboprophylaxis are discussed below. More recently, MVs incorporating new technologies (i.e., pyrolytic carbon fiber coating all valve parts that come in contact with blood) have been shown to render a lower thrombogenic potential. In those instances, their required target INR was only between 1.5 and 2.0 [33]. Adolescents receiving the same prosthetic devices (e.g., On-X® prosthetic valve, On-X® Life Technologies Inc., Austin, TX, USA) follow similar target INR laboratory parameters.

Recommended thromboprophylaxis for pediatric prosthetic valves is based on adult guidelines and suggests VKA for MVs (target 2.0–3.0 for

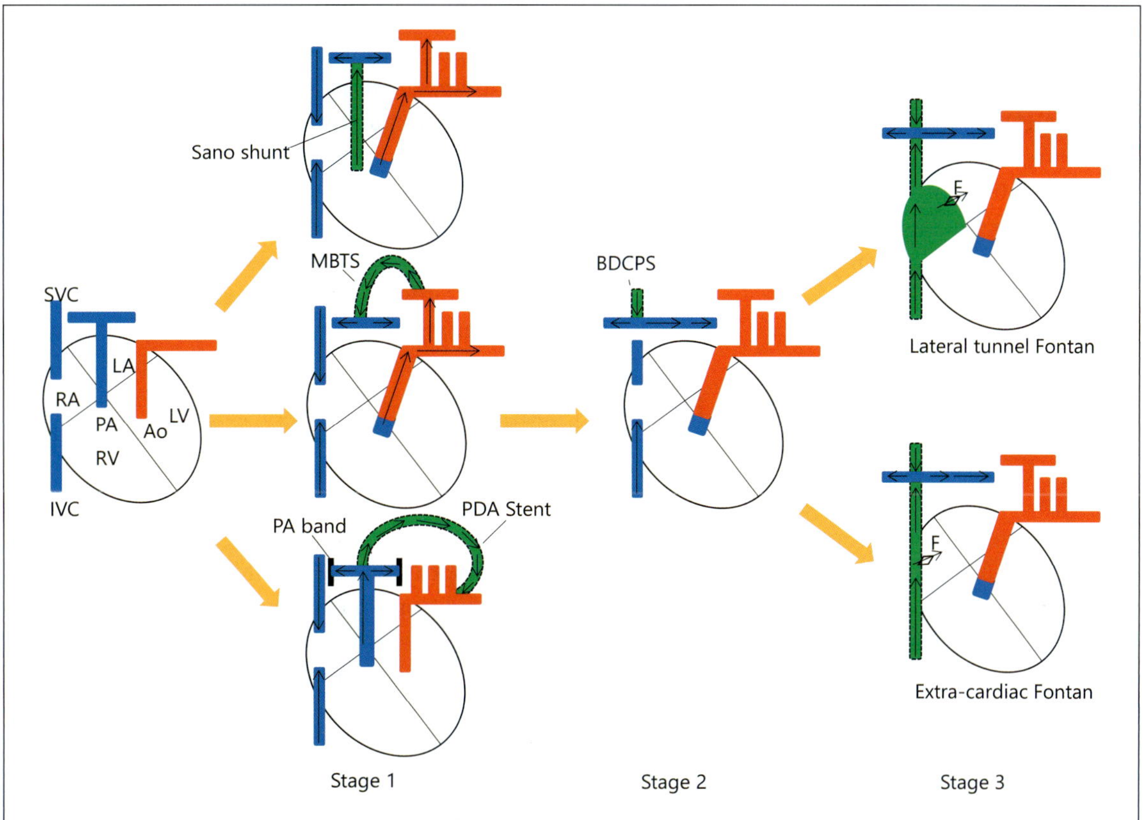

Fig. 1. Staged palliations for single-ventricle physiology. Surgery for CHD with single-ventricle physiology, such as hypoplastic left heart syndrome, consists of three stages. *Stage 1* is performed in the neonatal period (Norwood procedure) with the purpose of providing balanced systemic and pulmonary blood flow. In this first stage, the origin of the PA is connected to the aorta allowing the RV to pump blood to the systemic circulation, and a Gore-Tex graft connecting right innominate/subclavian artery and the right PA is created, i.e., MBTS (in "Sano modification," the Gore-Tex graft connects the RV to the PA). Atrial septectomy is also performed during Norwood procedure to ensure an unobstructed connection between the pulmonary venous return and the systemic RV. Alternatively, in some high-risk patients, a hybrid procedure is sometimes performed in the first stage in which percutaneous PDA stenting and surgical bilateral PA banding are performed off bypass. *Stage 2* is performed at 4–6 months of age (Glenn procedure) in which a bidirectional cavopulmonary shunt is fashioned via an end-to-side anastomosis between the cranial end of the SVC and right PA. *Stage 3* is performed at 2–3 years of age (Fontan procedure) in which the IVC is connected to the right PA either by placement of a Gore-Tex baffle along the lateral aspect of the right atrium, which conveys IVC blood to the SVC orifice (lateral tunnel Fontan), or via a Gore-Tex conduit (extracardiac Fontan). A small fenestration is often also placed in the baffle or conduit to prevent the systemic venous pressure from reaching intolerably high levels during the intraoperative and early postoperative period. The end result is creation of a system with a single ventricle pumping blood into separate, in-series systemic and pulmonary circulations with the entire systemic venous return flowing passively into the pulmonary arteries. Ao, aorta; F, fenestration; LA, left atrium; LV, left ventricle; MBTS, modified BT shunt; PA, pulmonary artery; RA, right atrium; RV, right ventricle.

aortic MVs, 2.5–3.5 for mitral MVs, 1.5–2.0 for On-X® aortic valve [On-X® Life Technologies Inc., Austin, TX, USA]), ASA (with or without clopidogrel) for 3 months for aortic BVs, and VKA (target INR = 2.0–3.0) for 3 months for mitral BVs, followed by long-term ASA for either aortic BVs or mitral BVs [34]. Thromboprophylaxis regimens used for prosthetic valves at SickKids are detailed in Table 1.

Single-Ventricle Heart Palliation

The three stages of single-ventricle palliation, from Norwood to superior cavopulmonary anastomosis (superior cavopulmonary connection [SCPC]/Glenn) to total cavopulmonary anastomosis with or without fenestration (Fontan) remain high-risk circulations for both bleeding and thrombosis.

Across the multiple stages of single-ventricle palliations, published guidelines for thromboprophylaxis recommend intraoperative UFH followed by ASA or no further antithrombotic therapy after the Norwood procedure, postoperative UFH after SCPC (Glenn procedure), and therapeutic UFH followed by VKA (target INR = 2.0–3.0) or ASA only after the Fontan procedure [5]. That said, the emergence of multiple trials examining DOACs in this population will certainly reshape future guidelines.

The UNIVERSE study evaluated the efficacy and safety of rivaroxaban vs. ASA for 1-year primary prophylaxis immediately following Fontan procedure and determined similar safety profile with fewer TEs in children treated with rivaroxaban (overall event rate of 3% in rivaroxaban vs. 9% in ASA), albeit not statistically significant [35]. The SAXOPHONE study examined the safety and efficacy of apixaban against the standard of care (SOC) (VKA/low-molecular-weight heparin [LMWH]) for the primary prevention of TEs in children with a broader range of acquired heart disease and CHD, of which many children had single-ventricle palliations, primarily Fontan [36]. The study has completed enrollment with publication of results derived from 192 randomized children (apixaban [129], SOC [63]), legitimizing apixaban as an alternative option to the SOC in this patient population (major/clinically relevant bleeding; apixaban [<1%], SOC [4.8%]). A second study, a large single-center retrospective cohort study of apixaban in 219 children, of whom 45% (98) had single-ventricle physiology, demonstrated a low adverse event rate of 2.9 serious bleeding events per 100 patient-years of apixaban exposure. This study also reported on the use of apixaban for treatment of TEs, with 95% improvement in thrombosis in 39 children, including intracardiac, arterial, and venous TEs [37]. The ENNOBLE-ATE trial evaluated the use of edoxaban against the SOC (VKA/LMWH) for thromboprophylaxis in children with various cardiac conditions, including single-ventricle palliations [38]. The study investigators found similar adverse event rate (46.8% edoxaban vs. 41.4% with SOC); among the 147 children who continued treatment with edoxaban, there was 1 clinically relevant bleeding event and 4 TEs. Overall, these studies highlight the interest in alternative antithrombotic agents for children with single ventricle, with promising results pertaining to their safety profiles and efficacy. Importantly, potential advantages of DOACs in contrast to SOC anticoagulants include the lack of need for laboratory monitoring, fewer drug-drug/drug-diet interactions, and a likely improved drug safety profile (see Chapter 20). The combination of the recently published/upcoming prospective randomized trials, registry-based, and single-center studies will complement each other, hopefully confirming the expected beneficial DOAC effects in children.

Currently, thromboprophylaxis practices for single-ventricle palliations continue to vary considerably between centers. For example, the thromboprophylaxis regimen employed at SickKids was recently found to be associated with a reduction in early and long-term TE complications, suggesting that routine thromboprophylaxis across all three palliative stages may be warranted [39]. Primary thromboprophylaxis with ASA was reported to lower the risk of shunt thrombosis after Norwood procedure in a non-randomized observational study [40]. There is no consensus regarding routine primary thromboprophylaxis for children after Fontan procedure. For children with a fenestrated Fontan circuit, continued anticoagulation until fenestration closure, either spontaneously or by transcatheter techniques, is advocated by some because of the theoretical risk of paradoxical cardioembolic stroke. While data from a dual center randomized controlled study suggested that there was no significant difference between ASA and warfarin as primary thromboprophylaxis in the first 2 years after Fontan surgery, long-term data from SickKids indicate that warfarin may be associated with a superior outcome, specifically if the INR can be maintained in the target range [39, 41]. Moreover, new data on alternative antiplatelet strategies, such as the use of the parenteral glycoprotein IIb/IIIa inhibitor eptifibatide or the parenteral $P2Y_{12}$ platelet receptor inhibitor agent cangrelor, are emerging [42, 43].

Primary Pulmonary Hypertension

Evidence has suggested that a prothrombotic state exists in children with pulmonary hypertension related to an increase in shear force on RBCs and platelets traversing the pulmonary vascular bed [44]. This altered rheological state has also been associated with an increased risk of bleeding secondary to AVWS [45]. While anticoagulation prophylaxis has historically been the SOC with VKA (target INR = 1.7–2.5 or 2–3) in addition to other medical therapies, there has been a shift toward no anticoagulation prophylaxis given additional risks of bleeding and unclear benefit. The formation of acute or acute on chronic pulmonary embolism (PE) warrants aggressive treatment to prevent right ventricle strain, failure, and, in the setting of massive PE, cardiovascular collapse [46].

Chronic Thromboprophylaxis: Lifelong Considerations

Many children with cardiac disease will "grow up" requiring lifelong anticoagulation. Beyond the myriad of known risks of bleeding, osteopenia, gastritis, and hair loss, described with long-term use of VKA and LMWH, there is the unknown but significant psychological stress associated with anticoagulation management [47, 48]. Increasing awareness is directed toward the impact of anticoagulation treatment and monitoring on quality of life with focused interventions to improve coping with long-term care requirements. Additionally, providers are seeking to evaluate not only the safety and efficacy of DOACs for cardiac disease but also the impact of DOACs on anxiety and quality of life as compared with SOC, given that these agents come with less interactions and lability, less monitoring, and easy to administer oral route. Ongoing attention toward the psychosocial impact of antithrombotic therapy on children and their families is paramount.

Thromboembolic Events

Pediatric cardiac disease represents an important risk factor for TE in children. Importantly, TE complications in this population are associated with increased mortality, significant morbidity, increased hospital stay, and overall suboptimal clinical outcomes compared with children without cardiac disease. Venous thromboembolism (VTE) in the setting of pediatric cardiac surgery is observed in 19–40% of children, depending on the severity of the congenital heart defect, surgical/procedural complexity, and overall level of disease acuity, with a 7% thrombosis-associated mortality, 15% recurrent VTE, and 8–30% post-thrombotic syndrome (PTS) frequency [49]. Up to a third of AIS in children result from cardiac disease with up to 26% mortality, 27% recurrence rate, and persistent neurologic deficits in 72% of

Table 2. Thromboembolic events in children with acquired or congenital heart disease

TE location	Presentation
Extrathoracic venous thrombosis	
Cerebral venous sinuses	Seizures, focal and nonspecific neurological deficits, headaches
Neck, upper extremity veins (internal/external jugular, brachiocephalic, and subclavian)	Upper extremity, facial swelling, catheter dysfunction, and chylous effusions
Intra-abdominal veins (portal/renal)	Abdominal swelling, specific organ dysfunction, and protein-losing enteropathy
Lower extremity veins (iliac, femoral, and others)	Lower extremity swelling and catheter dysfunction
Extrathoracic arterial thrombosis	
Cerebral arterial circle of Willis (cardioembolic stroke)	Seizures, focal, and nonspecific neurological deficits, headaches
Neck (internal/external carotid artery)	Seizures and neurological deficits
Lower extremity (iliac, femoral)	Color change (pallor to purple to black), decreased pulse, and decreased temperature
Intrathoracic thrombosis	
IVC, SVC	Bilateral lower extremity swelling (IVC), hepatic, renal and/or mesenteric dysfunction related to decreased perfusion pressure from IVC venous hypertension, facial swelling (SVC), SVC syndrome, low cardiac output related to reduced venous return
Cardiac chambers/valves	Cardiac dysfunction, arrhythmia
Pulmonary veins/pulmonary arteries	Cardiac/respiratory dysfunction
Aorta	Same as peripheral arterial thrombosis above except potentially bilateral, discrepant upper and lower extremity blood pressures, hypertension (if the renal artery is involved)
Fetal and surgically created shunts	Inadequate systemic or pulmonary perfusion
Mechanical valves	Acute pulmonary edema, cardiogenic shock, systemic embolism, and hemolysis
VAD/ECMO circuit	Visible circuit clots, circuit dysfunction, and embolic phenomena

See also Chapters 13–17 for further clinical presentations of TEs. ECMO, extracorporeal membrane oxygenation; IVC, inferior vena cava; SVC, superior vena cava; TE, thromboembolism/thromboembolic event; VAD, ventricular assist device.

survivors [50]. CHD and mechanical support are associated with a higher risk for AIS (see Chapter 19) in children after pediatric heart transplantation [51]. CHD is also a major risk factor for non-central nervous system arterial TE (see Chapter 15). Strikingly, up to 28% of TEs in the setting of pediatric cardiac disease are extremely serious events (i.e., cardioembolic AIS, cerebral sinovenous thrombosis, PE, superior vena cava [SVC] syndrome) often requiring thrombectomy/thrombolytics, or leading to cardiopulmonary arrest or death [49]. Table 2 illustrates the variable presentation of TE in children with cardiac disease.

Thromboembolism in Children with CHD

The reported frequency of TE in children with CHD ranges from as low as 3% to as high as 30–40%, depending on study design, imaging modality, and patient population investigated [49]. Neonatal age, baseline oxygen saturation <85%, previous thrombosis, heart transplantation, use of deep hypothermic circulatory arrest, longer cumulative time with central lines, and postoperative use of extracorporeal membrane oxygenation (ECMO) support are factors associated with increased risk of thrombosis. Conversely, inherited thrombophilia does not seem to play a role in short-term central line-induced thrombosis [52].

Clinical Presentation

The presentation of TE in children with cardiac disease is highly variable depending on the location and extent of the thrombus, i.e., occlusive vs. nonocclusive and long vs. short segment. While most TEs present acutely in the early postoperative or postprocedural phase, children with prosthetic valves or shunts or post-Fontan procedure can present with both early and/or late TE complications. The development of chylous effusions should prompt evaluation of the upper venous system to rule out central vein thrombosis [53]. Similarly, the presence of acute ascites may suggest the presence of infradiaphragmatic venous obstruction following surgical intervention, catheterization, or in the setting of lower extremity central venous lines. Some children with less extensive thrombi may have a late presentation with delayed sequelae such as PTS, portal hypertension, and long-term complications associated with arterial thrombosis (see Chapter 15). Chronic arterial or venous occlusions have significant implications for future cardiovascular procedures, limiting access to cardiac catheterization and peripheral cannulation of ECMO or CPB. As such, it is important to delineate vascular occlusions prior to invasive procedures that may necessitate vascular access. The burden of clinically unsuspected TE in children with cardiac disease is not well elucidated, as many thrombi may be discovered incidentally on radiological studies performed for other reasons [54, 55].

Diagnosis

It is important to maintain a high index of suspicion for TEs in children having undergone cardiac surgery or cardiac catheterization, given their increased propensity, variable and nonspecific presentation, and significant short-term and long-term complications. Confirmation of clinical suspicion requires radiological evidence, and the choice of the radiologic modality (Doppler ultrasound, venography/angiography, echocardiography, neuroimaging) depends on the location of the thrombus (see Chapters 13, 14, 16, and 17). New imaging modalities such as contrast-enhanced magnetic resonance venography (MRV) and multidetector computerized tomography angiography are emerging as useful imaging techniques for evaluation of TE. While MRV/magnetic resonance angiography is ideal for image quality and lack of radiation, its use in palliated CHD may be narrowed because of the presence of prosthetic material that is either not magnetic resonance imaging compatible and/or generates artifact, limiting the interpretability of the acquired images.

Management

The management of TEs in children with CHD does not differ substantially from TE in other children, and the clinician should follow published guidelines as discussed elsewhere (see Chapters 14–17 and 19–20). Anticoagulation alone is sufficient in most TEs and should be continued beyond the standard treatment duration if the primary trigger for TE has not been eliminated (e.g., uncorrected CHD in a child with cardioembolic AIS). Some cardiac TEs can be life threatening and may require more aggressive therapeutic approaches (i.e., thrombolysis, catheter, or

18

surgical interventions). These treatment modalities should be considered individually, balancing the risks and benefits [56].

Specific Thromboembolic Events in CHD

Mechanical Valve Thrombosis

MV thrombosis occurs at a rate of 0.1% per patient-year with the highest incidence in the first year after implantation and in children with a mechanical tricuspid/mitral valve replacement. Left-sided MV thrombosis in the mitral position or aortic position can present with obstructive (low cardiac output, left atrial hypertension, and acute pulmonary edema) or nonobstructive TE signs and symptoms. Almost 50% of MV thromboses are asymptomatic. The diagnosis of MV thrombosis can be confirmed in most children by the combination of transthoracic or transesophageal echocardiography and fluoroscopy. Current recommendations for acute treatment of MV thrombosis favor the use of systemic thrombolytic therapy as first-line treatment. Surgery is reserved for children who have a contraindication for or who fail thrombolysis [57]. Subsequently increasing the anticoagulation intensity (i.e., to a target INR 3.0–4.0) or adding ASA to VKA to prevent further events may be required for children who develop MV thrombosis while on adequate anticoagulation.

Blalock-Taussig Shunt Thrombosis

Thrombotic occlusion of the Blalock-Taussig (BT) shunt occurs in up to 17% of children and can compromise pulmonary blood flow requiring immediate intervention. Diagnosis is usually clinical, supported by echocardiographic and/or angiographic findings. Therapeutic options for children who develop acute BT shunt occlusion include systemic anticoagulation (bivalirudin/argatroban over UFH) [58], catheter-directed thrombolytic therapy, and/or angioplasty with stenting and reoperation. Moreover, children with BT shunts may have reduced peripheral pulses in the ipsilateral arm and may have measurably reduced growth of the arm. This can be of significance when assessing for PTS, which may also occur in the upper limbs secondary to VTE [59].

Increasingly, right ventricle to pulmonary artery conduits are being utilized. A study conducted in Birmingham, UK, involving approximately 1,000 children found that pulmonary and aortic homografts had superior durability in comparison to xenograft conduits in children weighing between 5 and 20 kg. Furthermore, homograft conduits had less dysfunction and replacement in comparison to xenografts in children of this weight range, in contrast to having similar durability in children with other weights. Judicious oversizing can also improve the conduit durability [60].

Another practice being considered often as an alternative to a surgical shunt in neonates with duct-depended pulmonary perfusion is stenting of their PDA (i.e., original bare metal CA stents). In those instances, loading doses of UFH immediately prior to stent placement, followed by switching to LMWH for at least 48 h before it can be transitioned to ASA (3 to 5 mg/kg per day), is recommended [61]. In children with ≤2.5 kg, re-interventions may be required [62].

Thromboembolism after Superior Cavopulmonary Connection (Glenn Procedure)

Although TEs are thought to be relatively uncommon in infants after SCPC (Glenn procedure), TEs were recently reported to occur in 28% after SCPC, suggesting that TEs are likely underappreciated [39]. There are, additionally, several considerations related to the vascular anatomy after SCPC (Glenn procedure; Fig. 1) that could justify more aggressive antithrombotic therapy in case of TE (i.e., thrombolysis or surgery). First, following SCPC (Glenn procedure), blood flows directly from the SVC into the pulmonary vasculature;

hence, any reduction in SVC flow to the lungs, because of thrombotic occlusion, will dramatically reduce pulmonary blood flow. Second, increased pulmonary vascular resistance, because of PE, is of concern since this might make the child unsuitable for future Fontan surgery. Third, thrombus in the lower venous system or from collaterals (i.e., SVC → IVC → pulmonary veins) can give rise to paradoxical emboli, as blood flow from the IVC is directed toward the systemic ventricle and the arterial circulation. Finally, collaterals around thrombosis of central thoracic veins may interfere with the ability to complete the Fontan surgery.

Thromboembolism after Fontan Procedure

TEs remain a major complication after Fontan surgery. In a prospective, open label, randomized study comparing the efficacy of thrombosis prevention between warfarin and ASA, the cumulative thrombosis rate (symptomatic and asymptomatic) was 23% in the first 2 years after surgery despite thromboprophylaxis with either warfarin or ASA [41]. The UNIVERSE study, a randomized multicenter two-part open label study of rivaroxaban vs. ASA for 1-year post-Fontan, led to the approval of this medication by the Food and Drug Administration (FDA) for children aged 2 years or older at the end of 2021 [35].

While the immediate postoperative period is high risk, TEs may occur any time following the Fontan procedure but often present months to years later. Factors associated with higher risk of TE include pulmonary atresia with intact ventricular septum, pulmonary artery distortion, lower pre-operative unconjugated bilirubin, use of central venous lines for >10 days or until hospital discharge, suboptimal VKA monitoring, and lower FiO_2 24 h after the procedure [63]. Similar to SCPC (Glenn) and Norwood procedures, TEs after a Fontan procedure can have several important implications and may warrant an aggressive antithrombotic strategy in case of thrombosis, i.e., thrombolysis and surgery. First, the risk for paradoxical emboli continues to be a concern because of the presence of right to left communication. Second, because the pulmonary pressure cannot be increased in Fontan circuits, PE has an accentuated impact on pulmonary blood flow. Third, the Fontan circuit makes it difficult to obtain full lung perfusion during imaging, rendering the radiological confirmation of PE particularly challenging.

Following Fontan surgery, children are sensitive to VKA and will require lower doses than what is recommended for other children. This sensitivity to VKA is thought to be due to subclinical hepatic dysfunction that likely results from chronically elevated systemic venous pressure because of the absence of a right-sided pumping chamber in children with Fontan physiology [64].

Long-term systemic venous hypertension related to Fontan circulation leads to progressive congestive hepatopathy and associated acquired thrombophilia. Protein C, protein S, and factor VII are lower in children post-Fontan. These coagulation abnormalities have also been demonstrated in children with Glenn physiology (SCPC) and ventricular dysfunction prior to Fontan conversion, suggesting that the presence of high systemic venous pressures and liver congestion is a major provoking factor [65–67].

Intracardiac Thrombosis

Intracardiac thrombosis can be encountered as a complication of CHD surgery, ECMO/ventricular-assisted devices, cardiomyopathy, or acquired cardiac disease. Right-sided and left-sided intracardiac TE can lead to PE and AIS, respectively. Any cardiac chamber may be involved in children with CHD, including hypoplastic chambers and blind stumps (right ventricle), aortic atresia, critical aortic stenosis, mitral atresia, pulmonary atresia with intact ventricular septum and Ebstein's anomaly. Right atrial thrombosis is most commonly because of indwelling central venous catheters [68]. It may be rarely encountered in children with Eisenmenger syndrome (secondary

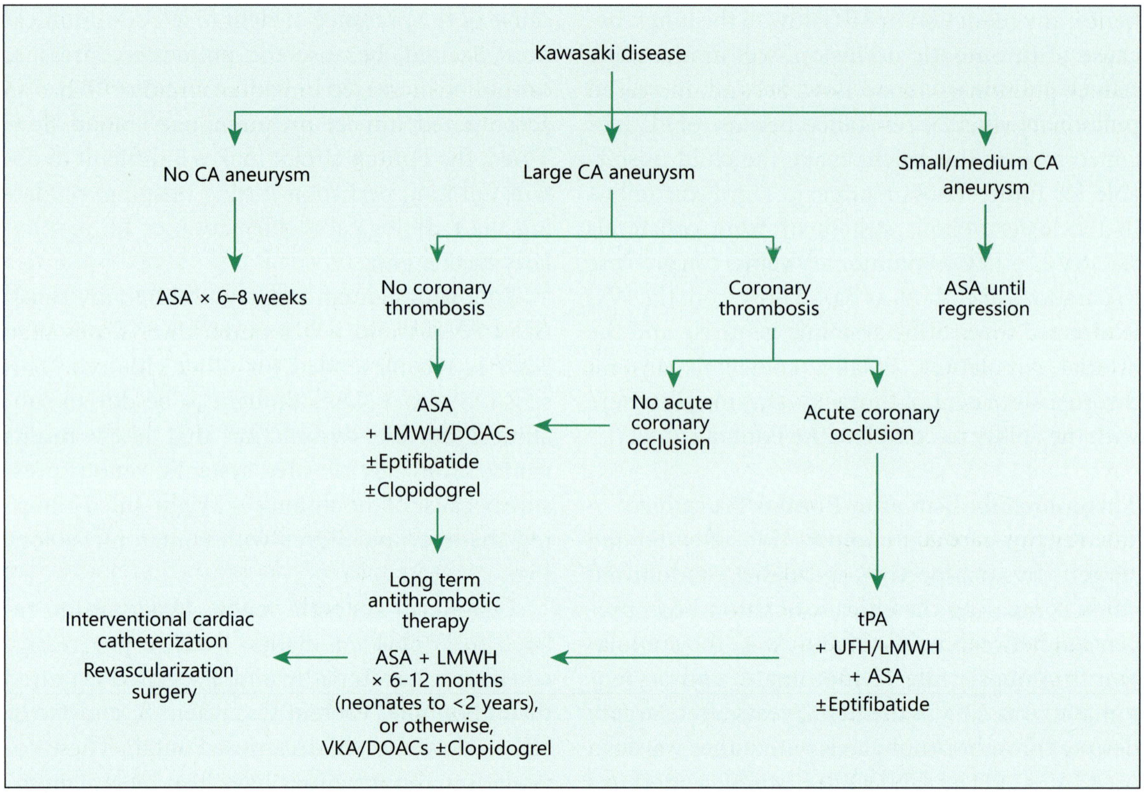

Fig. 2. Antithrombotic therapy in Kawasaki disease. Eptifibatide is an intravenous glycoprotein IIb/IIIa receptor antagonist given as a bolus (180 µg/kg; maximum 22.6 mg) followed by infusion (2 µg/kg/min; maximum 15 mg/h). A second bolus of the same dose can be administered 10 min after the first bolus. Infusion can continue up to 18–24 h. Catheter interventions, including balloon angioplasty, rotational ablation, and stent placement, may be considered in children presenting with ischemic symptoms, children without ischemic symptoms but with reversible ischemia on stress test, and children without ischemia but with ≥75% stenosis in the left anterior descending CA. Surgical revascularization may be considered in severe occlusion of the main trunk of the left main CA, severe occlusion of ≥1 major CA, severe occlusion in the proximal segment of the left anterior descending CA, if collateral coronary arteries in jeopardy, severe left ventricular dysfunction, or recurrent myocardial infarction. ASA, acetylsalicylic acid; CA, coronary artery; DOAC, direct oral anticoagulant; LMWH, low-molecular-weight heparin; tPA, tissue plasminogen activator; UFH, unfractionated heparin; VKA, vitamin K antagonist.

pulmonary hypertension because of development of pulmonary vascular obstructive disease associated with prolonged pulmonary arterial pressure and volume overload). Left atrial TE has been seen in children with restrictive cardiomyopathy and resultant dilated left atrial appendage that acts as a windsock for thrombus development. Left-sided cardiac catheterization ablation procedures performed for arrhythmia treatment have also been associated with postprocedural TE. Thrombi in either atrium have been reported after a Fontan procedure as well as within the Fontan connection. Although some authors have suggested that small nonmobile intracardiac right atrial thrombosis do not require any therapy [68], anticoagulation is the main therapy for most cases of uncomplicated intracardiac thrombosis; however, thrombolytic therapy or surgical thrombectomy may be considered in selected cases of intracardiac thrombi causing flow obstruction, valvular dysfunction, cardiac failure, or serious embolic phenomena [6].

Thromboembolism in Children with Acquired Heart Disease

Kawasaki Disease

Kawasaki disease is the leading cause of pediatric acquired cardiac disease in North America. Up to 25% of untreated children (5% of treated children) develop CA aneurysms, which significantly increases the risk of CA thrombosis and consequently myocardial infarction (MI). Recommendations for management of children with Kawasaki disease depend on the timing of presentation (acute phase vs. chronic phase), appearance, location, and size of any CA aneurysm and signs of CA aneurysm thrombosis [69, 70]. In the acute phase, a single high dose of intravenous immunoglobulin is recommended to be given within 10 days of the onset of symptoms. All children are started on low-dose ASA or medium-dose ASA followed by low dose once afebrile. For children with evolving CA involvement, pre-emptive escalation of thromboprophylaxis is warranted in anticipation that the involvement will progress. Once involvement is at maximum and stable, a decision regarding ongoing thromboprophylaxis can be made based on current involvement. In the long-term children with any size, CA aneurysm at any time are indicated for long-term low-dose ASA. Only children with current large or giant aneurysms are recommended for additional anticoagulation. At SickKids, children with large or giant CA aneurysms are given therapeutic doses of LMWH for 6–12 months before switching to VKA if clinically stable and free from TE based on data suggesting an association between use of LMWH and favorable vascular remodeling in Kawasaki disease [71]. The antithrombotic management after the acute phase is outlined in Fig. 2. When comparing efficacy of LMWH vs. VKA in children treated in the International Kawasaki Disease Registry, the positive impact of LMWH, initially detected in the SickKids cohort, was not confirmed, though there was an overall benefit of anticoagulation [72]. Caution should be exercised, given the limitations and potential biases relevant to nonrandomized comparisons. Challenges related to use of SOC anticoagulants highlight the need to further evaluate the impact of DOACs in this clinical context (i.e., SAXOPHONE and ENNOBLE-ATE trials). Alternatively, from a safety perspective in the setting of a resolving CA aneurysm and when excessive mucocutaneous bleeding occurs while the child receives combined anticoagulant and single antiplatelet therapy, consideration to changing the anticoagulation to dual antiplatelet therapy may be warranted.

Infective Endocarditis

IE is characterized by vegetations that typically involve native or prosthetic valves but can also affect other cardiac structures such as shunts, conduits, VSD, and PDA. Vegetations consist of a mass of platelets, fibrin, microcolonies of microorganisms and inflammatory cells, which can cause significant damage to the involved structure. Embolic complications can occur, including AIS, cerebral mycotic aneurysms, PE, renal and splenic infarcts, retinal Roth spots, and osteomyelitis [73]. Risk factors for TEs include larger size vegetations (>10 mm), mitral valve location of vegetations, and Staphylococcal and fungal infections. Most embolic episodes occur within the first 2–4 weeks after therapy.

The role of antithrombotic therapy in IE remains controversial given the risk of intracranial hemorrhage resulting from hemorrhagic transformation of ischemic infarcts, septic erosion of inflamed arteries, or rupture of mycotic aneurysms. For children with IE without a separate indication for anticoagulation or antiplatelet therapy, empiric initiation of anticoagulant therapy or

Table 3. Suggested strategy to antithrombotic therapy in IE

	Mechanical valve IE	Native/bioprosthetic valve IE
No clinical evidence of stroke	Continue anticoagulation and convert from VKA to intravenous UFH. Restart VKA when it is clear that invasive procedures will not be required, and the patient has stabilized without signs of central nervous system involvement[a]	Antithrombotic therapy is not indicated
Clinical evidence of stroke		
No radiological evidence for ICH	Hold VKA, resume anticoagulation with intravenous UFH within 1 week with serial brain imaging to exclude hemorrhagic transformation or ICH	
Radiological evidence of ICH	Withhold anticoagulation, exclude mycotic aneurysms	

ICH, intracranial hemorrhage; IE, infective endocarditis; UFH, unfractionated heparin; VKA, vitamin K antagonist. [a]Discontinuing anticoagulation until blood cultures are negative and the clinical signs of sepsis have resolved can be considered in patients with *Staphylococcus aureus* IE.

antiplatelet therapy is not indicated [73]. In other cases, it should be considered individually based on the assumed embolic risk, potential need for surgery, and bleeding risk, as exemplified in the historical cohort reported by SickKids, noting approximately 20% of 113 children with IE received either antiplatelet or anticoagulation therapy for different indications (i.e., stents, MVs), not complicated by bleeding [74]. A suggested strategy for the management of anticoagulation in children with valve-related IE is presented in Table 3.

Cardiomyopathy

Cardiomyopathy encompasses a heterogeneous group of diseases of the myocardium associated with cardiac dysfunction (systolic and/or diastolic) that can be primary, acquired (e.g., viral myocarditis), or part of a multisystem disorder. Cardiomyopathies are classified according to cardiac physiology into dilated, hypertrophic, restrictive, mixed, arrhythmogenic right ventricular, and left ventricular noncompaction. Dilated cardiomyopathy is the most common type.

TEs, i.e., intraventricular thrombosis and cardioembolic strokes, are reported in up to 16% of children with dilated cardiomyopathy. These events can occur at any time in the clinical course and are not related to clinical features or transplantation-free survival [75]. For children with dilated cardiomyopathy and severe dysfunction (generally ejection fraction ≤20% or shortening fraction <10%), VKA (target INR 2.0–3.0) is initiated no later than their activation on a cardiac transplantation waiting list [5]. DOACs may also be considered for thromboprophylaxis in the setting of severe ventricular dysfunction. Anticoagulation should also be considered for children with evident TE, cardiomyopathy with arrhythmia, previous TEs, thrombophilic conditions, or shortening fraction <10% or ejection fraction ≤20% [6]. The risk of TE is also increased in restrictive cardiomyopathy and in left ventricular noncompaction cardiomyopathy [76]. At SickKids, both primary and secondary thromboprophylaxis is prescribed to selected children with cardiomyopathy (Table 1).

Special Consideration

Myocardial Infarction

Although rare in children, MI is a serious condition that results from critical decrease in CA perfusion. See Chapter 20 for use of fibrinolytic therapy in MI management in children. Treatment of MI depends on the underlying cause, with percutaneous or surgical revascularization, in addition to pharmacological therapy with catheter-directed thrombolysis, antiplatelet, and anticoagulant, having an expanding role in children as they do in adults [77].

Causes for MI in children include:

1. CA anomalies (anomalous origin of left CA from the pulmonary artery, origin of a CA from the wrong aortic sinus with its course between the aorta and the pulmonary artery)
2. CA complications associated with CHD, cardiac surgeries, or catheterization (CA obstruction after arterial switch operation for D-transposition of the great arteries, CA complication after repair of tetralogy of Fallot, CA ostial stenosis associated with supravalvular aortic stenosis, CA obstruction associated with pulmonary atresia with intact ventricular septum, CA compression from epicardial pacing wires, and CA compression from surgical or transcatheter valve replacement)
3. CA sequelae of Kawasaki disease (thrombotic occlusion of large CA aneurysm, CA stenosis at ends of large aneurysm, and obliterative coronary arteritis without large aneurysm [rare])
4. Myocardial ischemia associated with hypertrophic cardiomyopathy, particularly in the setting of a myocardial bridge [78]
5. Myocardial ischemia associated with cocaine use
6. Atherosclerotic CA disease in children with homozygous familial hypercholesterolemia
7. Coronary allograft vasculopathy; an accelerated form of arteriopathy affecting the coronary arteries of heart transplant recipients.

Children with MI rarely manifest with classic pressure-like chest pain, particularly younger children. Presentation is more often nonspecific, such as unusual irritability, nausea and vomiting, abdominal pain, shock, syncope, seizure, sudden unexpected cardiac arrest, or even silent infarcts. Diagnosis of clinically suspected cases can be confirmed by elevated cardiac enzymes (creatinine phosphokinase subfractions and high-sensitivity troponin), ischemic changes on ECG and segmental wall motion abnormalities on echocardiography. The gold-standard diagnostic test remains coronary angiography. Management requires early recognition and involvement of a pediatric cardiologist and should be tailored depending on the underlying etiology (see Fig. 2 for management of CA thrombosis in Kawasaki disease). Furthermore, it is important to recognize clinical nuances related to child's age, type of fibrinolytic agents and mode of administration, and underlying conditions to optimize therapy [77, 79].

Cyanosis, Erythrocytosis, Hemolysis, and Secondary Thrombocytosis

In addition to secondary erythrocytosis, infants with cyanotic CHD are at increased risk for iron deficiency anemia, which can increase the risk for cerebral thrombosis because of the poor deformability of the iron-deficient RBC, which further increases blood viscosity. To prevent this complication and to allow for maximal tissue oxygenation, all infants should have adequate dietary iron intake and should receive iron replacement therapy as needed to normalize RBC indices.

Hemolysis can be present in a multitude of underlying palliated and unpalliated congenital heart lesions, such as restrictive VSD, stenotic native or artificial valves, valvar regurgitation, paravalvar leaks, and most notably in mechanical circulatory support/CPB. Hemolysis is defined by increasing level of plasma free-hemoglobin, lactate dehydrogenase, and decreasing haptoglobin. The sequela of hemolysis may extend beyond the destruction of RBC and anemia, resulting in multiorgan involvement of the renal, hepatic, pulmonary, and cerebrovascular systems. The release of free hemoglobin into the plasma scavenges nitric oxide from the endothelium, resulting in pulmonary and systemic vasoconstriction through basal and stress-mediated control of smooth muscle relaxation and vasomotor tone. This vasoconstriction further increases RBC shear and propagates intravascular hemolysis. Early identification of hemolysis and causative factors is imperative to halt the cascade of multiorgan failure. Treatment of hemolysis is primarily targeted at the underlying cause. There are currently no available treatments for removing free hemoglobin apart from whole volume exchanges or plasmapheresis.

Reactive thrombocytosis is also seen in critically ill children, related to multiple factors, including infection, medications, postsplenectomy, and iron deficiency anemia [80]. While the rise in platelets can be alarming, it does not appear to be a thrombotic risk [81]. Addressing the underlying cause of the thrombocytosis is the most effective treatment strategy, be it treatment of sepsis, discontinuation of offending medication, or repletion of iron. Conversely, elevation of platelets in the setting of inflammation, such as seen with Kawasaki disease, mechanical circulatory support, and ventricular-assisted devices, as well as post-CBP, may increase thrombotic risk and needs to be addressed by intensifying antiplatelet strategies and reducing inflammation (please, see Chapter 19). Similarly, if associated with myeloproliferative neoplasm, platelet monitoring, as well as consideration for antiplatelet or cytoreductive therapy, may be required as it is associated with increased thrombotic risk.

Conclusion

Both bleeding complications and TEs are significant morbidities in children with cardiac disease. While there remains limited pediatric data for the prevention and treatment for many of the complex and heterogenous cardiac conditions, there have been many pediatric-specific trials in the last decade. As we continue to focus studies on the pediatric population and cardiac indications, we will strengthen the evidence base supporting future recommendations. Despite considerable practice variation between and within institutions, learning collaboratives, registries, and consensus guidelines will help in understanding how this practice variation impacts outcomes. The management approaches presented here are based on available published data and the institutional experience at SickKids of managing a large number of children with cardiac disease over a span of several decades.

Acknowledgment

The authors express their appreciation for the continuous guidance provided by the late Dr. Patricia M. Massicotte (Edmonton, AB, Canada), in addition to the previous collaborations by Dr. Yaser Diab (Children's National Hospital, Washington, DC, USA).

Conflict of Interest Statement

Dr. Christina VanderPluym is a paid consultant for Merck and AstraZeneca. Dr. Brian McCrindle is a paid consultant for Amryt Pharm, Chiesi, Esperion, and Ultragenyx. Dr. Leonardo R. Brandão reports receiving consultancy and speaker fees from Astra Zeneca, Inari Medical, and Takeda. He was a member of the pediatric expert group for Boehringer Ingelheim (Dabigatran studies). He is recipient of an educational grant from Inari Medical. He is meeting co-chair for the not-for-profit organization named Thrombosis & Hemostasis Societies of North America (THSNA).

Author Contributions

Dr. Christina VanderPluym contributed by writing content, formatting, and editing. Dr. Brian McCrindle contributed by writing content and editing. Dr. Leonardo R. Brandão contributed by writing content, formatting, and editing.

Abbreviations

AIS	Arterial ischemic stroke
aPTT	Activated partial thromboplastin time
ASA	Acetylsalicylic acid
AVWS	Acquired von Willebrand syndrome
BT	Blalock-Taussig
BV	Bioprosthetic valve
CA	Coronary artery
CHD	Congenital heart disease
CPB	Cardiopulmonary bypass
DDAVP	1-Deamino-8-D-arginine vasopressin (desmopressin)
ECMO	Extracorporeal membrane oxygenation
FFP	Fresh frozen plasma
FP	Frozen plasma
FIX	Factor IX
IE	Infective endocarditis
INR	International normalized ratio
IVC	Inferior vena cava
LMWH	Low-molecular-weight heparin
MI	Myocardial infarction
MRV	Magnetic resonance venography
MV	Mechanical valve
PCC	Prothrombin complex concentrate
PDA	Patent ductus arteriosus
PE	Pulmonary embolism
PT	Prothrombin time
PTS	Post-thrombotic syndrome
RBC	Red blood cell
rFVIIa	Recombinant activated factor VII
SCPC	Superior cavopulmonary connection
SOC	Standard of care
SVC	Superior vena cava
TE	Thromboembolism/thromboembolic event
UFH	Unfractionated heparin
VKA	Vitamin K antagonist
VSD	Ventricular septal defect
VTE	Venous thromboembolism/thromboembolic event
VWF	von Willebrand factor
VWF:CBA	VWF collagen binding activity
VWF:RCo	VWF activity (ristocetin cofactor assay)

18

References

1 Dolbec K, Mick NW. Congenital heart disease. Emerg Med Clin North Am. 2011;29(4):811–27.

2 Paediatric multisystem inflammatory syndrome temporally associated with COVID-19 (PIMS) – guidance for clinicians | RCPCH. Accessed on November 2023. https://www.rcpch.ac.uk/resources/paediatric-multisystem-inflammatory-syndrome-temporally-associated-covid-19-pims-guidance

3 Multisystem inflammatory syndrome in children - Information for Healthcare Providers about Multisystem Inflammatory Syndrome in Children (MIS-C) - Centers for Disease Control and Prevention. Accessed on April 2024. http://www.cdc.gov/mis/mis-c/hcp_cstecdc/index.html.

4 Godfred-Cato S, Bryant B, Leung J, Oster ME, Conklin L, Abrams J, et al. COVID-19-associated multisystem inflammatory syndrome in children – United States, March-July 2020. MMWR Morb Mortal Wkly Rep. 2020;69(32):1074–80.

5 Monagle P, Chan AKC, Goldenberg NA, Ichord RN, Journeycake JM, Nowak-Göttl U, et al. Antithrombotic therapy in neonates and children: antithrombotic therapy and prevention of thrombosis, 9th ed: American College of Chest Physicians Evidence-Based Clinical Practice Guidelines. Chest. 2012;141(2 suppl): e737S-801S.

6 Giglia TM, Massicotte MP, Tweddell JS, Barst RJ, Bauman M, Erickson CC, et al. Prevention and treatment of thrombosis in pediatric and congenital heart disease a scientific statement from the American Heart Association. Circulation. 2013;128(24):2622–703.

7 Henderson LA, Canna SW, Friedman KG, Gorelik M, Lapidus SK, Bassiri H, et al. American College of Rheumatology clinical guidance for multisystem inflammatory syndrome in children associated with SARS-CoV-2 and hyperinflammation in pediatric COVID-19: version 3. Arthritis Rheumatol. 2022; 74(4):e1–20.

8 Sochet AA, Morrison JM, Jaffray J, Godiwala N, Wilson HP, Thornburg CD, et al. Enoxaparin thromboprophylaxis in children hospitalized for COVID-19:a phase 2 trial. Pediatrics. 2022;150(1): e2022056726.

9 Bansal N, Azeka E, Neunert C, Kim JS, Murray J, May L, et al. Multisystem inflammatory syndrome associated with COVID-19 anti-thrombosis guideline of care for children by action. Pediatr Cardiol. 2021;42(7):1635–9.

10 Rychik J, Atz AM, Celermajer DS, Deal BJ, Gatzoulis MA, Gewillig MH, et al. Evaluation and management of the child and adult with Fontan circulation: a scientific statement from the American Heart Association. Circulation. 2019; 140(6):E234–84.

11 Briggs BJ, Dickerman JD. Bleeding disorders in Noonan syndrome. Pediatr Blood Cancer. 2012;58(2):167–72.

12 Manlhiot C, McCrindle BW, Menjak IB, Yoon H, Holtby HM, Brandão LR, et al. Longer blood storage is associated with suboptimal outcomes in high-risk pediatric cardiac surgery. Ann Thorac Surg. 2012;93(5):1563–9.

13 Whitworth H, Amankwah EK, Betensky M, Castellucci LA, Cuker A, Goldenberg NA, et al. Updated guidance for efficacy and safety outcomes for clinical trials in venous thromboembolism in children: communication from the ISTH SSC Subcommittee on Pediatric and Neonatal Thrombosis and Hemostasis. J Thromb Haemost. 2023;21(6):1666–73.

14 Arnold P. Treatment and monitoring of coagulation abnormalities in children undergoing heart surgery. Paediatr Anaesth. 2011;21(5):494–503.

15 Bortot M, Ashworth K, Sharifi A, Walker F, Crawford NC, Neeves KB, et al. Turbulent flow promotes cleavage of VWF (von Willebrand factor) by ADAMTS13 (a disintegrin and metalloproteinase with a thrombospondin type-1 motif, member 13). Arterioscler Thromb Vasc Biol. 2019;39(9):1831–42.

16 Wesley MC, McGowan FX, Castro RA, Dissanayake S, Zurakowski D, DiNardo JA. The effect of milrinone on platelet activation as determined by teg® platelet mapping™. Anesth Analg. 2009; 108(5):1425–9.

17 Elbatarny M, Mollah S, Grabell J, Bae S, Deforest M, Tuttle A, et al. Normal range of bleeding scores for the ISTH-BAT: adult and pediatric data from the merging project. Haemophilia. 2014; 20(6):831–5.
18 Tiede A, Rand JH, Budde U, Ganser A, Federici AB. How I treat the acquired von Willebrand syndrome. Blood. 2011; 117(25):6777–85.
19 Marlar RA, Potts RM, Marlar AA. Effect on routine and special coagulation testing values of citrate anticoagulant adjustment in patients with high hematocrit values. Am J Clin Pathol. 2006; 126(3):400–5.
20 Murray JM, Hellinger A, Dionne R, Brown L, Galvin R, Griggs S, et al. Utility of a dedicated pediatric cardiac anticoagulation program: the Boston children's hospital experience. Pediatr Cardiol. 2015;36(4):842–50.
21 Newall F, Jones S, Bauman M, Bruce A, Massicotte MP, Monagle P. Recommendations for the development of a dedicated pediatric anticoagulation service: communication from the SSC of the ISTH. J Thromb Haemost. 2015;13(1): 155–9.
22 Romlin BS, Wåhlander H, Berggren H, Synnergren M, Baghaei F, Nilsson K, et al. Intraoperative thromboelastometry is associated with reduced transfusion prevalence in pediatric cardiac surgery. Anesth Analg. 2011;112(1):30–6.
23 Cholette JM, Willems A, Valentine SL, Bateman ST, Schwartz SM. Recommendations on RBC transfusion in infants and children with acquired and congenital heart disease from the pediatric critical care transfusion and anemia expertise initiative. Pediatr Crit Care Med. 2018;19(9S suppl 1):S137–48.
24 Faraoni D, Willems A, Melot C, De Hert S, Van der Linden P. Efficacy of tranexamic acid in paediatric cardiac surgery: a systematic review and meta-analysis. Eur J Cardiothorac Surg. 2012; 42(5):781–6.
25 McQuilten ZK, Barnes C, Zatta A, Phillips LE. Off-label use of recombinant factor VIIa in pediatric patients. Pediatrics. 2012;129(6):e1533–40.
26 Song HK, Tibayan FA, Kahl EA, Sera VA, Slater MS, Deloughery TG, et al. Safety and efficacy of prothrombin complex concentrates for the treatment of coagulopathy after cardiac surgery. J Thorac Cardiovasc Surg. 2014;147(3): 1036–40.
27 Noga T, Bruce AAK, Blain H, Nahirniak S. Four-factor prothrombin complex concentrates in paediatric patients – a retrospective case series. Vox Sang. 2016;110(3):253–7.
28 Jalal Z, Gewillig M, Boudjemline Y, Guérin P, Pilati M, Butera G, et al. Transcatheter interventions in patients with a Fontan circulation: current practice and future developments. Front Pediatr. 2022;10:965989.
29 Okubo M, Benson LN. Intravascular and intracardiac stents used in congenital heart disease. Curr Opin Cardiol. 2001; 16(2):84–91.
30 O'Laughlin MP, Perry SB, Lock JE, Mullins CE. Use of endovascular stents in congenital heart disease. Circulation. 1991;83(6):1923–39.
31 Otto CM, Nishimura RA, Bonow RO, Carabello BA, Erwin JP III, Gentile F, et al. 2020 ACC/AHA guideline for the management of patients with valvular heart disease: a report of the American College of Cardiology/American Heart Association Joint Committee on Clinical Practice Guidelines. J Thorac Cardiovasc Surg. 2021;162(2):e183–353.
32 Henaine R, Roubertie F, Vergnat M, Ninet J. Valve replacement in children: a challenge for a whole life. Arch Cardiovasc Dis. 2012;105(10):517–28.
33 Puskas J, Gerdisch M, Nichols D, Quinn R, Anderson C, Rhenman B, et al. Reduced anticoagulation after mechanical aortic valve replacement: interim results from the prospective randomized on-X valve anticoagulation clinical trial randomized Food and Drug Administration investigational device exemption trial. J Thorac Cardiovasc Surg. 2014;147(4): 1202–10.
34 Otto CM, Nishimura RA, Bonow RO, Carabello BA, Erwin JP III, Gentile F, et al. 2020 ACC/AHA guideline for the management of patients with valvular heart disease: executive summary – a report of the American College of Cardiology/American Heart Association Joint Committee on Clinical Practice Guidelines. J Am Coll Cardiol. 2021;77(4): 450–500.
35 McCrindle B, Michelson AD, Van Bergen AH, Horowitz ES, Sandoval JP, et al. Thromboprophylaxis for Children Post-Fontan Procedure: Insights From The UNIVERSE Study. J Am Heart Assoc. 2021;10:e021765.
36 Payne RM, Burns KM, Glatz AC, Male C, Donti A, Brandao LR, et al. Apixaban for Prevention of Thromboembolism in Pediatric Heart Disease. J Am Coll Cardiol. 2023;82:2296–2309.
37 VanderPluym C, Esteso P, Ankola A, Hellinger A, Ventresco C, Hawkins B, et al. Real-world use of apixaban for the treatment and prevention of thrombosis in children with cardiac disease. J Thromb Haemost. 2023 Jun;21(6):1601–9.
38 Portman MA, Jacobs JP, Newburger JW, Berger F, Grosso MA, Duggal A, et al. Edoxaban for thromboembolism prevention in pediatric patients with cardiac disease. J Am Coll Cardiol. 2022; 80(24):2301–10.
39 Manlhiot C, Brandão LR, Kwok J, Kegel S, Menjak IB, Carew CL, et al. Thrombotic complications and thromboprophylaxis across all three stages of single ventricle heart palliation. J Pediatr. 2012;161(3):513–9.
40 Li JS, Yow E, Berezny KY, Rhodes JF, Bokesch PM, Charpie JR, et al. Clinical outcomes of palliative surgery including a systemic-to-pulmonary artery shunt in infants with cyanotic congenital heart disease: does aspirin make a difference? Circulation. 2007;116(3): 293–7.
41 Monagle P, Cochrane A, Roberts R, Manlhiot C, Weintraub R, Szechtman B, et al. A Multicenter, Randomized Trial Comparin Heparin/Warfarin and Acetylsalicylic Acid as Primary Thromboprophylaxis for 2 Years After the Fontan Procedure in Children. J Am Coll Cardiol. 2011;58(6):645–51.
42 Emani S, Pereira LM, Piekarski BL, Diallo F, Chu E, Wesley MC, et al. Platelet inhibition with IV glycoprotein IIb/IIIa inhibitor to prevent thrombosis in pediatric patients undergoing aortopulmonary shunting. Pediatr Crit Care Med. 2020;21(6):e354–61.
43 Anton-Martin P, Matherne E, Kramer J, Joseph N, Rayburn M. Cangrelor dosing and monitoring for prevention of acute systemic-to-pulmonary artery shunt thrombosis in neonates. J Pediatr Pharmacol Ther. 2022;27(8):707–14.
44 Johnson SR, Granton JT, Mehta S. Thrombotic arteriopathy and anticoagulation in pulmonary hypertension. Chest. 2006;130(2):545–52.

45 Pelland-Marcotte MC, Humpl T, James PD, Rand ML, Bouskill V, Reyes JT, et al. Idiopathic pulmonary arterial hypertension – a unrecognized cause of high-shear high-flow haemostatic defects (otherwise referred to as acquired von Willebrand syndrome) in children. Br J Haematol. 2018;183(2):267–75.
46 Ross C, Kumar R, Pelland-Marcotte MC, Mehta S, Kleinman ME, Thiagarajan RR, et al. Acute management of high-risk and intermediate-risk pulmonary embolism in children: a review. Chest. 2022; 161(3):791–802.
47 Lancaster TR, Singer DE, Sheehan MA, Oertel LB, Maraventano SW, Hughes RA, et al. The impact of long-term warfarin therapy on quality of life: evidence from a randomized trial. Arch Intern Med. 1991;151(10):1944–9.
48 Ng DL, Gan GG, Chai CS, Chee KH, Tan KL, Tan SB, et al. Comparing quality of life and treatment satisfaction between patients on warfarin and direct oral anticoagulants: a cross-sectional study. Patient Prefer Adherence. 2019;13: 1363–73.
49 Manlhiot C, Menjak IB, Brandão LR, Gruenwald CE, Schwartz SM, Sivarajan VB, et al. Risk, clinical features, and outcomes of thrombosis associated with pediatric cardiac surgery. Circulation. 2011;124(14):1511–9.
50 Rodan L, McCrindle BW, Manlhiot C, MacGregor DL, Askalan R, Moharir M, et al. Stroke recurrence in children with congenital heart disease. Ann Neurol. 2012;72(1):103–11.
51 Morgan CT, Manlhiot C, McCrindle BW, Dipchand AI. Outcome, incidence and risk factors for stroke after pediatric heart transplantation: an analysis of the International Society for Heart and Lung Transplantation Registry. J Heart Lung Transplant. 2016;35(5):597–602.
52 Thom K, Male C, Mannhalter C, Quehenberger P, Mlczoch E, Luckner D, et al. No impact of endogenous prothrombotic conditions on the risk of central venous line-related thrombotic events in children: results of the KIDCAT study (KIDs with Catheter Associated Thrombosis). J Thromb Haemost. 2014;12(10): 1610–5.
53 Deogaonkar G, Sinha MD, Jones M, Calder F, Karunanithy N, Qureshi SA. Percutaneous venous reconstruction for central thrombosis-associated chylothorax: a safe and efficacious option. JACC Case Rep. 2021;3(14):1569–75.
54 Jones S, Butt W, Monagle P, Cain T, Newall F. The natural history of asymptomatic central venous catheter-related thrombosis in critically ill children. Blood. 2019;133(8):857–66.
55 Manlhiot C, McCrindle BW, Williams S, Menjak IB, O'Shea S, Chan AK, et al. Characterization of post-thrombotic syndrome in children with cardiac disease. J Pediatr. 2019;207:42–8.
56 Manlhiot C, Brandão LR, Schwartz SM, Sivarajan VB, Williams S, Collins TH, et al. Management and outcomes of patients with occlusive thrombosis after pediatric cardiac surgery. J Pediatr. 2016;169:146–53.
57 Sun JC, Davidson MJ, Lamy A, Eikelboom JW. Antithrombotic management of patients with prosthetic heart valves: current evidence and future trends. Lancet. 2009;374(9689):565–76.
58 Young G, Tarantino MD, Wohrley J, Weber LC, Belvedere M, Nugent DJ. Pilot dose-finding and safety study of bivalirudin in infants. J Thromb Haemost. 2007;5(8):1654–9.
59 Monagle P. Thrombosis in children with BT shunts, Glenns and Fontans. Prog Pediatr Cardiol. 2005;21:17–21.
60 Willetts RG, Stickley J, Drury NE, Mehta C, Stumper O, Khan NE, et al. Four right ventricle to pulmonary artery conduit types. J Thorac Cardiovasc Surg. 2021; 162(5):1324–33.
61 Wespi R, Callegari A, Quandt D, Logoteta J, von Rhein M, Kretschmar O, et al. Favourable short- to mid-term outcome after PDA-stenting in duct-dependent pulmonary circulation. Int J Environ Res Public Health. 2022;19(19):12794.
62 Nasef MA, Shahbah DA, Batlivala SP, Darwich R, Qureshi AM, Breatnach CR, et al. Short- and medium-term outcomes for patent ductus arteriosus stenting in neonates ≤2.5 kg with duct-dependent pulmonary circulation. Catheter Cardiovasc Interv. 2022;100(4):596–605.
63 McCrindle BW, Manlhiot C, Cochrane A, Roberts R, Hughes M, Szechtman B, et al. Factors associated with thrombotic complications after the fontan procedure: a secondary analysis of a multicenter, randomized trial of primary thromboprophylaxis for 2 years after the fontan procedure. J Am Coll Cardiol. 2013;61(3):346–53.
64 Streif W, Andrew M, Marzinotto V, Massicotte P, Chan AK, Julian JA, et al. Analysis of warfarin therapy in pediatric patients: a prospective cohort of 319 patients. Blood. 1999;94:3007–14.
65 Odegard KC, McGowan FX Jr, DiNardo JA, Castro RA, Zurakowski D, Connor CM, et al. Coagulation abnormalities in patients with single-ventricle physiology precede the Fontan procedure. J Thorac Cardiovasc Surg. 2002;123(3):459–65.
66 Rosenthal DN, Friedman AH, Kleinman CS, Kopf GS, Rosenfeld LE, Hellenbrand WE. Thromboembolic complications after Fontan operations. Circulation. 1995;92(9 suppl):II287–93.
67 Jahangiri M, Shore D, Kakkar V, Lincoln C, Shinebourne E. Coagulation factor abnormalities after the Fontan procedure and its modifications. J Thorac Cardiovasc Surg. 1997;113(6):989–92.
68 Yang JYK, Williams S, Brandão LR, Chan AKC. Neonatal and childhood right atrial thrombosis: recognition and a risk-stratified treatment approach. Blood Coagul Fibrinolysis. 2010;21(4): 301–7.
69 McCrindle BW, Rowley AH, Newburger JW, Burns JC, Bolger AF, Gewitz M, et al. Diagnosis, treatment, and long-term management of Kawasaki disease: a scientific statement for health professionals from the American Heart Association. Circulation. 2017;135(17):e927–99.
70 McCrindle BW, Manlhiot C, Newburger JW, Harahsheh AS, Giglia TM, Dallaire F, et al. Medium-term complications associated with coronary artery aneurysms after Kawasaki disease: a study from the International Kawasaki Disease Registry. J Am Heart Assoc. 2020;9(15): e016440.
71 Manlhiot C, Brandão LR, Somji Z, Chesney AL, MacDonald C, Gurofsky RC, et al. Long-term anticoagulation in Kawasaki disease: initial use of low molecular weight heparin is a viable option for patients with severe coronary artery abnormalities. Pediatr Cardiol. 2010; 31(6):834–42.
72 Manlhiot C, Newburger JW, Low T, Dahdah N, Mackie AS, Raghuveer G, et al. Low-molecular-weight heparin vs warfarin for thromboprophylaxis in children with coronary artery aneurysms after Kawasaki disease: a pragmatic registry trial. Can J Cardiol. 2020; 36(10):1598–607.

73 Baltimore RS, Gewitz M, Baddour LM, Beerman LB, Jackson MA, Lockhart PB, et al. Infective endocarditis in childhood: 2015 update – a scientific statement from the American Heart Association. Circulation. 2015;132(15):1487–515.
74 Thom K, Hanslik A, Russell JL, Williams S, Sivaprakasam P, Allen U, et al. Incidence of infective endocarditis and its thromboembolic complications in a pediatric population over 30years. Int J Cardiol. 2018;252:74–9.
75 McCrindle BW, Karamlou T, Wong H, Gangam N, Trivedi KR, Lee KJ, et al. Presentation, management and outcomes of thrombosis for children with cardiomyopathy. Can J Cardiol. 2006; 22(8):685–90.
76 Williams GD, Hammer GB. Cardiomyopathy in childhood. Curr Opin Anaesthesiol. 2011;24(3):289–300.
77 El-Sabrout H, Ganta S, Guyon P, Ratnayaka K, Vaughn G, Perry J, et al. Neonatal myocardial infarction: a proposed algorithm for coronary arterial thrombus management. Circ Cardiovasc Interv. 2022;15(5):e011664.
78 Yetman AT, McCrindle BW, MacDonald C, Freedom RM, Gow R. Myocardial bridging in children with hypertrophic cardiomyopathy–a risk factor for sudden death. N Engl J Med. 1998;339(17): 1201–9.
79 Paredes N, Mondal T, Brandão LR, Chan AKC. Management of myocardial infarction in children with Kawasaki disease. Blood Coagul Fibrinolysis. 2010; 21(7):620–31.
80 Dame C, Sutor AH. Primary and secondary thrombocytosis in childhood. Br J Haematol. 2005;129(2):165–77.
81 Denton A, Davis P. Extreme thrombocytosis in admissions to paediatric intensive care: no requirement for treatment. Arch Dis Child. 2007;92(6):515–6.

Published online: December 5, 2024

Blanchette VS, Brandão LR, Carcao MD, Kumar R, Rand ML, Revel-Vilk S (eds): SickKids Handbook of Pediatric Thrombosis and Hemostasis, ed 3, rev. and ext. Basel, Karger, 2024, pp 359–384 (DOI: 10.1159/000539148)

Hemostasis Management during Mechanical Circulatory Support

Alyssa Power[a] Mark Todd[b] Mariella Vargas-Gutierrez[c] Gail Annich[b] Aamir Jeewa[a] Anne-Marie Guerguerian[b] Leonardo R. Brandão[d]

[a]Division of Cardiology, The Hospital for Sick Children, University of Toronto, Toronto, ON , Canada; [b]Department of Critical Care Medicine, Extracorporeal Life Support Program, The Hospital for Sick Children, University of Toronto, Toronto, ON, Canada; [c]Department of Pediatric Critical Care Medicine, Children's Hospital of Eastern Ontario, University of Ottawa, Ottawa, ON, Canada; [d]Division of Haematology/Oncology, The Hospital for Sick Children, University of Toronto, Toronto, ON, Canada

Introduction

Mechanical circulatory support (MCS) is the use of medical devices to support heart and/or lung function in severe heart or lung failure refractory to conventional care.

This technology, also alluded to under the broad term extracorporeal life support (ECLS), was initially applied to children with congenital heart disease (CHD) undergoing cardiac surgery (i.e., cardiopulmonary bypass [CPB]). In CPB (Fig. 1), priming of the circuit and circuit/patient anticoagulation happen at the same time, prior to cardiac intervention. During the procedure, blood is drained from the venous system, passed to a reservoir, pumped through an oxygenator, and reinfused distal to the heart and/or site of surgery. Shed blood is aspirated through suckers in the surgical site and, after a few processing steps such as filtering or washing, is collected in the venous reservoir. A cardioplegic solution is typically added to venous reservoir blood, and the mix is refrigerated to 4°C and applied to the heart through the cardioplegia line. At the end of the procedure, rapid anticoagulation reversal is achieved by administration of an effective anticoagulant antidote (Table 1).

Historical Background

Starting in the 1950s, several medical centers developed the then-called heart-lung machines. One successful example was the atrial septal defect repair in an 18-year-old patient reported by Dr. John H. Gibbon in May 6, 1953. This report paved the way for other centers to continue their pursuit on conducting open heart surgery [1, 2]. In the same decade, Dr. William T. Mustard, an originally trained pediatric orthopedic surgeon, was hired by The Hospital for Sick Children (SickKids) to help develop the cardiovascular sur-

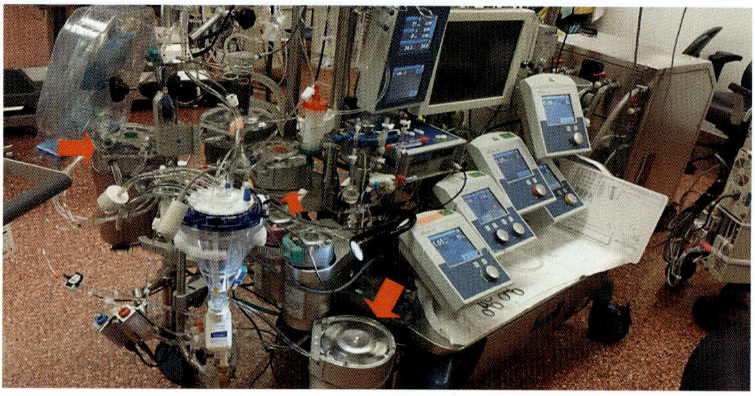

Fig. 1. CPB console with rotor pumps (red arrows). CPB, cardiopulmonary bypass. SickKids ECLS Copyright ©.

Table 1. Unfractionated heparin and protamine management protocol during CPB[a]

	Age		
	<1 month	1 month to 1 year	>1 year
Prime UFH	4 U/mL prime solution	3 U/mL prime solution	3 U/mL prime solution
Bolus UFH	Adjusted to target heparin concentration to 4.0 U/mL	Adjusted to target heparin concentration to 3.5 U/mL	300 U/kg
CPB UFH	Maintain UFH concentration at 3.0 U/mL (maximum total dose: 1,500 U/kg, <1 month; 900 U/kg, 1 month to 1 year)		150 U/kg if ACT <400 s; 100 U/kg if ACT <400–480 s
Protamine reversal	Total (patient + pump) protamine dose as calculated by the hemostasis management system × 1.5		3 mg/kg; administer an additional 1 mg/kg if ACT remained prolonged after the initial protamine dose

ACT, activated coagulation time; CPB, cardiopulmonary bypass; UFH, unfractionated heparin. [a]Current practice at The Hospital for Sick Children, Toronto, Ontario, Canada.

gery program, as he had been experimenting as to how to perfect extracorporeal circuits in preclinical models [3, 4]. It must be highlighted that all these advances were largely possible because of the discovery of heparin, which propelled the evolution of cardiac/cardiovascular surgery and MCS. Heparin was accidentally discovered in 1916 by a second-year medical student, Jay McLean, working under the supervision of Dr. William Henry Howell at the John Hopkins Medical School in Baltimore [5]. However, the original compound was toxic. Its clinical use became feasible only after further heparin purification happened in Toronto between 1933 and 1936, from collaborative work involving Drs. Charles Best and Gordon Murray, and the Connaugh Laboratories [6, 7].

Despite the relatively fast evolution of CPB, which allowed offering more complex and lengthy surgical interventions to children with congenital or acquired cardiopathies, devices capable of delivering prolonged cardiac support were still lacking. This gap started to be filled with the implantation of assisted circulatory devices in the 1960s

[8]. Further research started to improve extracorporeal circulatory systems by incorporating technologies that facilitated gas exchange through an interface between blood and air while maintaining sustainable anticoagulation. At the University of Michigan (Ann Arbor), Dr. Robert Bartlett, a pioneer in the ECLS field, was instrumental in the development of extracorporeal membrane oxygenation (ECMO) devices before they became widely adopted to treat critically ill neonates and children [9, 10]. Today, children with cardiac or cardiorespiratory failure have access to ECMO and/or ventricular assist devices (VADs). Furthermore, in instances of ensuing respiratory failure with a stable cardiovascular state requiring exclusive respiratory support, circuits may be simplified, particularly in patients with acute or chronic hypercapnic respiratory failure.

Knowledge Gaps

One of the main challenges in patients under ECLS are hemostatic complications like bleeding, thrombosis, and hemolysis. Anticoagulation is necessary to prevent circuit thrombo-occlusion, with bleeding as a common side effect. Anticoagulation during ECMO is complex due to the interactions between the patient and the ECMO circuit and to the patient's inflammatory responses to critical illness and to the ECMO circuit that collectively contribute to an imbalance in normal pediatric hemostasis. Comparable challenges exist in patients requiring VAD support. With the evolution of VAD technology and development of different devices, it became increasingly obvious that VAD-specific anticoagulant adjustments are required to optimize anticoagulant prophylactic regimens.

This chapter will provide an up-to-date overview of the hemostatic management of patients on ECLS, focusing on ECMO and VAD, reflecting the practices of our local institutional protocols at SickKids.

Extracorporeal Membrane Oxygenation

The ECMO circuit consists of three primary components: pump, gas exchange device (called membranes), and heat exchanger; those components are connected by a circuit. The circuit may include cannulas for vascular access, blood sampling access sites, monitors, safety devices, circuit shunts (i.e., bridges, recirculation lines), bubble and flow detectors, and oxygen measurement systems [11, 12]. At SickKids, we use a circuit that includes a bridge in young infants and is represented in Figure 2.

The pumps are essential to maintain adequate blood flow within the ECMO circuit, being basically of two types: roller and centrifugal pumps. In the former, rotating rollers compress a section of the tubing propelling blood forward, whereas in the latter, a spinning rotor generates flow and pressure to move blood through the circuit.

Gas exchange devices contain microporous membranes permeable to gas and impermeable to blood that promote blood exposure to oxygen resulting in increased oxygen saturation in exchange to carbon dioxide removal. A recent systematic review has shown that over time, silicone rubber and polypropylene hollow fiber devices have fallen in disfavor to polymethylpentene, polyvinylchloride, or polyurethane hollow fiber devices [13].

Circuit tubing is made of polyvinyl chloride-based plastic compound. The tubing can be coated with biocompatible lining to reduce the inflammatory reaction, platelet and coagulation cascade activation that results from the contact of blood with nonendothelialized circuit tubing surfaces [14]. One of the more commonly used biocompatible tubing relies on heparin-bonded surfaces that dampen cellular interactions related to the inflammatory response alluded herein. For example, the SickKids ECLS team has been using the CARMEDA® bioactive surface, a heparin-based coating tubing system shown to decrease fibrinogen activation in a neonatal ECMO animal

19

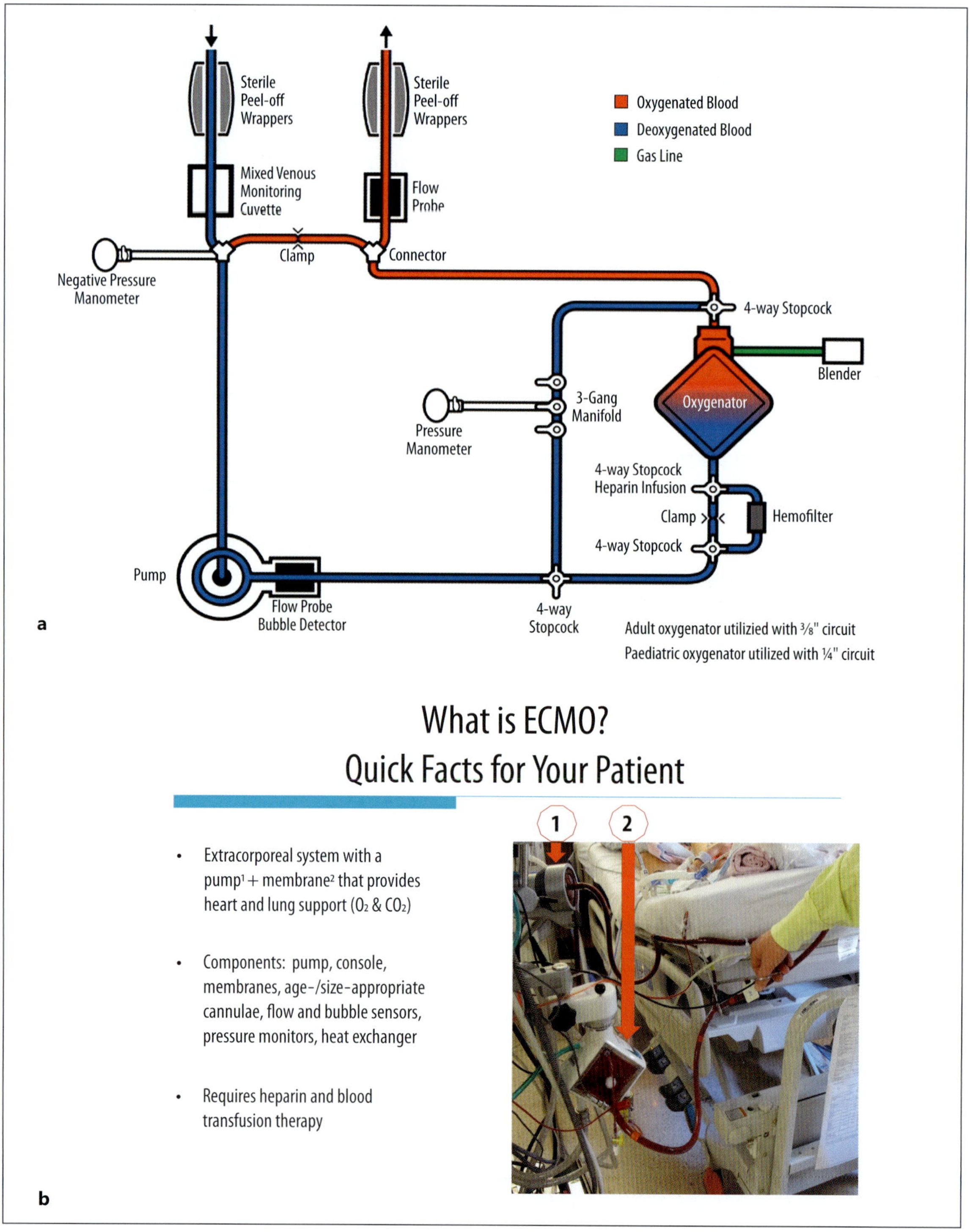

Fig. 2. **a** Schematic representation of ECMO Circuit at SickKids. **b** Picture of an ECMO Circuit Console at SickKids. ECLS, extracorporeal life support; ECMO, extracorporeal membrane oxygenation. SickKids ECLS Copyright ©.

model [15]. Nevertheless, similar to the findings reported in the experimental model, patient/circuit anticoagulation is still required to control the coagulation response to CARMEDA®-based ECMO circuits. A second biocompatible circuit tubing lining consists of nitric oxide (NO)-bonding circuitry, which has an inhibitory platelet activation effect [16], but it still required anticoagulation in animal models to keep coagulopathy at bay [17]. A different tubing strategy relies on circuitry lining with nonreactive surfaces (i.e., biopassive materials), such as phosphorylcholine, poly-2-methoxyethylacrylate, or with an experimental air-liquid membrane, but these techniques remain to be tested in clinical trials [18]. In addition, purely experimental strategies consist of in vitro circuit coating with endothelium or tubing exposure to endothelial progenitor cells, when a neoendothelial layer will coat the tubing [19, 20]. While promising, these in vitro techniques also require further clinical testing.

There are two main ECMO modalities: venoarterial (VA) and venovenous (VV). VA ECMO is the modality used for patients requiring cardiac or cardiorespiratory support where deoxygenated blood is drained from the venous circulation, oxygen and carbon dioxide are exchanged, and then blood is pumped back into the patient's arterial circulation. VV ECMO is the modality used for patients who require only respiratory or oxygenation support and are of sufficient size to accommodate the appropriate cannula. In this modality, deoxygenated blood is drained from a major vein and returned to another major vein (or to the same vein with a double lumen cannula) after gas exchange.

The site of cannulation for ECMO will depend mainly on the size of the patient. As a general rule at SickKids, peripheral VA ECMO in all neonates, infants, and children up to 15–20 kg are cannulated in the cervical region, whereas adolescents and patients who weigh >30–40 kg are cannulated via femoral vessels. Cannulation in patients weighing between 15 and 30 kg is less well established and will depend on the clinical situation and vessel size. Central VA cannulation is done on patients with open chest in the early postoperative period, on postcardiotomy patients (closed chest) <10 days to 2 weeks after surgery, and on those with difficult peripheral access or failed peripheral cannulation.

For VV ECMO, cannulation is determined case by case as it may have potential limitations for drainage depending on the cannula size and type (i.e., double lumen cannula) and also carries risk for venous congestion if placed via femoral vessels. Cannulas are available in sizes ranging from 8 French (Fr) gauge (3 Fr, equivalent to 1 mm) diameter to 27 Fr.

One must recognize that there are many variations in ECMO, even within those broad modalities. Variations in cannulation site, circuit set up, the presence or absence of bridges in the circuit, types of pumps, and in ancillary treatments such as NO or prostacyclin have an enormous influence on the blood flow and thrombin generation and, hence, in bleeding and patient- or circuit-related thrombotic complications.

ECMO-Induced Coagulation and Inflammatory Responses

Exposure of blood to the nonendothelial surface of the extracorporeal tubing activates von Willebrand factor (VWF), platelets, tissue factor (i.e., extrinsic pathway of the coagulation cascade), factor XII and the kallikrein-kinin system (i.e., contact system), fibrinolysis, and inflammation. Contemporary studies have continued to improve our understanding of clinical and laboratory phenotypes pertaining to different clinical settings in children supported by MCS/ECMO [21].

An observational single-center study of children aged 1 day to 19 years recruited over a decade investigated the presence of acquired von Willebrand syndrome (AVWS) in 30 patients supported by different MCS modalities, including 5 patients on ECMO. All patients developed

19

Table 2. Evolution of coagulation phases according to ECMO duration in neonates and children

	Immediate	First phase	Second phase	Third phase
Duration (tentative estimates)	6–48 h	2–10 days	7–14 days	2nd week onward
Clinical	Hemodilution (in case of CPB)	Small clots within the circuit	Increasing number and volume of clots	Patient and circuit bleeding and/or clotting
Laboratory	Prolonged PT/INR/aPTT Low platelet count and/or fibrinogen level	Stable ACTs Stable aPTT, normal coagulation parameters, UFH anti-Xa levels within target ranges	UFH resistance On/off blood product replacement pfHb↑ Antithrombin↓ D-dimers↑	Overt disseminated intravascular coagulopathy
Phase modulators: age, anticoagulation, and clotting within the circuit				

ACT, activated clotting time; aPTT, activated partial thromboplastin time; CPB, cardiopulmonary bypass; INR, international normalized ratio; pfHb, plasma free hemoglobin; PT, prothrombin time; UFH, unfractionated heparin; ↑, elevated values; ↓, lower than normal values.

AVWS early on during the MCS/ECMO run, and almost 2/3 had nonfatal bleeding complications, of which half required surgical re-exploration [22]. All the ECMO patients included in this study received unfractionated heparin (UFH)-based anticoagulation monitored by activated clotting time (ACT). A more recent prospective study evaluating neonates and children on VA ECMO that were serially tested for VWF activity and antigen was undertaken. Twenty-five patients with median age of 73 days (interquartile range [IQR] 3 days to 1 year) and median ECMO duration of 4 days (IQR 3 to 8 days) were enrolled. The study confirmed a decreased percentage of high-molecular-weight VWF levels during the entire ECMO run duration, which normalized within 24 hours postdecannulation. Sixty percent of patients had at least one major bleeding event, but VWF levels were not predictive of bleeding. Of note, the anticoagulation protocol included UFH (ACT and activated partial thromboplastin time [aPTT] monitoring), together with epoprostenol (prostaglandin) and NO. Therefore, a question remains if their study findings are generalizable to patients treated with different anticoagulant strategies or in other ECMO settings.

Turbulent flow and shear stress from the pump, tubing, and cannula contributes to cellular damage and platelet activation, seemingly shifting toward a hypercoagulable state [22–24]. A recent study exploring the role of platelet function laboratory tests (i.e., whole blood platelet flow cytometry) in a pediatric VA ECMO setting described the temporal changes of different platelet phenotypes in 87 children (median age 65 days [IQR 7 days to 4 years] and median ECMO duration 5 days [IQR 3 to 8 days]) [25]. Overall, the study confirmed a progressive loss of platelet responsiveness during the ECMO course duration. Furthermore, distinct platelet molecule expression such as increased CD63 expression at ECMO day 1 (finding reflective of increased lysosome exocytosis [e.g., platelet activation]) was associated with at least one major bleeding event during the ECMO run. Conversely, an increased platelet response reflected by excessive monocyte platelet aggregates, a robust marker of platelet activity and monocyte inflammation in cardiovascular disease, was associated with at least one thromboembolic event (TE) during the period the patients were supported by ECMO [26].

Besides the coagulation derangements that ensue during the ECMO run (Table 2), an inflammatory response that mirrors a systemic inflammatory response syndrome-like cascade, encompassing humoral and cellular response unfolds. There is crosstalk between the coagulation cascade and the complement system, which also involves endothelial cells and other cellular elements, resulting in abnormal cytokine response [27]. Nevertheless, the clinical prognostic value of the inflammatory, endothelial, and fibrinolytic derangements in this patient population is still unknown. Investigators from Baltimore, United States, conducted a two-center prospective observational study enrolling 99 patients, from infancy to adolescence. Three separate biomarker panels were drawn in a sequential manner on days 1, 2, 3, 5, 7 and at every third day thereafter until decannulation. The biomarker panels included an inflammatory panel (interferon gamma, interleukins-6 [IL-6] and 1 beta [IL-1β], and tumor necrosis factor alpha); an endothelial panel (E- and P-selectin, intercellular adhesion molecule-3, and thrombomodulin); and a fibrinolytic panel (tissue plasminogen activator and plasminogen activator inhibitor type 1). The study showed that all inflammatory biomarkers obtained on day 1 were elevated in ECMO patients, which were not predictive of brain hemorrhage at the end of ECMO support. Moreover, ECMO day 1 and peak levels for both IL-6 and PAI-1 were survival predictors, but no biomarkers were associated with long-term abnormal neurobehavioral outcomes [28].

Anticoagulation

A detailed review of anticoagulant agents and anticoagulant laboratory monitoring is shown elsewhere (see Chapter 20). In the context of ECMO patients, a brief pertinent drug and laboratory test comparison evaluating their respective pros and cons will be addressed.

To date, UFH is still the standard anticoagulant for children placed on ECMO due to its parenteral intravenous form and full reversibility with protamine. Of note, this recommendation was endorsed by the 2021 Extracorporeal Life Support Organization (ELSO) Adult and Pediatric Anticoagulation Guidelines [29]. The ELSO guidelines also recognized the increasing impact that direct thrombin inhibitors (DTIs), particularly bivalirudin, may have given its improved predictability and its independence from antithrombin to exert its anticoagulation effect (Table 3).

A systematic review compared safety and efficacy outcomes in children on ECMO receiving either heparin or bivalirudin anticoagulation. In total, 196 patients received UFH and 117 bivalirudin. Favorable findings for bivalirudin included less bleeding, thrombosis, and transfusion requirements, but these findings merit scrutiny since all included studies were retrospective and no risk of bias assessment was reported. Given the potential need for antithrombin replacement to optimize UFH, bivalirudin was cost-effective [30].

Anticoagulation Monitoring

Traditional monitoring for heparin during ECMO varies and usually includes single or combination testing including point-of-care testing with ACT and laboratory testing with aPTT and anti-Xa assay. Of note, the ACT continues to be the most widely used test because of its ease of use. For a detailed description of laboratory monitoring methods, refer to Chapter 20 and for antithrombin replacement, refer to Appendix III. For bivalirudin, the aPTT is the test classically applied

19

Table 3. Comparison of pros and cons between UFH and bivalirudin in the context of ECMO

	Unfractionated heparin	Bivalirudin
UFH disadvantages	Half-life: 30–90 min	25–30 min
	Nonspecific protein binding (i.e., acute phase reactants, PF4)	–
	Antithrombin dependency	–
	Inhibitory effect: soluble thrombin	Inhibitory effect: soluble + fibrin-bound thrombin
	Weak platelet aggregation	No interaction
	Variable bioavailability	–
	HIT	–
UFH advantages	Protamine reversal	–
		Not cleared in the setting of blood stasis
	Fast elimination by the reticuloendothelial system	Kidney (20%) + proteolysis

HIT, heparin-induced thrombocytopenia; PF4, platelet factor 4.

with target ranges varying between 60 and 100 s. However, the same limitations posed to UFH monitoring and aPTT apply to bivalirudin, and alternative methods can be considered. A comparison of several different testing methods conducted at the Texas Children's Hospital in Houston evaluated 17 patients receiving bivalirudin during MCS. In addition to the aPTT, the aPTT using heparinase (to minimize heparin sample contamination), the 1:4 dilute thrombin time (dTT1:4), the dTT1:10, and the ecarin chromogenic assay were evaluated. Ultimately, the dTT1:10 was the test with excellent correlation with ecarin chromogenic assay and less sensitive to interfering factors (i.e., heparin or hyperfibrinogenemia) [31].

One of the main challenges in monitoring anticoagulation during ECMO is that these methods do not take into consideration endothelial responses and interaction between blood and artificial surfaces. Most tests used to monitor anticoagulation are plasma-based assays that measure partial functional measures of coagulation and that do not account for platelet function or clot strength. In contrast, whole blood tests like ACT and viscoelastic methods (thromboelastography [TEG] or rotational thromboelastometry [ROTEM]) incorporate platelet function and clot strength, but they are not always routinely performed or available at ECMO institutions.

Approximately a decade ago, Bembea et al. [32] surveyed ELSO clinical directors, showing a great degree of variability in anticoagulation management in this patient population. Three quarters of all participating centers (n = 117) had a written institutional anticoagulation protocol, and only <10% were using DTIs at that time. The vast majority of centers relied on ACT and antithrombin testing, followed by anti-Xa and TEG.

As previously mentioned, neonates undergoing ECMO are at particular high risk for both bleeding and TEs. A single-center study, including approximately 250 neonates, revealed that the traditional coagulation laboratory profile failed to predict acute bleeding or arterial ischemic stroke (AIS). Similarly, a retrospective 5-year single-center study conducted at the Boston Children's Hospital enrolling 133 patients (78 neonates and 55 children) showed that neither ACT and aPTT nor anti-Xa levels were predictive of bleeding or thrombotic events [33]. Conversely, other researchers showed benefits in expanding the anticoagulation laboratory monitoring panel beyond ACT, as certain (i.e., anti-Xa levels) or several coagulation tests (i.e., ACT, fibrinogen level) better correlated with heparin dosing and thrombus prevention or prediction of bleeding [34, 35]. At SickKids, our approach has been to combine the ACT, aPTT, and anti-Xa levels in addition to a platelet count, fibrinogen level, and hemolysis markers to evaluate circuit patency and disease/systemic drug/circuit-induced coagulation derangement states, interpreting the results and projecting their evolution by placing them in clinical context.

Thrombosis and Bleeding

Despite several circuitry, pump, oxygenator, anticoagulant, and coagulation laboratory monitoring improvements, TE and bleeding continue to happen, affecting patient outcomes and survival. A retrospective cohort leveraging ELSO data from 8 tertiary critical care centers collected between 2005 and 2011 included 2,036 patients, of which 13% had congenital diaphragmatic hernia. Excluding those patients (*n* = 1,773 remaining), bleeding and TE complications were associated with decreased survival by 40% (relative risk: 0.59; 95% confidence interval [CI]: 0.53–0.66) and 33% (odds ratio: 0.67; 95% CI: 0.53–0.66), respectively. Most common bleeding complications included surgical related (17%), cannulation site (14%), and intracranial (11%). TEs were more commonly located within circuit (15%) or oxygenator (12%) or identified by excessive hemolysis (10%) [36].

A systematic review that gathered data from 10,659 critically ill children from 37 studies reported the overall prevalence of hematologic complications in children on ECMO. The reported pooled prevalence for bleeding, TEs, and hemolysis was 43.7% (95% CI: 28.6–58.9), 27.6% (95% CI: 20.4–34.8), and 34.3% (95% CI: 22.9–45.7), respectively [37].

Histological composition of thrombi within the circuitry proved to be heterogeneous and independent of their location (i.e., pump, oxygenator, tubing), consisting of two basic types, red blood cell-rich and fibrin-rich types. Surprisingly, neutrophil extracellular traps were reported to not play a major role in thrombus composition [38].

Blood Transfusion Practices

Blood transfusion practices vary widely, as demonstrated in a cross-sectional survey of centers participating in ELSO. Ozment et al. showed how transfusion thresholds, particularly for platelets, vary among centers. The same authors also reported centers using a variety of therapies to treat bleeding in patients on ECMO receiving UFH; 78% use aminocaproic acid, 53% use recombinant activated factor VII, and 38% reported the use of tranexamic acid. When used in combination, the most common therapies included aminocaproic acid and recombinant activated factor VII in 43% [40].

Titrating systemic anticoagulation is complicated by coagulation factor consumption, variable metabolism of therapeutic agents, and the dynamic nature of the patients' hemostatic hypercoagulable and hypocoagulable states, often necessitating transfusion of blood, platelets, or other blood products. In addition, studies demonstrated increased mortality associated with volume of transfusion on ECMO [39]. Currently, no evidence-based strategy exists to optimize anticoagulation and transfusion thresholds [40].

Ventricular Assist Devices

VADs are durable mechanical circulatory devices used for cardiac support in children with end-stage heart failure. They can support the left ven-

Table 4. VAD characteristics

Characteristic	Berlin Heart EXCOR®	PediMag/ CentriMag	HeartMate 3™	Impella®	SynCardia Total Artificial Heart
Location	Paracorporeal	Paracorporeal	Intracorporeal	Intracorporeal	Intracorporeal
Flow type	Pulsatile	Continuous	Continuous	Continuous	Pulsatile
Lower limit patient size	3–5 kg	3–5 kg	20–25 kg	20–25 kg	0.9 m^2 BSA
Duration	Long term	Short term[a]	Long term	Short term	Long term
Placement	Median sternotomy and CPB	Median sternotomy and CPB	Median sternotomy and CPB	Cardiac catheterization (± surgical support, but no bypass)	Median sternotomy and CPB
Potential for discharge	No	No	Yes	No	Yes
Anticoagulation/ antiplatelet goals	Bivalirudin infusion, typical aPTT target 70–90 s; ASA 3–5 mg/kg per day	Bivalirudin infusion, typical aPTT target 70–90 s; ASA 3–5 mg/kg per day	VKA, INR 2–3; ASA 81–325 mg daily	Intracatheter UFH + systemic UFH infusion, ACT 160–200 s	VKA, INR 2.5–3.5; ASA 81–325 mg daily

ACT, activated clotting time; aPTT, activated partial thromboplastin clotting time; ASA, acetylsalicylic acid; BSA, body surface area; CPB, cardiopulmonary bypass; INR, international normalized ratio; VAD, ventricular assist device; VKA, vitamin K antagonist. [a]Some centers use this device for this long-term therapy.

tricle assist device (LVAD), right ventricle assist device (RVAD), or both ventricles (biventricular assist device [BiVAD]) by unloading the failing chamber and returning blood to either the aorta (LVAD), pulmonary artery (RVAD), or both (BiVAD). Additionally, VADs can be used to support patients with single ventricle CHD (single ventricle assist device). A rising number of children are bridged to heart transplant with MCS. In 2017, 37% of children were bridged to transplant on MCS, the vast majority of whom were on VAD support [41].

VADs can be subdivided by several key aspects (Table 4). They differ in their predominant location, with *intracorporeal* (intrathoracic) devices housed within the body and *paracorporeal* devices housed outside the body. They differ in their flow characteristics, with *continuous flow* devices providing blood flow throughout the cardiac cycle and *pulsatile* devices providing intermittent flow with distinct times for device filling and emptying. Devices can also differ in duration of support provided, from short-term (days to weeks) to long-term (weeks to years) support. Currently, the most widely used pediatric VADs are the HeartMate 3™, an intracorporeal continuous-flow device with excellent hemocompatibility profile though limited by patient size constraints, and the Berlin Heart EXCOR®, a paracorporeal pulsatile device that offers the opportunity to support small infants but with increased complication burden.

Important potential complications on VAD support include bleeding, TE (including embolic AIS), and hemolysis. In the first 2 weeks of VAD implant, non-gastrointestinal (GI) bleeding is the most common complication (14%) followed by infection (12%) and neurologic dysfunction (11%) [42]. Beyond 2 weeks of support, the most frequent adverse events are infection (21%), non-

GI bleeding (9%), and neurologic dysfunction (14%). The overall incidence of stroke is 11%, with most being ischemic [42]. To reduce the risk of TE phenomenon, centers implement protocolized use of antiplatelet and anticoagulation therapies supported by consistent anticoagulation monitoring.

Advanced Cardiac Therapies Improving Outcomes Network (ACTION) is a collaborative learning network established in December 2017 that includes 55 pediatric hospitals in North America [43]. It was created with the purpose of improving outcomes for children with heart failure on VAD support. The Pediatric Interagency Registry for Mechanical Circulatory Support (Pedimacs) is a North American registry that captures and analyzes data on children on VAD support to advance care of this challenging population.

Preimplant Considerations

Prior to VAD implantation, patients should have coagulation evaluation that includes complete past medical and family history for relevant TE and bleeding events as well as baseline laboratory investigation (complete blood count [CBC], aPTT, prothrombin time [PT]/international normalized ratio [INR], and fibrinogen level). Besides conducting clinical and laboratory investigations for potential inherited or acquired ensuing coagulopathy (see Chapter 4), given that impending or de facto cardiac failure may be present, additional end organ damage assessment of renal, brain, and other organs should be pursued according to the patient's clinical context. Some centers also elect to send additional evaluations including protein C/S, TEG, and platelet mapping, and evaluation for factor V Leiden or prothrombin gene variant. However, the role of sending a thrombophilia panel in this context merits further clarification; as a result, interpretation could be challenging due to both acquired abnormalities or the absence of comparable literature in the context of abnormal blood rheology in contact with metallic devices.

Pediatric VAD support can be used for patients with cardiomyopathy (most commonly dilated cardiomyopathy, in which one or both ventricles are dilated with systolic dysfunction resulting in heart failure), myocarditis (acute inflammation of the myocardium resulting in systolic dysfunction and sometimes arrhythmias), CHD, or for heart transplant recipients with graft failure. Children with CHD can be biventricular (have two functional ventricles) or single ventricle (have one functional ventricle). In the Pedimacs cohort, cardiomyopathy is the most common underlying etiology (59%) followed by CHD (25%) and myocarditis (9%) [42].

19

Thrombosis and Bleeding

Similar to what happens in patients placed on CPB or ECMO, the interaction between the device material and whole blood affects the balance of the coagulation system, resulting in two common complications of VAD support: thrombosis and bleeding. While distinct from the pathophysiology of deep venous thrombosis, a modified version of the Virchow's triad can be applied to the VAD microenvironment to understand the increased predisposition to thrombus formation: bioreactive surfaces, activated platelets, and abnormal flow patterns [44]. Particularly in children, in whom the coagulation system evolves with age (i.e., quantitative and qualitative changes), identifying the ideal anticoagulant that offers maximal protection against thrombosis and minimal bleeding risk is modulated by the patient's age (for developmental hemostasis, see Chapter 2 and Appendix II), device characteristics, and device implantation duration [45].

At the time of VAD implant, there are several provoking factors that can increase the risk of either bleeding or TE, such as tissue injury, residual effects from CPB (see Chapter 18), and blood contact with artificial material. The risk of TE can be mitigated by the use of anticoagulation and antiplatelet therapy protocols tailored to the risk profile imposed by the device type and patient-specific factors. These therapies, however, interfere with the body's response to achieve hemostasis and increase bleeding risk.

Establishing effective control of any early bleeding is crucial in the immediate postoperative period. Initiation of anticoagulation is often delayed for at least several hours to establish that there are no surgical or clinical concerns toward bleeding. Except for the Impella®, all patients with a newly implanted VAD will have chest tubes in place allowing for external drainage of intrathoracic blood. The volume and appearance of chest tube losses are followed closely. Anticoagulation is generally not commenced until the volume of chest tube losses has fallen significantly, the appearance of the chest tube output improves from sanguineous to serosanguinous, and the coagulation tests and platelet count are within an acceptable range. Conversely, high volume of bleeding based on chest tube losses is managed with replacement (fresh frozen plasma, cryoprecipitate, platelets, or packed red blood cells; see Appendix III). Occasionally, surgical re-exploration is needed when chest tube output remains high despite improvement of coagulopathy in the postoperative setting. Of note, blood product replacement for bleeding may be accompanied by deleterious consequences, with increased risk of TE, hemolysis (worsening renal dysfunction and anemia), and fluid overload (particularly in the context of right ventricular dysfunction, which can worsen renal function and lead to prolonged intubation and prolonged inotropic support). Therefore, achieving an optimal hemostatic balance is a key clinical challenge to optimize the postoperative period, with potential end organ damage implications, as summarized above, in addition to the more obvious need for an immediate bleeding control that allows the initiation of effective anticoagulation in a timely manner, given the higher thrombotic risk period occurs immediately post-VAD implantation.

Frequent hematologic assessments form one of the cornerstones of VAD management and are performed throughout a patient's VAD course. Anticoagulation and antiplatelet regimens vary based on device type as well as institutional practice, and the SickKids approach will be outlined in the device subsections below. Notably, in light of very limited literature available, there is not yet a role for direct oral anticoagulants in the VAD population [46].

It is crucial that the anticoagulation/antiplatelet regimen is tailored to the individual patient's coagulation profile at that moment in time. For example, if the patient's laboratory or clinical profile indicates a predisposition to bleeding (such as decreased platelet count, decreased fibrinogen level, prolonged aPTT or PT/INR, active bleeding from mucosa, stool, urine, or chest tubes, bruising, or petechiae), then they will be managed by decreasing anticoagulation/antiplatelet therapy and sometimes administering blood-derived products and/or hemostatic agents to reverse the coagulopathic state. If the patient's laboratory or clinical profile indicates a predisposition to TE (acute phase reaction with marked elevated fibrinogen levels, shortened aPTT, device thrombosis, and significant schistocytosis), then they may be managed by anticoagulation/antiplatelet therapy escalation (i.e., increased dosing intensity or added antiplatelet agent) and sometimes, initiation of concomitant anti-inflammatory therapy (such as steroids). Patients with either increased thrombosis risk or evidence of consumptive coagulopathy should also have evaluation for infectious or for inflammatory states.

A global perspective of the patient's clinical condition is crucial to the comprehensive hematologic assessment. For example, one must consider how evolving renal impairment can reduce bivalirudin clearance (necessitating more frequent than usual aPTT surveillance), how changes in vitamin K intake can alter PT/INR in a patient on vitamin K antagonist (VKA), or how postoperative chylothorax can result in a hypercoagulable state from loss of antithrombin and intravascular volume (see Chapter 20).

Stroke

The Pedimacs registry reported that 9% of patients had one AIS, and 2% had two or more AIS. The occurrence of multiple strokes was associated with worse overall survival [42]. The most common etiology is an AIS secondary to TE phenomenon [47]. A careful reduction in anticoagulation is typically implemented to decrease the risk of hemorrhagic conversion, balanced with concerns of precipitating further thrombotic phenomenon. Close engagement with Neurology and Neurointerventional services and serial brain imaging is critical in management of AIS in VAD patients.

Bleeding Subtypes

In the Pedimacs cohort, 54% of patients had no bleeding on VAD support, while 17% had 1 bleeding episode, 13% had 2 bleeding episodes, and 17% had 3 or more bleeding episodes [42]. The occurrence of multiple bleeding events was associated with increased mortality risk, especially for patients on paracorporeal continuous-flow devices.

GI Bleeding

Pedimacs reported a 6% incidence of GI bleeding in pediatric VAD recipients, with similar incidence across all device types [42]. Minor bleeding in the absence of a concerning thrombotic history is often managed by minimizing anticoagulation/antiplatelet therapy. The first line change in our institution is to decrease or discontinue acetylsalicylic acid (ASA) therapy. More significant GI bleeding would be an indication to consult Gastroenterology. Little is published on GI bleeding in children with VAD. Conversely, the problem is well documented in adults on VAD support, with particular risk noted in the "destination therapy" patients who are on VAD support for an extended duration, in which it can become a recalcitrant long-term complication with an incidence of over 20% [48]. Some of this increased risk may also be related to intestinal health (i.e., the presence of angiodysplasia and diverticulitis), and it appears to be particularly common in patients on continuous-flow devices [49].

Heavy Menstrual Bleeding

In postmenarchal females on VAD support, menstruation is an important consideration. Heavy menstrual bleeding has been described in about 40% of menstruating patients on VAD support [50]. Intrauterine devices provide the most success at menstrual suppression but are not effective to manage acute bleeding and are ideally not placed when a patient is acutely coagulopathic. Acute bleeding management selection depends on the clinical situation but can include norethindrone acetate (oral progestin-based contraceptive pill), intravenous estrogen, combined hormonal contraceptive pill, and intracavitary foley in the uterus as a tamponade. Consultation with Gynecology or Adolescent Medicine is crucial to guide management of both acute, heavy menstrual bleeding, and long-term menstrual control (see Chapter 5).

Epistaxis

Epistaxis is a common post-VAD complication, described in 75% of patients [51]. Mild anterior epistaxis can be managed conservatively. Otolaryngology (ENT) should be consulted for significant or recurrent epistaxis. Management options include decreasing anticoagulation (where feasible depending on a patient's hematologic assessment), nasal packing, local vasoconstrictors (such as oxymetazoline), local hemostatic agents (such as thrombin), or cauterization with silver nitrate.

Acquired Bleeding Disorders while on VAD Support (see Chapters 7 and 11)

AVWS can develop in patients on VAD support and can predispose to bleeding. It has been demonstrated that patients on VAD support have loss of high-molecular-weight VWF multimers, which normalize after transplant [52]. Shear forces created by the VAD are postulated to cause

19

proteolysis of the VWF multimers [53]. Heilmann et al. [54] described that most of the patients on continuous flow VAD developed AVWS within 1 day.

Additionally, impaired platelet aggregation can contribute to bleeding predisposition in VAD recipients. Klovaite et al. [55] found that about 70% patients had impairment of VWF-dependent ristocetin-induced platelet aggregation, likely due to a combination of decreased high-molecular-weight VWF multimers and attenuated platelet function.

Hemolysis

Clinically significant hemolysis is an important complication of VAD therapy and is caused by increased shear stress on red blood cells as they pass through the mechanical components of the device. The presence of a hyperdynamic circulation (such as increased pump speed, aortic regurgitation, dehydration, or sepsis) can worsen this shear stress. Pump thrombosis and hemolysis are complications linked in a bidirectional way: device thrombosis can trigger hemolysis through erythrocyte membrane injury [56]. Conversely, the byproducts released from hemolysis can have prothrombotic consequences. Hemolysis results in increased carbon monoxide and iron, both of which have hypercoagulable and hypofibrinolytic properties [57]. Additionally, plasma-free hemoglobin (pfHb) scavenges circulating NO, and erythrocyte arginase depletes L-arginine (a substrate for NO synthesis), which reduces NO bioavailability and decreases its inhibitory action on platelet adhesion and activation [58]. Finally, pfHb inhibits the enzyme responsible for cleaving ultralarge VWF multimers, namely, a disintegrin and metalloproteinase with a thrombospondin type 1 motif, member 13 (ADAMTS 13). As the main function of ADAMTS 13 is to control the effects of the most adhesive forms of VWF, its inhibition in normal physiologic manner protects active VWF from degradation [59]. Conversely, individuals who become severely deficient of this protease can develop an abnormal platelet adhesive response leading to thrombotic microangiopathy (see Chapter 11).

The incidence of hemolysis varies (5–18%) depending on the VAD type: the risk is higher with continuous-flow devices than with pulsatile devices [60]. The risk may be as high as 60% in patients on Impella® support [61]. Close clinical screening for hemolysis and timely implementation of therapeutic maneuvers is crucial to minimize the consequences of hemolysis, which include device thrombosis, progressive anemia, and acute renal failure due to pigmentary deposition in the proximal tubule. In studies of adult patients on long-term VAD support, hemolysis is associated with a marked increase in mortality rate [59, 62–64].

There are no widely approved diagnostic criteria for hemolysis on VAD support. Most centers employ routine laboratory evaluation to screen for hemolysis, including pfHb, lactate dehydrogenase (LDH), and unconjugated bilirubin. Unfortunately, false elevation of pfHb is frequently noted, especially if there is difficulty with sample collection or if the sample is not centrifuged within 2 h of collection, both of which can result in artifactual red blood cell lysis. Serial increases in LDH are more helpful than the absolute LDH value in isolation [56]. Threshold LDH levels are affected by patient age and additionally prone to interlaboratory variability. Second-tier findings that can be more suggestive of clinically significant hemolysis include a decrease in hemoglobin, a decrease in haptoglobin, or the presence of hemoglobin or urobilinogen in the urine.

Management includes determining the underlying cause. Ruling out device thrombosis (with clinical examination, review of VAD parameters, and occasionally echocardiography or computed tomography scan) and evaluating for a hyperdynamic circulation (such as recent increase in pump speed or new or progressive aortic regurgitation) are important first steps. If thrombosis is identified, it may require augmented pharmacologic therapy or surgical intervention. In the ab-

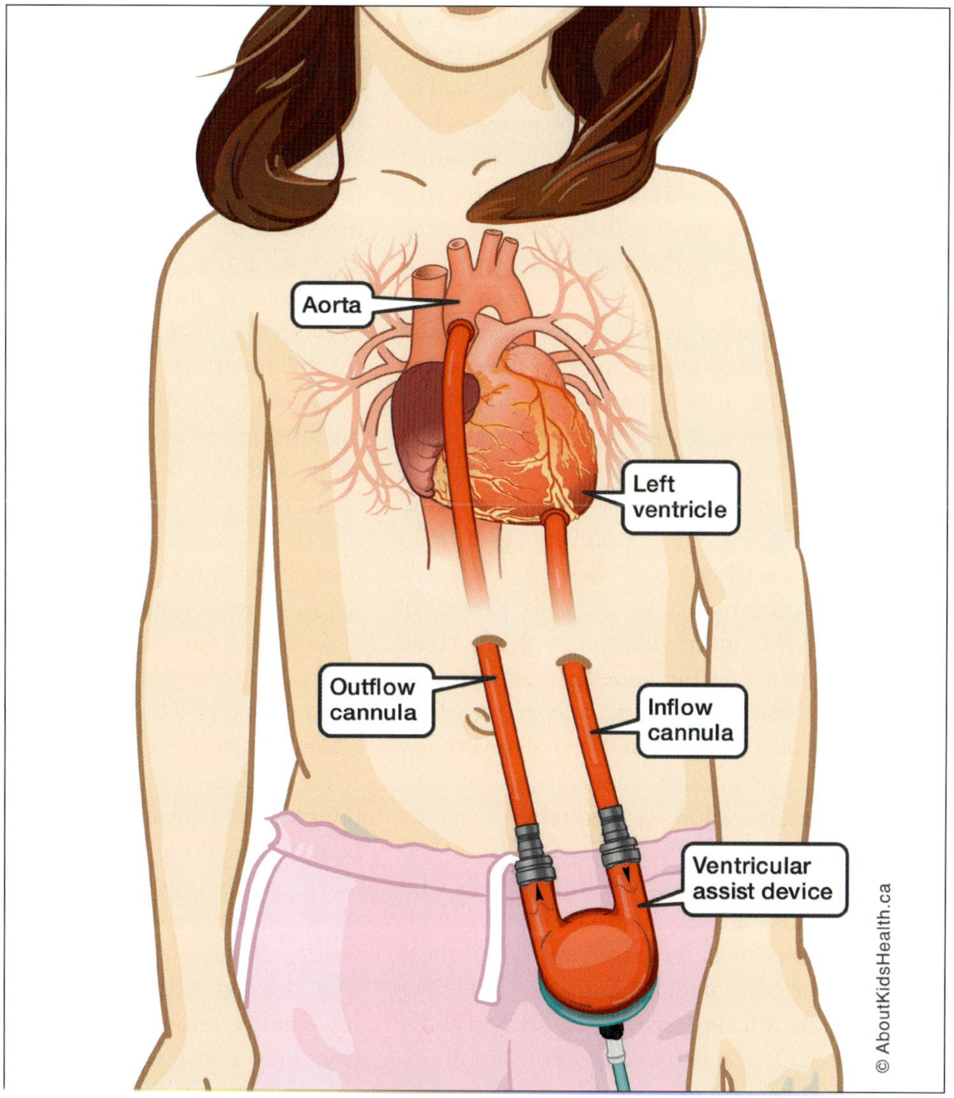

Fig. 3. Berlin Heart. Reprinted with permission from AboutKidsHealth. Source: https://www.aboutkidshealth.ca/Article?contentid=1586&language=English.

sence of a suspicion for device thrombosis, decreasing the device speed (if possible) can decrease the shear stress on the red blood cells and improve hemolysis. Regardless of the etiology of hemolysis, augmenting antithrombotic therapy can be beneficial to counteract the prothrombotic consequences of hemolysis.

Device-Specific Characteristics

Berlin Heart EXCOR®

The Berlin Heart EXCOR® (Berlin Heart AG, Berlin, Germany) is a durable paracorporeal and pulsatile VAD that can provide long-term support for pediatric heart failure (Fig. 3). In the classic LVAD configuration, the inflow cannula is secured within the apex of the left ventricle and is tunneled through the anterior abdominal wall to connect to the blood chamber of the pump, while the outflow cannula is connected to the blood chamber of the pump and is tunneled through the abdominal wall to connect to the ascending aorta. The pump sits outside the body and consists of two chambers that are separated by a membrane: a blood chamber (connected to the inflow and outflow cannula) and an air chamber (connected to the pneumatic driving unit). The pneumatic driving unit alternately sucks air into and out of the air chamber at a rate programmed by the clinician, thus delivering pulsatile flow. Inflow and outflow valves ensure that blood moves only in the intended direction.

Different pump sizes are available (from 10 mL up to 60 mL pump volume), with the small pump sizes allowing for neonatal support. The pump casing and cannula are transparent, which allows for visual inspection of fibrin deposits and thrombi. In the Pedimacs cohort, at 6 months after VAD implantation, a favorable outcome (transplantation, recovery, or alive on device) was achieved in 84% of patients on Berlin Heart support [42].

Though previously managed on UFH, more recently, centers have found improved outcomes on bivalirudin infusion (see ECMO section above and Chapter 20). It is delivered via continuous intravenous infusion with a rapid onset of action (approximately 2 min) and short half-life (26 min in the setting of normal renal function). Steady state is achieved within 4 h. Dose titration is based on aPTT. ACTION has released a standardized protocol for bivalirudin administration and monitoring – this harmonization practice document has been adopted by most pediatric VAD centers in North America [65].

At SickKids, we consider it reasonable to initiate bivalirudin once postsurgical bleeding has resolved (<2 mL/kg per hour of chest tube output for 4 h), platelet count >100,000 × 10^9/mL, fibrinogen >2.0 g/L, INR <1.3, and aPTT within 15 s of baseline. The initial goal aPTT in the first 24 h will be 50–70 s given increased bleeding risk, with the intent to increase the goal toward 70–90 s thereafter with the specific target chosen depending on the individual patient's bleeding/thrombosis profile. In the presence of normal renal function, initial dosing is 0.3 mg/kg per hour, while a lower starting dose should be chosen in the setting of renal dysfunction. The dose can subsequently be titrated up or down to maintain aPTT within the target range. An aPTT should be checked 2 h after bivalirudin initiation – if there has been a dramatic increase, then bivalirudin infusion should be decreased by 50% and aPTT rechecked in 2 h. If a mild increase is noted, typically no adjustment is made and a repeat aPTT is performed in 2 h as the level will continue to rise as steady state is achieved.

In the early phase of a patient's course, once steady state aPTT within target range has been achieved, levels are typically checked once daily. After the patient has proven clinical stability and their hematologic assessments are stable (no concerns for bleeding/thrombosis, relative stability of aPTT values, and stable renal function), then some centers choose to space the levels to once weekly. Bivalirudin primarily undergoes proteolytic cleavage with approximately 20% undergoing renal excretion. Hence, changes in renal function may affect bivalirudin concentration and should prompt increased frequency of aPTT monitoring. After dose adjustment, aPTT should be rechecked (often 4–6 h after dose adjustment, but in stable patients, the clinical team may consider rechecking in 1–3 days instead). Levels are ideally checked through a peripheral venipuncture or drawn from a dedicated vascular access that has not been contaminated by UFH. If neither option is feasible, then the bedside nursing team should ensure that sufficient waste has been performed prior to taking the sample to minimize risk of a falsely elevated aPTT value. Finally, when the patient has demonstrated a good period of stability on bivalirudin infusion and has tolerated initiation of enteral nutrition, ASA is started at a target dose of 3–5 mg/kg per day. At some centers, additional antiplatelet therapy (such as clopidogrel and/or dipyridamole) is also used, and TEG/platelet mapping are used to ensure adequate antiplatelet therapy.

In the first week after Berlin Heart implantation, daily monitoring is performed including coagulation assessment (aPTT, PT/INR, fibrinogen level, and platelet count), renal assessment (creatinine, blood urea nitrogen [BUN]), hemolysis assessment (pfHb, LDH, ± bilirubin), and inflammatory assessment (C-reactive protein and D-dimer). When in the maintenance phase, these laboratory tests can be transitioned to a weekly panel (CBC, creatinine, BUN, aPTT, PT/INR, and fibrinogen level), and when further stabilized, these labs can be done every 2–4 weeks (though aPTT typically drawn at least once weekly). Additional clinical monitoring including monitoring for bleeding (GI bleeding, mucosal bleeding, and chest tube output) and inspecting the cannula and pump for fibrin deposition or thrombus formation.

An inflammatory response post-Berlin Heart insertion, colloquially termed "VAD-itis", has been described in the first few weeks after implant. Inflammatory markers are trended after implantation, including CRP, fibrinogen, and D-dimer. This inflammation is increased in patients on BiVAD support (perhaps due to increased contact with artificial surfaces) and in patients on increased inotropic support (which may be related to upregulation of inflammatory pathways triggered by myocardial damage) [66]. The presence of inflammation shifts the hemostatic balance in favor of hypercoagulability, and many centers elect to treat with steroids to decrease the inflammation and taper its procoagulant impact [67].

The AIS rate was previously about 30% [68]. In the last decade, the AIS rate has improved to 12% (6% in the first 2 weeks postimplant and 8% beyond the first 2 weeks), and the true incidence in the modern era is likely lower [42, 65]. The improvement in AIS rate reflects several changes including use of bivalirudin for primary anticoagulation, use of steroids to alleviate inflammation, implementation of a consistent team to manage anticoagulation, improved blood pressure management, and standardized quality improvement bundles created by the ACTION learning network [65, 69, 70].

PediMag/CentriMag

The PediMag/CentriMag Blood Pump (Abbott, Lake Bluff, IL, USA) is a paracorporeal, continuous flow device with fully magnetically levitated pump rotors (Fig. 4). As with the Berlin Heart, for a classic LVAD configuration, the inflow and outflow cannulas are secured within the apex of the left ventricle and the aorta, respectively, and these cannulas are tunneled through the anterior abdominal wall to connect to the pump, which sits outside the body. The PediMag is the smaller device with a priming volume of 14 mL, allowing for support of neonates, infants, and young children, while the CentriMag has a priming volume of 31 mL allowing for support for older children and adolescents. The pump is connected to a motor driver and a console with a flat screen control monitor. The clinician can set the rotor speed (up to 5,500 revolutions per minute [RPM]). As with the Berlin Heart, the pump housing and cannula are transparent, allowing for visual inspection of fibrin deposits and thrombi. Unlikely the Berlin Heart, the PediMag/CentriMag system allows for incorporation of an oxygenator, which allows the system to function closer to central ECMO. Centers vary on their use of the PediMag/CentriMag system, with some using it as a mode of short-term support before transitioning to another durable system while others use it for long-term support.

In the Pedimacs cohort, worse outcomes are seen in patients supported on paracorporeal continuous flow compared to paracorporeal pulsatile

19

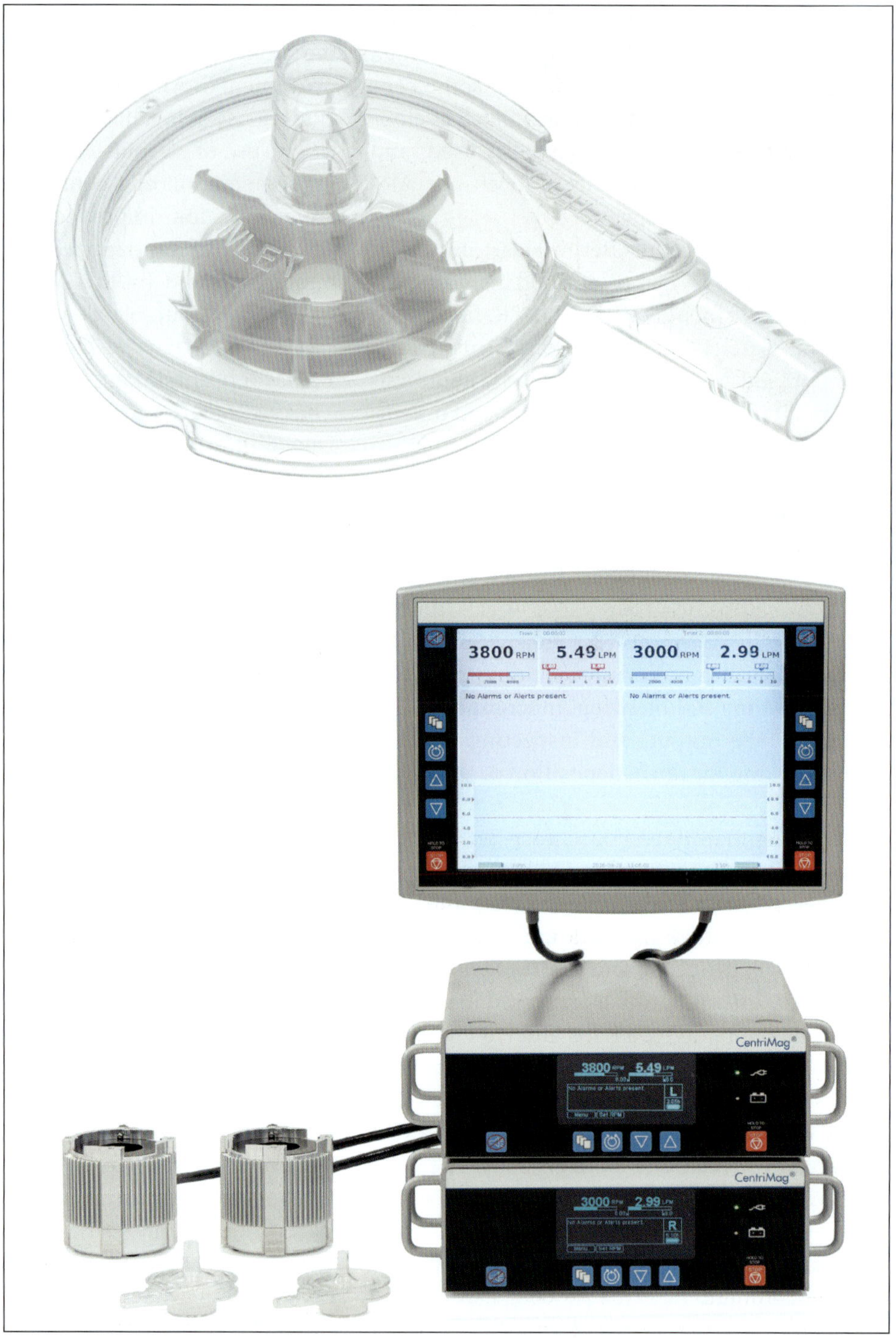

Fig. 4. CentriMag™ Blood Pumps, CentriMag™ Acute Circulatory Support System. CentriMag is a trademark of Abbott or its related companies. Reproduced with permission of Abbott,

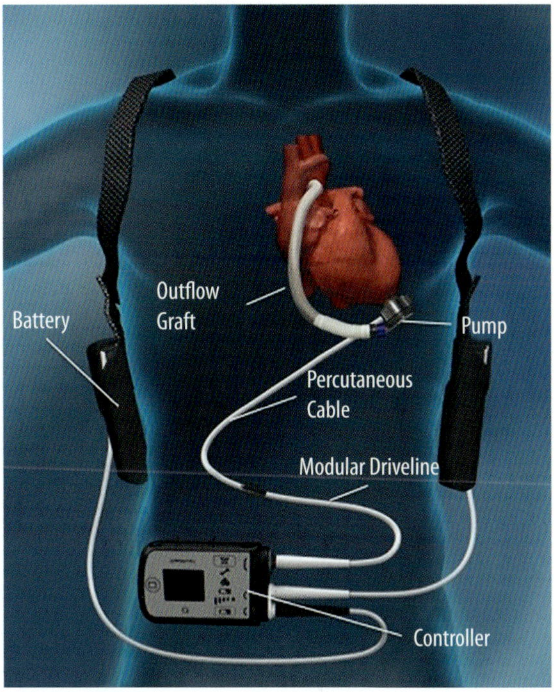

Fig. 5. HeartMate 3™ LVAD. Reprinted with permission from Heatley et al. [83]. Copyright Elsevier.

flow. At 6 months after VAD implantation, a favorable outcome (transplantation, recovery, or alive on device) is achieved in 69% of patients on paracorporeal continuous flow support compared to 84% of patients on paracorporeal pulsatile flow [42]. The cerebrovascular accident rate was also higher (6.4 vs. 11.1 events/100 patients) in the paracorporeal continuous flow group compared to the paracorporeal pulsatile group [71]. Notably, these results must be interpreted in the setting of different patient selection factors.

Anticoagulation management is generally similar between the Berlin Heart and the PediMag/CentriMag system, though given the increased thrombus formation described in patients on PediMag/CentriMag support consideration is given for higher anticoagulation and antiplatelet targets.

HeartMate 3™

The HeartMate 3™ (Abbott Laboratories, Chicago, IL, USA) is an intracorporeal VAD in which the motor is housed within the intrathoracic cavity and a driveline travel from the device, through the skin, and out to a controller and external battery pack (Fig. 5). The VAD is a continuous-flow device with a centrifugal pump, which spins at a rate set by the clinician (from 3,000 to 9,000 RPM). This durable device permits long-term support and patients can be discharged home with a Heartmate 3™ in situ. Notably, due to a pump diameter of 50.3 mm and height of 55.8 mm, patient selection is dependent on having sufficient intrathoracic space to safely house the device. Though increasingly the boundaries of lower patient size are being explored, this remains an important limitation to device use with the smallest report patient weighing 19 kg with a body surface area of 0.78 m^2 [72].

Several features make the HeartMate 3™ the most hemocompatible VAD on the market, including a fully magnetically levitated, self-centering rotor (no hydrodynamic or mechanical bears), large blood flow pathways, and intrinsic pulsatility (the "artificial pulse" or rotor speed modulation occurring every 2 s with a 2,000 RPM decrease in rotor speed followed by a 4,000 RPM increase in speed before returning to baseline, within the span of 350 ms). These unique features work together to reduce stasis, minimize thrombus, and decrease shear stress [73–75]. The HeartMate 3™ has an impressively low rate of in-pump thrombosis (0% and 1.1% at 6 and 24 months after implant, respectively) [76]. At 6 months after VAD implantation in the Pedimacs cohort, a favorable outcome (transplantation, recovery, or alive on device) was achieved in over 90% of patients with an intracorporeal VAD [77]. In an adult cohort, the HeartMate 3™ had very low pump thrombosis rate (1%) and low AIS rate (10%) at 2 years.

Unlike the paracorporeal devices, device thrombus cannot be directly visualized. Instead,

19

changes in device functioning parameters are used as surrogate markers to suspect thrombus, which then must be investigated with cross-sectional imaging.

For outpatients, a hematologic assessment is performed at each clinical encounter or if a patient has concerns (such as bleeding from the driveline site). Frequency of INR monitoring will vary based on individual patient level variability but at minimum will typically be checked weekly through the first month, then monthly for several months, then every 3 months.

The initial anticoagulation agent of choice after HeartMate 3™ implant, at SickKids, is bivalirudin within target aPTT between 50 and 70 s. When the patient's oral intake has improved, then warfarin is initiated (without a loading dose) with a goal INR of 2–3. Therapy is initiated with the expected daily dose of warfarin, and daily INR is obtained during the period of coadministration of bivalirudin and warfarin (given potential for combined effects on INR). Bivalirudin can be discontinued when a therapeutic INR is achieved. ASA will also be started during the initial hospitalization, typically dosed at 81 mg daily.

Impella®

The Impella® (Abiomed, Danvers, MA, USA) is an intracorporeal VAD that is placed percutaneously (via the femoral artery or axillary artery) by the cardiac interventional team with or without support from the cardiovascular surgery team (for chimney graft placement for device securement) (Fig. 6). In an LVAD configuration, the device is positioned into the left ventricle across the aortic valve. In cases of RVAD support, it is placed via the femoral vein and positioned across the pulmonary valve. It is a continuous-flow microaxial pump that is designed for short-term support. It is most often used to manage acute cardiogenic shock secondary to myocarditis, cardiac allograft rejection, or dilated cardiomyopathy [78]. Due to device sizing limitations, this therapy is limited to large children and adolescents.

During device insertion, an UFH bolus is administered to target an ACT of 250 s or longer. Thereafter, the goal ACT is 160–200 s depending on the clinical context. Impella® anticoagulation is unique as there are two sources of heparin delivery. The Impella® has a "purge solution," which is automatically regulated by the device controller. The purge fluid acts as a "rinsing fluid" to keep blood from entering the motor. UFH is added to the purge solution as soon as possible after device placement to decrease the risk of device thrombosis. Though not primarily intended to provide therapeutic anticoagulation, the purge solution naturally provides some systemic heparin exposure. A systemic UFH infusion is usually needed to maintain the ACT within goal and can be titrated by the clinical team (whereas the purge flow is adjusted by the controller). The total UFH delivered to the patient is the combination of the purge UFH and the systemic UFH infusion. Significant changes in the purge flow rate can occur in response to changes in purge pressure, and the bedside team must be vigilant in monitoring changes in the rate to decrease the risk of bleeding and TE. In cases of overanticoagulation despite discontinuation of systemic UFH, the concentration of UFH in the purge solution may be decreased.

The Impella® operates at very high RPMs, and thus, hemolysis is an important risk while on Impella® support. Monitoring for increases in LDH and pfHb as well as changes in urine color are useful monitoring tools. If there is concern for hemolysis, an echocardiogram is obtained to check for device malposition. One adult study described a cumulative incidence of hemolysis of over 60%, which highlights the importance of monitoring for hemolysis parameters at frequent intervals [61]. This risk is increased in patients who have additional extracorporeal technologies such as continuous renal replacement therapy and ECMO.

Total Artificial Heart

The SynCardia Total Artificial Heart (TAH, SynCardia Systems, LLC, Tucson, AZ, USA) is an in-

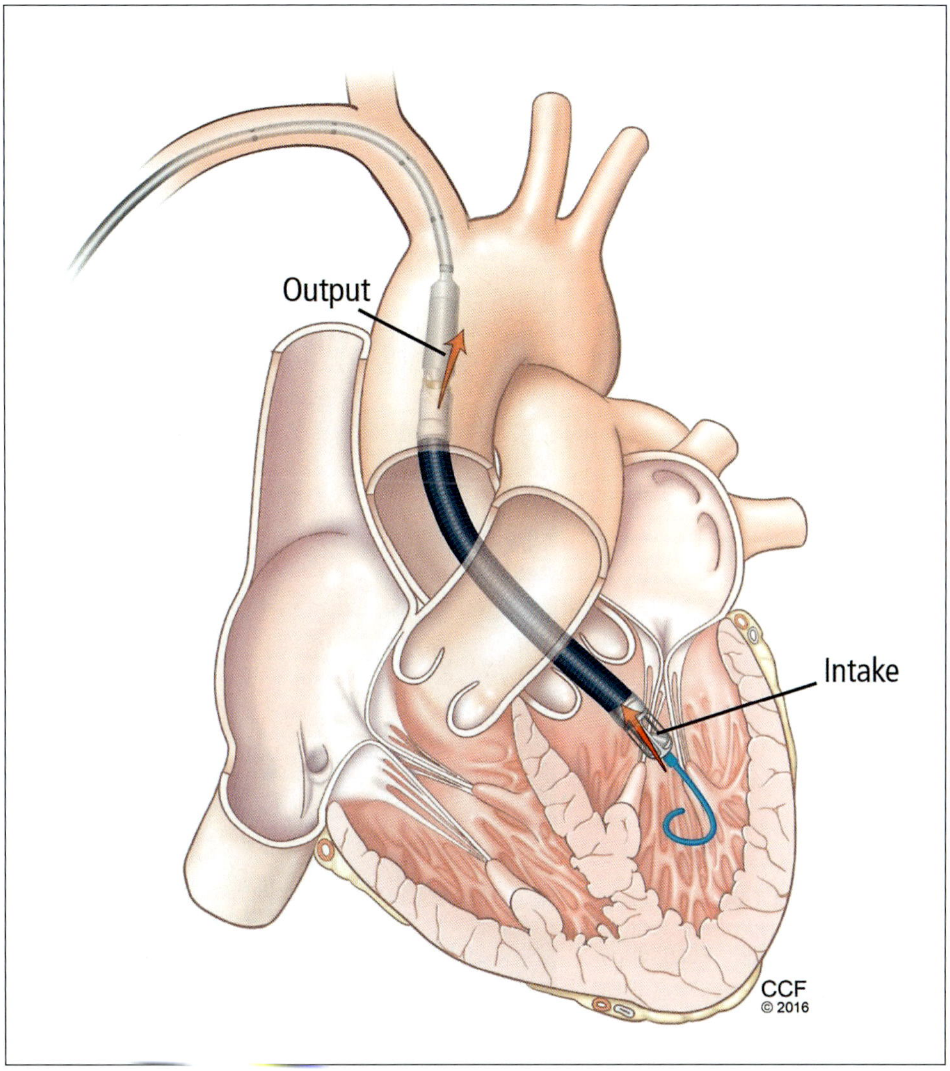

Fig. 6. Impella®. The Impella® device withdraws blood from the left ventricle and ejects it into the ascending aorta. Reprinted with permission from Shishehbor et al. [84]. Copyright © 2017 The Cleveland Clinic Foundation. All rights reserved.

tracorporeal and pneumatically driven pulsatile device that replaces the native ventricles and four cardiac valves in cases of end-stage biventricular heart failure (Fig. 7) [79]. The device consists of two artificial ventricles and comes in two sizes (50 and 70 mL). As with the Berlin Heart, each ventricle has a multilayer diaphragm separating the blood chamber from the air chamber. Artificial disc valves are mounted in the inflow and outflow ports of each artificial ventricle to control the direction of blood flow. Each ventricle is connected to the external pneumatic driver via a cannula tunneled through the chest wall, which acts as a pneumatic conduit to permit pulsatile flow. Patients have the opportunity when clinically stable to switch to the Freedom Portable Driver, a rela-

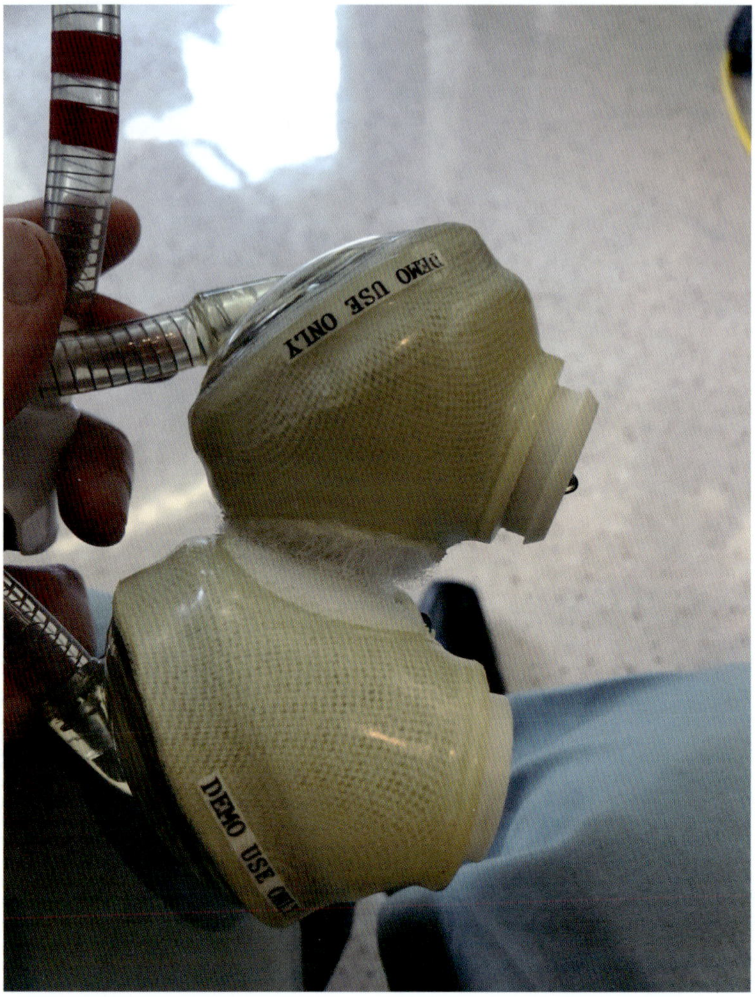

Fig. 7. SynCardia TAH. ECLS, extracorporeal life support; TAH, total artificial heart. SickKids ECLS Copyright ©.

tively small and light (~6.8 kg) pneumatic pump allowing for increased mobility (can be carried in a shoulder bag or backpack) and the opportunity for discharge home. Though included in this chapter for completeness, the TAH is not strictly a VAD because it is a temporary ventricular *replacement* device rather than a VAD.

Unfortunately, due to device sizing, the TAH is limited to older children and adolescents. Centers have been able to implant in children as young as 10 years and as small as 0.9 m^2 body surface area [80, 81].

Bivalirudin is used in the early postoperative period for anticoagulation, while VKA and ASA are the mainstays of long-term therapy. The anticoagulation and antiplatelet targets vary by center. At SickKids, an INR target of 2.5–3.5 is the goal and ASA is dosed between 81 and 325 mg daily.

Conclusions

Hemostatic management for children on ECLS is complex and challenging. The main goal for anticoagulation is to prevent thrombi while minimizing bleeding. UFH is the first-line anticoagulant despite variable pharmacodynamics and pharmacokinetics. Bivalirudin has been gaining terrain, but there is room for improvement in terms of its monitoring. Having a local strategy for anticoagulation in patients during MCS is important given the different availability and monitoring tests between centers. To date, it has been difficult to compare interventional approaches considering the lack of MCS standardized definitions as well as MCS-related outcomes [82]. This chapter provides a summary of the current practices at SickKids.

Acknowledgment

The authors express their appreciation for the previous collaborations by Dr. Yaser Diab (Children's National Hospital, Washington DC, USA).

Conflict of Interest Statement

Leonardo R. Brandão reports receiving consultancy and speaker fees from Takeda and Inari Medical. He is recipient of a research grant from Takeda and an educational grant from Inari Medical. Aamir Jewa is chair of the Berlin Heart EXCOR® Driver trial, and he is recipient of an unrestricted educational grant from Abbott Industries. Gail Annich, Anne-Marie Guerguerian, Alyssa Power, and Mariella Vargas-Gutierrez report no conflicts of interest. Dr. Annich is a member of the strategic advisory counsel for ELSO. Dr. Guerguerian participates on an ad hoc basis in the ELSO guidelines and as a volunteer for the American Heart Association and the Heart and Stroke Foundation of Canada. Mr. Mark Todd reports no conflicts of interest.

Author Contributions

All authors contributed to the review of data and the writing of this manuscript. All authors have read and approved the final version.

Abbreviations

ACT	Activated clotting time
ACTION	Advanced Cardiac Therapies Improving Outcomes Network
ADAMTS 13	A disintegrin and metalloproteinase with a thrombospondin type 1 motif, member 13
AIS	Arterial ischemic stroke
aPTT	Activated partial thromboplastin time
ASA	Acetylsalicylic acid
AVWS	Acquired von Willebrand syndrome
BiVAD	Biventricular assist device
BUN	Blood urea nitrogen
CBC	Complete blood count
CHD	Congenital heart disease
CPB	Cardiopulmonary bypass
DTI	Direct thrombin inhibitor
dTT	Dilute thrombin time
ECLS	Extracorporeal life support
ECLSO	Extracorporeal Life Support Organization
ECMO	Extracorporeal membrane oxygenation
GI	Gastrointestinal
IL-6	Interleukin-6
LDH	Lactate dehydrogenase
LVAD	Left ventricular assist device
MCS	Mechanical circulatory support
NO	Nitric oxide
PAI-1	Plasminogen activator inhibitor type 1
Pedimacs	Pediatric Interagency Registry for Mechanical Circulatory Support
pfHb	Plasma-free hemoglobin
PT/INR	Prothrombin time/international normalized ratio
ROTEM	Rotational thromboelastometry
RPM	Revolutions per minute
RVAD	Right ventricle assist device
SVAD	Single ventricle assist device
TAH	Total artificial heart
TE	Thromboembolism/thromboembolic event
TEG	Thromboelastography
UFH	Unfractionated heparin
VA	Venoarterial
VAD	Ventricular assist device
VV	Venovenous
VWF	von Willebrand factor

19

References

1 Gibbon JH. Application of a mechanical heart and lung apparatus to cardiac surgery. Minn Med. 1954;37:171–85.

2 Lillehei CW, Cohen M, Warden HE, Varco RL. The direct-vision intracardiac correction of congenital anomalies by controlled cross circulation; results in thirty-two patients with ventricular septal defects, tetralogy of Fallot, and atrioventricular communis defects. Surgery. 1955;38(1):11–29.

3 Mustard WT, Chute AL, Keith JP, Sirek A, Rowe RD, Vlad P. A surgical approach to transposition of the great vessels with extracorporeal circuit. Surgery. 1954;36:31–51.

4 Mustard WT, Thomson JA. Clinical experience with the artificial heart-lung preparation. Can Med Assoc J. 1957;76: 265–9.

5 Howell WH, Holt E. Two new factors in blood coagulation—heparin and proantithrombin. Am J Physiol. 1918;47: 328–41.

6 Charles AF, Scott DA. Studies on heparin: observations on the chemistry of heparin. The Biochem J. 1936;30:1927–33.

7 Murray DW, Jaques LB, Perrett TS, Best CH. Heparin and vascular occlusion. Can Med Assoc J. 1936;35:621–2.

8 Liotta D. Early clinical application of assisted circulation. Tex Heart Inst J. 2002;29(3):229–30.

9 Bartlett RH, Kittredge D, Noyer BS Jr, Willard RH III, Drinker PA. Development of a membrane oxygenator: overcoming blood diffusiolimitation. J Thorac Cardiovasc Surg. 1969;58(6):795–800.

10 Bartlett RH, Gazzaniga AB, Toomasian J, Coran AG, Roloff D, Ricker R. Extracorporeal membrane oxygenation (ECMO) in neonatal respiratory failure. 100 cases. Ann Surg. 1986;204(3):236–45.

11 Brogan T, ed. *Extracorporeal Life Support: The ELSO Red Book*. 5th ed. Extracorporeal Life Support Organization; 2017.

12 Lequier L, Horton SB, Mcmullan DM, Bartlett RH. Extracorporeal membrane oxygenation circuitry. Pediatr Crit Care Med. 2013;14(5 suppl 1):S7–12.

13 Cai T, Swaney E, Van Den Helm S, Brown G, MacLaren G, Horton S, et al. The evolution of extracorporeal membrane oxygenation circuitry and impact on clinical outcomes in children: a systematic review. ASAIO J. 2023;69(3):247–53.

14 Ontaneda A, Annich GM. Novel surfaces in extracorporeal membrane oxygenation circuits. Front Med (Lausanne). 2018;5:321.

15 Palmer K, Enhreb H, Benz R, Frenckner B. Carmeda surface heparinization in neonatal ECMO systems: long-term experiments in a sheep model. Perfusion. 1995;10(5):307–13.

16 Radomski MM, Zakar T, Salas E. Nitric oxide in platelet. Methods Enzymol. 1996;269:88–107.

17 Skrzypchak AM, Lafayette NG, Bartlett RH, Zhou Z, Frost MC, Meyerhoff ME, et al. Effect of varying nitric oxide release to prevent platelet consumption and preserve platelet function in an in vivo model of extracorporeal circulation. Perfusion. 2007;22(3):193–200.

18 Leslie DC, Waterhouse A, Berthet JB, Valentin TM, Watters AL, Jain A, et al. A bioinspired omniphobic surface coating on medical devices prevents thrombosis and biofouling. Nat Biotechnol. 2014;32(11):1134–40.

19 Liu T, Liu S, Zhang K, Chen J, Huang N. Endothelialization of implanted cardiovascular biomaterial surfaces: the development from in vitro to in vivo. J Biomed Mater Res A. 2014;102(10): 3754–72.

20 Pang JH, Farhatnia Y, Godarzi F, Tan A, Rajadas J, Cousin BC, et al. In situ endothelialization: bioengineering considerations to translation. Small. 2015;11(47): 6248–64.

21 Hensch LA, Hui SKR, Teruya J. Coagulation and bleeding management in pediatric extracorporeal oxygenation: clinical scenarios and review. Front Med. 2018;5:361.

22 Kubicki R, Stiller B, Kroll J, Siepe M, Beyerdorf F, Benk C, et al. Acquired von Willebrand syndrome in paediatric patients during mechanical circulatory support. Eur J Cardiothorac Surg. 2019;55:1194–1201.

23 Fortenberry JD, Bhardwaj V, Niemer P, Cornish JD, Wright JA, Bland L. Neutrophil and cytokine activation with neonatal extracorporeal membrane oxygenation. J Pediatr. 1996;128:670–8.

24 Meyer AD, Gelfond JA, Wiles AA, Freishtat RJ, Rais-Bahrami K. Platelet-derived microparticles generated by neonatal extracorporeal membrane oxygenation systems. ASAIO J. 2015;1: 37–42.

25 Van Den Helm S, Yaw HP, Letunica N, Barton R, Weaver A, Newall F, et al. Platelet phenotype and function changes with increasing duration of extracorporeal membrane oxygenation. Crit Care Med. 2022;50(8):1236–45.

26 Allen N, Barrett T, Guo Y, Nardi M, Ramkhelawon B, Rockman CB, et al. Circulating monocyte-platelet aggregates are a robust marker of platelet activity in cardiovascular disease. Atheroscler. 2019;282:11–8.

27 Foley JH, Conway EM. Cross talk pathways between coagulation and inflammation. Circ Res. 2016;118:1392–408.

28 Caprarola SD, Ng DK, Carroll MK, Tekes A, Felling RJ, Salorio CF, et al. Pediatric ECMO: unfavorable outcomes are associated with inflammation and endothelial activation. Pediatr Res. 2022;92:549–56.

29 McMichael ABV, Ryerson LM, Ratano D, Faraoni D, Annich GM. 2021 ELSO adult and pediatric anticoagulation guidelines. ASAIO J. 2022;68(3):303–10.

30 Valdes CA, Sharaf OM, Bleiweis MS, Jacobs JP, Mumtaz M, et al. Heparin-based versus bivalirudin-based anticoagulation in pediatric extracorporeal membrane oxygenation: A systematic review. Front Med (Lausanne). 2023;10: 1137134.

31 Teruya J, Bruzdoski K, Hensch L, Hui SKR, Kostousov. How to best monitor bivalirudin anticoagulant effect for ECMO and VAD—Comparison of four assay methods. Int J Lab Hematol. 2022;44:589–94.

32 Bembea MM, Annich G, Rycus P, Oldenburg G, Berkowitz I, Pronovost P. Variability in anticoagulation management of patients on extracorporeal membrane oxygenation: an international survey. Pediatr Crit Care Med. 2013; 14(20):e77.

33 Deshpande SJ, Vitali S, Thiagarajan R, Brediger S, McManus M, Geva A. Coagulations studies do not correlate with each other or with hematologic complications during pediatric extracorporeal membrane oxygenation. Pediatr Crit Care Med. 2021;22(6):542–52.

34 Liveris A, Bello RA, Friedmann P, Duffy MA, Manwani D, Killinger JS, et al. Anti-factor Xa assay is a superior correlate of heparin dose than activated partial thromboplastin time or activated clotting time in pediatric extracorporeal membrane oxygenation. Pediatr Crit Care Med. 2014;15:e72–9.
35 Bailly DK, Reeder RW, Muszynski JA, Meert KL, Ankola AA, Alexander PMA, et al. Anticoagulation practices associated with bleeding and thrombosis in pediatric extracorporeal membrane oxygenation; a multi-center secondary analysis. Perfusion. 2023;38(2):362–72.
36 Dalton HJ, Garcia-Filion PG, Holubkov R, Moler FW, Shanley T, Heideman S, et al. Association of bleeding and thrombosis with outcome in extracorporeal life support. Pediatr Crit Care Med. 2015;16(2):167–74.
37 Tang W, Zhang WT, Zhang J, Jiang KH, Ge YW, Zheng AB, et al. Prevalence of hematologic complications on extracorporeal membrane oxygenation in critically ill pediatric patients: a systematic review and meta-analysis. Thromb Res. 2023;222:75–84.
38 Staessens S, Moussa MD, Pierache A, Rauch A, Rousse N, Boulleaux E, et al. Thrombus formation during ECMO: insights from a detailed histological analysis of thrombus composition. J Thromb Haemost. 2022;20:2058–69.
39 Bembea MM, Cheifetz IM, Fortenberry JD, Bunchman TE, Valentine SL, Bateman ST, et al. Recommendations on the indications for RBC transfusion for the critically ill child receiving support from extracorporeal membrane oxygenation, ventricular assist, and renal replacement therapy devices from the pediatric critical care transfusion and anemia expertise initiative: Pediatr Crit Care Med. 2018;19:S157–62.
40 Ozment CP, Scott BL, Bembea MM, Spinella PC, For the Pediatric ECMO (PediECMO) subgroup of the Pediatric Acute Lung Injury and Sepsis Investigators (PALISI) Network and the Extracorporeal Life Support Organization (ELSO). Anticoagulation and transfusion management during neonatal and pediatric extracorporeal membrane oxygenation: a survey of medical directors in the United States. Pediatr Crit Care Med. 2021;22(6):530–41.
41 Rossano JW, Singh TP, Cherikh WS, Chambers DC, Harhay MO, Hayes D Jr, et al. The International Thoracic Organ Transplant Registry of the International Society for Heart and Lung Transplantation: twenty-second pediatric heart transplantation report—2019;Focus theme: donor and recipient size match. J Heart Lung Transplant. 2019;38(10):1028–41.
42 Adachi I, Peng DM, Hollander SA, Simpson KE, Davies RR, Jacobs JP, et al. Sixth annual pediatric interagency registry for mechanical circulatory support (Pedimacs) report: the Society Of Thoracic Surgeons Pedimacs annual report. Ann Thorac Surg. 2023;115(5):1098–1108.
43 Peng DM, Rosenthal DN, Zafar F, Smyth L, VanderPluym CJ, Lorts A. Collaboration and new data in ACTION: a learning health care system to improve pediatric heart failure and ventricular assist device outcomes. Transl Pediatr. 2019;8(4):349–55.
44 De Biasi AR, Manning KB, Salemi A. Science for surgeons: understanding pump thrombogenesis in continuous-flow left ventricular assist devices. J Thorac Cardiovasc Surg. 2015;149:667–73.
45 Attard C, van der Straaten T, Karlaftis V, Monagle P, Ignjatovic V. Developmental hemostasis: age-specific differences in the levels of hemostatic proteins. J Thromb Haemost. 2013;11: 1850–4.
46 VanderPluym C, Esteso P, Arkola A, Hellinger A, Ventresco C, Hawkins B, et al. Real-world use of apixaban for the treatment and prevention of thrombosis in children with cardiac disease. J Thromb Haemostat. 2023;21(6):1601–9.
47 Adachi I, Fraser CD Jr. Berlin heart EXCOR Food and Drug Administration Investigational device exemption trial. Semin Thorac Cardiovasc Surg. 2013; 25(2):100–6.
48 Aggarwal A, Pant R, Kumar S, Sharma P, Gallagher C, Tatooles AJ, et al. Incidence and management of gastrointestinal bleeding with continuous flow assist devices. Ann Thorac Surg. 2012;93(5): 1534–40.
49 Crow S, John R, Boyle A, Shumway S, Liao K, Colvin-Adams M, et al. Gastrointestinal bleeding rates in recipients of nonpulsatile and pulsatile left ventricular assist devices. J Thorac Cardiovasc Surg. 2009;137(1):208–15.
50 Heith C, McHugh K, Phimister A, Clipp M, Steiner M, Ameduri R. Menorrhagia and menstrual bleeding in patients supported with ventricular assist devices. Cardiovasc Dis. 2019;155(4):55A.
51 Brown CS, Abi-Hachem R, Jang DW. Management of epistaxis in patients with ventricular assist device: a retrospective review. J Otolaryngol Head Neck Surg. 2018;47:48.
52 Uriel N, Pak SW, Jorde UP, Jude B, Susen S, Vincentelli A, et al. Acquired von Willebrand syndrome after continuous-flow mechanical device support contributes to a high prevalence of bleeding during long-term support and at the time of transplantation. J Am Coll Cardiol. 2010;56(15):1207–13.
53 Rauch A, Susen S, Zieger B. Acquired von Willebrand syndrome in patients with ventricular assist device. Front Med. 2019;6:7.
54 Heilmann C, Geisen U, Beyersdorf F, Nakamura L, Benk C, Berchtold-Herz M, et al. Acquired von Willebrand syndrome in patients with ventricular assist device or total artificial heart. Thromb Haemost. 2010;103(05):962–7.
55 Klovaite J, Gustafsson F, Mortensen SA, Sander K, Nielsen LB. Severely impaired von Willebrand factor-dependent platelet aggregation in patients with a continuous-flow left ventricular assist device (HeartMate II). J Am Coll Cardiol. 2009; 53(23):2162–7.
56 Tchantchaleishvili V, Sagebin F, Ross RE, Hallinan W, Schwarz KQ, Massey HT. Evaluation and treatment of pump thrombosis and hemolysis. Ann Cardiothorac Surg. 2014;3:490–5.
57 Nielsen VG, Pretorius E. Iron and carbon monoxide enhance coagulation and attenuate fibrinolysis by different mechanisms. Blood Coagul Fibrinolysis. 2014; 25:695–702.
58 Ataga KI. Hypercoagulability and thrombotic complications in hemolytic anemias. Haematologica. 2009;94:1481–4.
59 Cowger JA, Romano MA, Shah P, Shah N, Mehta V, Haft JW. Hemolysis: a harbinger of adverse outcome after left ventricular assist device implant. J Heart Lung Transplant. 2014;33:35–43.
60 Papanastasiou CA, Kyriakoulis KG, Theochari CA, Kokkinidis DG, Karamitsos TD, Palaiodimos L. Comprehensive review of hemolysis in ventricular assist devices. World J Cardiol. 2020 Jul 26; 12(7):334–41.

19

61 Badiye AP, Hernandez GA, Novoa I, Chaparro SV. Incidence of hemolysis in patients with cardiogenic shock treated with impella percutaneous left ventricular assist device. ASAIO J. 2016;62(1): 11–4.
62 Katz JN, Jensen BC, Chang PP, Myers SL, Pagani FD, Kirklin JK. A multicenter analysis of clinical hemolysis in patients supported with durable, long-term left ventricular assist device therapy. J Heart Lung Transplant. 2015;34:701–9.
63 Ravichandran AK, Parker J, Novak E, Joseph SM, Schilling JD, Ewald GA, et al. Hemolysis in left ventricular assist device: a retrospective analysis of outcomes. J Heart Lung Transplant. 2014; 33:44–50.
64 Xia Y, Forest S, Friedmann P, Chou LC, Patel S, Jorde U, et al. Factors associated with prolonged survival in left ventricular assist device recipients. Ann Thorac Surg. 2019;107:519–26.
65 Villa CR, VanderPluym CJ, on behalf of the ACTION Investigators. ABCs of stroke prevention. Improving stroke outcomes in children supported with a ventricular assist device in a quality improvement network. Circ Cardiovasc Qual Outcomes. 2020;13:e006663.
66 Yu X, Larsen B, Rutledge J, West L, Ross DB, Rebeyka IM, et al. The profile of the systemic inflammatory response in children undergoing ventricular assist device support. Interact Cardiovasc Thorac Surg. 2012 Sep;15(3):426–31.
67 Byrnes JW, Bhutta AT, Rettiganti MR, Gomez A, Garcia X, Dyamenahalli U, et al. Steroid therapy attenuates acute phase reactant response among children on ventricular assist device support. Ann Thorac Surg. 2015;99:1392–8.
68 Fraser CD Jr, Jaquiss RDB, Rosenthal DN, Humpl T, Canter CE, Blackstone EH, et al. Prospective trial of a pediatric ventricular assist device. N Engl J Med. 2012;367:532–41.
69 Byrnes JW, Prodhan P, Williams BA, Schmitz ML, Moss MM, Dyamenahalli U, et al. Incremental reduction in the incidence of stroke in children supported with the Berlin EXCOR ventricular assist device. Ann Thorac Surg. 2013;96: 1727–33.
70 Peng DM, Shezad MF, Lorts A, Gajarski RJ, VanderPluym C, Murray JM, et al. Decreased risk of strokes in children with ventricular assist devices within ACTION. Pediatr Cardiol. 2022;43(6): 1379–82.
71 Niebler RA, Amdani S, Blume B, Cantor RS, Deng L, Kirklin JK, et al. Stroke in pediatric ventricular assist device patients-a pedimacs registry analysis. J Heart Lung Transplant. 2021;12:S1053-2498(21)02229-4.
72 O'Connor MJ, Lorts A, Davies RR, Fynn-Thompson F, Joong A, Maeda K, et al. Early experience with the HeartMate 3 continuous-flow ventricular assist device in pediatric patients and patients with congenital heart disease: a multicenter registry analysis. J Heart Lung Transplant. 2020;39(6):P573–9.
73 Mehra MR, Uriel N, Naka Y, Cleveland JC Jr, Yuzefpolskaya M, Salerno CT, et al. A fully magnetically levitated left ventricular assist device—final report. N Engl J Med. 2019;380(17):1618–27.
74 Bourque K, Cotter C, Dague C, Harjes D, Dur O, Duhamel J, et al. Design rationale and preclinical evaluation of the HeartMate 3 left ventricular assist system for hemocompatibility. ASAIO J. 2016;62:375–83.
75 Bourque K, Dague C, Farrar D, Harms K, Tamez D, Cohn W, et al. In vivo assessment of a rotary left ventricular assist device induced artificial pulse in the proximal and distal aorta. Artif Organs. 2006;30:638–42.
76 Mehra MR, Goldstein DJ, Uriel N, Cleveland JC, Yuzefpolskaya M, Salerno C, et al. Two-year outcomes with a magnetically levitated cardiac pump in heart failure. N Engl J Med. 2018;378:1386–95.
77 Morales DLS, Rossano JW, Vander-Pluym C, Lorts A, Cantor R, St Louis JD et al. Third annual pediatric interagency registry for mechanical circulatory support (Pedimacs) report: preimplantation characteristics and outcomes. Ann Thorac Surg. 2019;107(4):993–1004.
78 Parekh D, Jeewa A, Tume SC, Dreyer WJ, Pignatelli R, Horne D, et al. Percutaneous mechanical circulatory support using impella devices for decompensated cardiogenic shock: a pediatrÃic heart center experience. ASAIO J. 2018;64:98–104.
79 Chung JS, Emerson D, Megna D, Arabia FA. Total artificial heart: surgical technique in the patient with normal cardiac anatomy. Ann Cardiothorac Surg. 2020 Mar;9(2):81–8.
80 Villa CR, Moore RA, Morales DL, Lorts A. The total artificial heart in pediatrics: outcomes in an evolving field. Ann Cardiothorac Surg. 2020;9(2):104–9
81 Beasley GS, Allen K, Pahl E, Jackson L, Eltayeb O, Monge M, et al. Successful bridge to transplant in a pediatric patient using the SynCardia 50 cc total artificial heart. ASAIO J. 2020;66:e33–5.
82 Alexander PMA, Habet V, Barbaro RP. Realizing potential: pediatric extracorporeal membrane oxygenation needs common adverse event definitions to improve outcomes. Pediatr Crit Care Med. 2023;24(6):528–30.
83 Heatley G, Sood P, Goldstein D, Uriel N, Cleveland J, Middlebrook D, et al. Clinical trial design and rationale of the Multicenter Study of MagLev Technology in Patients Undergoing Mechanical Circulatory Support Therapy With HeartMate 3 (MOMENTUM 3) investigational device exemption clinical study protocol. J Heart Lung Transplant. 2016;35(4):528–36.
84 Shishehbor M, Moazami N, Zhen-Yu Tong M, Unai S, Wilson Tang W, Soltesz E. Cardiogenic shock: from ECMO to Impella and beyond. Cleve Clin J Med. 2017;84(4):287–95.

Published online: December 5, 2024

Blanchette VS, Brandão LR, Carcao MD, Kumar R, Rand ML, Revel-Vilk S (eds): SickKids Handbook of Pediatric Thrombosis and Hemostasis, ed 3, rev. and ext. Basel, Karger, 2024, pp 385–410 (DOI: 10.1159/000538193)

Antithrombotic Therapy

Tina Biss[a] Christoph Male[b] Jennifer Vincelli[c] Paul Monagle[d]

[a]Department of Haematology, The Newcastle upon Tyne Hospitals NHS Trust, Newcastle upon Tyne, UK; [b]Department of Pediatrics/Division of Pediatric Cardiology, Medical University of Vienna, Vienna, Austria; [c]Division of Hematology/Oncology, The Hospital for Sick Children, Toronto, ON, Canada; [d]Department of Clinical Haematology, The Royal Children's Hospital, Melbourne, VIC, Australia

Introduction

The requirement for antithrombotic therapy for the treatment and prevention of thromboembolism (TE) in children is increasing. This increase is likely multifactorial but certainly involves the improvement in survival from complex diseases being complicated by a rising incidence of thromboembolic complications [1].

Antithrombotic therapy has many specific challenges in infants and children, related to the changes that occur in the hemostatic system during normal development (see Chapter 2), the difficulty in administering anticoagulant therapy that arises from the lack of suitable preparations and the often small doses required, and the difficulties in monitoring because of physiologically different baseline tests and problematic venipuncture.

There is also a relative lack of evidence to guide dosing and monitoring of antithrombotic therapy in children. Prior to studies of the direct oral anticoagulants (DOACs), there were only a handful of small randomized controlled studies of antithrombotic therapy in children, in absolute contrast to the adult situation. Thus, much of the guidance for dosing and monitoring in children and adolescents is extrapolated from data obtained from adult studies. Treatment is often led by the experience of the treating physician and individualized according to the child being treated. The most comprehensive and globally accepted guidelines currently available are those published by the American College of Chest Physicians [2], although the American Society of Hematology (ASH) has published venous thromboembolism (VTE) treatment guidelines more recently [3].

Unfractionated Heparin

Mechanism of Action and Pharmacokinetics

Heparin acts as an anticoagulant by binding to and potentiating the effect of antithrombin (AT; see Chapter 2). Unfractionated heparin (UFH) is usually administered intravenously by continuous infusion but can also be given subcutaneously. UFH is metabolized by the liver and is renally excreted. If a bolus dose of heparin is administered, followed by a continuous infusion, the anticoagulant effect plateaus after 4 h. Without a bolus dose, it plateaus after 6 h. The half-life of UFH is short (although the actual half-life seems age and dose dependent), meaning that reversal of the anticoagulant effect is rapid if the infusion of either a prophylactic dose or a therapeutic dose is stopped.

Indications

UFH, administered by continuous infusion, is the anticoagulant of choice for situations where rapid onset of anticoagulant effect and/or rapid reversal are required, e.g., for postoperative anticoagulation or anticoagulation in patients with a high risk of bleeding because of other causes. UFH is also useful as a short-term anticoagulant agent, such as during renal dialysis or cardiopulmonary bypass (CPB) surgery.

Dosing

The use of a loading dose and the choice of initial maintenance dose mainly depend on clinical situation and age. A loading dose should be avoided or reduced in neonates, children with stroke, or if the risk of bleeding is high. Similarly, the initial maintenance dose may need to be reduced if the risk of bleeding is high. Further dose reduction is required if significant renal disease is present.

Loading dose: 75 U/kg as an intravenous (IV) infusion over 10 min.

Initial maintenance dose: <1 year of age, 28 U/kg/h; ≥1 year of age, 20 U/kg/h.

Laboratory Monitoring

UFH treatment requires monitoring to ensure that the anticoagulant effect is within the desired range. Monitoring classically should occur 6 h after commencing a heparin infusion and 4 h after any change in infusion rate, although in children this is often not feasible. Additionally, in children treated without boluses or reduced initial doses, monitoring tests may be more appropriate after 8 or even 12 h. A blood sample for monitoring should be taken at least every 24 h once therapeutic levels are achieved. UFH can be monitored using several different laboratory assays.

Activated Clotting Time

This is a bedside test that measures the time taken for whole blood to clot after the addition of kaolin or celite, often used for heparin monitoring during CPB surgery or extracorporeal membrane oxygenation (ECMO). The target range is analyzer dependent. The activated clotting time (ACT) may be prolonged by other factors, such as thrombocytopenia, hypothermia, and hemodilution.

Activated Partial Thromboplastin Time or Activated Partial Thromboplastin Ratio

The activated partial thromboplastin time (aPTT) measures clotting via the intrinsic pathway (see Chapter 2) and is prolonged by UFH. The target range is analyzer and reagent dependent, and clinicians should be aware of the target ranges in their individual health services. The aPTT is the most commonly used monitoring test of UFH and potentially the one that best correlates with the risk of bleeding, although further research is required [4]. The activated partial thromboplastin ratio (aPTR) is a ratio of patient aPTT/normal aPTT for age, and an aPTR of 1.5–2.5 is usually the desired range, although there have been specific recommendations against using aPTR in children (see Table 1 for details of UFH infusion adjustment according to aPTT/aPTR). Levels of aPTT/aPTR may be difficult to monitor in the presence of a prolonged baseline aPTT such as might be due to physiological factor deficiency in infants <6 months of age, the presence of a coagulation inhibitor (e.g., lupus anticoagulant), or a consumptive coagulopathy.

Table 1. Adjustment of heparin infusion according to monitoring of aPTT, aPTR, and anti-Xa levels

aPTT	aPTR	Anti-Xa level, IU/mL[a]	Bolus, U/kg	Hold, min	Rate change, %
<50 s	<1.2	<0.1	50	0	↑10
50–59 s	1.2–1.4	0.1–0.34	0	0	↑10
60–85 s	1.5–2.5	0.35–0.70	0	0	no change
86–95 s	2.6–3.0	0.71–0.89	0	0	↓10
96–120 s	3.1–3.5	0.9–1.2	0	30	↓10
>120 s	>3.5	>1.2	0	60	↓15

aPTR, activated partial thromboplastin time ratio; aPTT, activated partial thromboplastin time.
[a]This assumes that the aPTT range of 60–85 s correlates to an anti-factor Xa level of 0.35–0.70 IU/mL. This will depend on the reagent and analyzer used in the laboratory.

20

Anti-Factor Xa Activity Assay

Anti-Xa activity assay measures the degree of inhibition of activated factor X by UFH. The target range is usually 0.35–0.7 IU/mL anti-Xa level (see Table 1 for details of UFH infusion adjustment according to anti-Xa levels). While correlation of anti-Xa with aPTT/aPTR is often used to determine if a prolonged aPTT/aPTR is due to heparin or another coagulopathy, discrepancies may be due to variation in the UFH anti-IIa effect with age and UFH dose. In addition, there are multiple anti-Xa methodologies on the market that for technical reasons give different results on the same samples. Thus, while monitoring of UFH therapy using anti-Xa levels is often advocated, there are no clinical outcome data to support one means of monitoring over another in a pediatric population [4].

When UFH therapy is being monitored, care must be taken to avoid heparin contamination of blood samples. Patients and parents prefer blood samples to be taken from central venous catheters (CVCs) rather than by peripheral venipuncture. However, available data suggest that discard volumes more than 8 mL are required to ensure accuracy of coagulation tests taken from a CVC. Such volumes may be impossible in small unstable infants and at the very least require the discard to be returned to the patient to reduce transfusion requirements. Institutional guidelines should be followed but, in general, drawing a blood sample from a peripheral vein in the contralateral arm to the heparin infusion is preferred.

Problems

AT Deficiency

Response to UFH can be reduced by the presence of AT deficiency. Infants <6 months have relative "heparin resistance" because of a physiological deficiency of AT. Thus, in infants who cannot reach the required level of anticoagulation with UFH therapy, there is some evidence to support the administration of AT concentrate as a means of increasing anti-factor Xa levels alongside a lower administered UFH dose [5]. It should be remembered that the therapeutic targets quoted are extrapolated from adult data and have never actually been validated in children compared with any other therapeutic range. No studies have demonstrated improved clinical outcomes from AT replacement therapy, rather just better attainment of "therapeutic levels." In addition, AT concentrate is expensive, not commonly available, and few safety data exist for its use in infants. In fact, some studies raise the possibility of AT concentrates in neonates causing harm [6, 7]. Acquired causes for AT deficiency, e.g., nephrotic syndrome, protein-losing enteropathy, l-asparaginase chemotherapy, or chylothorax, may also result in heparin resistance, which can respond to replacement of AT using AT concentrate. Again, it should be used with caution since safety is unproven and there can be a substantial increase in heparin effect with associated risk of bleeding. The ASH VTE guidelines specifically recommend against AT use purely to achieve therapeutic UFH levels and suggest consideration only if clinical thrombus extension despite adequate UFH dosing.

Heparin-Associated Thrombocytopenia
Heparin-associated thrombocytopenia is a benign fall in platelet count, rarely below 100×10^9/L. It is not associated with increased bleeding risk or thrombotic risk, usually happening within the initial days of heparin exposure.

Heparin-Induced Thrombocytopenia
Heparin-induced thrombocytopenia (HIT) is detailed in Chapter 7 but is rare in children.

Osteopenia
Osteopenia was reported secondary to prolonged administration of subcutaneous UFH in pregnant women. Only three cases of osteopenia have been reported in children treated with UFH.

Reversal
UFH can be rapidly reversed by stopping the infusion. Within 2–4 h, reversal will be adequate for the patient to undergo surgery. If more rapid reversal is required, e.g., major hemorrhage, protamine sulfate can be administered. This is given at a dose of 1 mg per 100 U of heparin received within the previous 2 h to a maximum of 50 mg, as a slow IV infusion. Care must be taken when giving protamine as high doses can have an anticoagulant effect rather than a procoagulant effect. Allergic reactions to the drug are not uncommon, particularly in children with fish allergy.

Low-Molecular-Weight Heparin

Mechanism of Action and Pharmacokinetics
Low-molecular-weight heparin (LMWH) has a similar mode of action to UFH, although they have a higher ratio of anti-factor Xa/IIa activity. They are given by subcutaneous (SC) injection, either once or twice daily, and peak levels occur at around 2–4 h after administration. The half-life is 2–4 h, i.e., longer than UFH. LMWH is excreted renally.

Indications
LMWH is often the agent of choice for stable children with a low bleeding risk who require relatively short-term anticoagulant therapy (up to 3 months' duration). LMWH may be preferred to oral vitamin K antagonists (VKAs) in children who have dietary problems, multiple interacting medications, need frequent reversal of anticoagulation for invasive procedures such as lumbar punctures and in infants who often have poor stability of VKA. It may be the preferred agent for patient groups who were excluded from the clinical studies of DOACs. Until recently, LMWH was the established therapy for adult cancer patients, but no specific evidence exists for children with malignancy. There are few safety data to support the use of LMWH for periods longer than 3 months in children, in contrast to VKAs that are established as long-term anticoagulant agents. Further, DOACs also have randomized controlled trial (RCT) data to support their use for up to 12 months' duration.

Dosing
The dose of LMWH differs according to the age of the child and the clinical indication, i.e., therapeutic or prophylactic (Table 2). Most safety data are available for twice daily dosing schedules. There remains some debate over the optimal doses of LMWH in neonates. Most of these data relate to enoxaparin dosing with some support from retrospective studies for initial doses of 2.0

Table 2. Therapeutic and prophylactic dosing of enoxaparin, tinzaparin, and dalteparin according to age

	Therapeutic dose	Prophylactic dose
Enoxaparin		
≤2 months of age	1.5 mg/kg SC BID	1.5 mg/kg SC OD
>2 months of age	1 mg/kg SC BID	1 mg/kg SC OD
Tinzaparin		
≤2 months of age	275 U/kg SC OD	75 U/kg SC OD
2–12 months of age	250 U/kg SC OD	75 U/kg SC OD
1–5 years	240 U/kg SC OD	75 U/kg SC OD
5–10 years	200 U/kg SC OD	75 U/kg SC OD
10–16 years	175 U/kg SC OD	50 U/kg SC OD
Dalteparin		
≤2 months of age	150 U/kg SC BID	150 U/kg SC OD
>2 months of age	100 U/kg SC BID	100 U/kg SC OD

BID, twice a day; OD, once a day; SC, subcutaneous.

and 1.7 mg/kg twice daily for preterm and term neonates, respectively, in order to achieve therapeutic levels more rapidly [8]. Changes in clinical outcomes and in particular, safety were not assessed, however. As for UFH, the target therapeutic ranges quoted have not been validated.

When children are switched from UFH infusion to LMWH injections, the UFH infusion should be stopped at the same time the first dose of LMWH is given.

Laboratory Monitoring

LMWH therapy is monitored using the anti-Xa activity assay. The recommended therapeutic target range is 0.5–1.0 IU/mL in a sample taken 4–6 h after SC injection or 0.5–0.8 IU/mL in a sample taken 2–6 h after SC injection [2]. The anti-Xa assay is taken after the first dose for once daily regimens and after the second dose for twice daily regimens. Monitoring frequency will vary according to the age of the child but will usually occur after every change in dose and at least once weekly while the child is in hospital and once monthly when he/she is an outpatient, although there are no specific recommendations available in terms of the frequency of monitoring. LMWH doses are increased or reduced by varying increments depending on the degree of deviation from the therapeutic target range (Table 3). Trough levels are monitored if there is a concern about accumulation of the drug, such as because of renal impairment, or to monitor efficacy in once daily dosing (trough level of ≥0.1 IU/mL) [9].

Problems

Renal Impairment

LMWH can accumulate in the presence of significant renal impairment, i.e., glomerular filtration rate <30 mL/min. A 25% reduction in LMWH dose and more frequent monitoring is recommended for adults with significant renal impairment (as defined above), and similar precautions are likely required for children.

Administration

Daily SC injections are poorly tolerated by some children. Bruising, hematoma formation, and skin infection may occur at the injection sites. Some centers recommend the use of an SC port, such as the Insuflon™ device, into which the

Table 3. Adjustment of LMWH according to monitoring of anti-Xa levels

Anti-Xa level	Withhold next dose?	Dose change	Timing of next anti-Xa level
<0.35 IU/mL	No	Increase by 25%	After next dose
0.35–0.49 IU/mL	No	Increase by 15%	After next dose
0.5–1.0 IU/mL	No	No	After 1 week if hospitalized, 1 month if outpatient
1.01–1.25 IU/mL	No	Decrease by 15%	After next dose
1.26–1.5 IU/mL	No	Decrease by 25%	After next dose
1.51–2.0 IU/mL	Yes	Decrease by 30%	When next dose is due; if >1.5, continue to withhold dose and repeat after 12 h
>2.0 IU/mL	Yes	Decrease by 40%	When next dose is due; if >1.5, continue to withhold dose and repeat after 12 h

LMWH is injected. This port can be replaced every 5–7 days, avoiding daily needles. The occurrence of hematomas at the Insuflon™ injection site in low birthweight neonates has led some to avoid their use in neonates <3 kg in weight [10].

Heparin-Induced Thrombocytopenia

HIT in the context of LMWH use is even rarer than with the use of UFH (see Chapter 7).

Reversal

Stopping LMWH therapy results in return to a nonanticoagulated state within 18–24 h of the last dose of tinzaparin (once daily dosing) and 8–12 h of the last dose of enoxaparin (twice daily dosing). If more rapid reversal is required, protamine sulfate may be given. LMWH is not as readily reversed by protamine sulfate as UFH (≈40–50%) and the effectiveness of this strategy is unproven. The dose of protamine sulfate is estimated according to the degree of reversal required and the time elapsed since the last LMWH dose was given. If protamine sulfate is given within 8 h of the LMWH, then the maximum neutralizing dose is 1 mg protamine sulfate per 100 U (or 1 mg) of LMWH given in the last dose. If more than 8 h have elapsed, the dose is 0.5 mg protamine sulfate per 100 U (or 1 mg) of LMWH given. Repeated measurements of anti-Xa activity may be necessary to monitor the efficacy of reversal using protamine sulfate, with further aliquots being given until the desired reduction in anti-Xa activity is achieved. The maximum dose of protamine sulfate is 50 mg.

Vitamin K Antagonists

Mechanism of Action and Pharmacokinetics

Coumarin derivatives produce an anticoagulant effect by interfering with the cyclic conversion of vitamin K to its reduced form (vitamin K hydroquinone). VKAs inhibit the regeneration of vitamin K hydroquinone from vitamin K epoxide by inhibiting the VKOR enzyme in the vitamin K cycle. Vitamin K hydroquinone is an essential cofactor for the post-ribosomal activation (γ-carboxylation) of coagulation factors II, VII, IX and X, and protein C and protein S without which they are unable to bind calcium and become active in the coagulation cascade.

Coumarin derivatives are given orally and are rapidly absorbed from the gastrointestinal tract. However, the anticoagulant effect takes several days to develop due to the time taken for the circulating γ-carboxylated coagulation factors to undergo degradation. Warfarin is given as a once daily dose, preferably in the evening to allow dose adjustments to be made in response to monitoring. Warfarin is metabolized by the

Table 4. Adjustment of warfarin dose according to INR during initiation and maintenance phases of therapy

	INR	Action
Initiation		
Day 1	If the baseline INR is 1.0–1.3, give 0.2 mg/kg orally (maximum 10 mg)	
Days 2–4	1.1–1.3	Repeat initial loading dose
	1.4–1.9	50% of initial loading dose
	2.0–3.0	50% of initial loading dose
	3.1–3.5	25% of initial loading dose
	>3.5	Hold until INR <3.5 then restart at 50% of initial loading dose
Maintenance	1.1–1.4	Increase dose by 20%
	1.5–1.9	Increase dose by 10%
	2.0–3.0	No change
	3.1–3.5	Decrease dose by 10%
	>3.5	Hold until INR <3.5 then restart at 20% less than previous dose

INR, international normalized ratio.

liver. The half-life of warfarin is approximately 40 h causing its anticoagulant effect to last for 3–5 days.

Indications

VKAs are used for children who require long-term anticoagulation therapy such as children with cardiac disease requiring chronic anticoagulation and children with a history of venous TE and persisting risk factors for recurrence. Warfarin is occasionally used for shorter-term anticoagulant therapy in those who prefer to receive treatment via an oral route particularly for those in whom anticoagulation with a DOAC is not suitable. Warfarin is the long-term anticoagulant of choice for children with prosthetic cardiac valves or that require anticoagulation for VTE in the setting of antiphospholipid syndrome.

Dosing

Warfarin is the most used VKA in children. Acenocoumarol and phenprocoumon are used in some European and South American countries. Guidelines for the administration of warfarin are presented in Table 4. Age-related loading doses of acenocoumarol are: 2 months–1 year, 0.2 mg/kg; 1–5 years, 0.09 mg/kg; 6–10 years, 0.07 mg/kg; 11–18 years, 0.06 mg/kg [11]. Regardless of weight, an initial loading dose should rarely be more than 5 mg. The international normalized ratio (INR) was developed for monitoring patients treated with a VKA (see below). The INR is the ratio of a patient's prothrombin time (PT) to a normal control sample, raised to the power of the International Sensitivity Index value for the analytical system used: (observed PT/control PT)^{ISI}, where ISI = international sensitivity index (sensitivity of thromboplastin). There is a marked variability between children in response to loading doses, and factors other than weight, such as liver disease, nutritional status, and concurrent medications, are often taken into consideration when deciding a starting dose as these may all influence response to a VKA. While some studies have suggested that the VKORC1 and CYP2C9 genotypes are significant determinants of VKA dose requirements, other studies have refuted this in children [12, 13].

In the case of a newly diagnosed TE or thromboprophylaxis for high risk of thrombosis, VKA dosing should begin when the child is on therapeutic doses of UFH or LMWH. UFH or LMWH therapy should be continued until the child has had two consecutive INRs that are within the desired therapeutic target range.

Monitoring

The anticoagulant effect of VKA is monitored using the PT which becomes prolonged when the levels of active coagulation factors II, VII, IX and X fall. The degree of prolongation is proportional to the degree of anticoagulant effect. When used for monitoring VKA therapy, the PT is expressed as the INR, which is a means of standardizing results from different laboratories that may use different thromboplastin reagents and equipment. The INR is maintained within a desired therapeutic range that is dependent upon the clinical indication for anticoagulation (see relevant chapters). VKAs have a narrow therapeutic window and a deviation from the desired INR target range can result in a reduction in efficacy (if the INR is too low) or a hemorrhagic event (if the INR is too high).

Children receiving a VKA have regular INR checks. These can be done at a hospital anticoagulant clinic or a private laboratory. However, many children use point-of-care (POC) INR monitors, such as the Coaguchek® monitor. This allows a child/parent/caregiver to test the INR on a capillary blood sample and receive an immediate result. Within a patient home testing program, the result is then telephoned or emailed to the anticoagulant management team who will advise on the warfarin dose required and when the INR should next be checked. Most studies in children have described home POC INR monitoring supported by anticoagulation clinics which support dosing adjustments. Recently self-management programs, where the child/parent/caregiver determine the dose and timing of next INR test have been reported as successful for motivated families. The anticoagulation service provides back up support if required. All home testing and home management programs require strong education components. The benefits of using a home monitoring device include less time taken off school/work and rapid response to situations that may result in deviation from target INR range, such as fever, diarrhea and interactions with other medications. The use of a POC device, alongside appropriate education of the child and family, has been shown to improve anticoagulation control in children [14]. Recent studies have demonstrated improvement in quality of life for parents using this approach in addition to economic benefit due to a reduction in the cost of monitoring [15, 16]. There are published recommendations for the management of POC testing programs which include guidance on the education of patient/parents and quality control of the POC INR testing device [17].

Interactions and Problems

Poor INR Control

Control of VKA in children is complicated by numerous factors such as complexity of the underlying health problem(s), multiple intercurrent viral illnesses and variation in the vitamin K content of the child's diet. In infants, additional problems include the challenge of accurate dosing (VKA is often only available in tablet form), increased sensitivity due to physiologically low levels of the vitamin-K dependent clotting factors and differences in vitamin K content of formula (more vitamin K) versus breast milk (less vitamin K). Adolescents can also experience variability in INR due to alcohol intake. VKAs interact with many medications and herbal remedies that may potentiate or reduce the anticoagulant effect [18].

These problems mean that maintenance of INR within target range in children is often poor, with as few as 50% of measurements within range in some studies. This can be improved by close monitoring and awareness of the described problems [2]. Home monitoring and home management programs may also help improve the time in therapeutic target.

Adolescent females taking a VKA should be aware of the risk of teratogenicity in the fetus

Table 5. Recommendations for the reversal of an oral vitamin K antagonist

Speed of reversal required	Clinical scenario(s)	Recommended action
EMERGENCY Immediate	Life-threatening bleeding or bleeding at a critical site[a] Immediate surgery required	Stop warfarin AND 2–5 mg IV vitamin K AND 25–50 U/kg PCC (use 15 mL/kg FP/FFP if PCC unavailable)
URGENT 4–6 h	Major non-life-threatening bleeding[b] Urgent surgery required	Stop warfarin AND 30 µg/kg IV vitamin K
NON-URGENT 24 h	Asymptomatic over-anticoagulation	Omit warfarin AND/OR 1–2 mg oral vitamin K

FP/FFP, fresh plasma/fresh frozen plasma; IV, intravenous; PCC, prothrombin complex concentrate. [a]e.g., intracranial hemorrhage, retroperitoneal hemorrhage, major gastrointestinal hemorrhage, retinal hemorrhage, pericardial hemorrhage. [b]Other significant hemorrhage with >2 g/dL fall in hemoglobin or hemodynamic instability.

should they become pregnant. This issue should be raised in a sensitive manner, but they should be aware that the VKA needs to be stopped immediately on discovery of pregnancy and that an alternative anticoagulant may be required.

Osteopenia

Long-term use of VKAs in children was associated with osteopenia in some studies. While many of these studies lacked adequate control groups, the true cause of the osteopenia (VKAs vs. underlying disease vs. multifactorial) remains unclear. However, a recent long-term follow-up study of Fontan patients with a control group receiving aspirin confirmed a significant effect of warfarin on bone density [19]. As such monitoring of bone mineral density with DEXA scanning on an annual or bi-annual basis in children receiving long-term VKA should be considered.

Reversal

The management needed for the reversal of a VKA depends on the INR, the presence or absence of bleeding symptoms and the indication for anticoagulant therapy.

The options for VKA reversal differ in the time of response (as detailed in Table 5):

- Stopping VKA: 3–5 days.
- Vitamin K: oral vitamin K, 24 h; IV vitamin K, 4–6 h. Doses of 30 µg/kg have been used IV in children [20]. Although there are no published data on the efficacy of VKA reversal using oral vitamin K in children, 1–2 mg as a single dose is often recommended, with a further dose 24 h later if the degree of reversal is inadequate. For children with active bleeding, particularly those who are unlikely to restart a VKA soon, 5 mg oral/IV vitamin K may be given.
- Fresh plasma/Fresh frozen plasma (FP/FFP): 15 mL/kg – immediate effect.

- Prothrombin complex concentrates (PCC): 25–50 IU/kg, dosing may vary depending on product (see Appendix III) – immediate effect.

For VKA associated with major hemorrhage or the need for urgent surgery, rapid reversal of VKA with PCC and IV vitamin K is indicated. If PCC is not available, FP/FFP should be used with IV vitamin K.

For VKA associated with minor hemorrhage – slower reversal with IV or oral vitamin K.

An elevated INR without hemorrhage is usually managed conservatively by omission of one or more VKA doses and monitoring of INR. However, vitamin K may be indicated in asymptomatic cases when there are significant risk factors for bleeding, challenging social circumstances or an anticipated further rise in INR, particularly with INR >9.

Direct Oral Anticoagulants

Introduction

In recent years, there has been much interest in the development of novel oral anticoagulants that directly inhibit specific coagulation factors without the need for an endogenous cofactor. These are broadly divided into two groups according to their target for inhibition: direct thrombin inhibitors (DTIs) and factor Xa (FXa) inhibitors. These agents have advantages over standard anticoagulant therapy in children with UFH, LMWH and VKAs, all of which can be problematic in this patient population for various reasons (refer to sections above). The major advantages are oral administration, predictable anticoagulation response when given as a fixed dose according to bodyweight that obviates the need for monitoring, and a wider therapeutic index. Other advantages include only few interactions with other drugs and a lack of influence of diet and alcohol.

Pediatric development programs have included pediatric studies of the direct thrombin inhibitor (DTI) dabigatran and the FXa antagonists rivaroxaban, apixaban and edoxaban, with some studies still ongoing.

Mechanism of Action and Pharmacokinetics

Dabigatran is a DTI that directly binds to and inhibits thrombin. It inhibits both thrombin that is within clot and circulating thrombin, in comparison to UFH and LMWH which only inhibit circulating thrombin.

Apixaban, betrixaban, edoxaban (removed from the market for business reasons in April 2020) and rivaroxaban, are highly selective inhibitors of FXa. They work independent of AT.

These agents have a rapid onset and relatively short half-life. Rapid absorption results in a peak concentration at 0.5–2 h after administration of dabigatran, 2–4 h after administration of rivaroxaban and 1–4 h for apixaban. Half-life is 12–17 h for dabigatran, 5–9 h for rivaroxaban and 8–15 h for apixaban.

Both classes of DOACs rely on renal elimination to a degree, meaning that the half-life is prolonged in individuals with renal impairment. This is more significant for dabigatran, with 80% renal elimination, than rivaroxaban with 36% or apixaban with 25% renal elimination (Table 6).

Initial pediatric studies used single-dose or short-duration therapy to establish pharmacokinetic characteristics and to assess safety and tolerability. These confirmed in all age groups that administration of a bodyweight-adjusted dose achieved DOAC concentrations that were comparable to adult plasma levels at therapeutic doses [21–25].

Indications

Pivotal clinical studies in pediatric populations have confirmed non-inferiority of rivaroxaban and dabigatran, when compared with standard of care, for the treatment and secondary prevention of VTE in children aged 0–17 years [26–28]. There are no pediatric data to support their use in the treatment of arterial thrombosis. To date, there is only one published study on thrombopro-

Table 6. Pharmacokinetic properties of direct oral anticoagulants

Pharmacokinetic parameter	Dabigatran	Rivaroxaban	Apixaban	Edoxaban	Betrixaban
Bioavailability	3–7%	≈80%	50%	62%	34%
Food dependency	pH dependent	✓	X	X	↓Fatty food
Time to peak, h	0.5–2	2–4	1–4	1–2	3–4
Protein binding	35%	95%	90%	55%	60%
Effect on CYP3A4/P-glycoprotein metabolism	X/✓	✓(33%)/✓	✓(25%)/✓	✓(minor)/✓	X/✓
Number of doses (per 24 h)	× 2	× 1–3	× 2	× 1	× 1
Half-life, h	12–17	5–9	8–15	10–14	19–27
Renal clearance	80%	36%	25%	50%	≈20%
Fecal clearance	82–88%	≈25%	47–56%	≈62%	≈85%

CYP3A4, cytochrome P450 3A4. Adapted from Huisman and Klok [49].

20

phylaxis with rivaroxaban for Fontan patients [29]. Further thromboprophylaxis studies with apixaban and edoxaban are not yet published.

Dosing

Based on the design of the clinical trials, at least 5 days of parenteral anticoagulation (with UFH, LMWH or fondaparinux) is given prior to starting a DOAC for the treatment of VTE in a child. Older children can be administered a DOAC in tablet or capsule form, using the commercially available strengths. Granules for oral suspension (rivaroxaban) and coated granules or powder for oral solution (dabigatran) can be administered to younger children. Dosing is weight-based with 1–3 times daily dosing, according to published schedules [26, 27] as shown in Tables 7 and 9. Dose regimes are also available for thromboprophylaxis with rivaroxaban for children 2 years and above shown in Table 8 [30, 31].

Monitoring

Due to the predictable dose-response relationship of the DOACs there is no requirement for routine monitoring of response in adults and children. Some dose adjustments based on monitoring levels were made in the pediatric dabigatran trials.

Basic coagulation screening is abnormal in the presence of a DOAC. DTIs result in prolonged aPTT and thrombin time (TT), where factor Xa antagonists result in a prolonged PT. DOACs also interfere with many other clotting tests, including those used for the measurement of blood clotting proteins and natural anticoagulants. A reagent, such as DOAC Stop (Haematex Research, Sydney, Australia), can be added to patient plasma to neutralize the effect of a DOAC.

The plasma concentration of DOAC can be measured using a Dilute Thrombin Test (dabigatran) or anti-factor Xa assay (calibrated for the specific FXa antagonist).

Interactions and Problems

Drug Interactions

There are relatively few drug interactions. However, there are some medications which can potentiate or reduce the anticoagulant effect of the DOAC so a full drug history should be taken. In particular concomitant use of strong inhibitors or inducers of both Cytochrome P450 3A4 (CYP3A4) and P-glycoprotein (P-gp) is not recommended, i.e., all human immunodeficiency virus protease inhibitors and azole-antimycotic agents (i.e. ketoconazole, itraconazole, voriconazole, posaconazole).

Table 7. Recommended dosing of rivaroxaban for pediatric therapeutic anticoagulation (birth to <18 years)[a]

Dosage form	Body weight	1 mg rivaroxaban = 1 mL suspension			
		Dosage			Total daily dose
		Once a day[b]	2 times a day[b]	3 times a day[b]	
Oral suspension only	2.6–2.9 kg			0.8 mg	2.4 mg
	3–3.9 kg			0.9 mg	2.7 mg
	4–4.9 kg			1.4 mg	4.2 mg
	5–6.9 kg			1.6 mg	4.8 mg
	7–7.9 kg			1.8 mg	5.4 mg
	8–8.9 kg			2.4 mg	7.2 mg
	9–9.9 kg			2.8 mg	8.4 mg
	10–11.9 kg			3 mg	9 mg
	12–29.9 kg		5 mg		10 mg
Oral suspension or tablets	30–49.9 kg	15 mg			15 mg
	≥50 kg	20 mg			20 mg

[a]Initiate rivaroxaban treatment following at least 5 days of initial parenteral anticoagulant therapy. Patients <6 months of age should meet the following criteria: at birth were at least 37 weeks of gestation, have had at least 10 days of oral feeding, and weigh ≥2.6 kg at the time of dosing. All doses should be taken with feeding or with food since exposures match that of 20 mg daily dose in adults. [b]Once a day: approximately 24 h apart; 2 times a day: approximately 12 h apart; 3 times a day: approximately 8 h apart. Adapted from Xarelto 1 mg/mL granules for oral suspension, Summary of Product Characteristics, European Medicines Agency.

Table 8. Recommended dosing of rivaroxaban for thromboprophylaxis in pediatric patients with congenital heart disease

Dosage form	Body weight	1 mg rivaroxban = 1 mL suspension		
		Dosage		Total daily dose[a]
		Once a day[b]	2 times a day[b]	
Oral suspension only	7–7.9 kg		1.1 mg	2.2 mg
	8–9.9 kg		1.6 mg	3.2 mg
	10–11.9 kg		1.7 mg	3.4 mg
	12–19.9 kg		2 mg	4 mg
	20–29.9 kg		2.5 mg	5 mg
	30–49.9 kg	7.5 mg		7.5 mg
Oral suspension or tablets	≥50 kg	10 mg		10 mg

Adapted from McCrindle et al [29]. [a]All doses can be taken with or without food since exposures match that of 10 mg daily dose in adults. [b]Once a day: approximately 24 h apart; 2 times a day: approximately 12 h apart.

Populations Excluded from Pediatric Clinical Trials

Some groups were excluded from the pediatric clinical trials, including premature and low birth weight infants, infants who had not had a defined period of oral feeding, children with a high risk of bleeding and/or thrombocytopenia, and those with significant renal or liver impairment. The

Table 9. Recommended dosing of dabigatran for pediatric therapeutic anticoagulation

<table>
<tr><th rowspan="2">Weight, kg</th><th colspan="10">Age, years</th></tr>
<tr><th>8 to <9</th><th>9 to <10</th><th>10 to <11</th><th>11 to <12</th><th>12 to <13</th><th>13 to <14</th><th>14 to <15</th><th>15 to <16</th><th>16 to <17</th><th>17 to <18</th></tr>
<tr><td>>81</td><td colspan="2"></td><td colspan="8" rowspan="3">300 mg as two 150 mg capsules
OR
four 75 mg capsules</td></tr>
<tr><td>71 to <81</td><td colspan="2"></td></tr>
<tr><td>61 to <71</td><td colspan="2"></td></tr>
<tr><td>51 to <60</td><td colspan="10">260 mg
as one 110 mg plus one 150 mg capsule
OR
one 110 mg plus two 75 mg capsules</td></tr>
<tr><td>41 to <50</td><td colspan="10">220 mg
as two 110 mg capsules</td></tr>
<tr><td>31 to <41</td><td colspan="10">185 mg
as one 75 mg plus one 110 mg capsule</td></tr>
<tr><td>26 to <31</td><td colspan="8" rowspan="2">150 mg
as one 150 mg capsule
OR
two 75 mg capsules</td><td colspan="2"></td></tr>
<tr><td>21 to <26</td><td colspan="2"></td></tr>
<tr><td>16 to <21</td><td colspan="6">One 110 mg capsule</td><td colspan="4"></td></tr>
<tr><td>13 to <16</td><td colspan="3"></td><td colspan="7"></td></tr>
<tr><td>11 to <13</td><td>One 75 mg capsule</td><td colspan="9"></td></tr>
</table>

Light green shading means that no dosing recommendation can be provided. Adapted from Pradaxa®, Summary of Product Characteristics, European Medicines Agency.

use of DOACs in the treatment of VTE in these populations is not currently supported by clinical trial data, must be done with caution and an alternative agent considered.

DOACs are not used to treat adults with artificial heart valves or antiphospholipid syndrome and current opinion is that they should also be avoided in children with these conditions.

Reversal

Specific antidotes have been developed for the reversal of DOAC anticoagulant effect, Idaracizumab for dabigatran reversal and andexanet alfa for FXa antagonist reversal [32, 33], but the safety and efficacy of these have not been evaluated in a pediatric population. Suggested approaches to the reversal of DOAC in the event of hemorrhage or the need for urgent surgery are as follows:

Stop the Drug

It is important to establish the timing of the most recent dose administered. Once stopped, the time taken for reversal of the anticoagulant effect depends on the half life of the agent and the presence or absence of renal impairment.

Treat Anatomical Causes of Bleeding

This may require endoscopy, invasive radiological procedures (such as vessel embolization) or surgery.

Antifibrinolytic Agents/1-Desamino-8-D-Vasopressin

Antifibrinolytic agents/1-desamino-8-D-vasopressin (DDAVP) may reduce bleeding.

Table 10. Recommended dosing and monitoring for parenteral anticoagulant agents in children

Anticoagulant agent	Mode of administration	Dose	Monitoring test	Target range
Bivalirudin	IV	0.125 mg/kg bolus, followed by 0.125 mg/kg/h infusion	aPTT	60–85 s
Argatroban	IV	0.75 µg/kg/min	aPTT	60–85 s
Fondaparinux	SC	0.1 mg/kg once daily	anti-Xa levels[a], although routine monitoring not required	0.5–1.0 IU/mL

aPTT, activated partial thromboplastin time; IV, intravenous; SC, subcutaneous. [a]This assay must be calibrated with fondaparinux.

Consider FFP/Recombinant Activated Factor VII/PCCs/Activated PCCs

Although these agents have no specific effect against the direct anticoagulant agents, they may be useful. PCCs and activated PCCs (aPCCs) (see Appendix III) are helpful in the reversal of DTIs but recombinant activated factor VII (rFVIIa) is not as its hemostatic effect relies on the generation of a 'thrombin burst'. Due to their high content of FX (see Appendix III), PCCs and aPCCs may be useful in the reversal of direct FXa inhibitors.

Activated Charcoal

Administration of activated charcoal may be effective if given within 6 h of ingestion.

Dialysis

Although this has not been well studied, hemodialysis probably adequately removes dabigatran from the circulation because it is the least protein bound of the oral DTIs.

Parenteral Direct Anticoagulants

These are divided into direct thrombin inhibitors and FXa inhibitors. These parenteral agents may have advantages over heparin with its risk of development of HIT and potential heparin resistance resulting from AT deficiency in infants.

Parenteral Direct Thrombin Inhibitors

Preparations

The two parenteral DTIs that have been used in children are bivalirudin and argatroban. Bivalirudin has been evaluated as an anticoagulant in children, and dosing recommendations are shown in Table 10 [34]. It has also been evaluated in the prevention of TEs during percutaneous coronary intervention, and safety was confirmed in children 0–16 years of age. Dose reduction is required in renal disease. Argatroban has been studied in children requiring alternative anticoagulation to heparin for HIT and was found to prevent VTEs: dosing guidance is shown in Table 10. The dose should be reduced in the presence of hepatic failure as argatroban is metabolized exclusively by the liver. For the parenteral DTIs, the half-life is short, particularly for bivalirudin which has a half-life of approximately 25 min.

Laboratory Monitoring

Bivalirudin and argatroban are monitored using the aPTT or aPTR in a similar way to UFH, although the correlation between laboratory results and drug concentration is poor, and further research is required to clarify the need for and optimal monitoring strategy [34]. Monitoring should occur 4 h after an initial bolus followed by an infusion or 6 h after starting an infusion without a bolus, should be repeated 4 h after each change in dose, and should be requested a minimum of 24 hourly.

Parenteral Factor Xa Inhibitor

Preparations

Fondaparinux is a synthetic pentasaccharide FXa inhibitor which is administered SC as a once daily dose. Fondaparinux acts by binding to and potentiating the effect of AT. There have been only a few reports of fondaparinux cross-reacting with HIT antibodies, so it can be safely used in patients with HIT or who are at risk of HIT. A prospective dose-finding and safety study of fondaparinux in children aged 1–18 years led to the dosing recommendations shown in Table 10. The half-life of fondaparinux is 17–21 h.

Antiplatelet Therapy

Mechanism of Action and Pharmacokinetics

Antiplatelet agents inhibit platelet aggregation and therefore prevent them from performing their role in primary hemostasis. The mechanism of action varies according to the specific agent. Typical antiplatelet agents and their mechanisms of action are listed below.

Acetylsalicylic Acid

Inhibition of the cyclooxygenase enzyme prevents the formation of thromboxane A_2 via the cyclooxygenase pathway (see Chapter 2). The enzyme is irreversibly inhibited, so the effect of acetylsalicylic acid (ASA) can last for 7–10 days after the last dose as this is the duration of time that it takes for new platelets to be generated.

Dipyridamole

Inhibition of adenosine deaminase and phosphodiesterase results in an accumulation of adenosine and cAMP, which causes a reduction in platelet aggregation in response to ADP (see Chapter 2). The effect of dipyridamole lasts for only 12–24 h after the last dose is given.

Clopidogrel/Prasugrel/Ticagrelor

Inhibition of the P2Y12 subtype of the ADP receptor inhibits platelet aggregation by blocking activation of the glycoprotein IIb/IIIa pathway (see Chapter 2). This inhibition is irreversible. Clopidogrel and Prasugrel are pro-drugs, so their effect can be seen for as long as 14 days after the last dose is given due to ongoing conversion of pro-drug to active drug. Ticagrelor is not a pro-drug but has an active metabolite which prolongs its antiplatelet effect. Prasugrel and Ticagrelor are more rapid-acting than Clopidogrel, have a greater anti-platelet effect and result in a higher risk of bleeding.

Other Antiplatelet Agents

There are other classes of antiplatelet agent that are currently in use in adult populations or under development. In general, those which have a more potent and sustained antiplatelet effect carry a higher risk of haemorrhagic complications.

Indications

Antiplatelet agents are usually used to treat and prevent arterial thrombosis. In children, they are most frequently used for the prevention of recurrent ischemic stroke, thrombosis of endovascular stents and for the treatment of Kawasaki disease. In some cases, dual antiplatelet therapy is used to prevent thrombosis of endovascular stents or ventricular assist devices.

Dosing

The doses for the common antiplatelet agents for children are: ASA, 1–5 mg/kg per day; dipyridamole, 2–5 mg/kg per day; clopidogrel, 0.2 mg/kg per day in children 0–24 months and 1 mg/kg per day for older children (rounded to one quarter or one half tablets [75 mg tablets]) [35]. All are given as a single daily dose.

Laboratory Monitoring

The efficacy of antiplatelet agents is usually monitored clinically, i.e., by the assessment of their ability to prevent TEs. The clinical utility of laboratory monitoring of antiplatelet therapy is debated. Platelet aggregation studies may be performed to demonstrate a reduction in platelet response to agonists, including arachidonic acid (inhibited in the presence of ASA) and ADP (inhibited in the presence of dipyridamole or P2Y12 antagonist). The platelet function analyser (PFA-100®) has been shown to be unreliable for the monitoring of aspirin or clopidogrel therapy [36, 37]. Other techniques include Platelet-mapping thromboelastography which uses a global hemostatic test (thromboelastography) to demonstrate inhibition of platelet response to arachidonic acid/ADP, and multiple electrode aggregometry (Multiplate®) to assess response to antiplatelet therapy. Both of these techniques perform analysis using whole blood samples.

Problems

Bleeding

Antiplatelet agents can result in hemorrhagic complications. These usually take the form of mucocutaneous bleeding, i.e., bruising, epistaxis, oral cavity bleeding, but can result in gastrointestinal bleeding and posttraumatic bleeding. Gastrointestinal bleeding is a particular problem with ASA due to its tendency to cause gastric inflammation and ulceration.

Reye's Syndrome

Reye's syndrome is a rare complication of ASA therapy in children usually associated with doses >40 mg/kg. This dose is much higher than that required for antiplatelet therapy and is more consistent with ASA doses when used as an anti-pyretic or analgesic. ASA should not be used for these indications in children. Reye's syndrome may be temporally associated with viral illness and results in hepatitis and encephalopathy with the potential for long-term morbidity and mortality in relation to brain damage.

Reversal

Stopping the antiplatelet agent will reverse the antiplatelet effect within 24 h for dipyridamole, 5–7 days for ASA, and 7–14 days for P2Y12 antagonists. In the case of ongoing or major hemorrhage associated with antiplatelet therapy or the need for urgent surgery, transfusion of platelet concentrate 15 mL/kg should be considered. Transfused platelets will not be sensitive to the effects of ASA or dipyridamole once the agent is stopped, but repeated platelet transfusions may be required for P2Y12 antagonist-related bleeding due to the ongoing production of active drug or metabolite. In life-threatening bleeding, administration of off label rFVIIa could be considered.

Thrombolysis

Mechanism of Action and Pharmacokinetics

The most frequently used thrombolytic agent in pediatric practice is recombinant tissue plasminogen activator (r-tPA, Alteplase®) [38]. r-tPA catalyzes the conversion of plasminogen to plasmin which in turn converts fibrin to fibrin degradation products (FDPs) (see Chapter 2). r-tPA is rapidly metabolized by the liver with a half-life of only 5 min.

Indications and Contraindications

Thrombolysis is reserved for cases of severe arterial or venous thrombosis in which rapid restoration of blood flow is likely to improve outcome either in the short-term or long-term, particularly where there is risk of loss of life, limb or organ (see relevant chapters).

Thrombolysis is contraindicated in the presence of active bleeding, head injury, recent trauma/surgery, recent childbirth, recent cardiopulmonary resuscitation, congenital bleeding disorder and uncontrolled systolic hypertension.

If there are concerns that there may be an intracranial hemorrhage, e.g., in a premature neonate, imaging must be performed to rule this out before commencing thrombolysis.

The decision to administer thrombolytic therapy is often a multidisciplinary one and should involve discussion with the child and/or their parents due to the risk of bleeding complications. Many of the contraindications are 'relative', and the potential benefits of thrombolysis may still outweigh the risks even if contraindications are present.

Dosing

Due to its short half-life, r-tPA is administered by continuous IV infusion.

Systemic Thrombolysis for Venous Thrombosis

While several dosing regimens have been reported, most commonly, r-tPA is administered at a dose of 0.5 mg/kg/h as a continuous infusion for 6 h. A low-dose UFH infusion is administered concurrently at 10 U/kg/h to prevent further thrombus formation. If the child was previously receiving full-dose UFH, the infusion rate must be reduced 30 min prior to starting thrombolytic therapy. The rate is increased to full dose 30 min after completion of a 6-h infusion of r-tPA.

Response to thrombolysis is assessed after 6 h using appropriate imaging, and the course may be repeated if indicated.

Due to physiological deficiency of plasminogen, children <1 year of age receiving thrombolytic therapy are pre-treated with 15 mL/kg FP/FFP to provide a source of plasminogen. Administration of FP/FFP can be considered for older children who fail to respond to thrombolysis.

Catheter-Directed Thrombolysis for Venous Thrombosis

This may be an option if the site of the thrombus can be accessed, e.g., placement of a catheter adjacent to the site of a vascular thrombus. The dose of r-tPA for local thrombolysis varies between centers and can range from 0.01 mg/kg/h to 0.05 mg/kg/h, and in general bleeding increases if the infusion is continued beyond 6 h duration. The dose may be increased if lysis is not achieved.

Systemic Thrombolysis for Stroke

A weight-based total dose of 0.9 mg/kg r-tPA is administered, with a loading dose of 0.1 mg/kg over 1 minute followed by 0.8 mg/kg over the next 1 h. The maximum recommended dose is 90 mg.

Systemic Thrombolysis for Myocardial Infarction

An initial bolus of 0.2 mg/kg r-tPA is administered (maximum 15 mg). This is followed by an infusion of 0.75 mg/kg over 30 min (maximum 50 mg) then an infusion of 0.5 mg/kg over the next 1 h (maximum 35 mg).

Preparation and Monitoring

Children receiving thrombolysis are frequently nursed on a pediatric intensive care unit. All staff should be made aware that thrombolytic therapy is being administered. Baseline bloods include complete blood count (CBC), PT, aPTT, fibrinogen, D-dimer. A crossmatch sample should be sent in case blood transfusion is required.

During thrombolysis, the risk of hemorrhage can be reduced by the avoidance of arterial puncture, catheterization, intramuscular injections, physiotherapy, excessive handling/personal care, ASA/nonsteroidal anti-inflammatory agents.

Most protocols suggest that the CBC, PT, aPTT, fibrinogen and D-dimer should be repeated after 4 h and every 8 h thereafter. The fibrinogen level is expected to fall, and the D-dimer levels are expected to rise. If this does not occur, it may mean that the lysis is not optimal. A platelet count of $>50 \times 10^9$/L should be maintained using infusions of 15 mL/kg platelet concentrate as appropriate (refer to Appendix III for details of platelet dosing).

Management of Thrombolysis-Related Bleeding

Major bleeding during thrombolytic therapy occurs in 10–30% of children. Management de-

Table 11. Assessment of risk of thrombosis and bleeding during interruption of anticoagulant therapy for surgery

Risk of thrombotic event whilst off anticoagulation	
High risk	Recent VTE (within the previous 6 weeks), recurrent VTE, metal prosthetic heart valve (especially mitral), major thrombophilic abnormality[a], antiphospholipid syndrome, stroke
Low risk	Fontan procedure, distant history of VTE, central venous catheter-associated DVT
Risk of bleeding from surgical procedure	
Major bleeding risk	Neuro-/spinal surgery (including lumbar puncture), intra-abdominal surgery, major orthopedic surgery
Minor bleeding risk	Dental extractions, excision of small skin lesion, grommet insertion

DVT, deep vein thrombosis; VTE, venous thromboembolism/thromboembolic event. [a]Antithrombin deficiency; protein S deficiency; protein C deficiency; combined thrombophilic defect, e.g., double heterozygosity for *FVL* variant and prothrombin gene variant.

pends on the severity of the bleeding. The following should be considered: stopping infusion of rt-PA and UFH; use of local measures to achieve hemostasis, such as pressure at wound site or nasal packing; administration of cryoprecipitate to reverse the thrombolytic effect of r-tPA and administration of protamine sulfate to reverse the UFH effect. In major life-threatening bleeding, administration of off label rFVIIa should be considered.

Management of Anticoagulant Therapy during Surgery

Introduction

Anticoagulation during the perioperative period can increase the risk of surgical bleeding. For all anticoagulated children undergoing a surgical procedure, it is essential that there is close communication between the hematology/thrombosis and surgical teams. Anticoagulated children and their parents/caregivers should be advised to inform the hematology/thrombosis team if a surgical or dental procedure is scheduled.

The perioperative management of anticoagulation prior to surgery will depend on the risk of TE whilst off anticoagulant therapy, the type of anticoagulant drug and the nature of the surgery in terms of the bleeding risk (Table 11).

These lists are not comprehensive, and clinical scenarios will often need to be assessed on an individual basis prior to deciding on a plan for the management of anticoagulation therapy during surgery.

Major Risk of Bleeding

Management of Anticoagulation during Surgery with a Major Risk of Bleeding and Low Risk of Thrombosis

Anticoagulant therapy can safely be stopped prior to surgery and restarted postoperatively when the bleeding risk is acceptable. The exact schedule will depend upon the type of anticoagulant therapy due to the variation in half-life between different agents.

Vitamin K Antagonist

In order to allow the INR to fall to <1.5, warfarin is stopped 4–5 days prior to the surgical procedure. The INR is checked on the morning of surgery to ensure that it is safe to proceed. VKA can be restarted within 24 h of surgery if the bleeding risk is felt to be low. In this situation, VKA is usually restarted at the child's usual maintenance dose.

Low-Molecular-Weight Heparin

The last therapeutic dose of tinzaparin or enoxaparin should be given at least 24 h prior to surgery. In patients who are not at excessive risk of thrombosis, it is usual practice to start a prophylactic daily dose of LMWH the evening following surgery (provided that there is no bleeding) and to continue this until the bleeding risk is felt to be low and therapeutic anticoagulation can be restarted.

Unfractionated Heparin

This is stopped 4 h prior to a major surgical procedure and is restarted once the bleeding risk is low, usually at least 24 h after surgery.

Direct Oral Anticoagulant

The last therapeutic dose of DOAC should be given at least 48 h prior to surgery. For children with renal impairment, it may be necessary for the last dose to be given 72 h or more prior to surgery.

Management of Anticoagulation during Surgery with a Major Risk of Bleeding and High Risk of Thrombosis

"Bridging anticoagulant therapy" is needed to ensure that the period of time that the child is not anticoagulated is as short as is safe in terms of the bleeding risk associated with surgery.

Vitamin K Antagonist

The INR should be measured 2–3 days after stopping the VKA and an alternative anti-coagulant agent administered if the INR is below the desired therapeutic INR range. This can be a therapeutic dose of LMWH up until 12–18 h prior to surgery or UFH as an infusion that is stopped 4 h prior to surgery. There are some data to support this approach in children requiring peri-procedural interruption of warfarin anticoagulation [39]. Postoperatively, a UFH infusion may be started 4–6 h after surgery if there is no active bleeding, and this is continued until it is safe to restart LMWH and/or VKA.

Low-Molecular-Weight Heparin

The last dose of LMWH should be given at least 12 h prior to surgery for a twice daily dosing regimen or 18 h prior to surgery for a once daily dosing regimen. A previous study of a small number of children on a twice daily dosing regimen with LMWH has showed residual anti-factor Xa activity was present 12 h after a dose in the majority of those children, so omission of LMWH for at least 24 h may be safer for procedures which carry a high risk of hemorrhage-associated morbidity/mortality, e.g. neuro-/spinal surgery, lumbar puncture [40]. Postoperatively, an UFH infusion may be started 4–6 h after surgery if there is no active bleeding, and this is continued until it is safe to restart the LMWH.

20

Unfractionated Heparin

The UFH infusion should be stopped 4 h prior to surgery and may be restarted 4–6 h after surgery if there is no active bleeding.

Direct Oral Anticoagulant

There are no published pediatric data for bridging anticoagulant therapy in children who are anticoagulated with a DOAC. A similar approach to that used for LMWH can be adopted, using knowledge of the clearance characteristics of the DOAC. Alternatively, switching from a DOAC to LMWH in the immediate pre-operative period may be preferred due to the data that support this approach [39].

In children with an extremely high risk of pulmonary embolism, e.g., in the case of a recent proximal DVT, who are undergoing a surgical procedure with a major risk of bleeding, e.g., brain tumor resection, it may not be safe to allow the child to remain without anticoagulant therapy for the duration of time that is required to prevent surgical bleeding. In this situation, it is appropriate to insert an inferior vena cava (IVC) filter in order to prevent further TE. Anticoagulation can be deferred for up to 14 days after IVC filter insertion. It is recommended that a temporary

IVC filter is inserted and that it is removed as soon as practical as long-term complications of IVC filters can include filter migration (to the heart or pulmonary vessels) and erosion of the IVC wall. Thrombus may form proximal and/or distal to the filter, resulting in PE or significant lower limb swelling. In most cases delaying surgery until anticoagulation can be reasonably withheld is a better option.

Minor Risk of Bleeding

Management of Anticoagulation during Surgery with a Minor Risk of Bleeding

Vitamin K Antagonist

It may not be necessary to stop VKA for some procedures, e.g., dental extraction. An INR measurement on the day of the procedure is advised to ensure that it is not above the desired therapeutic INR range. For other procedures, halving the warfarin dose for 2–3 days prior to the procedure will allow the INR to drift down to the lower part of the therapeutic range allowing the surgery to proceed safely. The usual maintenance dose is reinstated, or a loading dose is given on the evening following surgery.

Low-Molecular-Weight Heparin

It may not be necessary to stop LMWH therapy, but the timing of the dose should be altered so that surgery occurs at the trough level and the LMWH dose is given immediately after the procedure provided that there is no bleeding.

Direct Oral Anticoagulant

It may not be necessary to stop DOAC therapy when the bleeding risk is low but adjusting the timing of the DOAC dose to avoid peak levels at the time of the procedure, similar to LMWH therapy, is appropriate. Stopping a DOAC 24 h prior to a minor procedure and restarting 24 h after has been shown to result in low rates of bleeding and stroke in adults receiving a DOAC for atrial fibrillation [41] but no such data exist in a pediatric population.

Management of Antithrombotic Therapy in Children with Thrombocytopenia

Introduction

Children requiring anticoagulant, antiplatelet, or thrombolytic therapy may become thrombocytopenic for other reasons, most commonly chemotherapy or sepsis. The risk of continuing antithrombotic therapy in thrombocytopenic children is increased risk of bleeding. However, thrombocytopenia in itself is not protective in terms of thrombosis. Generally speaking, children with thrombocytopenia who require antithrombotic therapy fall into two categories: (a) those in whom antithrombotic therapy may be reduced or ceased in relation to the degree of thrombocytopenia as the risk of thrombosis is relatively low; (b) those in whom antithrombotic therapy must be continued due to a high risk of thrombosis and in whom a 'safe' platelet count may need to be maintained using transfusion of platelet concentrates. Management decisions will often need to be individualized according to the particular needs of the child. Published evidence on this topic is limited and recommendations are based on consensus opinion [42].

Anticoagulant Therapy

UFH or LMWH therapy may be given at a reduced intensity in children with thrombocytopenia. Doses are often halved when the platelet count is $<50 \times 10^9$/L and UFH/LMWH is stopped when the platelet count is $<20–30 \times 10^9$/L [42]. Daily monitoring of the platelet count allows for UFH/LMWH to be restarted at half or full dose once the platelet count recovers to the desired threshold. For children who are at a particularly high risk of a TE, e.g. recent TE (within the last 6 weeks), it may be necessary to continue therapeutic doses of UFH/LMWH. In this situation, platelet concentrates may be transfused in order to maintain a platelet count of $>50 \times 10^9$/L. VKA therapy is often avoided in children who are thrombocytopenic or who are likely to become thrombocytopenic, e.g. children receiving chemotherapy. LMWHs or DOACs are preferred due to their shorter half-life.

Thrombolytic Therapy

Thrombolytic therapy is usually reserved for a significant TE that threatens life, limb or organ. A platelet count threshold of $>50 \times 10^9$/L is sometimes recommended prior to thrombolysis. It may be necessary to transfuse platelet concentrates in order to achieve this prior to or concurrent to commencing thrombolytic therapy, depending on the clinical urgency of thrombolysis. In other cases a surgical approach, e.g., embolectomy, may be preferred in a child with thrombocytopenia and a high risk of bleeding.

Antiplatelet Therapy

A platelet count threshold of $>50 \times 10^9$/L is considered by some to be adequate for antiplatelet therapy. Children with a lower platelet count may continue antiplatelet therapy if the risk of thrombosis is considered to be higher than the risk of bleeding. These children should be monitored closely for the occurrence of hemorrhagic symptoms.

Supporting the Child on Anticoagulant Therapy

Anticoagulant therapy carries potential risks, such as bleeding. Anticoagulant medications are considered "high alert" due to the potential for harm when used clinically. Thus, children receiving these medications must be monitored closely.

Local/Regional Anticoagulation Management Service

Having a local or regional anticoagulation service is essential for providing safe and effective care regarding anticoagulation monitoring and dose adjustments, bridging/procedural management, and resumption of anticoagulation therapy after interruption. A multidisciplinary approach to management is recommended, including input from physicians, nurses, pharmacists and even psychologists. All health professionals who prescribe, dispense, and administer these medications must have the competence and knowledge to provide ongoing education to patients and their families and close clinical monitoring [43]. With support from a dedicated anticoagulation management team, patient self-monitoring or self-management of a VKA can be possible via home POC INR testing (refer to section on VKA above).

Safety Measures for Children on Anticoagulation

Sport and Activity Recommendations

Given the potential bleeding risks for children receiving anticoagulation, special consideration must be taken regarding participation in sports and activities. Children with known coordination or balance issues may also need a safety plan in place while on anticoagulant medications.

Contact sports are not recommended, such as ice hockey, American football, boxing and rugby. Children may bruise and bleed more easily from injuries related to these sports. Other activities such as downhill skiing, trampoline or extreme mountain biking are also not recommended. Head protection is important for sports such as cycling or skateboarding, and even tobogganing.

Theme park rides that spin children at high g forces or rapidly accelerate/decelerate should also be avoided due to an increased risk of intracranial hemorrhage in anticoagulated patients.

For children on DOACs or LMWHs, there is the potential for intermittent interruption of anticoagulation to allow for participation in sport (i.e., once weekly), or altering the timing of administration of an anticoagulant in order to avoid peak levels during sport. This is an especially important consideration for the overall management of the child, including both their physical and mental health. While not supported by trial data, the risk benefit of such practice should be discussed with individuals.

Surgical and Dental Considerations

Children undergoing any kind of surgery, including dental work, medical procedures or emergency treatment should disclose they are on anticoagulant medications so that bleeding complications can be avoided or minimized. See above for guidelines on anticoagulation reversal and bridging.

Vaccinations

Vaccines can be given while children are on anticoagulant medications. Due to the risk of intramuscular bleeding with intramuscular injections, consideration should be made to administer vaccines either at trough levels (LMWH) or when the INR is on the lower end of target range when possible. It is also recommended to apply firm pressure directly to the site for approximately 10 min continuously post injection. Many vaccinations can be given via a deep subcutaneous route rather than intramuscular. A small gauge needle should be used where possible.

Medications

Some anticoagulants, especially coumarin derivatives, may interact with several other common drugs including:

- Prescription and non-prescription drugs
- Inhalers
- Topical creams or ointments
- Natural health products
- Alternative therapies
- Herbal remedies
- Homeopathic medicines
- Probiotics
- Amino acids.

It is important for children/parents to disclose any medication changes to their anticoagulation management team prior to initiation to prevent adverse drug interactions. It is equally important to take all medications as prescribed, including anticoagulant medications, and to only follow the advice of the anticoagulation management team for dosing adjustments.

The use of nonsteroidal anti-inflammatory drugs should be avoided in anticoagulated children.

Managing Head Injuries

Head injuries are common among children. Any child taking an anticoagulant medication is at risk for developing significant intracranial hemorrhage from head injury mechanisms, including blunt force or fall from ground level height. Urgent assessment ± CT imaging must be considered for the following:

- Any loss of consciousness following head trauma
- Any mental status changes following head trauma
- Any other sign of concussion (vomiting, dizziness, severe headache)
- History of direct impact to head or neck
- Fall from one level to another.

Managing Frequent Bleeding Complications

While bleeding is a common side effect of anticoagulant medications, most bleeding events are non-life threatening and can be managed conservatively. The first step in managing any significant bleeding event is often to temporarily stop using the anticoagulant. Transfusion of blood products may be needed for more significant bleeding events [44].

Epistaxis

Local measures, such as manual compression, can be useful in the management of epistaxis. If epistaxis persists for greater than 15–20 min, children should seek the advice of the anticoagulant management team or visit the emergency department for further evaluation and intervention (i.e., packing) [45].

Heavy Menstrual Bleeding

Heavy menstrual bleeding (HMB) can also be a common side effect of anticoagulant therapy. Assessment of HMB should be conducted at onset of anticoagulation therapy in post-menarchal females and again after initiation of anticoagulant therapy. Management of HMB while on anticoagulation may include modification of anticoagulant medication, prescribing hormonal therapies or antifibrinolytics, of procedural therapies in severe cases. Females with HMB may be evaluated with periodic laboratory investigations including ferritin and CBC, as well as administration of a validated bleeding assessment tool (BAT) (see Appendix I) [46]. Joint consultations with a haematologist and a gynaecologist in a multi-specialty clinic can be helpful for managing HMB (see Chapter 5).

Emergency Medical Care

Most of the following side effects are uncommon but may be a sign of a serious problem. Families are encouraged to contact the anticoagulation service if any of the following occur:

- Unusual or severe bleeding (e.g., a very long nosebleed, blood in the urine or stools, coughing or throwing up blood or material that looks like coffee grounds, bleeding from cuts or wounds that does not stop
- Dizziness, light-headedness, or fainting
- Severe stomach pain
- Swelling in hands, ankles, or feet
- Numbness, tingling or weakness anywhere in the body, or problems with movement, swallowing or speech
- Signs of a life-threatening reaction including wheezing, shortness of breath, chest tightness or chest pain, swelling of face, lips, or tongue
- Purple discoloration of the toes or soles of the feet, or new pain in a leg, foot, or toes.

Quality of Life and Psychosocial Considerations for Anticoagulated Children

Both short-term and chronic anticoagulation use may impact quality of life and mental health for children and adolescents. For example, young athletes may be prohibited from participating in contact sports during anticoagulant therapy, which can cause psychological harm. Assessing and recognizing the impact of anticoagulants on activity participation should be evaluated so that early intervention can be implemented [47].

HEEADSSS screening (Home; Education & Employment; Activities; Drugs/Drinking; Sex; Self-harm, depression and Suicide; Safety) is also an important consideration for older children and adolescents receiving anticoagulation therapy [48]. This should be assessed at each clinic visit, and additional supports should be coordinated as required (i.e., adolescent medicine, psychology).

Conflict of Interest Statement

Tina Biss has received consultancies, honoraria and educational grant from Bayer, Boehringer Ingelheim and Leo Pharma; Christoph Male has received consultancies and honoraria from Anthos, Bayer, Bristol-Myers-Squibb, Chiesi, Janssen, Norgine, Pfizer and Stago. Jennifer Vincelli has no conflicts of interest to declare. Paul Monagle reports receiving no consultancy and speaker fees. He is recipient of peer reviewed grants (NBA, NHMRC and MRFF schemes within Australia). He is a member of Pedi-ATLAS, a not-for-profit consortium which supports antithrombotic trials in children, and serves as a member of advisory boards (no financial payment) for Bayer, Takeda and Janssen. He was a member of steering committees (no financial payments) for the Einstein junior studies (rivaroxaban/Bayer) and for the SAXOPHONE study (apixaban/Bristal Myer Squibb).

Author Contributions

All authors contributed to the review of data and the writing of this manuscript. All authors have read and approved the final version.

Abbreviations

ACT	Activated clotting time
ADP	Adenosine 5′-diphosphate
Anti-Xa	Anti-factor Xa

aPCC	Activated prothrombin complex concentrate
aPTR	Activated partial thromboplastin ratio
aPTT	Activated partial thromboplastin time
ASA	Acetylsalicylic acid
ASH	American Society of Hematology
AT	Antithrombin
BAT	Bleeding assessment tool
BID	Twice a day
cAMP	Cyclic adenosine monophosphate
CBC	Complete blood count
CPB	Cardiopulmonary bypass
CVC	Central venous catheter
CYP2C9	Cytochrome P450 2C9
CYP3A4	Cytochrome P450 3A4
DDAVP	1-Deamino-8-D-arginine vasopressin (desmopressin)
DOAC	Direct oral anticoagulant
DTI	Direct thrombin inhibitor
DVT	Deep vein thrombosis
ECMO	Extracorporeal membrane oxygenation
ELISA	Enzyme-linked immunosorbent assay
FDP	Fibrin degradation product
FEIBA	FVIII inhibitor bypass activity
FFP	Fresh frozen plasma
FP	Frozen plasma
FX	Factor X
GP	Glycoprotein
HEEADSSS	Home, education, eating, activities/employment, drugs, suicidality, sex, safety
HIT	Heparin-induced thrombocytopenia
HMB	Heavy menstrual bleeding
INR	International normalized ratio
IV	Intravenous
IVC	Inferior vena cava
LMWH	Low-molecular-weight heparin
OD	Once a day
PCC	Prothrombin complex concentrate
PF4	Platelet factor 4
P-gp	P-glycoprotein
PT	Prothrombin time
RCT	Randomized controlled trial
rFVIIa	Recombinant activated factor VII
r-tPA	Recombinant tissue plasminogen activator
SIC	Subcutaneous
TE	Thromboembolism/thromboembolic event
TT	Thrombin time
UFH	Unfractionated heparin
VKA	Vitamin K antagonist
VKOR	Vitamin K epoxide reductase
VKORC1	Vitamin K epoxide reductase complex subunit 1
VTE	Venous thromboembolism/thromboembolic event

References

1 Raffini L, Huang YS, Witmer C, Feudtner C. Dramatic increase in venous thromboembolism in children's hospitals in the United States from 2001 to 2007. Pediatrics. 2009;124(4):1001–8.

2 Monagle P, Chan AKC, Goldenberg NA, Ichord RN, Journeycake JM, Nowak-Göttl U, et al. Antithrombotic therapy in neonates and children: antithrombotic therapy and prevention of -thrombosis, ed 9—American College of Chest Physicians evidence-based clinical practice guidelines. Chest. 2012;141:e737S–801S.

3 Monagle P, Cuello CA, Augustine C, Bonduel M, Brandão LR, Capman T, et al. American Society of Hematology 2018 guidelines for management of venous thromboembolism: treatment of pediatric venous thromboembolism. Blood Adv. 2018;2(22):3292–316.

4 Newall F, Chan AK, Ignjatovic V, Monagle P. Perinatal and paediatric haemostasis Subcommittee of the Scientific and Standardization Committee of the International Society for Thrombosis and Haemostasis: recommendations for developing uniform laboratory monitoring of heparinoid anticoagulants in children. J Thromb Haemost. 2012;10(1):145–7.

5 Ryerson LM, Bauman ME, Kuhle S, Bruce AA, Massicotte MP. Antithrombin concentrate in pediatric patients requiring unfractionated heparin anticoagulation: a retrospective cohort study. Pediatr Crit Care Med. 2014; 15(8):e340–6.

6 Schmidt B, Gillie P, Mitchell L, Andrew M, Caco C, Roberts R. A placebo-controlled randomized trial of antithrombin therapy in neonatal respiratory distress syndrome. Am J Respir Crit Care Med. 1998;158:470–6.

7 Wong TE, Nguyen T, Shah SS, Brogan TV, Witmer CM. Antithrombin concentrate use in pediatric extracorporeal membrane oxygenation: a multicenter cohort study. Pediatr Crit Care Med. 2016;17(12):1170–8.

8 Hicks JK, Shelton CM, Sahni JK, Christensen ML. Retrospective evaluation of enoxaparin dosing in patients 48 weeks' postmenstrual age or younger in a neonatal intensive care unit. Ann Pharmacother. 2012;46(7–8):943–51.

9 Trame MN, Mitchell L, Krümpel A, Male C, Hempel G, Nowak-Göttl U. Population pharmacokinetics of enoxaparin in infants, children and adolescents during secondary thromboembolic -prophylaxis: a cohort study. J Thromb Haemost. 2010;8:1950–8.

10 Dix D, Andrew M, Marzinotto V, Charpentier K, Bridge S, Monagle P, et al. The use of low molecular weight heparin in pediatric patients: a prospective cohort study. J Pediatr. 2000;136:439–45.

11 Bonduel M, Sciuccati G, Hepner M, Feliu Torres A, Pieroni G, Frontroth JP, et al. Acenocoumarol therapy in pediatric patients. J Thromb Haemost. 2003;1: 1740–3.

12 Biss TT, Avery PJ, Brando LR, Chalmers EA, Williams MD, Grainger JD, et al. VKORC1 and CYP2C9 genotype and patient characteristics explain a large proportion of the variability in warfarin dose requirement among children. Blood. 2012;119:868–73.

13 Nowak-Göttl U, Dietrich K, Schaffranek D, Eldin NS, Yasui Y, Geisen C, et al. In pediatric patients, age has more impact on dosing of vitamin K antagonists than VKORC1 or CYP2C9 genotypes. Blood. 2010;116(26):6101–5.

14 Bauman ME, Black K, Kuhle S, Wand L, Legge L, Callen-Wicks D, et al. KIDCLOT©: the importance of validated educational intervention for optimal long-term warfarin management in children. Thromb Res. 2009;123:707–9.
15 Jones S, Monagle P, Manias E, Bruce AA. Quality of life assessment in children commencing home INR self-testing. Thromb Res. 2013;132(1):37–43.
16 Gaw JR, Crowley S, Monagle P, Jones S, Newall F. The economic costs of routine INR monitoring in infants and children – examining point-of-care devices used within the home setting compared to traditional anticoagulation clinic monitoring. Thromb Res. 2013;132(1):26–31.
17 Bauman ME, Bruce A, Jones S, Newall F. Recommendations for point-of-care home International Normalized Ratio testing in children on vitamin K antagonist therapy. J Thromb Haemost. 2013; 11(2):366–8.
18 Bonduel MM. Oral anticoagulation therapy in children. Thromb Res. 2012; 118:85–94.
19 Attard C, Monagle PT, d'Udekem Y, Mackay MT, Briody J, Cordina R, et al. ANZ Fontan Registry Research group. Long-term outcomes of warfarin versus aspirin after Fontan surgery. J Thorac Cardiovasc Surg. 2021;162(4):1218–28.
20 Bolton-Maggs P, Brook L. The use of vitamin K for reversal of over-warfarinisation in children. Br J Haematol. 2002; 118:924.
21 Kubitza D, Willmann S, Becka M, Thelen K, Young G, Brandao LR, et al. Exploratory evaluation of pharmacodynamics, pharmacokinetics and safety of rivaroxaban in children and adolescents: an EINSTEIN-Jr phase I study. Thromb J. 2018;16:31–43.
22 Monagle P, Lensing AWA, Thelen K, Martinelli I, Male C, Santamaria A, et al. EINSTEIN-Jr Phase 2 Investigators. Bodyweight-adjusted rivaroxaban for children with venous thromboembolism (EINSTEIN-Jr): results from three multicentre, single-arm, phase 2 studies. Lancet Haematol. 2019;6(10):e500–9.
23 Halton JM, Lehr T, Cronin L, Lobmeyer MR, Haertter S, Belletrutti M, et al. Safety, tolerability and clinical pharmacology of dabigatran etexilate in adolescents. An open-label phase IIa study. Thromb Haemost. 2016;116(3):461–71.
24 Halton JML, Albisetti M, Biss B, Bomgaars L, Brueckmann M, Gropper S, et al. Phase IIa study of dabigatran etexilate in children with venous thrombosis: pharmacokinetics, safety, and tolerability. J Thromb Haemost. 2017;15(11): 2147–57.
25 Halton JML, Picard AC, Harper R, Huang F, Brueckmann M, Gropper S, et al. Pharmacokinetics, pharmacodynamics, safety and tolerability of dabigatran etexilate oral liquid formulation in infants with venous thromboembolism. Thromb Haemost. 2017;117(11):2168–75.
26 Male C, Lensing AWA, Palumbo JS, Kumar R, Nurmeev I, Hege K, et al. EINSTEIN-Jr Phase 3 Investigators. Rivaroxaban compared with standard anticoagulants for the treatment of acute venous thromboembolism in children: a randomised, controlled, phase 3 trial. Lancet Haematol. 2020;7(1):e18–27.
27 Halton J, Brandão LR, Luciani M, Bomgaars L, Chalmers E, Mitchell LG, et al. DIVERSITY Trial Investigators. Dabigatran etexilate for the treatment of acute venous thromboembolism in children (DIVERSITY): a randomised, controlled, open-label, phase 2b/3, non-inferiority trial. Lancet Haematol. 2021; 8(1):e22–33.
28 Brandao LR, Albisetti M, Halton J, Bomgaars L, Chalmers E, Mitchell LG, et al. DIVERSITY Study Investigators. Safety of dabigatran etexilate for the secondary prevention of venous thromboembolism in children. Blood. 2020; 135(7):491–504.
29 McCrindle BW, Michelson AD, Van Bergen AH, Horowitz ES, Sandoval JP, Justino H, et al. Thromboprophylaxis for children post-Fontan procedure: insights from the UNIVERSE study. J Am Heart Assoc. 2021;10(22):e021765.
30 Zhu P, Willmann S, Zhou W, Yang H, Michelson AD, McCrindle BW, et al. Dosing regimen prediction and confirmation with rivaroxaban for thromboprophylaxis in children after the Fontan procedure: insights from the phase III UNIVERSE study. J Clin Pharmacol. 2022;62(2):220–31.
31 Willmann S, Ince I, Ahsman M, Coboeken K, Zhang Y, Thelen K, et al. Model-informed bridging of rivaroxaban doses for thromboprophylaxis in pediatric patients aged 9 years and older with congenital heart disease. CPT Pharmacometrics Syst Pharmacol. 2022; 11(8):1111–21.
32 Pollack CV, Reilly PA, van Ryn J, Eikelboom JW, Glund S, Bernstein RA, et al. Idarucizumab for dabigatran reversal – full cohort analysis. N Engl J Med. 2017;377(5):431–41.
33 Connolly SJ, Crowther M, Eikelboom JW, Gibson CM, Curnutte JT, Lawrence JH, et al. ANNEXA-4 Investigators. Full study report of andexanet alfa for bleeding associated with factor Xa inhibitors. N Engl J Med. 2019;380(14):1326–35.
34 O'Brien SH, Yee DL, Lira J, Goldenberg NA, Young G. UNBLOCK: an open-label, dose-finding, pharmacokinetic and safety study of bivalirudin in children with deep vein thrombosis. J Thromb Haemost. 2015;13(9):1615–22.
35 Li JS, Yow E, Berezny KY, Bokesch PM, Takahashi M, Graham TP, et al. PICOLO Investigators. Dosing of clopidogrel for platelet inhibition on infants and young children: primary results of the Platelet Inhibition in Children On cLOpidogrel (PICOLO) trial. Circulation. 2008; 117(4):553–9.
36 Schmugge M, Speer O, Kroiss S, Knirsch W, Kretschmar O, Rand ML, et al. Monitoring aspirin therapy in children after interventional cardiac catheterization: laboratory measures, dose response, and clinical outcomes. Eur J Pediatr. 2015; 174(7):933–41.
37 Bartels A, Sarpong Y, Coberly J, Hughes N, Litt J, Quick J, et al. Failure of the Platelet Function Assay (PFA)-100 to detect antiplatelet agents. Surgery. 2015;158(4):1012–9.
38 Williams MD. Thrombolysis in children. Br J Haematol. 2010;148:26–36.
39 Moruf A, Spyropoulos AC, Schardt TQ, Gibson E, Manco-Johnson JM, Wang M, et al. Peri-procedural bridging with low molecular weight heparin in patients receiving warfarin for venous thromboembolism: a pediatric experience. Thromb Res. 2012;130(4):612–5.
40 Dix D, Charpentier K, Sparling C, Massicotte MP. Determination of trough anti-factor Xa levels in pediatric patients on low molecular weight heparin (LMWH). J Pediatr Hematol Oncol. 1998;20:667.

41 Douketis JD, Spyropoulos AC, Duncan J, Carrier M, Le Gal G, Tafur AJ, et al. Perioperative management of patients with atrial fibrillation receiving a direct oral anticoagulant. JAMA Intern Med. 2019; 179:1469–78.
42 Sibson KR, Biss TT, Furness CL, Grainger JD, Hough RE, Macartney C, et al, on behalf of the British Society for Haematology. BSH guideline: management of thrombotic and haemostatic issues in paediatric malignancy. Br J Haematol. 2018;180:511–25.
43 Testa S, Paoletti O, Zimmermann A, Bassi L, Zambelli S, Cancellieri E. The role of anticoagulation clinics in the era of new oral anticoagulants. Thrombosis. 2012;2012:835356.
44 Hanigan S, Barnes GD. Managing anticoagulant-related bleeding in patients with venous thromboembolism. American College of Cardiology 2019. https://www.acc.org/Latest-in-Cardiology/Articles/2019/10/07/14/29/Managing-Anticoagulant-related-Bleeding-in-Patients-with-Venous-Thromboembolism [accessed 25 January 2024].
45 L'Huillier V, Badet C, Tavernier L. Epistaxis complicating treatment by antivitamin K and new oral anticoagulants. Eur Ann Otorhinolaryngol Head Neck Dis. 208;135(4):231–5.
46 Bannow B. Management of heavy menstrual bleeding on anticoagulation. Hematol Am Soc Hematol Educ Program. 2020;2020(1):533–7.
47 Bastas D, Vincelli J, De R, Benia E, Gairdner S, Brandao LR, Avila L. Impact of deep vein thrombosis on adolescent athletes: navigating an invisible disability. Res Pract Thromb Haemost. 2022; 6(5):e12779.
48 Jones S, Mertyn E, Alhucema P, Monagle P, Newall F. HEEADSSS assessment for adolescents requiring anticoagulation therapy. Arch Dis Child. 2012; 97(5):453.
49 Huisman MV, Klok FA. Pharmacological properties of betrixaban. Eur Heart J Suppl. 2018;20(suppl E):E12–5.

Published online: December 5, 2024

Blanchette VS, Brandão LR, Carcao MD, Kumar R, Rand ML, Revel-Vilk S (eds): SickKids Handbook of Pediatric Thrombosis and Hemostasis, ed 3, rev. and ext. Basel, Karger, 2024, pp 411–422 (DOI: 10.1159/000538203)

Genetic Testing and Counseling for Inherited Bleeding and Clotting Disorders

Riyana Babul-Hirji[a] Vanessa Bouskill[b] Jennifer Vincelli[b] Manuel D. Carcao[c]

[a]Department of Molecular Genetics and Department of Genetic Counselling, Hospital for Sick Children, Toronto, ON, Canada; [b]Department of Nursing, Hospital for Sick Children, Toronto, ON, Canada; [c]Division of Haematology/Oncology, Department of Paediatrics, Hospital for Sick Children, Toronto, ON, Canada

Introduction

Recent advances in genetic and genomic technologies have resulted in a dramatic increase in the availability of genetic testing for many hematological conditions. Some of the reasons for offering genetic testing to the patient and/or family include establishing or confirming a diagnosis, carrier testing, predictive/presymptomatic testing, and prenatal diagnosis. Because of the inherent complexities of genetic testing and the uniqueness of information that can be divulged (e.g., implications to other family members), obtaining informed consent is of paramount importance. The implications to other family members are particularly an issue when dealing with conditions, such as inherited thrombophilia, that simply increase the risk of, but do not necessarily cause disease states. This chapter elaborates on the aims of pursuing genetic testing, key aspects of various testing methodologies, the informed consent process, and the importance of obtaining family trees (pedigrees), and concludes with options that are currently available for prenatal diagnosis. Thrombophilia testing and hemophilia carrier testing are used to illustrate many of the issues pertaining to genetic testing for bleeding and clotting disorders.

Issues to Consider when Organizing Genetic Testing

The decision to offer genetic testing should consider its potential benefits as well as its limitations and risks. The clinical utility of genetic testing is reviewed in the next section. Equally important is the anticipation of potential downstream effects resulting from genetic testing including social, legal, and ethical implications to both the patient and/or their extended family. Examples of downstream effects include privacy/confidentiality of results in the family context, potential insurance discrimination, predictive testing of children/adolescents where such results would have no impact on their clinical management/treatment until adulthood, duty to (re)contact should new information arise regarding the disease, and unveiling of secondary findings, i.e., those findings not related to the indication for testing but clinically relevant (e.g., pathogenic variant in a breast cancer gene) [1, 2]. Such issues represent important topics of discussion during the informed consent process and decision-making regarding genetic testing. Ideally, an interdisciplinary team approach involving social worker, hematology specialists, and genetic counselors is optimal to facilitate best practices in patient and family centered care.

Once the potential benefits, as well as the limitations and risks of genetic testing, have been considered and if the decision is to proceed, the next steps in this process include deciding which type of test to order, what sample to obtain from the patient, and which specialized laboratory to utilize.

Deciding Which Type of Test to Order

When a particular clinical diagnosis is being considered and is known to be caused by one gene (e.g., hemophilia A or B, disorders of fibrinogen, Glanzmann thrombasthenia), then testing for variants within the relevant gene (vs. panel testing) is recommended. Such testing of a single gene is generally performed by Sanger sequencing. In Sanger sequencing, the laboratory looks for sequence alterations or pathogenic variants (i.e., mutations) within the suspected gene. For some disorders, where the mechanism of disease has been shown to be associated with a deletion or duplication of part of a gene, it may be worthwhile to request that the laboratory perform deletion/duplication analysis in addition to sequence analysis. Genetic testing can lead to three possible results: (1) the finding of a clearly pathogenic variant (which previously was generally referred to as a mutation), (2) the finding of normal sequencing, or (3) the discovery of variants that have not been previously reported as being pathogenic; these would be classified as variant(s) of unknown significance (VUS). Testing of parents and potentially of other affected and unaffected family members may be recommended to facilitate interpretation of the clinical significance of a VUS. The finding of a VUS can often be challenging, not only for the clinician but also for families trying to understand the relevance to their own/their child's condition. With the increasing availability of panel testing, more VUS are being identified. Occasionally with time, some VUS get reclassified as true disease-causing variants if more individuals with the condition are reported to have the same variant.

When multiple genes are known to cause a particular condition (e.g., familial thrombocytopenia), then a targeted gene panel approach using next-generation sequencing (NGS) technology may be more cost-effective, efficient, and likely to find a genetic explanation for the condition. Some panels contain many genes, whereas others contain a more limited repertoire. When both single gene and panel genetic testing fail to identify the underlying pathogenic variant(s), and depending on the clinical scenario, further testing may be considered. This can include a more expanded gene panel, whole exome sequencing (WES), or whole genome sequencing (WGS) [3]. WES analyzes the exonic (coding) regions of all the genes, whereas WGS evaluates not only the exonic regions but also the intronic (noncoding) regions (see Table 1 for the pros and cons of these different approaches). With the decreasing cost of WES/WGS and increasing clinical validity and utility, WES/WGS may become the test of choice over single gene or targeted gene panel testing for either complex genetic traits or conditions in which the precise genetic etiology is unclear.

Specific to children, the Canadian Paediatric Society has published a position statement outlining a number of recommendations when considering genetic testing in children, keeping in mind the best interests of the child [4]. In brief, the recommendation is to do single gene analysis or targeted gene panels, when possible, rather than WES or WGS.

Table 1. A comparison of genetic sequencing technologies

	Sanger[a]	Targeted panel	Whole exome	Whole genome
Uses	• Disorders caused by one gene (e.g., WAS, hemophilia A, hemophilia B)	• Genetically heterogeneous disorders (e.g., inherited thrombocytopenias)	• Genetically heterogeneous disorders and for gene discovery	• Used now in research setting mostly for gene discovery • Beginning to be used clinically
Pros	• Very accurate (gold standard in sequencing) • Inexpensive • Quick turnaround time	• Can adjust panel to add more genes as needed • Low chance of secondary findings • Cost-effective for disorders caused by many genes (e.g., Noonan syndrome)	• Looks at all genes (no bias) • Fairly cost-effective when a patient does not fit the typical presentation of a disorder (i.e., no good targeted panel available) • Easy to reanalyze patient results at a future date to look for new genes	• Looks at all genetic material, not just exons and therefore can find variants in noncoding regions
Cons	• Low diagnostic yield for genetically heterogeneous diseases • Slow turnaround time if looking at many genes (low throughput) • Expensive if looking at more than one gene	• Laboratory design and redesign required • Higher chance of finding VUS compared with Sanger	• Cannot detect disorders caused by trinucleotide repeats • Cannot look at noncoding regions • Risk of uncovering secondary findings	• Data analysis bottleneck • Difficult to interpret because of many variants found • Expensive and time-consuming • Risk of uncovering secondary findings

VUS, variant(s) of unknown significance; WAS, Wiskott-Aldrich syndrome. [a]For the purposes of this table, Sanger refers to the sequencing of a single gene.

21

Given that genomic testing is associated with complexities in data interpretation along with potential ethical/legal social implications, families should be made aware of the availability of genetic counseling, which would include a discussion of the informed consent process.

Informed Consent Process

Genetic testing results can potentially predict future health status and indicate potential health risks for the person being tested as well as for other family members. There is the possibility that such results may lead to discrimination/stigmatization and cause psychological harm. Thus, the pretest counseling session with the patient and family should include key elements as summarized in Table 2. This informed consent process empowers families to make educated decisions regarding testing. When a child/adolescent is not capable of making such decisions, then informed consent is obtained from the parents/legal guardians with the goal of supporting the best interests of the child [4]. However, the child/adolescent should be involved in the informed consent process where possible and depending on the decision-making capacity of the child/adolescent (i.e., assent).

Table 2. Discussion points to include in the pretesting counseling session

- Best testing strategy (i.e., single gene vs. targeted gene panel testing vs. WES/WGS dependent on the clinical scenario)
- Review of the risks/benefits/limitations/consequences and possible test outcomes (e.g., benign, likely benign, VUS, likely pathogenic, pathogenic)
- Turnaround time for results
- Testing to be undertaken by a clinical or a research laboratory
- Possible psychosocial ramifications
- Managing expectations
- Insurability
- Confidentiality of results

VUS, variant of unknown significance; WES, whole exome sequencing; WGS, whole genome sequencing.

Table 3. Resources to assist with locating a clinical laboratory for genetic testing

Global genetic testing resources	• Genetic Testing Registry: http://www.ncbi.nlm.nih.gov/gtr/ • Orphanet: https://www.orpha.net/en/diagnostic-tests/laboratories • Concert genetics (USA labs only): www.concertgenetics.com

Deciding What Type of Sample to Obtain from the Patient

Genetic testing can be undertaken on DNA extracted from blood, cells obtained from the inside of the cheek (i.e., buccal swab), cultured fibroblasts, and lymphoblasts. Certain conditions (e.g., vascular malformations – see Chapter 12) are usually caused by somatic pathogenic variants for which testing requires obtaining tissue from the affected area. Depending on the type of technology to be used for the genetic test in question, the laboratory may have specific sample requirements. The best approach is to directly contact the receiving genetic testing laboratory to confirm logistics or verify sample requirements from their website.

Selecting the Appropriate Laboratory

Many factors are involved in choosing the appropriate laboratory for testing. In some situations, testing may be done "in-house," or there may be a standing agreement to utilize specific laboratories. Depending on the rarity of the condition, there may only be one clinical laboratory worldwide offering the test (see Table 3). In general, factors to consider when selecting a laboratory are: (i) what technology is the laboratory using for the genetic test (e.g., sequencing only, sequencing and deletion/duplication); (ii) the specificity and sensitivity of the test; (iii) turn-around time for results; (iv) cost; and (v) whether the laboratory undertaking the test is a research or clinical laboratory. Clinical laboratories are always the preferred option as they are accredited facilities that must maintain rigorous standards of quality control and accuracy. However, when the test in question is not offered by a clinical laboratory but offered as part of a research study, then it is standard practice among genetics health care providers to replicate research results that may be used in the provision of delivering health care to individual patients.

Coverage for genetic testing may vary depending on geographic region. In some jurisdictions, testing may be covered through government-supported programs. In other jurisdictions, coverage may involve insurance companies or even the individual family being responsible for the cost of testing. Even when the cost of testing is covered through government health-care funding, there is likely still a need for application and prior approval to be done prior to the send out of the sample for testing.

Clinical Utility of Genetic Testing

In deciding whether to proceed with genetic testing, clinicians often evaluate if knowing the underlying genetic etiology would help with clinical decision-making, treatment, and/or management (i.e., direct patient care). However, the results of a genetic test may also be of benefit to patients/families for reproductive decision-making, psychosocial reasons, and cascade testing for other at-risk family members.

As genetic testing for diagnostic purposes is often done in young children, it is important that when an individual transitions from pediatric to adult care they receive information about their condition (clinical presentation, medical management, and genetics) [5, 6]. Although the results of genetic testing performed on a child would have been communicated to the parents, it likely occurred at a time when the child was too young to comprehend, and the child (now an adolescent) may have very little understanding of their genetic condition and its implications for their future and future reproductive planning.

Diagnosis/Management

Confirming or ruling out a known or suspected hematological disorder in a child with disease symptoms may be beneficial from a clinical management and treatment perspective. Some examples include the following:

1. *Genetic testing for hemophilia (F8 or F9 gene on the X chromosome).* This is particularly helpful in cases of mildly reduced factor VIII (FVIII) levels, which can be caused by mild hemophilia A, von Willebrand disease (VWD) subtype 2N (see Chapter 9), or by a combined deficiency of factor V and FVIII (see Chapter 10). In these settings, finding a pathogenic variant in the *F8* gene or *F9* gene may establish the diagnosis. Additionally, determining the causative variant for hemophilia is useful in predicting the severity of hemophilia and especially in estimating the risk of developing inhibitors against FVIII or factor IX (FIX) (see Chapter 8). Most importantly knowing the causative genetic variant allows for carrier detection in at-risk females within the extended family (discussed later).
2. *Genetic testing for VWD (VWF gene on chromosome 12).* This can help in differentiating between VWD subtypes with similar phenotypes (e.g., 2M vs. type 1) as well as differentiating subtypes of VWD that mimic other non-VWD disorders: type 2N VWD vs. mild hemophilia A and type 2B VWD vs. platelet-type VWD (see Chapter 9). It may also be important in determining the risk of inhibitor development to VWF in those with type 3 VWD (risk highest in those with a finding of a large deletion variants).
3. *Genetic testing for familial thrombocytopenias.* Determining the causative gene responsible for this may have significant implications as many inherited thrombocytopenias have additional nonplatelet pathologies, including hearing loss, cataracts, and renal failure (in MYH-9 macrothrombocytopenias) and predisposition to myeloid leukemias in thrombocytopenias caused by variants in the genes *RUNX*, *ANKRD26*, or *ETV6* (see Chapter 6).
4. *Genetic testing in syndromic disorders with bleeding symptoms.* Patients sometimes are referred to a hematologist because of bleeding symptoms in the setting of what appears to be a syndromic-type disorder (e.g., Noonan syndrome, Ehlers-Danlos syndrome (EDS), hereditary hemorrhagic telangiectasia (HHT), Hermansky-Pudlak syndrome (HPS), 22q11 deletion syndrome). In such settings, genetic testing may establish/confirm the suspected diagnosis. For a discussion on some of these conditions, please refer to Chapters 4, 6, and Appendix IV.

Predictive Testing

In addition to diagnostic testing, genetic testing has other uses, including predictive testing, where finding a variant can predict disease. An example of this is HHT, a condition associated with many features that only appear as the child ages: skin telangiectasias, arterial-venous fistulas in the brain, liver, and lungs, and bleeding symptoms (see Appendix IV). If a parent has the disorder and the causative pathogenic variant is known, given that the inheritance is autosomal dominant, testing the at-risk asymptomatic child is possible (i.e., predictive testing). However, careful consideration and preparatory discussion should be pursued with the family regarding the possible psychological impact (i.e., assigning a diagnosis prior to symptom presentation) and ramifications of a positive or negative result. In such cases, pretest counseling should include a review of possible problems and options regarding obtaining life insurance/disability insurance. For those conditions that present in adulthood rather than in childhood, published guidelines recommend against predictive testing in children if there is no effective treatment or medical benefit. Testing is typically deferred until such a time when the child/adolescent can participate in the decision-making process regarding genetic testing [4, 7].

Inherited thrombophilia (inherited predisposition to clotting) testing fits into this category of predictive testing. Children often undergo testing to determine if they carry an underlying genetic predisposition to thrombotic disease; this can be either because they have had a thrombotic event themselves or because of a family history of a thrombotic event with or without a known thrombophilia within the family (see Chapter 13). These thrombophilias are discussed in depth in Chapter 13. Below, we only discuss thrombophilia testing in asymptomatic children.

The decision to perform thrombophilia testing in asymptomatic children and adolescents in families with known thrombophilia or when first-degree relatives have experienced unprovoked clots should be made on an individual basis after discussion with the family. The final decision regarding whether to test is likely to vary depending upon the clinical situation and the family's preference [8]. For example, there are ethical issues and potential life insurance implications of genetic screening in children who may lack the understanding and maturity to make an informed decision. Additionally, with the lack of an identified thrombophilia trait in an affected family member, negative testing may provide false security.

It should be noted that finding a thrombophilia in a child can "open up a can of worms" as it raises the question: does one of the parents (who may be completely asymptomatic) carry the same thrombophilia variant and if so, do the child's sibling(s)? The same heightened concern may then extend to more distant family members: grandparents, uncles, aunts, and cousins. Therefore, when deciding whether to test or not, all this should be discussed with the family. Furthermore, finding a thrombophilia variant does not necessarily predict disease (thrombotic event) as many persons with an inherited thrombophilia may never experience a thrombotic event or if they do, not until late adulthood.

Carrier Testing

Identification of a pathogenic variant(s) in a child, depending on the inheritance, allows for carrier testing of the parent(s), which in turn facilitates the option of prenatal diagnosis. This information would especially be valuable for a couple whose child has an autosomal recessive disorder (e.g., severe rare factor deficiencies, type 3 VWD, afibrinogenemia) or an X-linked disorder (e.g., hemophilia, Wiskott-Aldrich syndrome [WAS]). In autosomal recessive disorders, both parents would likely be asymptomatic carriers, and for each of their pregnancies, there would be a 25% risk of the child being affected. In X-linked disorders, the child's mother is likely to be a carrier (she may or may not be symptomatic), and in such a scenario, each of her sons would have a

50% risk of being affected, whereas each of her daughters would have a 50% chance of being a carrier.

Regarding other at-risk family members, the option of familial variant targeted testing is available. Sharing of such information within and between families can sometimes be challenging because of familial relationships/dynamics and potential stigmatization (i.e., guilt, blame from self or partner). Some family members may wish not to know about their at-risk carrier status, and consequently, disclosure of such information may breach their right to autonomy (i.e., they have a right not to know). Additionally, carrier testing in children, for the sole purpose that this information may be useful for future reproductive planning of this child, should be deferred until the child can provide informed consent [9].

Importance of Family Trees

A pedigree (also known as family tree) is a diagram showing the relationships between people in several generations of a family. Taking a pedigree is an important consideration in the clinic setting as it can help to identify those at risk of being carriers or of being affected with the condition under consideration. A comprehensive discussion of how to construct pedigrees is beyond the scope of this textbook. Instead, the reader is referred to a recent paper by Bennett et al. [10]. However, some useful suggestions when obtaining pedigrees for disorders of hemostasis and thrombosis will be alluded to.

It is important to be systematic in drawing a pedigree. One should begin first with the proband, then move on to their siblings, followed by their parents and their parents' siblings, followed by the children of those siblings, followed by the next generation (i.e., grandparents and their siblings). Without a systematic approach, obtaining a family history can easily become confusing and convoluted.

For autosomal recessive disorders such as type 3 VWD and many other rare factor deficiencies inherited in the same manner, when obtaining a family history, determining if there is a history of consanguinity in parents is important. For X-linked disorders such as hemophilia, it is paramount to obtain an accurate family history on the maternal side. This should go far back enough to identify any potential carriers within the family and to possibly determine in whom did the "hemophilia variant first begin". Invariably, in families with hemophilia (particularly mild or moderate hemophilia), there are likely to be additional affected males who may be undiagnosed, and it should be recognized that for every male with hemophilia, it is hypothesized that there are likely to be two or three female carriers of hemophilia. Additionally, if patients are going to be followed for many years as most hemophilia patients are, it should be appreciated that pedigrees will change over time, and so it is useful to maintain a pedigree that can be altered as the family "grows." Given this, it is better to record the year of birth of individuals rather than age as age will change over time, whereas the year of birth will not.

Figure 1 gives an example of how a properly constructed pedigree can reveal individuals within the family who have remained undiagnosed and can identify carriers of hemophilia unaware of their status. In this case, a 2-year-old male presented with oral bleeding, and investigations showed mild hemophilia A (FVIII 6%). Further questioning revealed that the child's maternal grandfather had a history of bleeding suggesting a lifelong bleeding disorder. Additionally, the maternal grandfather's brother also had suffered from, and subsequently died from bleeding. Eventually, at age 68, the grandfather was tested and confirmed to have mild hemophilia A (FVIII 9%). Based on analysis of the pedigree, 10 female members within the family were identified to be obligate carriers, and additionally, a cousin of the proband at age 5 was also diagnosed with mild hemophilia A (FVIII 7%). Other female members

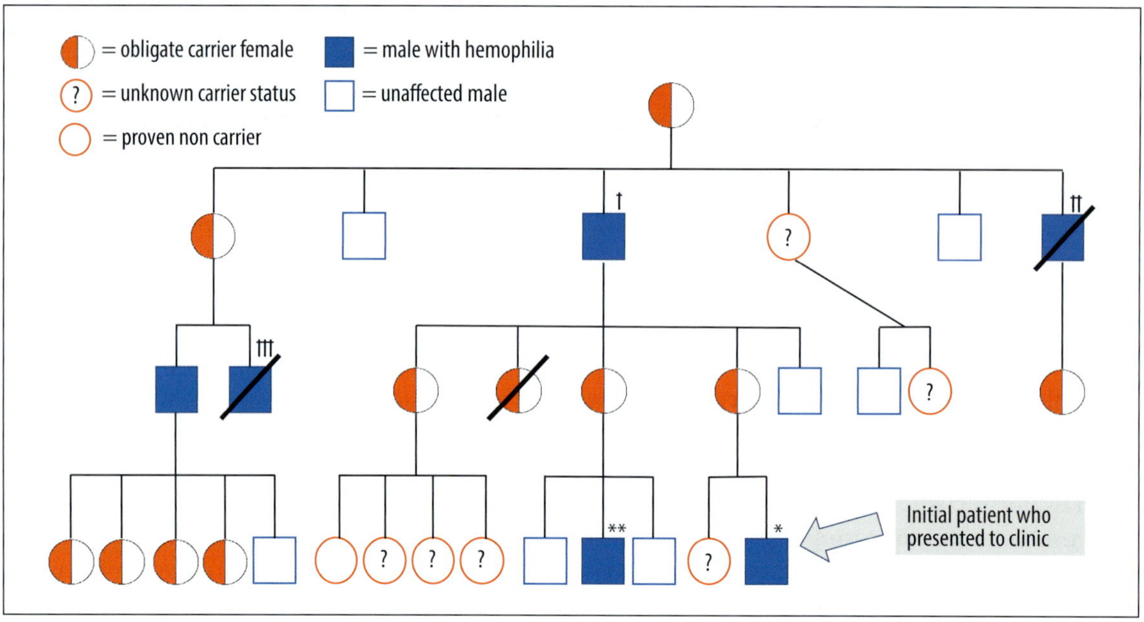

Fig. 1. Family tree of a family with mild hemophilia A (personal communication – M. Carcao). *Proband – diagnosed at age 2 with mild hemophilia A. **Subsequently diagnosed with mild hemophilia A. †History of significant bleeding with trauma; subsequently tested and diagnosed with mild hemophilia A at age 68. ††Died of a traumatic intracranial hemorrhage at age 21. †††Died at age 27 from bleeding.

within the family have a 50% chance of also being carriers, which raises several issues regarding hemophilia carrier testing (see below).

Hemophilia Carrier Testing

Determining carrier status in females can be done in several ways depending on whether there is a family history of hemophilia.

Determining Carrier Status in Women with a Family History of Hemophilia

Given that hemophilia is an X-linked disorder, taking a pedigree may make it obvious that certain female members in the family may be obligate carriers. This includes all daughters of a man with hemophilia and all women with an affected son as well as another first-degree male relative (another son, brother, uncle, or cousin) with hemophilia.

Women (e.g., mothers, grandmothers, or sisters of a boy with hemophilia) who have a family history of hemophilia (but are not obligate carriers) can be made aware of the availability of carrier testing if the familial pathogenic variant is known and provided that the woman herself can provide informed consent.

Other laboratory markers suggestive of carrier status, such as prolonged activated partial thromboplastin time (aPTT), low FVIII or FIX levels, or reduced ratio of FVIII to VWF, are useful but are not definitive to correctly diagnose carrier status [11].

Determining Carrier Status in Women with No Family History of Hemophilia

Very rarely, a woman with abnormal bleeding might be found to have a low FVIII or FIX level not explained by VWD, Vitamin K deficiency, or liver disease. In such cases, when no other obvious explanation for bleeding exists, then genetic testing for hemophilia may be indicated. The above scenario is rare as most carriers of hemophilia will either not have a lot of bleeding symptoms and hence are not likely to undergo testing, or if they do, their factor levels are not likely to be low enough to result in being identified as potential carriers. Therefore, carriers (in families without a family history of hemophilia) are likely to go undetected or may only be diagnosed if they have affected sons or grandsons with hemophilia. Until that occurs, they usually remain undiagnosed.

Being a carrier of hemophilia has implications for future reproductive planning, thus carrier testing should ideally only be offered when a woman is of the age to make decisions for herself, after genetic counseling. It should be noted that young girls suspected of being carriers of hemophilia can still undergo testing for factor levels (e.g., prior to surgery) if there is a concern that such a girl could be at risk of bleeding.

Prenatal Diagnosis

Prenatal diagnosis is available for couples who have a child with a hematological condition where the pathogenic variant causing the child's condition is known as well as for confirmed female carriers of an X-linked condition. Reasons why couples choose prenatal diagnosis are varied and can include preparing themselves psychologically for the birth of an affected child, for management purposes at delivery (e.g., a male fetus predicted by prenatal diagnosis to be affected with hemophilia), or for the purpose of terminating the pregnancy. Couples interested in prenatal diagnosis should be referred to a medical genetics service prior to embarking on a pregnancy for a discussion of their available options. In this way, if genetic testing has not yet been undertaken to identify the pathogenic variant(s), it can be organized prior to achieving a pregnancy. This would also provide the couple with an opportunity to receive anticipatory guidance or counseling, i.e., reviewing the various possible outcomes of prenatal diagnosis so that the couple can begin to explore their feelings. Initiating such discussions prior to undertaking a pregnancy and before the return of possible positive results may facilitate the process of decision-making for the couple. Prepregnancy counseling also provides an opportunity to explore with the couple their feelings regarding preimplantation genetic diagnosis (PGD).

Some couples may choose to terminate a pregnancy for a hematological condition even if treatment is available if the family's perception of the burden of the disease is overwhelming (e.g., time lost from work, cost of treatment, and stigma in certain ethnic groups). The burden of many bleeding disorders (particularly hemophilia) has lessened with newer therapies, and it is important that families have up-to-date information on the disease as part of their informed decision-making process. Regardless of what the family chooses, the provision of information to families by the clinician should be tailored to support the family's personal interests, beliefs, and values.

Invasive Prenatal Testing

Currently, there are two prenatal diagnostic procedures (chorionic villus sampling [CVS] and amniocentesis) available to couples who wish to know whether the fetus is affected with the condition that they are at risk for. Details of these options are presented in Table 4. These procedures differ in timing: amniocentesis is performed later in the pregnancy than CVS. If a family decides to proceed with amniocentesis for example, then results from the genetic testing on amniotic fluid/cultured cells would be available later in pregnancy, and this could influence the mode of termination that would be available to the family should they decide to abort an affected fetus (e.g., dilation and curettage vs. dilation and evacuation vs. induction of labor with medication). As the prenatal diagnosis procedures available and abortion options may vary depending on the center, a referral to the local medical genetics service is recommended for any family considering prenatal diagnosis.

Table 4. Prenatal diagnosis options: chorionic villus sampling and amniocentesis

Prenatal diagnosis procedure	Timing of procedure	Details	Risk of miscarriage	Reasons for choosing
Chorionic villus sampling	11.5–14 weeks of gestation	Under ultrasound guidance, sample of chorionic villus tissue is obtained either transvaginally or transabdominally depending on location of placenta	~1%	• Anxious to know if fetus affected, but results would not influence outcome of the pregnancy, i.e., would continue the pregnancy even if affected • Would consider terminating an affected fetus
Amniocentesis	After ~15.5 weeks of gestation	Under ultrasound guidance, amniotic fluid (~30 mL) is removed, which contains cells that the fetus has shed. Often, these cells need to be cultured (can take up to ~2 weeks) prior to DNA analysis, which may prolong time for return of results	~0.5–1%	• Anxious to know if fetus affected, but results would not influence outcome of the pregnancy, i.e., would continue the pregnancy even if affected • For management purposes, e.g., male fetus predicted to be affected with hemophilia. Delivery recommendations would take this information into account • Would consider terminating an affected fetus

Preimplantation Genetic Diagnosis

In simplistic terms, PGD is a test where after in vitro fertilization, cells from the developing embryo are obtained, and DNA testing is done for the genetic condition in question. Embryos free of the condition are transferred to the uterus. PGD can also be undertaken together with human leukocyte antigen (HLA) typing for choosing an HLA-matched sibling in relevant cases (e.g., a sibling needing hematopoietic stem cell transplantation for Fanconi anemia). Follow-up invasive prenatal testing, either by CVS or amniocentesis, is recommended to confirm the results obtained from PGD because of the possibility of a false result. As per recommendations by the Society of Obstetrics and Gynecologists in Canada, "before PGD is performed, genetic counseling must be provided by a certified genetic counselor to ensure that patients fully understand the risk of having an affected child, the impact of the disease on an affected child, and the benefits and limitations of all available options for preimplantation and prenatal diagnosis". Couples should be referred to their local medical genetics service to obtain further information and receive the appropriate counseling.

Noninvasive Prenatal Testing

Noninvasive prenatal testing (NIPT) is a screening test that analyzes cell-free fetal DNA in maternal blood. Quantitative differences in chromosome fragments in maternal blood can be used to screen for trisomy 13, 18, and 21 and for extra or missing sex (X or Y) chromosomes. A blood sample for NIPT can be obtained from the mother as early as 10 weeks of gestation. The use of NIPT to test for single gene disorders has been slow to develop due in part to technical challenges. However, specific to X-linked conditions, such as hemophilia or WAS, NIPT can be used to identify female bearing pregnancies (by detecting the absence of Y-chromosome fragments) with a high degree of accuracy, thereby eliminating the need for invasive testing. Conversely, if the results show the presence of Y-chromosome fragments, then the option of having CVS/amniocentesis to determine if the male fetus is affected or not with the X-linked disorder is available. Prior to NIPT, some couples choose to have an ultrasound to determine the fetal sex prior to deciding on invasive testing; however, with the availability of NIPT, the fetal sex can be determined at a much earlier gestational age compared with ultrasound. As NIPT is a screening test and has limitations to its clinical application, interested families should be referred to a medical genetics service for counseling.

Conclusions

As progress has continued to be made in the discovery of genes causing hematological conditions, genetic testing has become more widespread in the clinic setting. There are many reasons for initiating genetic testing, including making/confirming a diagnosis, carrier testing of at-risk individuals, predictive testing, and prenatal diagnosis. Given the multitude of genetic testing platforms available, careful consideration needs to be given to choosing the most appropriate test, whether it be a single gene test or a panel approach. As genetic testing has limitations, it is important that patients be made aware of the risks as well as the benefits so that their decision to proceed with testing is informed.

Conflict of Interest Statement

Riyana Babul-Hirji reports no conflict of interests. Vanessa Bouskill reports having received research support from Novo Nordisk and Roche and honoraria for speaking/participating in advisory boards from Bayer, Bioverativ/Sanofi, Novo Nordisk, Pfizer, Roche, and Shire/Takeda. Jennifer Vincelli reports no conflict of interests. Manuel Carcao reports having received research support from Bayer, Bioverativ/Sanofi, Novartis, Novo Nordisk, Pfizer, Roche, and Shire/Takeda and honoraria for speaking/ participating in advisory boards from Bayer, Bioverativ/Sanofi, CSL Behring, LFB, Novo Nordisk, Pfizer, Roche, and Shire/Takeda.

Author Contributions

All authors (Riyana Babul-Hirji, Vanessa Bouskill, Jennifer Vincelli, and Manuel Carcao) wrote different parts of this chapter, and all authors reviewed and revised the chapter and approved the final version for submission.

Abbreviations

aPTT	Activated partial thromboplastin time
CVS	Chorionic villus sampling
EDS	Ehlers-Danlos syndrome
FIX	Factor IX
FVIII	Factor VIII
HHT	Hereditary hemorrhagic telangiectasia
HLA	Human leukocyte antigen
HPS	Hermansky-Pudlak syndrome
NGS	Next-generation sequencing
NIPT	Noninvasive prenatal testing
PGD	Preimplantation genetic diagnosis
VUS	Variant(s) of unknown significance
VWD	von Willebrand disease
VWF	von Willebrand factor
WAS	Wiskott-Aldrich syndrome
WES	Whole exome sequencing
WGS	Whole genome sequencing

References

1 Scott J, Trotter T. Primary care and genetics and genomics. Pediatrics. 2013; 132(suppl 3):S231–7.
2 Clifton JM, VanBeuge SS, Mladenka C, Wosnik KK. The Genetic Information Nondiscrimination Act 2008:what clinicians should understand. J Am Acad Nurse Pract. 2010;22(5):246–9.
3 Boycott K, Hartley T, Adam S, Bernier F, Chong K, Fernandez BA, et al. The clinical application of genome-wide sequencing for monogenic diseases in Canada: position statement of the Canadian College of Medical Geneticists. J Med Genet. 2015;52(7):431–7.
4 Moore AM, Richer J. Genetic testing and screening in children. Paediatr Child Health. 2022;27(4):243–53.
5 Transition to adult care for youth with special health care needs. Paediatr Child Health. 2007;12(9):785–93.
6 Szybowska M, Hewson S, Antle BJ, Babul-Hirji R. Assessing the informational needs of adolescents with a genetic condition: what do they want to know? J Genet Couns. 2007;16(2):201–10.
7 Committee on Bioethics; Committee on Genetics; American College of Medical Genetics and Genomics Social, Ethical, and Legal Issues Committee. Ethical and policy issues in genetic testing and screening of children. Pediatrics. 2013; 131(3):620–2.
8 Raffini L, Thornburg C. Testing children for inherited thrombophilia: more questions than answers. Br J Haematol. 2009; 147(3):277–88.
9 Borry P, Fryns JP, Schotsmans P, Dierickx K. Carrier testing in minors: a systematic review of guidelines and position papers. Eur J Hum Genet. 2006; 14(2):133–8.
10 Bennett RL, French KS, Resta RG, Austin J. Practice resource-focused revision: standardized pedigree nomenclature update centered on sex and gender inclusivity: a practice resource of the National Society of Genetic Counselors. J Genet Couns. 2022;31(6):1238–48.
11 Labarque V, Perinparajah V, Bouskill V, Stain AM, Wakefield C, Manuel C, et al. Utility of factor VIII and factor VIII to von Willebrand factor ratio in identifying 277 unselected carriers of hemophilia A. Am J Hematol. 2017;92(6):E94–6.

Published online: December 5, 2024

Blanchette VS, Brandão LR, Carcao MD, Kumar R, Rand ML, Revel-Vilk S (eds): SickKids Handbook of Pediatric Thrombosis and Hemostasis, ed 3, rev. and ext. Basel, Karger, 2024, pp 423–430 (DOI: 10.1159/000538209)

Bleeding Assessment Tools

Margaret L. Rand[a, b] Sara J. Israels[c, d] Victor S. Blanchette[a, e] Paula D. James[f]

[a]Division of Haematology/Oncology, Research Institute, Hospital for Sick Children, Toronto, ON, Canada; [b]Department of Laboratory Medicine & Pathobiology, University of Toronto, Toronto, ON, Canada; [c]Department of Pediatrics and Child Health, University of Manitoba, Winnipeg, MB, Canada; [d]CancerCare Manitoba Research Institute, Winnipeg, MB, Canada; [e]Department of Pediatrics, University of Toronto, Toronto, ON, Canada; [f]Department of Medicine, Queen's University, Kingston, ON, Canada

Introduction

The assessment of subjects referred for evaluation of a possible inherited or acquired bleeding disorder should include three key elements: (1) a carefully obtained bleeding history from the subject and close relatives, including details of consanguinity; (2) a detailed physical examination with a focus on the identification of physical findings that may provide important clues regarding an underlying diagnosis (e.g., presence of cutaneous telangiectasia(s) in cases with recurrent epistaxis and hereditary hemorrhagic telangiectasia); and (3) selected laboratory tests (see Chapter 4).

With regard to obtaining a bleeding history, there have been significant advances over the past 15 years in the development and evaluation of standardized bleeding questionnaires targeted at the investigation of subjects with inherited hemostatic disorders such as von Willebrand disease (VWD) (see Chapter 9) and platelet function disorders (see Chapter 6) in which bleeding symptoms are predominantly mucocutaneous [1–5]. In this Appendix, we provide details of a general Bleeding Assessment Tool (BAT) developed through a consensus of international experts (International Society on Thrombosis and Haemostasis [ISTH]-BAT) and two organ-specific BATs (Pictorial Blood Loss Assessment Chart [PBAC] and an epistaxis score). For details on bleeding questionnaires/scores for acquired bleeding disorders such as immune thrombocytopenia (ITP) or inherited coagulation deficiencies such as hemophilia, the reader is referred to Chapters 7 and 8.

The ISTH/SSC BAT

The ISTH-BAT is a standardized BAT developed by members of an ISTH/SSC Joint von Willebrand factor (VWF) and Perinatal/Pediatric Hemostasis Subcommittee Working Group (Table 1) [5]. The goal of the Working Group was to develop a standardized bleeding questionnaire with a well-defined interpretation grid allowing for the

Table 1. International Society on Thrombosis and Haemostasis-Bleeding assessment tool (ISTH-BAT) scoring key, with permission from Elsevier [5]

Symptom	0[a]	1[a]	2	3	4
Epistaxis	No/trivial	>5/year or more than 10 min	Consultation only[b]	Packing, cauterization, or antifibrinolytics	Blood transfusion or replacement therapy (use of hemostatic blood components and rFVIIa), or desmopressin
Cutaneous	No/trivial	For bruises 5 or more (>1 cm) in exposed areas	Consultation only[b]	Extensive	Spontaneous hematoma requiring blood transfusion
Bleeding from minor wounds	No/trivial	>5/year or more than 10 min	Consultation only[b]	Surgical hemostasis	Blood transfusion, replacement therapy, or desmopressin
Oral cavity	No/trivial	Present	Consultation only[b]	Surgical hemostasis or antifibrinolytics	Blood transfusion, replacement therapy, or desmopressin
GI bleeding	No/trivial	Present (not associated with ulcer, portal hypertension, hemorrhoids, angiodysplasia)	Consultation only[b]	Surgical hemostasis or antifibrinolytics	Blood transfusion, replacement therapy, or desmopressin
Hematuria	No/trivial	Present (macroscopic)	Consultation only[b]	Surgical hemostasis, iron therapy	Blood transfusion, replacement therapy, or desmopressin
Tooth extraction	No/trivial or none done	Reported in ≤25% of all procedures, no Intervention[c]	Reported in >25% of all procedures, no Intervention[c]	Resuturing or packing	Blood transfusion, replacement therapy, or desmopressin
Surgery	No/trivial or none done	Reported in ≤25% of all procedures, no intervention[c]	Reported in >25% of all procedures, no intervention[c]	Surgical hemostasis or antifibrinolytics	Blood transfusion, replacement therapy, or desmopressin
Menorrhagia	No/trivial	Consultation only[b] or Changing pads more frequently than every 2 h or Clot and flooding or PBAC score >100[d]	Time off work/ school >2/year or Requiring antifibrinolytics or hormonal or iron therapy	Requiring combined treatment with antifibrinolytics and hormonal therapy or Present since menarche and >12 months	Acute menorrhagia requiring hospital admission and emergency treatment or Requiring blood transfusion, replacement therapy, desmopressin or Requiring dilatation and curettage or endometrial ablation or hysterectomy
Postpartum hemorrhage	No/trivial or no deliveries	Consultation only[b] or Use of syntocin or Lochia >6 weeks	Iron therapy or Antifibrinolytics	Requiring blood transfusion, replacement therapy, desmopressin or Requiring examination under anesthesia and/or the use of uterine balloon/ package to tamponade the uterus	Any procedure requiring critical care or surgical intervention (e.g., hysterectomy, internal iliac artery legation, uterine artery embolization, uterine brace sutures)
Muscle hematomas	Never	Post-trauma, no therapy	Spontaneous, no therapy	Spontaneous or traumatic, requiring desmopressin or replacement therapy	Spontaneous or traumatic, requiring surgical intervention or blood transfusion

Table 1 (continued)

Symptom	0[a]	1[a]	2	3	4
Hemarthrosis	Never	Post-trauma, no therapy	Spontaneous, no therapy	Spontaneous or traumatic, requiring desmopressin or replacement therapy	Spontaneous or traumatic, requiring surgical intervention or blood transfusion
CNS bleeding	Never	–	–	Subdural, any intervention	Intracerebral, any intervention
Other bleedings[e]	No/trivial	Present	Consultation only[b]	Surgical hemostasis, antifibrinolytics	Blood transfusion, replacement therapy, or desmopressin

The full questionnaire is available online at http://www1.wfh.org/docs/en/Resources/Assessment_Tools_ISTHBAT.pdf.
CNS, central nervous system; GI, gastrointestinal; PBAC, Pictorial Blood Loss Assessment Chart; rFVIIa, recombinant activated factor VII.
[a]Distinction between 0 and 1 is of critical importance. Score 1 means that the symptom is judged as present in the patient's history by the interviewer but does not qualify for a score of 2 or more. [b]Consultation only: the patient sought medical evaluation and was either referred to a specialist or offered detailed laboratory investigation. [c]Example: 1 extraction/surgery resulting in bleeding (100%): the score to be assigned is 2; 2 extractions/surgeries, 1 resulting in bleeding (50%): the score to be assigned is 2; 3 extractions/surgeries, 1 resulting in bleeding (33%): the score to be assigned is 2; 4 extractions/surgeries, 1 resulting in bleeding (25%): the score to be assigned is 1. [d]If already available at the time of the collection. [e]Include: umbilical stump bleeding, cephalohematoma, cheek hematoma caused by sucking during breast/bottle feeding, conjunctival hemorrhage, or excessive bleeding following circumcision or venipuncture. Their presence in infancy requires detailed investigation independently from the overall score.

calculation of a total bleeding score (BS) that could be used in the assessment of children and adults referred for evaluation of a possible inherited bleeding disorder such as VWD or a platelet function disorder. In their report [5], members of the Working Group stressed the following:

1. "Administration of the questionnaire will require some degree of assessor training (typically performed by a physician or other health professional) to ensure reliability and to reduce time load";
2. "To improve the predictive value of the BAT (for the diagnosis of bleeding disorders), only symptoms reported before and at the time of diagnosis should be included";
3. "The validity, reliability, and predictive power of the new BS will need to be tested prospectively".

The Working Group was assisted in their task by previously published standardized bleeding questionnaires in children and adults with suspected or proven VWD and inherited platelet function disorders; in children, this was the Pediatric Bleeding Questionnaire (PBQ), which included pediatric-specific bleeding symptoms [1–4].

An important consideration in the clinical use of a standardized BS is the "cutoff" score that should be used to differentiate between normal and abnormal, adjusted for age (the pediatric population) and sex (adult females vs. males). An abnormal ISTH-BAT BS for children younger than 18 years of age (male or female) is ≥3; it is ≥6 for adult females and ≥4 for adult males [6]. A recognized limitation of BSs in the pediatric population is that the subject under consideration may have had limited experience with hemostatic challenges that would result in abnormal bleeding and indicate the possibility of an underlying bleeding disorder. In the pediatric population, the importance of a detailed family history with a focus on abnormal bleeding cannot be overemphasized.

Recent guidelines from the American Society of Hematology (ASH), ISTH, National Hemophilia Foundation (NHF), and World Federation of Hemophilia (WFH) on the diagnosis of VWD [7] strongly recommend that for patients with a low probability of VWD (e.g., seen in the primary care setting), a validated BAT be used as an initial screening test to determine whether they require

Date of start: ____________________ Month / Day / Year **Score:** ____________

Pad	Days 1	2	3	4	5	6	7	8
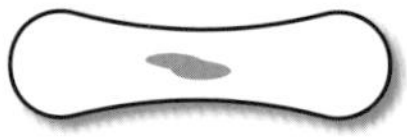								
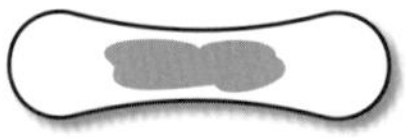								
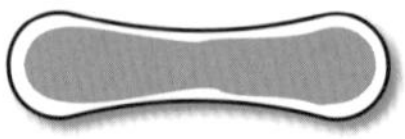								
Clots (size)								

Tampon	Days 1	2	3	4	5	6	7	8
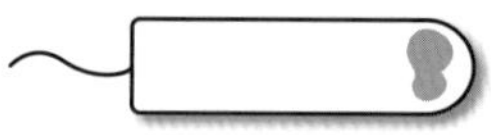								
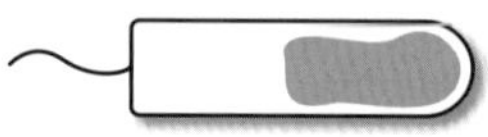								
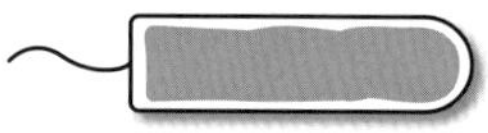								
Clots (size)								

Fig. 1. Pictorial Blood Loss Assessment Chart (PBAC), adapted from Higham et al. [14]. A mark is to be made in the appropriate box for each item of sanitary protection used. Then, using the scales below, the total score is calculated by adding up the sum of all scores for the tampons or sanitary napkins used in the menstrual cycle. For pads (sanitary napkins; towels): 1 for lightly stained, 5 for moderately soiled, and 20 for completely saturated pads. For tampons: 1 for lightly stained, 5 for moderately soiled, and 10 for completely saturated tampons. Passage of clots is also recorded, with a score of 1 for small and 5 for large clots. The possible range of the total score is completely dependent on the quantitative and qualitative amount of bleeding during menstruation. Abnormal PBAC BS ≥100, which correlates with menorrhagia, defined as >80 mL of menstrual blood loss. App version "Sisterhood" can be downloaded for free from App store/Google Play.

specific laboratory testing. For patients with an intermediate probability of VWD (e.g., referred to a hematologist), the guidelines suggest against relying on a BAT to decide whether to order specific laboratory testing; for patients with a high probability of VWD (e.g., with an affected first-degree relative), this is a strong recommendation. In these latter cases, BATs can be used to assess and document the severity of bleeding and can be used in conjunction with specific laboratory testing as part of the initial diagnostic approach.

To inform on the evolution of bleeding in a patient, the BAT can be repeated at follow-up visits but should only include interval bleeding, i.e., bleeding that has occurred since the previous assessment [8].

A practical consideration with any assessment tool is the average time taken to administer the tool by a trained health care professional. For the ISTH-BAT, an estimated average time of 10 min (range: 5–20 min) is required. To allow bleeding questionnaire self-completion (i.e., completion by the patient/parent or guardian) rather than expert administration, Casey et al. [9] generated, optimized, and validated the Self-PBQ, as distinguished from the Self-BAT, validated for completion by adult patients [10]. In addition, an electronic self-administered pediatric BAT (eBAT) has now been validated [11].

A free on-line version of the Self-BAT is available on the Let's Talk Period website (http://letstalkperiod.ca); it provides a BS and indicates whether it is normal/abnormal according to the ISTH-BAT "cutoffs," i.e., for children up to 18 years of age, an abnormal score is ≥3.

Versions of (pediatric) BATs are available in French (http://letstalkperiod.ca), German, Italian, Norwegian, Spanish, and Thai [12, 13].

Pictorial Blood Loss Assessment Chart

The PBAC is a validated semiobjective tool to measure menstrual blood loss (Fig. 1) [14]. A score ≥100 has a sensitivity and specificity of ≥80% for a diagnosis of heavy menstrual bleeding, defined as blood loss of ≥80 mL for the whole menstrual cycle [14]. The chart allows detailed recording of sanitary material (tampons/towels) graded as lightly stained, moderately soiled, or completely saturated. In addition, passage of blood clots (graded as small or large) and episodes of flooding are recorded. The chart is to be completed by the patients prospectively for the next menstrual cycle. If completed for the most recent menstrual cycle during an interview with a health care professional, the average time taken to administer the PBAC is estimated to be 10 min (range: 7–20 min). The sanitary materials for which the PBAC was originally validated (in 1990) have been discontinued, and recently, it has been validated using newer products with different absorbencies to ensure accuracy when scoring blood loss (Fig. 2a, b) [15].

Given the wide variety of sanitary material that is available commercially and used by women during the menstrual cycle, reference gynecology/bleeding disorders clinics are required to establish local well-defined interpretation guides for use when administering the PBAC. Attention should also be paid to cultural sensitivities when selecting the health care professional to administer the PBAC.

The period tracking app, WeThrive (https://play.google.com/store/apps/details?id=com.iwk.wethrive&pcampaignid=web_share), developed for teenagers younger than 18 years of age, identifies heavy menstrual bleeding by recording the duration of bleeding and the number of sanitary products used along with their staining pattern. Most other period tracking apps provide a general indication of menstrual blood loss only.

Epistaxis Score

A simple-to-administer questionnaire for recurrent epistaxis (five or more spontaneous nose bleeds per year) was reported by Katsanis et al. [16]

a

Pad	Type	New PBAC score
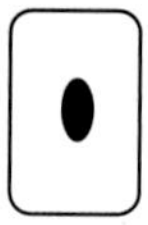	Regular	2
	Heavy	3
	Night	4
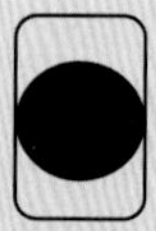	Regular	9
	Heavy	13
	Night	20
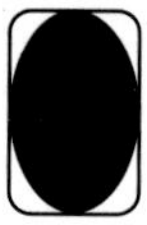	Regular	18
	Heavy	24
	Night	40
Flooding	Regular	25
	Heavy	34
	Night	55

b

Tampon	Type	New PBAC score
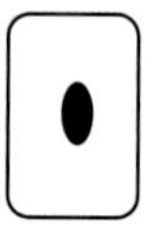	Regular	1
	Super	1
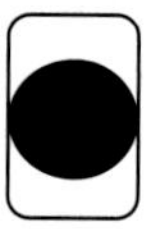	Regular	2
	Super	3
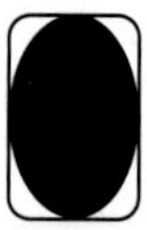	Regular	3
	Super	4
Flooding	Regular	4
	Super	7

Fig. 2

(For legend see next page.)

Table 2. Epistaxis scoring system, with permission from Elsevier [16]

Component	Score[a]
Frequency	
5–15/year	0
16–25/year	1
>25/year	2
Duration	
<5 min	0
5–10 min	1
>10 min	2
Amount[b]	
<15 mL	0
15–30 mL	1
>30 mL	2
Epistaxis history/age[c]	
<33%	0
33–67%	1
>67%	2
Site	
Unilateral	0
Bilateral	2

Available online at http://www1.wfh.org/docs/en/Resources/Assessment_Tools_Epistaxis.pdf.
[a] Sum of scores for all components: mild = 0–6; severe = 7–10. [b] Estimation of average blood loss per episode, based on fractions or multiples of teaspoons, tablespoons, or cups. [c] Proportion of the child's life that nosebleeds have been recurrent (>5/year).

Fig. 2. Pictorial Blood Loss Assessment Chart (PBAC) for modern sanitary products of different absorbencies, with permission from Wiley [15]. **a** The original scoring system from Higham et al. [14] was adjusted for use of the All-Nighter® Extra Heavy CleanWear® Ultra Thin Heavy Flow and CleanWear® Ultra Thin Regular Flow (U by Kotex®; Kimberly-Clark, Mississauga, ON) products. The new validated PBAC scores for each pad were adjusted so that 80 mL of blood loss corresponded with a PBAC score of 100. **b** The original scoring system from Higham et al. [14] was adjusted for use of the Click® Tampons Regular and Super Compact (U by Kotex®; Kimberly-Clark, Mississauga, ON). The pictograms above do not look like tampons as the same pictograms were used for pads and tampons when participants scored. The new validated PBAC scores for each tampon were adjusted so that 80 mL of blood loss corresponded with a PBAC score of 100.

in 1988 (Table 2). It includes questions related to the frequency, duration, and amount of blood loss with each episode of epistaxis, duration of epistaxis over the patient's life span, and site (unilateral vs. bilateral). Each element scores from 0 to 2 with a total score that ranges from 0 to 10 (worse affected). This epistaxis score has not been formally studied with regard to its measurement properties, i.e., reliability, validity, and responsiveness to change (e.g., interventions such as nasal cautery). It is attractive because of its ease of administration (<5 min) and its focus on a bleeding symptom that appears early in life and is not sex specific.

Closing Remarks

General and organ-specific standardized BATs are useful for the assessment of subjects referred for evaluation of an underlying bleeding disorder. Common symptoms in children younger than 18 years of age with these disorders include recurrent epistaxis and, in adolescent females who have started menstruation, heavy menstrual bleeding. Careful attention should be paid to the age at onset of abnormal bleeding symptoms; children with severe epistaxis starting early in life, or adolescent females with a history of excessive menstrual bleeding for 6–12 months postmenarche, are more likely to have an underlying bleeding disorder as compared with others without such a history.

Conflict of Interest Statement

Margaret L. Rand has no conflicts of interest to declare. Sara J. Israels has no conflicts of interest to declare. Victor S. Blanchette reports receiving consultancy and speaker fees from Bayer HealthCare, Novo Nordisk, Pfizer, Roche, Takeda, and Spark Therapeutics. He is recipient of research grants from Sanofi-Genzyme, Bayer HealthCare, and Takeda and serves as a member of Data Safety Monitoring Boards for Octapharma and Takeda. He is Chair of a nonprofit organization, the International Prophylaxis Study Group (IPSG). Paula

D. James receives research funding from Bayer and has performed consultant work for Band Therapeutics and Star Therapeutics.

Author Contributions

Margaret L. Rand drafted the Appendix, critically revised the Appendix, and approved the final version. Sara J. Israels critically revised the Appendix and approved the final version. Victor S. Blanchette critically revised the Appendix and approved the final version. Paula D. James critically revised the Appendix and approved the final version.

Abbreviations

ASH	American Society of Hematology
BAT	Bleeding Assessment Tool
BS	Bleeding score
eBAT	Electronic self-administered pediatric BAT
ISTH	International Society on Thrombosis and Haemostasis
ITP	Immune thrombocytopenia
NHF	National Hemophilia Foundation
PBAC	Pictorial Blood Loss Assessment Chart
PBQ	Pediatric Bleeding Questionnaire
SSC	Scientific and Standardization Committee
VWD	von Willebrand disease
VWF	von Willebrand factor
WFH	World Federation of Hemophilia

References

1 Rodeghiero F, Castaman G, Tosetto A, Batlle J, Baudo F, Cappelletti A, et al. The discriminant power of bleeding history for the diagnosis of type 1 von Willebrand disease: an international, multicenter study. J Thromb Haemost. 2005; 3(12):2619–26.

2 Tosetto A, Rodeghiero F, Castaman G, Goodeve A, Federici AB, Batlle J, et al. A quantitative analysis of bleeding symptoms in type 1 von Willebrand disease: results from a multicenter European study (MCMDM-1 VWD). J Thromb Haemost. 2006(4);4:766–73.

3 Bowman M, Riddel J, Rand ML, Tosetto A, Silva M, James PD. Evaluation of the diagnostic utility for von Willebrand disease of a pediatric bleeding questionnaire. J Thromb Haemost. 2009;7(8): 1418–21.

4 Biss TT, Blanchette VS, Clark DS, Bowman M, Wakefield CD, Silva M, et al. Quantitation of bleeding symptoms in children with von Willebrand disease: use of a standardized pediatric bleeding questionnaire. J Thromb Haemost. 2010; 8(5):950–6.

5 Rodeghiero F, Tosetto A, Abshire T, Arnold DM, Coller B, James P, et al. ISTH/SSC bleeding assessment tool: a standardized questionnaire and a proposal for a new bleeding score for inherited bleeding disorders. J Thromb Haemost. 2010;8(9):2063–5.

6 Elbatarny M, Mollah S, Grabell J, Bae S, Deforest M, Tuttle A, et al. Normal range of bleeding scores for the ISTH-BAT: adult and pediatric data from the merging project. Haemophilia. 2014(6); 20:831–5.

7 James PD, Connell NT, Ameer B, Di Paola J, Eikenboom J, Giraud N, et al. ASH ISTH NHF WFH 2021 guidelines on the diagnosis of von Willebrand disease. Blood Adv. 2021;5(1):280–300.

8 Lavin M, Christopherson P, Grabell J, Abshire T, Flood V, Haberichter SL, et al. Longitudinal bleeding assessment in von Willebrand disease utilizing an interim bleeding score. J Thromb Haemost. 2022;20(10):2246–54.

9 Casey LJ, Tuttle A, Grabell J, Hopman W, Moorehead PC, Blanchette VS, et al. Generation and optimization of the self-administered pediatric bleeding questionnaire and its validation as a screening tool for von Willebrand disease. Pediatr Blood Cancer. 2017;64(10): e26588.

10 Deforest M, Grabell J, Albert S, Young J, Tuttle A, Hopman WM, James PD. Generation and optimization of the self-administered bleeding assessment tool and its validation as a screening test for von Willebrand disease. Haemophilia. 2015; 21(5):e384–8.

11 Kaur D, Kerlin BA, Stanek JR, O'Brien SH. Use of electronic self-administered bleeding assessment tool in diagnosis of paediatric bleeding disorders. Haemophilia. 2021;27(5):710–6.

12 James PD, Mahlangu J, Bidlingmaier C, Mingot-Castellano ME, Chitlur M, Fogarty PF, et al. Evaluation of the utility of the ISTH-BAT in haemophilia carriers: a multinational study. Haemophilia. 2016; 22(6):912–8.

13 Pakdeeto S, Natesirinilkul R, Komwilaisak P, Rand ML, Blanchette VS, Vallibhakara SA, et al. Development of a Thai version of the paediatric bleeding assessment tool (Thai paediatric-BAT) suitable for use in children with inherited mucocutaneous bleeding disorders. Haemophilia. 2017;23(6):e539–42.

14 Higham JM, O'Brien PMS, Shaw RW. Assessment of menstrual blood loss using a pictorial chart. Br J Obstet Gynaecol. 1990(8);97:734–9.

15 Spence M, de Repentigny K, Bowman M, Hopman W, Thibeault L, James P. Validation of the pictorial blood loss assessment chart using modern sanitary products. Haemophilia. 2021;27(5): e632–5.

16 Katsanis E, Luke KH, Hsu E, Li M, Lillicrap D. Prevalence and significance of mild bleeding disorders in children with recurrent epistaxis. J Pediatr. 1988;113(1 Pt 1):73–6.

Appendix II

Published online: December 5, 2024

Blanchette VS, Brandão LR, Carcao MD, Kumar R, Rand ML, Revel-Vilk S (eds): SickKids Handbook of Pediatric Thrombosis and Hemostasis, ed 3, rev. and ext. Basel, Karger, 2024, pp 431–446 (DOI: 10.1159/000538189)

Reference Ranges for Common Tests of Bleeding and Clotting

Ahmad Al-Huniti[a] Rajiv K. Pruthi[b] Margaret L. Rand[c] Laura Avila[c] Paul Monagle[d]

[a]Pediatric Hematology Oncology, Mayo Clinic, Rochester, MN, USA; [b]Hematology, Mayo Clinic, Rochester, MN, USA; [c]Division of Hematology/Oncology, The Hospital for Sick Children, Toronto, ON, Canada; [d]Division of Clinical Hematology, The Royal Children's Hospital Melbourne, Melbourne, VIC, Australia

Any laboratory test is only of value in distinguishing health from disease if the clinician knows what is normal for that particular individual and whether the parameter is affected by the disease in question. Therefore, having accurate reference ranges for the individuals in question is a critical first step in being able to interpret any laboratory assay. There are several concepts that medical providers should be aware of when applying reference ranges in clinical practice.

First, a reference range encapsulates only 95% of the normal population. A reference range is usually defined as the 95% confidence interval for the specific analyte on a specific analyzer in a specific population; there are multiple methodologies used in determining reference ranges. One approach consists of testing relatively small numbers of healthy subjects (presumed to be representative of a given population); in this approach, the testing laboratory verifies reference ranges provided by the manufacturer or established by a different laboratory. A second approach consists of determining means and standard deviations from very large numbers of clinically collected samples from healthy donors. Careful selection of donors is important to ensure the absence of disease states or use of medications that affect the analyte being studied. In addition, the reference range determination requires some statistical assumptions about the distribution of normal values. Normally distributed and skewed variables will require different methodologies in calculating accurate reference ranges. By definition, 2.5% of subjects will be below a reference range and 2.5% above the reference range and yet be normal. These subjects may have results within the ranges that signify disease in other subjects. For example, a mildly elevated activated partial thromboplastin time (aPTT) can be found in children without bleeding symptoms and normal coagulation factor levels. However, in other children, a slightly elevated aPTT may indicate an inherited bleeding disorder, such as hemophilia.

Second, abnormal laboratory results could be due to factors not related to the test in question. Preanalytical variables are crucial in all laboratory testing but especially in coagulation testing in children. Prolonged attempts at drawing up of the blood sample, high suction pressures because of small gauge needles, or failure to mix the blood with the anticoagulant in the tube adequately upon collection, or overfilling/underfilling of the tubes such that there is inadequate/increased anticoagulation will all lead to spurious results. Similar processes may lead to cell hemolysis within the sample. Blood clots may or may not be visible to the naked eye on initial inspection. Another frequent problem is contamination of the samples, most frequently with heparin if samples are collected from previously inserted vascular access devices. Patients undergoing platelet aggregation studies should ideally have not ingested any medications affecting platelet function for 10 days prior to testing (see Chapter 6). Preanalytical variables commonly lead to test results being outside the reference range, and careful attention to these factors is required to avoid misdiagnosis. For example, platelet function testing may be inaccurate because of thrombocytopenia and/or anemia, and von Willebrand factor (VWF) and factor VIII (FVIII) can be falsely elevated because of physiological stress at the time of blood collection as both are acute phase reactants. In general, repeated consistent abnormalities are required in laboratory tests, in conjunction with the family history and patient history before abnormalities in the hemostatic system can be reliably diagnosed.

Third, medical providers must be aware of the type of coagulation testing (antigen vs. activity levels; clot-based vs. chromogenic assays), as well as analyzer/reagent combinations, and are encouraged to consult with the local coagulation laboratory to have a solid understanding of the coagulation testing available together with local reference ranges and how these reference ranges were generated. Very few laboratory assays are absolute measurements of a physiological entity, and this is certainly true of the common tests for bleeding and clotting. Coagulation assays should not be considered physiological measurements but rather as artificial constructs that, hopefully, have been shown in clinical studies to correlate with the clinical outcome of the patient. There are many different types of coagulation tests. Immunological assays measure the amount of protein actually present but do not address the functionality of the protein. Measurements of the same protein will vary according to the different antibodies used and the sensitivity of the antibody detection method. Functional assays may be chromogenic, in which a light-emitting substrate to a specific enzyme reaction is incubated with the patient's plasma, and then the emitted light is measured using a luminometer. Different versions of these tests can vary in the rate and intensity of light emission and the sensitivity of detection amongst other things. True coagulation (clot)-based functional assays measure the ability for clot formation within the plasma under a variety of conditions. Consider the physiological mechanisms by which blood clots in vivo and then contrast that to clot-based assays, where the plasma is separated from endothelium and cells and is artificially activated to form a clot at a uniform arbitrary temperature of 37 °C. In this context, the assay mechanisms are critical to the result, and different laboratory analyzers have major differences in methods of detecting clot formation (optical vs. electromechanical), let alone slight variations in the remaining test conditions. Reagents vary in their binding and activation capacity. The results from immunological, chromogenic, and coagulation-based assays are not directly comparable. Even within the same assay type, every different analyzer/reagent combination will require determination of a reference range specific to that test situation. The same holds true for platelet testing in which aggregation stimulated by varying concentrations of different agonists is measured in suspension by an increase in light transmission through a rapidly stirred sample of citrated platelet-rich plasma (light transmission aggregometry). Alternatively, agonist-stimulated aggregation on electrodes placed into in a rapidly stirred sample of diluted anticoagulated whole blood is measured as an increase in electrical impedance (impedance aggregometry). The use of generic reference ranges, without attention to the specifics of the laboratory, is a common source of error and misdiagnosis [1].

Fourth, reference ranges are even more important in children, because there is well-documented age-related variation in reference ranges of most blood parameters. The concept of "developmental hemostasis" was first published by Dr. Maureen Andrew in the late 1980s, and this was a landmark step in improving the use of the coagulation laboratory in children (see Chapter 2) [2–5]. However, the data in these publications cannot be used as the gold-standard reference ranges for every laboratory, unless the identical analyzer reagent combination used in the Andrew publications is also used in the laboratory in question. As was shown by Monagle et al. [6], while the trends described by Andrew have been consistent over a number of studies, the absolute values certainly do vary with analyzer and reagent combinations. The major studies that have documented reference ranges for coagulation assays in children are outlined in Table 1. Table 2 helps readers find the published reference range for different analyzer/reagent combinations. Tables 3–13 show published reference ranges that are only applicable to the appropriate analyzer/reagent combinations [6]. In contrast, for platelet aggregation testing, there is little evidence indicating that reference ranges for different age groups are necessary since platelet aggregation responses are similar in children and adults. Only in newborns do platelet responses differ, i.e., aggregation is decreased [7].

Fifth, although reference ranges are presented as discrete groups based on age, coagulation test results are continuous variables that gradually change over time. This becomes important when evaluating children who are close to the lower limit or upper limit of each age group for which reference ranges are quoted. For example, a child might have an abnormal coagulation test result based on an appropriate reference range for his/her age group, but the test result will shift to normal within as short a time interval as 1 month as the child moves into older age group.

Sixth, the interpretation of laboratory data in children is even more complex than just having determined age-appropriate reference ranges. There is a second step in diagnosing disease. Having a laboratory level below the 2.5th percentile or above the 97.5th percentile is not enough to diagnose a disease (see Chapter 4). For example, if the lower limit of the reference range for FVIII in a child is 0.57 IU/mL (57%) based on a population study, and a subject of appropriate age presents who, when using the same analyzer and reagent, has an FVIII level of 0.52 IU/mL (52%), then it is unlikely that the subject has even mild hemophilia. This is because, by definition, we define hemophilia by arbitrary plasma levels (<0.4 IU/mL [40%] for mild hemophilia) or at least plasma levels that are thought to be associated with an increased risk of bleeding. In addition, there is increasing recognition of the effect of race on what is considered abnormal. As an example, it has been shown that a VWF variant prevalent in African Americans affects the results of the ristocetin cofactor activity such that carriers of that variant have lower average VWF levels yet no bleeding tendency. In the absence of genetic studies, the definition of heterozygote states remains difficult. For the laboratory tests to be clinically useful, we need to understand the level at which results define clinically relevant disease, probably more so than the levels at which the results are outside the 95% confidence limits of the healthy population, especially remembering the earlier point that reference ranges by definition only encapsulate 95% of the normal population.

The need to match clinical acumen with laboratory data can be further illustrated with a specific example: in a critically unwell child in pediatric intensive care, an aPTT result that is 1 or 2 s above the upper limit of the reference range is of no particular consequence. The rationale for doing a coagulation screen in the child was to determine the presence or absence of coagulopathy and the need for intervention, and in a nonbleeding child, a result that is slightly abnormal will not change the clinical decision process. This is why, for example, major pediatric hospitals have coped in the absence of properly established reference ranges for premature infants (note that only few publications listed in Table 1 have included pre-30 week ex utero infants). Hemostatic tests are usually only ordered in this population to assist in the management of clinical coagulopathy, and so accuracy of the reference ranges is less important. However, the implication of an aPTT result 1 or 2 s above the designated reference range has totally different consequences if the test was performed in an otherwise well child from the community in whom the question of a bleeding disorder has been raised. This could easily signify clinically significant von Willebrand disease or mild hemophilia, and an accurate diagnosis is essential. The use of the wrong reference range could have adverse consequences for the child.

In summary, an understanding of the principles behind reference range determination and the clinical significance of reference ranges (and, by default, test results that are outside reference ranges) is fundamental to the clinical care of children with bleeding and clotting disorders. Moreover, a specific knowledge of the reference ranges used in the laboratory providing the results to the clinician is also critical. Clinicians should demand that laboratories to which they send tests are transparent and clear about how their reference ranges were generated and, in particular, the age appropriateness of the ranges in question. Laboratories should not perform assays for which they do not have appropriate reference ranges if they have the opportunity to forward the sample to a laboratory that can provide the test result in the context of a properly established reference range. There remains much more research to be done to improve our knowledge of reference ranges in children and our ability to accurately define clinically significant hemostatic disease across all age groups.

Table 1. Studies reporting age-related differences in coagulation assays during childhood

Author, year	Assays reported	Age-groups
Perlman and Dvilansky, 1975 [8]	PT, TT, aPTT, fibrinogen, FDP, FV, FVIII, plasminogen	Healthy newborns Small-for-dates newborns Post-mature newborns
Beverley et al., 1984 [9]	aPTT, FII, FVII, FX, fibrinogen, α2-AP, plasminogen	Cord blood Newborns (48 h)
Andrew et al., 1987 [3]	PT, aPTT, TT, fibrinogen, FII, FV, FVII, FVIII, VWF, FIX, FX, FXI, FXII, PK, HMWK, FXIIIa, FXIIIb, plasminogen, antithrombin, α_2-macroglobulin, α_2-AP, C_1-esterase inhibitor, α1-AT, heparin cofactor II, protein C, protein S	Day 1, 5, 30 newborns Day 90, 180 infants Adult
Andrew et al., 1988 [5]	PT, aPTT, TT, Fibrinogen, FII, FV, FVII, FVIII, VWF, FIX, FX, FXI, FXII, PK, HMWK, FXIIIa, FXIIIb, plasminogen, antithrombin, α_2-macroglobulin, α_2-AP, C_1-esterase inhibitor, α1-AT, heparin cofactor II, protein C, protein S	Premature (30–36 weeks gestation) Day 1, 5, 30 newborns Day 90, 180 infants Adult
Boos et al., 1989 [10]	PIVKA, FVII, FII, FII:antigen	Day 1, 2, 3 newborns
Andrew et al., 1990 [4]	PT, aPTT, fibrinogen, FII, FV, FVII, FVIII, VWF, FIX, FX, FXI, FXII, PK, HMWK, antithrombin, heparin cofactor II, protein C	Premature (19–27 and 28–31 weeks gestation) At birth

(Table continued on next page.)

Table 1 (continued)

Author, year	Assays reported	Age-groups
Andrew et al., 1992 [2]	PT/INR, aPTT, bleeding time, fibrinogen, FII, FV, FVII, FVIII, VWF, FIX, FX, FXI, FXII, PK, HMWK, FXIIIa, FXIIIs, plasminogen, TPA, PAI-1, antithrombin, α_2-macroglobulin, α_2-AP, C_{1-} esterase inhibitor, α1-AT, Heparin cofactor II, protein C, protein S (total and free)	1–5 years 6–10 years 11–16 years Adults
Reverdiau-Moalic et al., 1996 [11]	PT/INR, aPTT, TT, thrombin, FII, FVII, FVII, FIX, FX, FV, FVIII, FXI, FXII, PK, HMWK, antithrombin, heparin cofactor II, TFPI, protein C, protein S	Premature newborns 19–23 weeks gestation 24–29 weeks gestation 30–38 weeks gestation Mature newborns Adults
Ries et al., 1997 [12]	TAT, F1+2, PAP, D-dimer	1–6 years 7–12 years 13–18 years Adults
Carcao et al., 1998 [13]	PFA-100®	Neonates Children Adults
Salonvaara et al., 2003 [14]	FII, FV, FVII, FX, aPTT, PT/INR	Premature newborns 24–27 weeks gestation 28–20 weeks gestation 31–33 weeks gestation 34–36 weeks gestation
Flanders et al., 2005 [15]	PT, aPTT, FVIII, FIX, FXI, antithrombin, VWF:Rco, VWF:Ag, protein C, protein S	7–9 years 10–11 years 12–13 years 14–15 years 16–17 years Adults
Monagle et al., 2006 [6]	aPTT (4 reagents), PT/INR, fibrinogen, TT, FII, FV, FVII, FVIII, FIX, FX, FXI, FXII, antithrombin, protein C, protein S, D-dimers, TFPI (free and total), endogenous thrombin potential	Day 1, 3 newborns <1 year 1–5 years 6–10 years 11–16 years Adults
Chan et al., 2007 [16]	Thromboelastography Multiple parameters	<1 year 1–5 years 6–10 years 11–16 years Adults
Sosothikul et al., 2007 [17]	PT, aPTT, fibrinogen, TAT, protein C, TF, FVIIa, sTM, VWF:Ag, VWF:RCo, D-dimer, tPA, PAI-1, TAFI	1–5 years 6–10 years 11–18 years Adults
Mitsiakos et al., 2009 [18]	INR, PT, aPTT, fibrinogen, FII, FV, FVII, FVIII, FIX, FX, FXI, FXII, antithrombin, protein C, protein S, aPCR, tPA, PAI-1, VWF	Small for age newborns Appropriate for age newborns
Newall et al., 2009 [19]	PF4 and vitronectin	<1 year 1–5 years 6–10 years 11–16 years Adults
Appel et al., 2012 [20]	PT, aPTT, fibrinogen, thrombin time, FII, FV, FVII, FVIII, FIX, FX, FXI, FXII, FXIII, VWF, plasminogen, protein C, protein S, antithrombin, D-dimer, α_2-AP	1–6 months 7–12 months 1–5 years 6–10 years 11–18 years >19 years

(Table continued on next page.)

Table 1 (continued)

Author, year	Assays reported	Age-groups
Attard et al., 2013 [21]	Immunological FII, FV, FVII, FVIII, FIX, FX, FXI, FXII, FXIII, plasminogen, protein C total and free protein S	Day 1, 3, 28 newborns 1 year 1–5 years 6–10 years 11–16 years Adults
Toulon et al., 2016 [22]	PT, aPTT, fibrinogen, FII, FV, FVII, FVIII, FIX, FX, FXI, FXII, FXIII, VWF, plasminogen, protein C, protein S, antithrombin, D-dimer	2–4 weeks 1–5 months 6–12 months 1–5 years 6–10 years 11–17 years
Nowak-Göttl et al., 2017 [23]	aPTT, fibrinogen, FII, FV, FVII, FVIII, FIX, FX, FXI, FXII, FXIII, VWF, plasminogen, protein C, protein S, protein Z, antithrombin, D-dimer, α_2-AP, TFPI, α_2-macroglobulin, α1-AT	5–30 days 1.1–5.9 months 6–12 months 1–5 years 5.1–10 years 10.1–≤18 Adults
Liu et al., 2018 [24]	PT, aPTT, TT, fibrinogen	0–≤15 days >15 days–≤1 month >1 month–≤6 months >6 months–≤11 years >11 years–15 years Adults
Zhang et al., 2020 [25]	PT, aPTT, TT, fibrinogen	≥29 days–<1 year ≥1 year–<3 years ≥3 years–<6 years ≥6 years–<12 years
Sung et al., 2021[26]	PT, aPTT, fibrinogen	Different age cut off for each coagulation test
Nielsen et al., 2022 [27]	PT, aPTT	At birth At 2 months

α1-AT, α1-antitrypsin; α2-AP, α2-antiplasmin; aPCR, activated protein C resistance; aPTT, activated partial thromboplastin time; F1+2, prothrombin fragment 1+2; FDP, fibrin degradation product; FII, factor II; FV, factor V; FVII, factor VII; FVIIa, activated factor VII; FVIII, factor VIII; FIX, factor IX; FX, factor X; FXI, factor XI; FXII, factor XII; FXII, factor XIII; FXIIIa, factor XIIIa; FXIIIb, factor XIIIb; HMWK, high-molecular-weight kininogen; INR, international normalized ratio; PAI, plasminogen activator inhibitor; PAI-1, plasminogen activator inhibitor type 1; PAP, plasmin-antiplasmin complex; PF4, platelet factor 4; PFA-100®, platelet function analyzer-100®; PIVKA, proteins induced by vitamin K absence; PK, Prekallikrein; PT, prothrombin time; sTM, soluble thrombomodulin; TAFI, thrombin activatable fibrinolysis inhibitor; TAT, thrombin-antithrombin complex; TF, tissue factor; TFPI, tissue factor pathway inhibitor; tPA, tissue plasminogen activator; TT, thrombin time; VWF, von Willebrand factor; VWF:Ag, von Willebrand factor:antigen; VWF:RCo, von Willebrand factor:ristocetin cofactor.

Table 2. Published reference ranges for specific analyzer-reagent combinations (to find reference ranges for a specific test, first, choose the appropriate *test* from the table; second, find the *analyzer-reagent* combination that you are looking for; this combination will direct you to the *table number* where you can find the published reference ranges; lastly, go to the specified table and find the test you are looking for and the appropriate reference range for the age group in mind)

Analyzer	Reagent	Table No. [reference]
Activated partial thromboplastin time (aPTT)		
ACL (IL)	Actin FS	Tables 3–5 [2–4]
STA-R (Stago)	STA-PTT A	Tables 6–7 [6, 15]
BCS (Siemens)	Pathromtin SL	Table 9 [20]
CA-1500 (Sysmex)	Dade Actin FS	Table 9 [20]
ACL top 700/500 (IL)	HemosIL SynthASil	Table 11 [22]
ACL top 700/500 (IL)	HemosIL APTT SP	Tables 11, 13 [22, 25]
STA-R (Stago)	CK Prest	Table 6 [6]
STA-R (Stago)	Actin FSL	Table 6 [6]
STA-R (Stago)	Platelin L	Table 6 [6]
Prothrombin time (PT)		
ACL (IL)	Thromborel S	Tables 3–5 [2–4]
STA-R (Stago)	Neoplastin CI	Tables 6, 7 [6, 15]
BCS (Siemens)	Thromborel S	Table 9 [20]
CA-1500 (Sysmex)	Dade Innovin	Table 9 [20]
ACL top 700/500 (IL)	HemosIL RecombiPlasTin 2G	Tables 11, 13 [22, 25]
Fibrinogen		
STA-R (Stago)	STA-Fibrinogen (Stago)	Tables 6, 7 [6, 28]
BCS (Siemens)	Multifibren U	Tables 9, 12 [20, 23]
CA-1500 (Sysmex)	Dade Thrombin Reagent	Table 9 [20, 23]
ACL top 700/500 (IL)	HemosIL Fibrinogen C (IL)	Table 11 [22]
ACL top 700/500 (IL)	HemosIL QFA (IL)	Tables 11, 13 [22, 25]
Factor levels (II, V, VII, VIII, IX, X, XI, XII, XIII)		
ACL (IL)	OSA/in house and commercial deficient plasma	Tables 3–5 [2–4]
STA-R (Stago)	OSA/deficient plasmas (HRF Inc)	Table 8 [18]
STA-R (Stago)	OSA/STA-deficient plasmas (Stago)	Table 6 [6]
BCS (Siemens)	OSA/coagulation factor deficient plasmas and Pathromtin Sl/ Thromborel S	Tables 9, 12 [20, 23]
CA-1500 (Sysmex)	OSA/coagulation factor deficient plasmas and Dade Actin/ Dade Innovin	Table 9 [20]
Microplate reader	Elisa Asserachrom (Stago)	Table 10 [21]
Microplate reader	Affinity Bioogicals	Table 10 [21]
ACL top 700/500 (IL)	OSA/HemosIL Deficient plasmas (IL)	Table 11 [22]
Antithrombin		
ACL (IL)	Antigen (radial immunodiffusion)	Tables 3, 5 [3, 4]
ACL (IL)	Chromogenic antigen (radial immunodiffusion)	Table 3 [2]
STA-R (Stago)	Stachrom ATIII (chromogenic, Stago)	Tables 6, 7 [6, 15]
BCS (Siemens)	Innovance Antithrombin (chromogenic, Siemens)	Tables 9, 12 [20, 23]
CA-1500 (Sysmex)	Behrichrom Antithrombin III (chromogenic, Siemens)	Table 9 [20]
ACL top 700/500 (IL)	HemosIL Liquid Antithrombin (chromogenic, IL)	Table 11 [22]

(Table continued on next page.)

II

Table 2 (continued)

Analyzer	Reagent	Table No. [reference]
Protein C		
ACL (IL)	Asserachrom Protein C (ELISA, Stago)	Tables 3–5 [2–4]
ACL (IL)	Chromogenic (Siemens)	Table 3 [2]
STA-R (Stago)	Staclot Protein C (clotting, Stago)	Tables 6, 7 [6, 15]
STA-R (Stago)	Stachrom Protein C (chromogenic, Stago)	Table 6 [6]
BCS (Siemens)	Protein C reagenz (clotting, Siemens)	Tables 9, 12 [20, 23]
CA-1500 (Sysmex)	Behrichrom Protein C (chromogenic, Siemens)	Table 9 [20]
Microplate reader	ELISA (Affinity Bioogicals)	Table 10 [21]
Microplate reader	Asserachrom Protein C (ELISA, Stago)	Table 10 [21]
ACL top 700/500 (IL)	HemosIL Protein C (chromogenic, IL)	Table 11 [22]
ACL top 700/500 (IL)	HemosIL Protein ProClot (clotting, IL)	Table 11 [22]
Protein S		
ACL (IL)	Total antigen (immunoelectrophoresis)	Tables 3, 5 [3, 4]
ACL (IL)	Total and free antigen (ELISA, Affinity Biologicals)	Table 3 [2]
STA-R (Stago)	Staclot Protein S (clotting, Stago)	Tables 6, 7 [6, 15]
BCS (Siemens)	Protein S Ac (Siemens)	Tables 9, 12 [20, 23]
CA-1500 (Sysmex)	Protein S Ac (Siemens)	Table 9 [20]
Microplate reader	Asserachrom free/total Protein S (ELISA, Stago)	Table 10 [21]
ACL top 700/500 (IL)	HemosIL Protein S Activity (clotting, IL)	Table 11 [22]
ACL top 700/500 (IL)	HemosIL Free Protein S (latex agglutination, IL)	Table 11 [22]
D-dimer		
STA-R (Stago)	STA-Liatest D-dimer (latex agglutination, Stago)	Table 6 [6]
BCS (Siemens)	Innovance D-dimer (Siemens)	Tables 9, 12 [20, 23]
CA-1500 (Sysmex)	Innovance D-dimer (Siemens)	Table 9 [20]
ACL top 700/500 (IL)	HemosIL D-dimer HS 500 (latex agglutination, IL)	Table 11 [22]
von Willebrand factor (VWF)		
ACL (IL)	Asserachrom VWF (ELISA, Stago)	Table 3–5 [2–4]
STA-R (Stago)	STA-Liatest VWF:Ag (latex agglutination, Stago)	Table 7 [15]
BCS (Siemens)	BC von Willebrand (VWF:RCo, Siemens)	Table 9, 12 [20, 23]
CA-1500 (Sysmex)	BC von Willebrand (VWF:RCo, Siemens)	Table 9 [20]
ACL top 700/500 (IL)	HemosIL von Willebrand Factor Ristocetin Cofactor Activity (IL)	Table 11 [22]
ACL top 700/500 (IL)	HemosIL von Willebrand Factor Activity (latex agglutination, IL)	Table 11 [22]
ACL top 700/500 (IL)	HemosIL von Willebrand Factor Antigen (latex agglutination, IL)	Table 11 [22]
Plasminogen		
ACL (IL)	Chromogenic Stago	Table 3 [2]
ACL (IL)	Unspecified	Table 5 [3, 4]
STA-R (Stago)	STA-Stachrom Plasminogen (chromogenic, Stago)	Table 7 [28]
BCS (Siemens)	Behrichrom Plasminogen (chromogenic, Siemens)	Table 12 [23]
CA-1500 (Sysmex)	Behrichrom Plasminogen (chromogenic, Siemens)	Table 9 [20]
Microplate reader	ELISA (Affinity Bioogicals)	Table 10 [21]
ACL top 700/500 (IL)	HemosIL Plasminogen (chromogenic, IL)	Table 11 [22]
Thrombin time (TT)		
STA-R (Stago)	STA-Thrombin Test Kit (Diagnostica Stago)	Table 6 [6]
CA-1500 (Sysmex)	Thromboclotin	Table 9 [20]
ACL top 700 /500 (IL)	HemosIL Thrombin	Table 13 [25]

(Table continued on next page.)

Table 2 (continued)

Analyzer	Reagent	Table No. [reference]
α2-Antiplasmin (α2-AP)		
ACL (IL)	Rabbit Antihuman Antibody (Atlantic Antibodies, NCS Diagnostics)	Tables 3, 5 [3, 4]
STA-R (Stago)	STA-Stachrom Antiplasmin	Table 7 [28]
CA-1500 (Sysmex)	Berichrom α2-Antiplasmin	Table 9 [20]
BCS (Siemens)	Berichrom α2-Antiplasmin	Table 12 [23]

ELISA, enzyme-linked immunosorbent assay; OSA, one-stage assay; VWF:Ag, von Willebrand factor:antigen; VWF:RCo, von Willebrand factor:ristocetin cofactor.

Table 3. Using the ACL (IL) analyzer, the reference ranges for coagulation tests in healthy full-term infants and healthy children, compared to values for adults

Assay	Age								Adults
	Day 1	Day 5	Day 30	Day 90	Day 180	1–5 years	6–10 years	11–16 years	
PT, s	10.1–15.9	10.0–15.3	10.0–14.3	10.0–14.2	10.7–13.9	10.6–11.4	10.1–12.1	10.2–12.0	11.0–14.0
aPTT, s	31.3–54.5	25.4–59.8	32.0–55.2	29.0–50.1	28.1–42.9	24–36	26–36	26–37	27–40
Fibrinogen, g/L	1.67–3.99	1.62–4.62	1.62–3.78	1.50–3.79	1.50–3.87	1.70–4.05	1.57–4.0	1.54–4.48	1.56–4.00
FII, IU/mL	0.26–0.70	0.33–0.93	0.34–1.02	0.45–1.05	0.60– 1.16	0.71–1.16	0.67–1.07	0.61–1.04	0.70–1.46
Factor V, IU/mL	0.34–1.08	0.45–1.45	0.62–1.34	0.48–1.32	0.55–1.27	0.79–1.27	0.63–1.16	0.55–0.99	0.62–1.50
Factor VII, IU/mL	0.28–1.04	0.35–1.43	0.42–1.38	0.39–1.43	0.47–1.27	0.55–1.16	0.52–1.20	0.58–1.15	0.67–1.43
Factor VIII, IU/mL	0.50–1.78	0.50–1.54	0.50–1.57	0.50–1.25	0.50–1.09	0.59–1.42	0.58–1.32	0.53–1.31	0.50–1.49
VWF:antigen, IU/mL	0.50–2.87	0.50–2.54	0.50–2.46	0.50–2.06	0.50–1.97	0.60–1.20	0.44–1.44	0.46–1.53	0.50–1.58
Factor IX, IU/mL	0.15–0.91	0.15–0.91	0.21–0.81	0.21–1.13	0.36–1.36	0.47–1.04	0.63–0.89	0.59–1.22	0.55–1.63
Factor X, IU/mL	0.12–0.68	0.19–0.79	0.31–0.87	0.35–1.07	0.38–1.18	0.58–1.16	0.55–1.01	0.50–1.17	0.70–1.52
Factor XI, IU/mL	0.10–0.66	0.23–0.87	0.27–0.79	0.41–0.97	0.49–1.34	0.56–1.50	0.52–1.20	0.50–0.97	0.67–1.27
Factor XII, IU/mL	0.13–0.93	0.11–0.83	0.17–0.81	0.25–1.09	0.39–1.15	0.64–1.29	0.60–1.40	0.34–1.37	0.52–1.64
Prekallikrein, IU/mL	0.18–0.69	0.20–0.76	0.23–0.91	0.41–1.05	0.56–1.16	0.65–1.30	0.66–1.31	0.53–1.45	0.62–1.62
HMWK, IU/mL	0.06–1.02	0.16–1.32	0.33–1.21	0.30–1.46	0.36–1.28	0.64–1.32	0.60–1.30	0.63–1.19	0.50–1.36
Factor XIII_a, IU/mL	0.27–1.31	0.44–1.44	0.39–1.47	0.36–1.72	0.46–1.62	0.72–1.43	0.65–1.51	0.57–1.40	0.55–1.55
Factor XIII_b, IU/mL	0.30–1.22	0.32–1.80	0.39–1.73	0.48–1.84	0.50–1.70	0.69–1.56	0.77–1.54	0.60–1.43	0.57–1.37
Plasminogen (CTA), IU/mL	1.25–2.65	1.41–2.93	1.26–2.70	1.74–3.22	2.21–3.81	0.78–1.18	0.75–1.08	0.68–1.03	0.77–1.22
Antithrombin antigen, IU/mL	0.39–0.87	0.41–0.93	0.48–1.08	0.73–1.21	0.84–1.24				0.79–1.31
Antithrombin chromogenic, IU/mL						0.82–1.39	0.90–1.31	0.77–1.32	0.74–1.26
α2-AP, IU/mL	0.55–1.15	0.70–1.30	0.76–1.24	0.76–1.40	0.83–1.39	0.93–1.17	0.89–1.10	0.78–1.18	0.68–1.36
Protein C, IU/mL	0.17–0.53	0.20–0.64	0.21–0.65	0.28–0.80	0.37–0.81	–	–	–	0.64–1.28
Protein S, IU/mL	0.12–0.60	0.22–0.78	0.33–0.93	0.54–1.18	0.55–1.19	–	–	–	0.60–1.24
Protein C chromogenic, IU/mL	–	–	–	–	–	0.40–0.92	0.45–0.93	0.55–1.11	0.64–1.28
Protein S total, IU/mL	–	–	–	–	–	0.54–1.18	0.41–1.14	0.52–0.92	0.60–1.13
Protein S free, IU/mL	–	–	–	–	–	0.21–0.69	0.22–0.62	0.26–0.55	0.27–0.61

Modified from Andrew et al. [2–4]. α2-AP, α2-antiplasmin; aPTT, activated partial thromboplastin time; CTA, Committee on Thrombolytic Agents; HMWK, high-molecular-weight kininogen; PT, prothrombin time; VWF, von Willebrand factor.

Table 4. Using the ACL (IL) analyzer, reference ranges for coagulation tests in healthy fetuses (19–27 weeks gestational age) and premature infants at birth (28–31 weeks gestational age)

Assay	Gestational age	
	19–27 weeks, 95% CI	28–31 weeks, range
PT, s	–	14.6–16.9
aPTT, s	–	80–168
Fibrinogen, g/L	0.14–1.86	1.60–5.50
Factor II, IU/mL	0.08–0.16	0.19–0.54
Factor V, IU/mL	0.21–0.61	0.43–0.80
Factor VII, IU/mL	0.20–0.36	0.24–0.76
Factor VIII, IU/mL	0.11–0.67	0.37–1.26
VWF:antigen, IU/mL	0.38–0.90	0.83–2.23
Factor IX, IU/mL	0.08–0.12	0.17–0.20
Factor X, IU/mL	0.15–0.27	0.25–0.64
Factor XI, IU/mL	–	0.11–0.33
Factor XII, IU/mL	0.16–0.28	0.05–0.35
Prekallikrein, IU/mL	–	0.15–0.32
HMWK, IU/mL	–	0.19–0.52
Antithrombin, IU/mL	0.18–0.30	0.20–0.38
Heparin cofactor II, IU/mL	0.17–0.37	–
Protein C, IU/mL	0.05–0.17	–

Modified from Andrew et al. [4]. aPTT, activated partial thromboplastin time; CI, confidence interval; HMWK, high-molecular-weight kininogen; PT, prothrombin time; VWF, von Willebrand factor.

Table 5. Using the ACL (IL) analyzer, reference ranges for coagulation tests in the healthy premature infant (30–36 weeks gestation) during the first 6 months of life, compared to those in adults

Assay	Gestational age 30–36 weeks					Adults
	Day 1	Day 5	Day 30	Day 90	Day 180	
PT, s	10.6–16.2	10.0–15.3	10.0–13.6	10.0–14.6	10.0–15.0	10.8–13.9
aPTT, s	27.5–79.4	26.9–74.1	26.9–62.5	28.3–50.7	27.1–53.3	26.6–40.3
Fibrinogen, g/L	1.50–3.73	1.60–4.18	1.50–4.14	1.50–3.52	1.50–3.60	1.56–4.00
Factor II, IU/mL	0.20–0.77	0.29–0.85	0.36–0.95	0.30–1.06	0.51–1.23	0.70–1.46
Factor V, IU/mL	0.41–1.44	0.46–1.54	0.48–1.56	0.59–1.39	0.58–1.46	0.62–1.50
Factor VII, IU/mL	0.21–1.13	0.30–1.38	0.21–1.45	0.31–1.43	0.47–1.51	0.67–1.43
Factor VIII, IU/mL	0.50–2.13	0.53–2.05	0.50–1.99	0.58–1.88	0.50–1.87	0.50–1.49
VWF:antigen, IU/mL	0.78–2.10	0.72–2.19	0.66–2.16	0.75–1.84	0.54–1.58	0.50–1.58
Factor IX, IU/mL	0.19–0.65	0.14–0.74	0.13–0.80	0.25–0.93	0.50–1.20	0.55–1.63
Factor X, IU/mL	0.11–0.71	0.19–0.83	0.20–0.92	0.35–0.99	0.35–1.19	0.70–1.52
Factor XI, IU/mL	0.08–0.52	0.13–0.69	0.15–0.71	0.25–0.93	0.46–1.10	0.67–1.27
Factor XII, IU/mL	0.10–0.66	0.09–0.69	0.11–0.75	0.15–1.07	0.22–1.42	0.52–1.64
Prekallikrein, IU/mL	0.09–0.57	0.25–0.75	0.31–0.87	0.37–1.21	0.40–1.16	0.62–1.62
HMWK, IU/mL	0.09–0.89	0.24–1.00	0.16–1.12	0.32–1.24	0.41–1.25	0.50–1.36
Factor XIII_a, IU/mL	0.32–1.08	0.57–1.45	0.51–1.47	0.71–1.55	0.65–1.61	0.55–1.55
Factor XIII_b, IU/mL	0.35–1.27	0.68–1.58	0.57–1.57	0.75–1.67	0.67–1.63	0.57–1.37
Antithormbin, IU/mL	0.14–0.62	0.30–0.82	0.37–0.81	0.45–1.21	0.52–1.28	0.79–1.31
Protein C, IU/mL	0.12–0.44	0.11–0.51	0.15–0.59	0.23–0.67	0.31–0.83	0.64–1.28
Protein S, IU/mL	0.14–0.38	0.13–0.61	0.22–0.90	0.40–1.12	0.44–1.20	0.60–1.24
Plasminogen, IU/mL	1.12–2.48	1.21–2.61	1.09–2.53	1.58–3.18	1.91–3.59	2.48–4.24
α2-AP, IU/mL	0.40–1.16	0.49–1.13	0.55–1.23	0.64–1.48	0.77–1.53	0.68–1.36

Modified from Andrew et al. [4]. α2-AP, α2-antiplasmin; aPTT, activated partial thromboplastin time; HMWK, high-molecular-weight kininogen; PT, prothrombin time; VWF, von Willebrand factor.

Table 6. Using the STA-R (Stago) analyzer, reference ranges for coagulation tests

Assay	Age						Adults
	Day 1	Day 3	1 month–1 year	1–5 years	6–10 years	11–16 years	
aPTT, s							
PTT-A	34.3–44.8	29.5–42.2	35.1–46.3	33.6–43.8	31.8–43.7	33.9–46.1	28.6–38.2
CK Prest	–	–	31.1–36.6	29.8–35.0	30.8–34.8	29.4–40.4	25.7–31.5
Actin FSL	–	–	33.4–41.4	31.8–42.8	30.1–40.4	32.2–42.2	27.1–34.3
Platelin L	–	–	33.6–40.4	32.5–43.8	31.0–39.3	32.6–49.2	27.2–35.4
PT, s	14.4–16.4	13.5–16.4	11.5–15.3	12.1–14.5	11.7–15.1	12.7–16.1	11.5–14.5
Thromin time, s	–	–	16.3–17.6	16.5–18.2	16.1–18.5	16.2–17.6	16.2–17.2
Fibrinogen, g/L	1.92–3.74	2.83–4.01	0.82–3.83	1.62–4.01	1.99–4.09	2.12–4.33	1.9–4.3
Factor II, IU/mL	41–69	50–73	62–103	70–109	67–110	61–107	78–138
Factor V, IU/mL	64–103	92–154	94–141	67–127	56–141	67–141	78–152
Factor VII, IU/mL	52–88	67–107	83–160	72–150	70–156	69–200	61–199
Factor VIII, IU/mL	105–329	83–274	54–145	36–185	52–182	59–200	52–290
Factor IX, IU/mL	35–56	44–97	43–121	44–127	48–145	64–216	59–254
Factor X, IU/mL	46–67	46–75	77–122	72–125	68–125	53–122	96–171
Factor XI, IU/mL	7–41	24–79	62–125	65–162	65–162	65–139	67–196
Factor XII, IU/mL	43–80	14–80	20–135	36–135	26–137	14–117	35–207
Antithrombin, IU/mL	58–90	60–89	72–134	101–131	95–134	96–126	66–124
Protein C chromogenic, IU/mL	24–44	28–54	31–112	65–127	71–129	66–118	74–164
Protein C clotting, IU/mL	24–40	24–51	28–124	50–134	64–125	59–112	54–166
Protein S clotting, IU/mL	28–47	33–67	29–162	67–136	64–154	65–140	54–103
D-dimers, mg/L	0.41–2.47	0.58–2.74	0.11–0.42	0.09–0.53	0.10–0.56	0.16–0.39	0.05–0.42

Modified from Monagle et al. [6]. aPTT, activated partial thromboplastin time; PT, prothrombin time.

Table 7. Using the STA-R (Stago) analyzer, reference ranges for coagulation tests

Assay	Age					Adults
	7–9 years	10–11 years	12–13 years	14–15 years	16–17 years	
PT, s	13.0–15.4	13.0–15.6	13.0–15.2	12.8–15.4	12.6–15.7	12.3–14.4
aPTT, s	27–38	27–38	27–39	26–36	26–35	26–38
Fibrinogen, g/L	1.98–4.13	1.97–4.10	2.15–3.78	2.04–3.92	2.08–4.38	2.11–4.41
Factor II, IU/mL	0.78–1.25	0.78–1.20	0.72–1.23	0.75–1.35	0.77–1.30	0.86–1.50
Factor V, IU/mL	0.69–1.32	0.66–1.36	0.66–1.35	0.61–1.29	0.65–1.31	0.62–1.40
Factor VII, IU/mL	0.67–1.45	0.71–1.63	0.78–1.60	0.74–1.80	0.63–1.63	0.80–1.81
Factor VIII, IU/mL	0.76–1.99	0.80–2.09	0.72–1.98	0.69–2.37	0.63–2.21	0.56–1.91
Factor IX, IU/mL	0.70–1.33	0.72–1.49	0.73–1.52	0.80–1.61	0.86–1.76	0.78–1.84
Factor X, IU/mL	0.74–1.30	0.70–1.34	0.69–1.33	0.63–1.46	0.74–1.46	0.81–1.57
Factor XI, IU/mL	0.70–1.38	0.66–1.37	0.68–1.38	0.57–1.29	0.65–1.59	0.56–1.53
VWF:activity, IU/mL	0.52–1.76	0.60–1.95	0.50–1.84	0.50–2.03	0.49–2.04	0.51–2.15
VWF:antigen, IU/mL	0.62–1.80	0.63–1.89	0.60–1.89	0.57–1.99	0.50–2.05	0.52–2.14
α2-AP, IU/mL	0.88–1.47	0.90–1.44	0.87–1.42	0.83–1.36	0.77–1.34	0.82–1.33
Antithrombin, IU/mL	0.90–1.35	0.90–1.34	0.90–1.32	0.90–1.31	0.87–1.31	0.76–1.28
Plasminogen, IU/mL	0.76–1.16	0.74–1.17	0.66–1.14	0.71–1.24	0.75–1.32	0.71–1.44
Protein C, IU/mL	0.70–1.42	0.68–1.43	0.66–1.62	0.69–1.70	0.70–1.71	0.83–1.68
Protein S, IU/mL, male	0.66–1.40	0.65–1.39	0.72–1.39	0.68–1.45	0.77–1.67	0.66–1.43
Protein S, IU/mL, female	0.62–1.51	0.65–1.42	0.70–1.40	0.55–1.45	0.51–1.47	0.57–1.31

Modified from Flanders et al. [15, 28]. α2-AP, α2-antiplasmin; aPTT, activated partial thromboplastin time; PT, prothrombin time; VWF, von Willebrand factor.

Table 8. Using the STA-R (Stago) analyzer, reference ranges for coagulation tests in healthy full-term small for gestational age (SGA) and appropriate for gestational age (AGA) newborns at birth

Assay	SGA newborns	AGA newborns
PT, s	13.3–23.6	13.4–19
aPTT, s	33–63	30–57
Fibrinogen, g/L	0.61–2.88	0.63–3.24
Factor II, IU/mL	0.22–0.60	0.29–0.60
Factor V, IU/mL	0.18–1.20	0.22–1.27
Factor VII, IU/mL	0.26–1.05	0.24–1.08
Factor VIII, IU/mL	0.42–4.38	0.40–4.20
Factor IX, IU/mL	0.17–0.86	0.22–0.94
Factor X, IU/mL	0.17–0.61	0.21–0.75
Factor XI, IU/mL	0.19–1.06	0.20–1.05
Factor XII, IU/mL	0.22–1.05	0.20–1.47
VWF:antigen, IU/mL	1.07–4.05	1.14–3.88
Antithrombin, IU/mL	0.30–1.20	0.30–0.83
Protein S free activity, IU/mL	0.21–0.52	0.25–0.53
Protein C activity, IU/mL	0.17–0.56	0.18–0.50

Modified from Mitsiakos et al. [18]. aPTT, activated partial thromboplastin time; PT, prothrombin time; VWF, von Willebrand factor.

Table 9. Using the BCS (Siemens) and CA-1500 (Sysmex) analyzers, reference ranges for coagulation tests

Assay	Analyzer	Reagents	Age					Adults
			1–6 months	7–12 months	1–5 years	6–10 years	11–18 years	
PT, s	BCS	Thromborel S	11.2–15.5	11.4–13.5	11.2–13.4	11.5–14.0	11.4–13.8	10.7–12.9
	CA-1500	Innovin	10.0–12.7	9.5–12.8	10.0–11.4	10.2–11.6	10.1–11.9	9.7–11.4
aPTT, s	BCS	Pathromtin SL	33–56	32–49	31–44	31–44	30–43	27–40
	CA-1500	Actin FS	21–33	24–33	24–30	25–32	25–30	22–28
Thrombin time, s	CA-1500	Thromboclotin	16.2–24.9	15.4–21.1	15.3–19.7	14.5–19.9	15.2–24.0	15.5–20.5
Fibrinogen, g/L	BCS	Multifibren U	1.5–3.8	1.8–4.8	1.9–3.9	2.0–3.9	1.9–3.7	2.1–4.2
	CA-1500	Dade Thrombin	1.3–3.3	1.6–4.0	1.7–3.5	1.8–3.6	1.8–3.3	2.0–3.9
Factor II, IU/mL	BCS	Thromborel S	0.66–1.12	0.83–1.32	0.85–1.26	0.78–1.21	0.78–1.32	0.96–1.47
	CA-1500	Innovin	0.60–1.09	0.77–1.34	0.81–1.26	0.77–1.16	0.70–1.20	0.93–1.51
Factor V, IU/mL	BCS	Thromborel S	0.82–1.45	0.97–1.48	0.85–1.53	0.80–1.23	0.76–1.32	0.84–1.49
	CA-1500	Innovin	0.56–1.48	0.66–1.41	0.68–1.43	0.62–1.27	0.55–1.19	0.57–1.28
Factor VII, IU/mL	BCS	Thromborel S	0.54–1.26	0.74–1.31	0.81–1.17	0.79–1.19	0.75–1.30	0.86–1.42
	CA-1500	Innovin	0.38–1.29	0.41–1.48	0.61–1.11	0.61–1.27	0.55–1.15	0.67–1.46
Factor VIII, IU/mL	BCS	Pathromtin SL	0.58–1.44	0.59-1.52	0.76–1.43	0.68–1.37	0.70–1.48	0.87–1.52
	CA-1500	Actin FS	0.67–1.41	0.70–2.13	0.83–1.70	0.75–1.63	0.80–1.66	0.96–2.16
Factor IX, IU/mL	BCS	Pathromtin SL	0.41–0.87	0.42–1.09	0.58–0.99	0.57–1.06	0.60–1.17	0.78–1.39
	CA-1500	Actin FS	0.44–0.78	0.46–1.14	0.63–0.97	0.60–1.08	0.72–1.16	0.87–1.74
Factor X, IU/mL	BCS	Pathromtin SL	0.66–1.32	0.74–1.24	0.84–1.29	0.74–1.20	0.73–1.28	0.90–1.49
	CA-1500	Actin FS	0.55–1.20	0.67–1.46	0.75–1.24	0.69–1.18	0.66–1.17	0.78–1.59
Factor XI, IU/mL	BCS	Pathromtin SL	0.54–1.01	0.65–1.25	0.72–1.34	0.75–1.27	0.72–1.22	0.77–1.30
	CA-1500	Actin FS	0.57–1.05	0.64–1.29	0.74–1.34	0.78–1.31	0.78–1.22	0.83–1.58
Factor XII, IU/mL	BCS	Pathromtin SL	0.29–1.12	0.35–1.13	0.44–1.27	0.41–1.22	0.44–1.16	0.52–1.40
	CA-1500	Actin FS	0.28–1.16	0.31–1.26	0.36–1.22	0.37–1.23	0.43–1.22	0.53–1.65
Factor XIII, IU/mL	BCS	Berichrom FXIII	0.63–1.52	0.42–1.28	0.71–1.39	0.76–1.33	0.64–1.33	0.68–1.56
VWF:antigen, IU/mL	BCS	VWF Ag	0.58–2.06	0.53–1.53	0.52–1.40	0.58–1.45	0.57–1.47	0.65–1.82
	CA-1500	VWF Ag	0.63–2.23	0.60–1.58	0.60–1.40	0.60–1.42	0.60–1.59	0.72–1.88

(Table continued on next page.)

Table 9 (continued)

Assay	Analyzer	Reagents	Age					Adults
			1–6 months	7–12 months	1–5 years	6–10 years	11–18 years	
VWF:activity, IU/mL	BCS	BC von Willebrand reagent	0.56–1.50	0.51–1.50	0.51–1.28	0.46–1.38	0.51–1.47	0.56–1.50
α2-AP, IU/mL	CA-1500	Berichrom α2-antiplasmin	1.03–1.39	1.00–1.51	1.07–1.45	1.03–1.40	0.97–1.26	1.03–1.33
Antithrombin, IU/mL	BCS	INNOVANCE AT	0.81–1.26	0.90–1.32	0.93–1.28	0.92–1.22	0.90–1.19	0.97–1.33
	CA-1500	Berichrom AT	0.78–1.29	0.88–1.32	0.97–1.29	0.97–1.22	0.93–1.22	0.98–1.31
Plasminogen, IU/mL	CA-1500	Berichrom Plasminogen	0.56–1.02	0.66–1.15	0.84–1.30	0.75–1.26	0.83–1.28	0.92–1.50
Protein C, IU/mL	BCS	Protein C reagent	0.41–1.15	0.60–1.17	0.63–1.33	0.62–1.34	0.71–1.44	0.78–1.48
	CA-1500	Berichrom Protein C	0.43–1.02	0.59–1.03	0.71–1.25	0.75–1.20	0.70–1.31	0.83–1.53
Protein S, IU/mL	BCS	Protein S Ac	0.60–1.03	0.61–0.95	0.65–0.99	0.63–0.97	0.69–1.19	0.83–1.30
	CA-1500	Protein S Ac	0.59–0.99	0.59–1.10	0.60–1.15	0.63–1.16	0.62–1.26	0.86–1.30
D-dimer, mg/L	BCS	INNOVANCE D-dimer	<0.17–2.81	<0.17–3.32	<0.17–0.64	<0.17–0.49	<0.17–0.99	<0.17–0.44
	CA-1500	INNOVANCE D-dimer	<0.19–3.49	<0.19–10.9	<0.19–0.65	<0.19–0.52	<0.19–0.75	<0.19–0.48

Modified from Appel et al. [20]. α2-AP, α2-antiplasmin; aPTT, activated partial thromboplastin time; PT, prothrombin time; VWF, von Willebrand factor.

Table 10. Using the Microplate reader analyzer, reference ranges for coagulation tests

Assay	Age						Adult
	Day 1	Day 3	1 month–1 year	1–5 years	6–10 years	11–16 years	
Affinity Biologicals, IU/mL							
Factor II	0.07–0.96	0.49–0.95	0.13–1.91	0.72–2.47	0.65–1.66	0.87–1.88	0.63–2.08
Factor V	0.05–0.48	0.19–0.34	0.10–0.85	0.05–0.89	0.12–0.58	0.02–0.35	0.06–0.46
Factor XI	0.01–0.14	0.05–0.25	0.08–0.64	0.18–0.70	0.14–0.62	0.10–0.36	0.27–0.61
Factor XII	0.03-0.15	0.07-0.17	0.04-0.36	0.04-0.39	0.06-0.38	0.10-0.52	0.08-0.4
Factor XIII	0.67–2.82	0.26–3.16	0.99–4.78	0.67–3.73	0.31–7.85	0.12–6.01	0.47–7.94
Protein C	0.18–0.36	0.16–0.48	0.18–0.96	0.32–1.09	0.38–1.13	0.41–1.18	0.37–2.25
Plasminogen	0.18–0.84	0.37–1.29	0.68–1.77	0.84–3.33	0.87–3.13	0.50–2.78	0.57–8.14
Diagnostica Stago, %							
Factor VII	21–57	23–77	40–101	53–92	38–114	48–174	30–146
Factor VIII	47–162	51–128	40–197	61–159	37–177	38–138	43–155
Factor IX	13–43	15–60	33–77	37–74	32–114	42–97	48–93
Factor X	30–71	28–89	28–164	48–322	58–265	26–277	42–467
Protein C	13–36	23–53	28–93	38–99	38–151	46–133	44–148
Total protein S	6–17	4–24	5–47	15–52	18–55	20–57	18–105
Free protein S	18–29	22–51	33–95	3–141	44–104	41–103	35–142

Modified from Attard et al. [21].

Table 11. Using the ACL top 700/500 (IL) analyzer, reference ranges for coagulation tests

Assay	Age						Adults
	15 days–4 weeks	1–5 months	6–11 months	1–5 years	6–10 years	11–17 years	
PT, s	9.5–12.6	9.7–12.8	9.8–13.0	9.9–13.4	10.0–14.6	10.0–14.1	9.2–12.2
aPTT SynthASil, s	27.6–45.6	24.8–40.7	25.1–40.7	24.0–39.2	26.9–38.7	24.6–38.4	27.8–36.3
aPTT APTT SP, s	33.2–45.6	25.0–43.3	31.7–45.3	25.7–38.4	25.5–42.4	26.1–47.4	26.9–39.5
Fibrinogen Fib C, g/L	1.43–4.02	1.50–3.76	1.57–3.60	1.88–4.13	1.89–4.75	1.77–4.20	2.17–3.42
Fibrinogen QFA, g/L	1.36–3.00	1.41–4.37	1.48–3.67	1.64–4.97	1.71–5.37	1.68–5.29	2.13–4.22
Factor II, %	44.8–74.3	46.7–110.6	73.9–117.2	49.4–130.0	68.4–132.0	47.6–119.2	75.2–132.0
Factor V, %	69.0–123.7	59.5–147.0	59.0–159.8	73.2–188.1	82.0–140.6	61.7–124.8	60.7–141.6
Factor VII, %	55.0–108.0	43.0–141.1	55.2–128.0	47.8–124.2	55.0–135.4	55.4–133.1	59.0–151.0
Factor VIII, %	65.2–153.4	50.3–187.3	53.4–132.2	59.0–167.0	60.6–154.4	42.8–154.6	56.0–145.9
Factor IX, %	30.0–77.0	29.0–105.1	50.5–106.8	52.6–128.9	55.3–156.0	60.2–138.4	69.5–131.0
Factor X, %	66.0–92.0	67.5–122.2	75.8–134.4	59.7–152.8	71.3–161.5	64.0–130.5	72.8–150.4
Factor XI, %	32.9–75.0	27.6–126.4	60.9–125.6	58.0–154.0	31.8–154.0	55.4–139.4	49.1–139.2
Factor XII, %	25.0–81.0	38.0–136.6	48.0–156.1	50.0–174.7	49.4–153.5	49.4–153.5	46.5–157.3
Factor XIII, %	78.4–100.0	55.3–133.2	51.1–136.8	49.4–137.2	53.5–142.4	64.4–133.1	68.1–138.2
Antithrombin, %	32.8–62.8	29.0–120.0	63.0–121.8	60.5–128.3	64.2–136.4	69.1–135.9	83.2–125.7
Protein C chromogenic, %	27.2–48.0	22.8–95.0	46.6–150.9	59.1–147.5	45.9–153.5	72.3–155.1	70.2–144.0
Protein C clot, %	29.7–114.6	28.1–127.8	43.7–151.3	61.0–143.5	39.3–170.3	65.8–126.6	68.8–149.0
Protein S free Ag, %	61.0–108.0	48.0–126.5	63.0–138.9	53.0–134.9	61.5–141.7	61.4–130.7	63.1–127.2
Protein S clot, %	29.0–115.2	33.3–153.9	51.8–138.4	60.2–148.8	66.5–161.5	52.5–147.1	57.9–137.5
Plasminogen, %	41.0–82.7	37.6–109.6	49.3–126.4	59.6–178.0	52.4–158.1	58.1–130.6	63.4–134.8
D-dimer, mg/L	0.45–1.20	0.09–0.88	0.13–0.84	0.09–0.78	0.06–0.57	0.07–0.58	0.11–0.56
VWF:GP1bR, %	87.8–121.5	33.2–154.1	37.1–118.6	40.8–131.8	42.1–162.6	45.0–139.1	46.8–131.4
VWF:activity, %	73.7–188.9	40.9–191.0	42.7–176.0	43.6–155.8	41.2–128.9	54.0–136.9	41.6–152.5
VWF:antigen, %	46.0–219.5	35.5–217.0	48.4–199.4	41.0–185.7	44.8–141.1	55.6–123.4	42.5–144.4

Modified from Toulon et al. [22]. aPTT, activated partial thromboplastin time; PT, prothrombin time; VWF, von Willebrand factor.

Table 12. Using the BCS (Siemens) analyzer, reference ranges for coagulation tests

Assay	Age					
	5–30 days	1.1–5.9 months	6–12 months	1–5 years	5.1–10 years	10.1–≤18 years
aPTT, s	25–60	30–55	28–41	25–41	25–39	25–38
Fibrinogen, g/L	0.50–2.85	0.50–2.06	0.50–1.97	0.44–1.45	0.44–1.45	0.44–1.45
Factor II, %	26–102	45–105	60–120	67–107	67–107	67–116
Factor V, %	34–134	48–132	55–130	70–140	72–140	72–140
Factor VII, %	28–143	39–143	47–130	52–120	52–140	52–140
Factor VIII, %	50–178	50–123	50–134	55–142	58–142	48–142
Factor IX, %	15–85	21–115	36–136	45–110	52–120	55–110
Factor X, %	12–87	35–107	38–136	53–120	53–120	55–140
Factor XI, %	23–87	40–97	49–134	55–140	52–120	55–130
Factor XII, %	11–83	25–109	39–115	55–130	55–140	55–150
Factor XIII, %	39–155	36–170	46–160	62–145	65–150	65–150
VWF:activity, %	50–285	50–206	50–197	44–145	44–145	44–145
Antithrombin, %	35–108	70–120	70–123	80–139	90–130	90–130
Protein S free Ag, %	15–93	54–118	55–120	54–118	48–105	48–105
Protein C, %	17–65	28–80	37–81	40–92	45–93	45–93
α2-AP, %	68–120	70–130	80–130	90–115	85–115	75–115
Plasminogen, %	39–70	54–95	65–110	79–120	76–110	70–104
D-dimer, mg/L	<0.79					

Modified from Nowak-Göttl et al. [23]. α2-AP, α2-antiplasmin; aPTT, activated partial thromboplastin time; VWF, von Willebrand factor.

Table 13. Using the ACL top 700/500 (IL) analyzer, reference ranges for coagulation tests

Assay	Age	
	≥29 days–<3 years	≥3 years–<12 years
PT, s	10.00–12.67	10.60–13.10
Assay	Age	
	≥29 days–<1 year	≥1 year–<12 years
aPTT, s	27.43–43.68	27.87–40.80
Thrombin time, s	15.40–21.27	14.42–18.90
Fibrinogen, g/L	1.34–2.94	1.73–3.36

Modified from Zhang et al. [25]. aPTT, activated partial thromboplastin time; PT, prothrombin time.

Acknowledgments

Our special thanks go to Vicky R. Breakey, Shoshana Revel-Vilk, and William Brien who were the authors of this appendix in the first or second editions of this Handbook, which provided a valuable background for this updated appendix.

Conflict of Interest Statement

Laura Avila holds official copyrights for CAPTSure©. Paul Monagle reports receiving no consultancy and speaker fees. He is recipient of peer-reviewed grants (NBA, NHMRC, and MRFF schemes within Australia). He is a member of Pedi Atlas, a not-for-profit consortium that supports antithrombotic trials in children, and serves as a member of advisory boards (no financial payment) for Bayer, Takeda, and Janssen. He was a member of steering committees (no financial payments) for the Einstein junior studies (rivaroxaban/Bayer) and for the saxophone (apixaban/Bristal Myer Squibb) study. Rajiv K. Pruthi has received consulting honoraria (for attending advisory boards) for CSL Behring; Genentech, Inc; Bayer Healthcare AG; HEMA biologics; and Instrumentation Laboratories (Werfen). Ahmad Al-Huniti and Margaret L. Rand have no conflicts of interest to declare.

Author Contributions

Ahmad Al-Huniti drafted the appendix and submitted the final version. Rajiv K. Pruthi, Margaret L. Rand, Laura Avila, and Paul Monagle contributed to the design of the appendix, critically revised it, and approved the final version for publication.

Abbreviations

aPTT	Activated partial thromboplastin time
FVIII	Factor VIII
VWF	von Willebrand factor

References

1 Ignjatovic V, Kenet G, Monagle P. Developmental hemostasis: recommendations for laboratories reporting pediatric samples. J Thromb Haemost. 2012; 10(2):298–300.

2 Andrew M, Vegh P, Johnston M, Bowker J, Ofosu F, Mitchell L. Maturation of the hemostatic system during childhood. Blood. 1992;80(8):1998–2005.

3 Andrew M, Paes B, Milner R, Johnston M, Mitchell L, Tollefsen DM, et al. Development of the human coagulation system in the full-term infant. Blood. 1987;70(1):165–72.

4 Andrew M, Paes B, Johnston M. Development of the hemostatic system in the neonate and young infant. Am J Pediatr Hematol Oncol. 1990;12(1):95–104.

5 Andrew M, Paes B, Milner R, Johnston M, Mitchell L, Tollefsen DM, et al. Development of the human coagulation system in the healthy premature infant. Blood. 1988;72(5):1651–7.

6 Monagle P, Barnes C, Ignjatovic V, Furmedge J, Newall F, Chan A, et al. Developmental haemostasis. Impact for clinical haemostasis laboratories. Thromb Haemost. 2006;95(2):362–72.

7 Israels SJ. Diagnostic evaluation of platelet function disorders in neonates and children: an update. Semin Thromb Hemost. 2009;35(2):181–8.

8 Perlman M, Dvilansky A. Blood coagulation status of small-for-dates and postmature infants. Arch Dis Child. 1975; 50(6):424–30.

9 Beverley DW, Inwood MJ, Chance GW, Schaus M, O'Keefe B. 'Normal' haemostasis parameters: a study in a well-defined inborn population of preterm infants. Early Hum Dev. 1984;9(3):249–57.

10 Boos J, Pollmann H, Dominick HC. Vitamin K-dependent coagulation parameters during the first six days of life: incidence of PIVKA II in newborns. Pediatr Hematol Oncol. 1989;6(2):113–9.

11 Reverdiau-Moalic P, Delahousse B, Body G, Bardos P, Leroy J, Gruel Y. Evolution of blood coagulation activators and inhibitors in the healthy human fetus. Blood. 1996;88(3):900–6.

12 Ries M, Klinge J, Rauch R. Age-related reference values for activation markers of the coagulation and fibrinolytic systems in children. Thromb Res. 1997; 85(4):341–4.

13 Carcao MD, Blanchette VS, Dean JA, He L, Kern MA, Stain AM, et al. The Platelet Function Analyzer (PFA-100): a novel in-vitro system for evaluation of primary haemostasis in children. Br J Haematol. 1998;101(1):70–3.

14 Salonvaara M, Riikonen P, Kekomäki R, Vahtera E, Mahlamäki E, Halonen P, et al. Effects of gestational age and prenatal and perinatal events on the coagulation status in premature infants. Arch Dis Child Fetal Neonatal Ed. 2003;88(4): F319–23.

15 Flanders MM, Crist RA, Roberts WL, Rodgers GM. Pediatric reference intervals for seven common coagulation assays. Clin Chem. 2005;51(9):1738–42.

16 Chan KL, Summerhayes RG, Ignjatovic V, Horton SB, Monagle PT. Reference values for kaolin-activated thromboelastography in healthy children. Anesth Analg. 2007;105(6):1610–3, table of contents.

17 Sosothikul D, Seksarn P, Lusher JM. Pediatric reference values for molecular markers in hemostasis. J Pediatr Hematol Oncol. 2007;29(1):19–22.

18 Mitsiakos G, Papaioannou G, Papadakis E, Chatziioannidis E, Giougi E, Karagianni P, et al. Haemostatic profile of full-term, healthy, small for gestational age neonates. Thromb Res. 2009;124(3): 288–91.

19 Newall F, Johnston L, Ignjatovic V, Summerhayes R, Monagle P. Age-related plasma reference ranges for two heparin-binding proteins – vitronectin and platelet factor 4. Int J Lab Hematol. 2009;31(6):683–7.

20 Appel IM, Grimminck B, Geerts J, Stigter R, Cnossen MH, Beishuizen A. Age dependency of coagulation parameters during childhood and puberty. J Thromb Haemost. 2012;10(11):2254–63.

21 Attard C, van der Straaten T, Karlaftis V, Monagle P, Ignjatovic V. Developmental hemostasis: age-specific differences in the levels of hemostatic proteins. J Thromb Haemost. 2013;11(10):1850–4.

22 Toulon P, Berruyer M, Brionne-Francois M, Grand F, Lasne D, Telion C, et al. Age dependency for coagulation parameters in paediatric populations. Results of a multicentre study aimed at defining the age-specific reference ranges. Thromb Haemost. 2016;116 (1):9–16.

23 Nowak-Gottl U, Limperger V, Kenet G, Degenhardt F, Arlt R, Domschikowski J, et al. Developmental hemostasis: a lifespan from neonates and pregnancy to the young and elderly adult in a European white population. Blood Cells Mol Dis. 2017;67:2–13.

24 Liu J, Dai Y, Yuan E, Li Y, Wang Q, Wang L, et al. Paediatric reference intervals for common coagulation assays in Chinese children as performed on the STA-R coagulation analyzer. Int J Lab Hematol. 2019;41(5):697–701.

25 Zhang H, Li J, Chen H, Wu X. Establishing reference intervals of coagulation indices based on the ACL Top 700 system for children in Southwestern Fujian, China. Clin Biochem. 2020;75:78–82.

26 Sung JY, Seo JD, Ko D-H, Park M-J, Hwang SM, Oh S, et al. Establishment of pediatric reference intervals for routine laboratory tests in Korean population: a retrospective multicenter analysis. Ann Lab Med. 2021;41(2):155–70.

27 Nielsen ST, Strandkjaer N, Juul Rasmussen I, Hansen MK, Lytsen RM, Kamstrup PR, et al. Coagulation parameters in the newborn and infant – The Copenhagen Baby Heart and COMPARE studies. Clinical Chemistry and Laboratory Medicine. 2022;60(2):261–70.

28 Flanders MM, Phansalkar AR, Crist RA, Roberts WL, Rodgers GM. Pediatric reference intervals for uncommon bleeding and thrombotic disorders. J Pediatr. 2006;149(2):275–7.

Published online: December 5, 2024

Blanchette VS, Brandão LR, Carcao MD, Kumar R, Rand ML, Revel-Vilk S (eds): SickKids Handbook of Pediatric Thrombosis and Hemostasis, ed 3, rev. and ext. Basel, Karger, 2024, pp 447–462 (DOI: 10.1159/000538210)

Common Products Used to Manage Disorders of Hemostasis and Thrombosis

Alexandra Zabeida[a] Alicia Koo[b] Victor S. Blanchette[a] Nancy Robitaille[c, d]

[a]Division of Hematology/Oncology, The Hospital for Sick Children, Toronto, ON, Canada; [b]Department of Pharmacy, The Hospital for Sick Children, Toronto, ON, Canada; [c]Héma-Québec, Montréal, QC, Canada; [d]Division of Hematology/Oncology, Department of Pediatrics, CHU Sainte-Justine, Montréal, QC, Canada

Disclaimer: Dosing guidelines are suggestions based on the current practices at the Hospital for Sick Children, Toronto, ON, Canada. Doses do not necessarily conform to the manufacturer's recommendations and not all products listed in this Appendix are licensed for use in children in all countries. It is essential that the reader be aware of the product mix available in their hospital and that they verify the indications, contraindications, and recommended doses in relevant product monographs in their country of practice. Licensed indications, commercial names, and availabilities vary by country.

For the purposes of this appendix, the term blood component will be used to describe red blood cell concentrates, plasma, cryoprecipitate, and platelet concentrates. Blood products is the term used for plasma protein products that are manufactured using pools of human plasma or recombinant technologies. In this appendix, we refer primarily to blood components and blood products that are currently available in Canada.

Blood Components: Transfusion Basics

Blood is collected as whole blood or apheresis donations. In most high- and middle-income countries, whole blood donations are then separated into components, i.e., red blood cell (RBC) concentrates and some combination of plasma (frozen plasma [FP], fresh frozen plasma [FFP]), platelets, cryoprecipitate, and cryosupernatant plasma (CSP). In lower-middle and low-income countries, some whole blood donations are not further processed into components. Apheresis technology utilizes an automated in-line process in which whole blood from the donor enters a collection chamber where flow patterns separate the component to be collected (plasma or cellular blood components, most often platelets), directing the desired component into a collection bag while the remaining constituents of the blood are returned to the donor [1].

In high-income countries, blood components are prepared exclusively from blood obtained through voluntary donations, which, except for

Table 1. Donor/unit testing in Canada (as of July 2022)

Donor/units tested for	Specific agents	Tests used
Immunohematology	ABO and Rh D group K phenotype Other phenotypes (some units)	Phenotypes
	RBC alloantibodies	Serology
Viruses	HIV	Antigen, antibody, and nucleic acid testing
	Hepatitis B	Hepatitis B surface antigen, antibody to hepatitis B core antigen, and nucleic acid testing
	Hepatitis C	Antibody and nucleic acid testing
	HTLV I and II	Antibody testing
	West Nile Virus (seasonal testing)	Nucleic acid testing
Bacteria	Syphilis Bacterial contamination	Serology Bacterial culture (platelets only)
Parasites	Chagas disease/*Trypanosoma cruzi* (at risk donors only)	Antibody testing

For all infectious disease testing, except bacterial cultures, the test result must be nonreactive for issue of the unit from the blood supplier; bacterial cultures of platelet units must be negative at the time of issue from the blood supplier. HIV, human immunodeficiency virus; HTLV-I and II, human T-lymphotropic virus I and II; RBC, red blood cell; Rh, Rhesus.

directed donations, are anonymous. This is also the case for many upper-/middle-income countries. However, in some lower-/middle- and low-income countries, more than half of blood donations are from family/replacement donors or paid donors. The World Health Organization (WHO) advocates for the development of national blood collection systems based on voluntary anonymous donors vs. family/replacement donors because this group tends to have fewer blood-borne infections, particularly in first-time donors [2, 3]. Before individuals can donate blood, they undergo an assessment for donor and recipient safety. This includes a screening questionnaire and a hemoglobin measurement. The screening questionnaire includes an assessment of the donor's general health and other elements, such as travel history, malaria exposure, medication, and vaccination history and behaviors at high risk of sexually transmitted diseases. Before being released for transfusion, immunohematologic and transmissible disease testing (TDT) are performed on the donated blood unit; with respect to TDT, the results must be negative. There is considerable variation internationally both with respect to donor eligibility as per the donor questionnaire and the testing, particularly the TDT that is performed. The testing performed in Canada (as of July 2022) is shown in Table 1.

Risks of Blood Component Transfusions

Transfusion carries risks, which vary depending on the blood component and its method of preparation, the donor population, the geographic location, and the testing used by the blood supplier. Users of this book are cautioned to check with their local blood supplier for information on the risks of transfusion where they practice. This information is needed to accurately assess the benefit:risk ratio in determining the indication

Table 2. Transfusion reactions/complications

Immediate reactions (<24 h)	Delayed reactions/complications (1 day to 4–6 weeks)	Late complications (>4–6 weeks to years)
Febrile nonhemolytic transfusion reactions	Alloimmunization (to red cells or platelets)	Transmission of infections (viruses, parasites, and other)
Minor allergic reactions – urticaria	Delayed hemolytic transfusion reactions	Iron overload (following multiple red cell transfusions)
Transfusion-associated circulatory overload (TACO)	Septic transfusion reactions	
Transfusion-related acute lung injury (TRALI)	Transfusion-associated graft-vs.-host disease (TA-GVHD)	
Transfusion-associated dyspnea	Post-transfusion purpura	
Acute hemolytic transfusion reactions	Transfusion-related alloimmune thrombocytopenia	
Major allergic reactions/ anaphylaxis	Transfusion-related alloimmune neutropenia	
Hypotension		
Septic transfusion reactions		
Metabolic reactions		

for transfusion and to obtain consent for transfusion.

Blood component transfusion carries risks at the time of transfusion as well as delayed risks. These complications are summarized in Table 2. There are common reactions (occurring in <1% to 3–5% of transfusions, depending on the component and the reaction), such as febrile nonhemolytic transfusion reactions and minor allergic reactions, which although bothersome, are not dangerous to the patient. Serious potentially life-threatening reactions are fortunately much less common. These include transfusion-associated circulatory overload (approximately 1 in 700 units), transfusion-related acute lung injury (approximate risk 1 in 5,000 transfusions), septic transfusion reactions (approximately 1 in 100,000 platelet transfusions), and acute hemolytic transfusion reactions (approximately 1 in 40,000 transfusions). Complications of a massive transfusion include dilutional coagulopathy, hypothermia, citrate toxicity (hypocalcemia and hypomagnesemia), metabolic acidosis, and hyperkalemia [4]. With respect to transfusion-transmitted viral diseases, the current estimated risks in Canada are human immunodeficiency virus, 1 in 21.4 million units; hepatitis B, 1 in 7.5 million units; and hepatitis C, 1 in 12.6 million units [5]. Vaccination against hepatitis B, where available, should be highly encouraged to prevent transfusion-transmitted hepatitis B. For further information on the description, prevention, and management of acute and delayed transfusion reactions, the reader is referred to references [4, 6].

Pathogen Reduction Technologies

In an effort to further reduce transfusion transmission of known infectious agents and emerging pathogens, a number of pathogen reduction technologies (PRTs) have been developed. Different PRT platforms for plasma and platelet components have reached commercial availability in many countries.

However, PRT for whole blood and RBCs are still in the early phase of development [7]. Technologies for plasma include solvent detergent (SD) treatment and methylene blue followed by ultraviolet A illumination. SD plasma is prepared from multiple (approximately 1,000) blood donations, whereas the other techniques are applied to single donations or in the case of buffy coat platelets (see below), donations from a few donors. SD plasma has been licensed and widely used for several years in a number of European countries. It is also licensed in Canada and USA, but its use is more limited.

Two other technologies, namely amotosalen (S59, a psoralen) plus ultraviolet A illumination and riboflavin plus ultraviolet light illumination, have also been applied to plasma and platelet units; ultraviolet C illumination alone has been used to inactivate platelets stored in additive solutions. Plasma and/or platelet components that have undergone pathogen reduction based on ultraviolet illumination in the presence or absence of photoactive chemicals are available in Europe and USA. They have been used for both adult and pediatric populations, though published evidence is limited for some technologies.

Blood Components: Composition, Indications, and Risks/Complications

Blood components include RBCs, FP, FFP, cryoprecipitate, CSP, and platelet concentrates. The indications that will be addressed in this appendix are those that pertain to the patients with the disorders that are the subject of this book (e.g., RBC transfusion indications in sickle cell disease or other disorders with specialized indications will not be discussed). In 2018, the Pediatric Critical Care Transfusion and Anemia Expertise Initiative published 102 recommendations to guide RBC transfusion and blood management practices in critically ill children [8]. In 2022, the Transfusion and Anemia Expertise Initiative-Control/Avoidance of Bleeding published expert-based consensus for pediatric intensivists for the administration of plasma and/or platelet transfusions in critically ill pediatric patients [9]. The WHO also has educational modules on clinical use of blood that are easily accessible electronically [10]. Readers are invited to consult these references for further information on blood components' indications.

A summary including information on dosing and component volumes and description is presented in Table 3. Acceptable ABO groups and Rhesus (Rh) type for each component are shown in Table 4. In Canada, all RBC and platelet concentrates are prestorage leukoreduced by the blood supplier (i.e., the white blood cell count per unit is less than 5×10^6). In most jurisdictions, leukoreduced units are considered "cytomegalovirus (CMV) safe" (i.e., do not require additional testing for CMV antibodies); in Canada, this is so for all transfusions (including those for hematopoietic stem cell transplant patients) except for intrauterine transfusions and for granulocyte transfusions to CMV-seronegative recipients [11].

Patients with hemostatic and thrombotic disorders would not usually require irradiation of cellular blood components (for the avoidance of transfusion-associated graft-vs.-host disease) unless they also had a congenital or acquired immunodeficiency disorder and/or they were receiving blood components from biologic relatives. Readers are referred to recent published irradiation guidelines/recommendation for further information [12–14]. In Canada, it is recommended that individuals 45 years and younger, with childbearing potential, be transfused with K (also known as K1 or Kell)-negative red cell units unless they are known to be K positive [11]. This is to prevent alloimmunization and potential hemolytic disease of the fetus and newborn.

RBC Concentrates

The primary indication for a RBC transfusion in patients who are actively bleeding or who have

Table 3. Blood components: dosage, component volumes, and constituents

Blood component	Dosage	Approximate volume/unit	Component description
RBC concentrates	Weight <20 kg: 10–15 mL/kg Weight ≥20 kg: 1 unit	250–350 mL	Nonadditive preservative solution: hematocrit 0.75; some plasma Additive solution: hematocrit 0.50–0.60; almost no plasma
FP/FFP	10–20 mL/kg	Depending on preparation methods 250–290 mL	Contains all coagulation and complement factors
Cryoprecipitate	1 unit/5–10 kg up to 10 units	10 mL	Contains fibrinogen, FVIII, FXIII, and VWF
Cryosupernatant plasma	10–20 mL/kg	300 mL	Plasma deficient in high-molecular-weight multimers of VWF and other factors removed in the preparation of cryoprecipitate
Platelet concentrates			
Whole blood derived (WBD)	5–10 mL/kg or one unit WBD/10 kg; up to 5 units WBD platelets	50–70 mL	>5.5 × 10^{10} platelets per unit
Apheresis	5–10 mL/kg; up to one unit apheresis platelets	225 mL	>2.4 × 10^{11} platelets per unit
Buffy coat (BC)	5–10 mL/kg; up to one unit BC platelets	350 mL	>2.4 × 10^{11} platelets per unit
BC-derived pathogen-reduced platelet	5–10 mL/kg; up to one unit BC pathogen-reduced platelets	180 mL	>2.0 × 10^{11} platelets per unit

FP/FFP, frozen plasma/fresh frozen plasma; FVIII, factor VIII; FXIII, factor XIII; RBC, red blood cell; VWF, von Willebrand factor.

bleeding disorders is increasing the blood's oxygen-carrying capacity [1]. Standard pediatric dosing in stable nonbleeding patients is 10–15 mL/kg, depending on the hematocrit of the RBC concentrates. Physicians should be aware of the nature of the concentrate available where they practice. RBC concentrates stored in nonadditive solutions (e.g., CPD, CPDA1, CP2A) have a hematocrit of approximately 0.75 and the usual dose in a stable nonbleeding patient is 10 mL/kg, whereas concentrates stored in additive solutions (e.g., SAGM, AS1, AS3, AS-5) have a hematocrit of approximately 0.50–0.60 and the standard dose is 15 mL/kg [4]. In Canada, RBC concentrates are stored in the additive solution SAGM. In USA, both additive and nonadditive solutions are used; in Europe, most RBC concentrates are stored in additive solutions.

In the actively bleeding patient, RBC transfusion dose depends more on the clinical status of the patient (and the extent and rate of bleeding) than the hemoglobin level.

Table 4. Blood group compatibility for red blood cell, plasma, or platelet transfusions

Patient's blood group	Compatible red blood cells	Compatible plasma	Compatible platelets
O	O	O, A, B, AB	O, A, B, AB
A	A, O	A, AB	A, AB, O[a]
B	B, O	B, AB	B, AB, O[a]
AB	AB, A, B, O	AB	ABO[a]
Rh positive	Rh positive or negative (Rh positive preferred[b])	n/a	Rh positive or negative (Rh positive preferred[b])
Rh negative	Rh negative (in extreme emergencies may use Rh positive)	n/a	Rh positive or negative[a] (Rh negative preferred)

Note: Cryoprecipitate does not need to be ABO or Rh compatible. Rh, Rhesus. [a]See section on platelet concentrates. [b]For inventory reasons, i.e., to preserve Rh-negative units for Rh-negative recipients.

Frozen Plasma/Fresh Frozen Plasma

In Canada and the USA, most of the plasma is FFP (frozen within 8 h of collection) or FP (frozen within 24 h of collection). FFP and FP contain all clotting factors. Factors V (FV) and VIII (FVIII) are generally considered "labile" coagulation factors, whereas the remaining coagulation factors are considered stable. Levels of FVIII may be slightly reduced in FP as compared with FFP (e.g., FVIII in apheresis FFP is 1.05 ± 0.37 IU/mL [mean ± SD] and in FP 0.88 ± 0.27 IU/mL), but FV in FFP and FP are essentially equivalent [12]. In Canada, FP and FFP are used interchangeably. Allowable use of thawed plasma varies by country. In Canada, thawed FP/FFP stored at 4°C may be used for up to 5 days after thawing. FV and FVIII concentrations in thawed plasma depend on the time from the initial thaw.

The current suggested indications for the use of FP/FFP [15] include:

1. The treatment of patients who are bleeding or undergoing invasive procedures who require replacement of multiple plasma coagulation factors.
2. The treatment of patients with single congenital or acquired coagulation factor deficiencies for which a more appropriate alternative therapy is not available.
3. Reversal of vitamin K antagonist (VKA) (e.g., warfarin) effect or immediate correction of vitamin K deficiency in patients with active bleeding, or prior to surgery, or an invasive procedure if a prothrombin complex concentrate (PCC; see below) is not available.
4. As the replacement fluid in plasma exchange for thrombotic microangiopathies (thrombotic thrombocytopenia purpura and atypical hemolytic uremic syndrome).
5. The treatment of patients with massive transfusion with clinically significant coagulation abnormalities.
6. Preparation of reconstituted whole blood for exchange transfusion in neonates.

SD plasma is occasionally used for patients requiring treatment with large volumes of plasma (e.g., repetitive exchange transfusions for thrombotic thrombocytopenia purpura) who have recurrent and/or severe allergic reactions with other plasma components.

For more information on the management of rare coagulation factor deficiencies, see Chapter 10; for thrombotic thrombocytopenia purpura and disseminated intravascular coagulation (DIC), see Chapter 11; and for VKA reversal, see Chapter 20.

Cryoprecipitate and CSP

Cryoprecipitate is prepared from slowly thawed plasma that is centrifuged to separate the insoluble cryoprecipitate from the remaining plasma (CSP). The insoluble cryoprecipitate and CSP are refrozen separately. Cryoprecipitate contains fibrinogen, fibronectin, FVIII, factor XIII (FXIII), as well as von Willebrand factor (VWF). In Canada, the fibrinogen content of one unit of cryoprecipitate is 366 ± 115 mg and the average volume of one unit is 10 ± 1.7 mL [15]. CSP contains all the remaining plasma proteins, including the remaining coagulation factors.

Cryoprecipitate may be useful in the management of patients requiring fibrinogen or FXIII supplementation (see Chapters 10 and 11). Fibrinogen and FXIII concentrates are available in some countries, including Canada. In general, in Canada, clotting factor concentrates are used for patients with single congenital coagulation factor deficiencies, whereas cryoprecipitate is used for acquired deficiencies (e.g., massive bleeding) [16]. If no clotting factor concentrates are available, cryoprecipitate may be used in the treatment of patients with hemophilia A and severe von Willebrand disease (VWD; see Chapters 8 and 9).

CSP may be used for the treatment of patients with thrombotic thrombocytopenic purpura or atypical hemolytic uremic syndrome undergoing plasma exchange. If a PCC (see below) is not available, CSP may also be used in patients on warfarin who are bleeding or need to undergo an invasive procedure, before vitamin K can reverse the warfarin effects [8] (see Chapter 20).

Platelet Concentrates

As described in this section, there are four different types of platelet components. In Canada (and several other countries), only the latter three types of platelet concentrates are produced, whereas in USA, buffy coat platelets are not available. Platelet additive solutions (PASs) may be used to improve platelet storage of either apheresis or buffy coat platelets. PAS-platelets contain approximately two-thirds less plasma than "standard" platelets. Availability from blood providers differs [17]. The average volume for each type of platelet components is described in Table 3.

1. Whole blood-derived platelets are a concentrate of platelets separated from a single unit of whole blood. One unit of whole blood-derived platelets should contain >5.5 × 10^{10} platelets. This component can be provided as a single unit for smaller recipients or can be pooled for larger recipients.
2. Apheresis platelets are prepared from a single donor via an automated in-line process, which separates the platelets from whole blood and directs them to a collection bag, whereas the remaining constituents of the blood are returned to the donor. In Canada, one unit contains >2.4 × 10^{11} platelets [11, 18].
3. A buffy coat platelet pool is a platelet concentrate prepared by the separation of the buffy coat layer (which contains white blood cells and platelets) from 4 to 6 ABO identical whole blood units. The platelet concentrates are pooled in the residual plasma from one of the whole blood units and then leukoreduced by filtration. One unit contains >2.4 × 10^{11} platelets [11, 18].
4. Pooled psoralen-treated platelets were introduced in Canada in 2022. They have been used in Europe and USA for several years. This platelet concentrate is prepared by separation of the buffy coat layer (which contains white blood cells and platelets) from 7 ABO identical whole blood units and pooled in 280 mL of platelet additive solutionE (PAS-E). This double dose pool is leukocyte reduced by filtration and then pathogen reduced using the INTERCEPT® DS Blood System for Platelets. The pathogen-reduced double dose is split into two single transfusion units (mean platelet count: 1,363 ± 188 × 10^9/unit) [19].

Platelet transfusions may be given to patients with thrombocytopenia or dysfunctional platelet disorders (congenital, metabolic, or medication induced) who have active bleeding or are at serious risk of bleeding (i.e., prophylactic use) related to their thrombocytopenia/platelet dysfunction [20] (See Chapters 6 and 7).

Dosing of platelets at 5–10 mL/kg (of any of the four platelet component types) should increase the circulating platelet count by at least 15–25 × 10^9/L in patients without platelet refractoriness caused by platelet alloantibodies or conditions, such as fever, septicemia, or DIC [4]. The presence of clinically significant splenomegaly will also decrease the expected platelet increment immediately following a platelet transfusion.

ABO-identical platelets are preferred for platelet transfusion to children whenever possible. ABO plasma-incompatible platelets (e.g., group O platelets given to a group A patient) may result in clinically significant hemolysis of the patient's red cells. To the extent possible, group O platelets should not be transfused to non-group O pediatric recipients, particularly if the child is not bleeding or undergoing an emergency invasive procedure. If ABO-identical platelets or plasma-compatible platelets are not available for a non-group O pediatric recipient, then to the extent possible, low anti-A/B titer or plasma-reduced units should be used.

Platelet concentrates may contain small amounts of erythrocytes; the residual amount depends on the manufacturing process. Therefore, in general, it is recommended that female children and females of child-bearing age/potential, who are Rh D-negative should receive Rh immunoglobulin before, immediately after, or within 72 h of receiving an RhD-positive platelet component. Males and females who are not of child-bearing age/potential, who are RhD-negative, and are transfused with RhD-positive platelet components probably do not require Rh immunoglobulin. For further discussion of these recommendations and dosing guidelines, the reader is referred to reference [19].

Patients who are refractory to platelet transfusions and have human leukocyte antigen (HLA), class 1 antibodies, or human platelet antigen (HPA) antibodies should receive HLA, class 1-selected or HPA-selected, or cross-match compatible platelets [4, 15].

Plasma Protein Products

Plasma protein products (PPPs) encompass a broad variety of products used in the field of hemostasis and thrombosis. They may be derived from human plasma or made by recombinant technology. New products are constantly being developed, and their availability and licensed indications for use vary widely between countries. Since the commercial name may differ according to the production method and country of administration, only generic names are used for the PPPs discussed in this section.

Human-derived PPPs are derived from pools of plasma from whole blood or apheresis donations of both volunteer and paid donors. Donors are screened and must meet eligibility criteria. Their donations undergo TDT as required by the fractionation facility and the regulatory authorities in the countries where a company operates and where the products are used. In general, the TDT for the individual donations contributing to the pools is similar to the TDT for whole blood and apheresis donations for blood components as described above (Table 1). In addition, depending on the product, there may be additional testing requirements for the plasma pools (e.g., hepatitis A and parvovirus B19 testing).

Current fractionation technology largely relies on a backbone process encompassing cryoprecipitation and cold ethanol precipitation steps. This process involves successive processing steps at defined ethanol concentrations, associated with shifts in pH, temperature, and osmolality that result in selective precipitation of proteins. Precipitates are separated by centrifugation or filtration. In the past 2–3 decades, the addition of large-scale chromatography and monoclonal affinity columns have further improved the purity, diversity, and yield of extracted products [21, 22].

Besides rigorous screening of candidate blood/plasma donors and TDT of donations, PPP safety is further ensured by a variety of pathogen reduction techniques including SD treatment, heat treatment, and/or nanofiltration [21–24], and hepatitis B and hepatitis C testing of most plasma products. Of note, nonenveloped viruses such as hepatitis A and parvovirus B19 are not inactivated by SD treatment; hence, these viruses are tested for in blood/plasma donations used for the production of commercially available PPPs. Heat treatment, including pasteurization, is used to inactivate both enveloped and nonenveloped viruses. Nanofiltration is used to complement the core viral inactivation process and to provide enhanced safety against nonenveloped viruses or other resistant infectious agents [21, 22].

Recombinant PPPs are synthesized in vitro from isolated genes expressed in cell cultures using recombinant DNA techniques. They may contain small amounts of human albumin depending on the product.

Despite the measures described above, PPPs (either human plasma derived or recombinant) carry a theoretical risk of transmitting infectious agents such as viruses, prions (e.g., such as the variant Creutzfeldt-Jakob disease agent), or emerging pathogens. However, to date, no cases of transmission of viral diseases or variant Creutzfeldt-Jakob disease have been reported in the literature with the use of PPP in Canada [22]. Other risks specific to each product are discussed in the individual product sections.

Fibrinogen Concentrates

Human fibrinogen concentrate is indicated for use in prophylaxis and/or management of hemorrhage in adults and children with congenital fibrinogen disorders (afibrinogenemia, hypofibrinogenemia, dysfibrinogenemia, or hypodysfibrinogenemia; see Chapter 10). Human fibrinogen concentrates may also be used to treat major bleeding in patients with acquired hypofibrinogenemia; licensing of human fibrinogen concentrate for this indication varies among products and countries. A recent randomized clinical trial demonstrated noninferiority of fibrinogen concentrates to cryoprecipitate in patients with acquired hypofibrinogenemia [25]. In some countries (e.g., the United Kingdom), cryoprecipitate rather than human fibrinogen concentrate is used for acquired hypofibrinogenemia, whereas in others (e.g., many European countries), human fibrinogen concentrate has entirely replaced the use of cryoprecipitate. In Canada and USA, jurisdictions differ in their use of human fibrinogen concentrates vs. cryoprecipitate for the treatment of acquired hypofibrinogenemia. Fibrinogen concentrates are purified and pathogen reduced, whereas cryoprecipitate does not undergo viral inactivation treatment [25].

Factor VII Concentrates

Purified plasma-derived factor VII (FVII) concentrates are indicated for the treatment of congenital FVII deficiency (see Chapter 10). Recombinant activated FVII (rFVIIa) is indicated for the treatment of bleeding in patients with congenital FVII deficiency (see Chapter 10) and for the prophylaxis and management of acute bleeding in patients with hemophilia A or B, who have developed neutralizing antibodies ("inhibitors") to FVIII or factor IX (FIX) (see Chapter 8). It may also be used in patients with platelet dysfunction, e.g., Glanzmann thrombasthenia, to minimize the need for platelet transfusions (see Chapter 6).

It is important to note that rFVIIa concentrates are associated with an increased risk of thrombosis (much higher in the elderly than in children), which increases when coadministered with activated prothrombin complex concentrates (APCCs) [26]. Recommended doses of rFVIIa depend on the indication (see relevant chapters for detail).

Factor VIII Concentrates

FVIII concentrates are indicated for the treatment of bleeding episodes, perioperative prophylaxis, as well as routine prophylaxis in patients with hemophilia A (see Chapter 8). Plasma-derived and recombinant FVIII products are available. Recombinant FVIII products are either full-length or B-domain-deleted molecules. Longer acting (extended half-life) recombinant FVIII concentrates have recently been developed. See Chapter 8 for further details regarding dosage recommendations for these products. Emicizumab is discussed below, in the section "Other Agents for Achieving Hemostasis."

Factor IX Concentrates

FIX concentrates are indicated for the treatment of bleeding episodes, perioperative prophylaxis, as well as routine prophylaxis in patients with hemophilia B (see Chapter 8). There are recombinant and plasma-derived concentrates available. Longer acting FIX factor concentrates have recently been developed. See Chapter 8 for further details regarding dosage recommendations for FIX concentrates.

VWF Concentrates

VWF concentrates are available for the treatment and prophylaxis of bleeding in patients with severe VWD. In general, treatment with VWF concentrates is not required in patients with mild forms of VWD as these patients can be treated with desmopressin (1-deamino-8-D-arginine vasopressin [DDAVP]) (see Chapter 9). For patients with severe VWD, treatment is necessary to prevent operative bleeding or bleeding associated with invasive procedures, to prevent/manage bleeding during childbirth or miscarriage and in the event of excessive mucosal bleeding such as heavy menstrual bleeding (HMB) or epistaxis. Both plasma-derived (human and porcine) and recombinant products exist, where available (see Chapter 9) [27]. Plasma-derived products contain VWF in combination with FVIII. See Chapter 9 for further details regarding dosage and treatment recommendations.

Factor XI Concentrates

Factor XI (FXI) concentrate is indicated for the treatment of clinically significant bleeding and for perioperative prophylaxis in high-risk surgical procedures in patients with FXI deficiency. A plasma-derived product is available. Details on the treatment of FXI deficiency and the risk of thrombosis associated with the use of FXI concentrate is discussed in Chapter 10.

Factor XIII Concentrates

FXIII concentrate is indicated for the treatment and prophylaxis of patients with congenital FXIII deficiency. Both human plasma-derived and recombinant FXIII products are available. Factor FXIII deficiency is discussed in Chapter 10.

Prothrombin Complex Concentrates

PCCs are human plasma-derived products containing a mixture of vitamin K-dependent coagulation factors (II, IX, and X and protein S and protein C [3-factor products]). A few 4-factor products also contain FVII but usually at lower amounts than other factors. Some also contain antithrombin and heparin. All these products are labeled according to their FIX content.

PCC is indicated for the treatment of bleeding episodes and perioperative bleeding prophylaxis in acquired deficiencies of the prothrombin complex coagulation factors, such as deficiency caused by treatment or overdose with VKAs (see Chapter 20). The second licensed indication for the use of PCC is for the treatment of bleeding and perioperative prophylaxis in patients with congenital deficiencies of coagulation factors II and X when purified specific factor concentrates are not available (see Chapter 10). These products carry a risk of thrombosis and should be used with caution. Because of the different PCCs available internationally, it is recommended to consult the drug monograph for specifics of administration and dosing. PCCs are contraindicated in patients with heparin-induced thrombocytopenia as they contain heparin. They are not generally recommended for the elective reversal of direct oral anticoagulants, treatment of an elevated international normalized ratio (INR) without bleeding or need for surgical intervention, massive transfusion, coagulopathy of liver disease, or for patients with a recent history of thrombosis, myocardial infarction, or DIC [28].

Activated Prothrombin Complex Concentrate

APCC is a human plasma-derived factor complex that contains mainly nonactivated factors II, IX, and X and mainly activated FVII, as well as trace levels of FVIII. The main source of APCC in Canada is FEIBA, Baxalta. APCC bypasses FVIII activity in patients who cannot respond normally to FVIII because of the presence of FVIII inhibitors. It is indicated for the treatment and prophylaxis of bleeding episodes in patients with hemophilia A or B with inhibitors to FVIII or FIX, respectively, and in nonhemophiliac patients with acquired inhibitors to FVIII, FIX, and/or FXI. Importantly, APCC should be avoided in patients on emicizumab because of the increased risk of thrombosis with this combination. For specific recommendations on the management of hemophilia patients with inhibitors, see Chapter 8, and for acquired inhibitors, see Chapter 11.

Protein C Concentrate

Protein C concentrate is indicated for pediatric patients with severe congenital protein C deficiency for the prevention and treatment of venous thrombosis and purpura fulminans (see Chapter 13).

Antithrombin Concentrate

Antithrombin concentrates may be indicated for patients with acquired or congenital antithrombin deficiency for thrombosis prophylaxis or treatment [29] (see Chapters 14, 16, 19, and 20 for discussion on the use of antithrombin concentrates in children with acquired antithrombin deficiency [i.e., asparaginase-related, renal, cardiac] and heparin resistance]). Antithrombin concentrates are available in plasma-derived and recombinant formulations and should be used judiciously, as bleeding risk may increase when it is coadministered with heparin.

Intravenous Immunoglobulins

Intravenous immunoglobulins (IVIGs) have several licensed indications (which may vary with the preparation and among countries) including immune thrombocytopenia (ITP) (see Chapter 7). There are several IVIG preparations available; all are plasma derived. Headache, minor allergic reactions, and febrile nonhemolytic reactions are common complications of all IVIG preparations; other less common complications include aseptic meningitis, alloimmune hemolysis, anaphylaxis, and rarely, thromboembolic events or renal failure [4]. There is a potential association between anaphylaxis and anti-IgA antibodies in patients with absent or very low IgA levels; however, the role of anti-IgA antibodies in causing anaphylaxis in IgA-deficient patients receiving IVIG remains controversial [30]. The mechanism of hemolysis involves passive transfer of anti-A and anti-B isohemagglutinins that react with the RBC antigens. Mild hemolysis is not uncommon and may result in transient anemia with reticulocytosis. A direct antiglobulin test (previously called Coombs test) may be positive but can also be negative because of rapid clearance of antibody-sensitized RBCs. Acute severe intravascular hemolysis is reported to occur in 1.6% of patients and may result in hemoglobinuria, hemoglobinemia, and renal insufficiency [31–33]. The onset of hemolysis ranges from 12 h to 10 days following infusion of IVIG. Risk factors include higher IVIG doses, female sex, and non-O blood group.

Rh Immune Globulin

Rh immune globulin (RhIG) is used to prevent RhD hemolytic disease of the newborn, RhD alloimmunization in RhD-negative persons who have received RhD-positive blood transfusion (see above), and in the treatment of ITP in D-positive patients who have not undergone splenectomy (see Chapter 7). RhIG is prepared from pooled human plasma. Some formulations can only be administered intramuscularly, whereas others can be given either intramuscularly or intravenously. For ITP, only the intravenous formulation is used. As the doses of RhIG used in the treatment of ITP are large, there is a risk of RBC hemolysis, thus patients' hemoglobin should be monitored after administration. Given the risk of intravascular hemolysis associated with RhIG, there is a strong recommendation against its use in ITP if other alternatives exist [34]. ITP management is discussed in Chapter 7.

Other Agents for Achieving Hemostasis

Topical Agents for Maintaining Hemostasis

Topical hemostatic agents are various biological products that can be applied directly to a surgical site to achieve or maintain hemostasis. In some centers, such agents are used routinely for hemostatic support in patients with bleeding disorders who are undergoing major dental procedures, circumcision, or orthopedic surgery. Mechanical topical hemostatic agents provide a physical matrix to assist in the clotting process. These agents include gelatin foams, collagen, cellulose sheets, and polysaccharide spheres. Adhesive hemostatic agents participate in the late stages of the coagulation cascade to promote fibrin clot formation. They are usually comprised of human-purified fibrinogen and/or thrombin concentrates, with possible other additions, such as FXIII, fibronectin, or antifibrinolytic agents (e.g., tranexamic acid) [35]. High fibrinogen concentration enhances clot strength, whereas high thrombin concentration shortens clotting time [35]. Commercial products prepared from pooled plasma are now widely available, with viral inactivation incorporated into the manufacturing process. Topical thrombins are derived from human thrombin or bovine thrombin, and in some countries may be available as a recombinant product. The use of products containing bovine thrombin may lead to the development of antibodies to bovine thrombin or FV, which may cross-react with human clotting factors and cause an immune-related coagulopathy with potentially fatal bleeding or thrombosis [36] (see Chapter 11). Given the risk of neurotoxicity (seizures), adhesives with tranexamic acid must be avoided in cases of cerebrospinal fluid leakage or dura mater tear [35]. Topical hemostatic agents should be used upon consultation between a hematologist and a surgeon with expertise in their use (indications and precautions).

Desmopressin

DDAVP is a synthetic analog of vasopressin that elevates plasma VWF and FVIII levels and increases platelet adhesiveness. Formulations include intravenous, subcutaneous, and intranasal. Patients with type I VWD, some forms of type 2 VWD, and patients with mild hemophilia A (particularly those with baseline FVIII coagulant activity >10%) with minor bleeding can usually be managed with DDAVP. A DDAVP challenge test is usually recommended for VWD and hemophilia A patients prior to its use in the clinical setting (see Chapters 8 and 9). DDAVP may also be used for mild-to-moderate bleeding in patients with inherited platelet function disorders (see Chapter 6) and acquired hemophilia or VWD (see Chapter 11).

Intravenous dosing of DDAVP may cause hyponatremia and a severe drop in plasma osmolality, especially in infants, which can lead to coma, seizures, and death. For this reason, DDAVP should not be used in children younger than 3 years of age. Fluid restriction 12–24 h following

Table 5. Desmopressin/DDAVP dosing[a]

Intravenous/subcutaneous
0.3 µg/kg (maximum 20 µg/dose)
Slow (over 20–30 min) intravenous infusion in 50 mL normal saline
Subcutaneous dosing is given undiluted
One dose per day for up to 2–3 days
Fluid restriction (<2/3 maintenance intravenous fluids)
Check sodium level prior to subsequent dose if using >1 dose
If used preoperatively, to be administered 30 min before procedure
Intranasal
Weight <50 kg: 150 µg (1 spray)/24 h
Weight ≥50 kg: 300 µg (1 spray in each nostril)/24 h
No more than 3 doses over 3 days
Repeat use is determined based on the patient's clinical status and laboratory investigations
If used preoperatively, to be administered 2 h before procedure

[a]Do not use in children younger than 3 years of age.

administration and close monitoring of serum sodium levels and urine output are necessary, particularly if more than one dose is administered, for patients of all ages. Patients on intravenous solutions should only receive isotonic solutions (e.g., normal saline) in the 24 h following DDAVP administration. Serial doses are also associated with tachyphylaxis. Mostly commonly, only one dose is given although second and third doses may be given after 24-h intervals. DDAVP dosing is summarized in Table 5.

Antifibrinolytic Agents

Antifibrinolytic agents are drugs that exert their effect through inhibition of fibrinolysis. Tranexamic acid and ε-aminocaproic acid are synthetic derivatives of the amino acid lysine. They bind to specific sites on both plasminogen and plasmin and inhibit their ability to degrade fibrin. They are used to stop excessive bleeding, particularly mucosal, such as epistaxis, dental, or HMB. They can be administered orally, intravenously, or topically. These drugs are contraindicated in patients with active or history of thrombosis and are to be used with caution in patients with DIC (usually contraindicated, except for uncontrolled bleeding with marked hyperfibrinolysis, e.g., in acute promyelocytic leukemia), and in patients with gross hematuria [37]. Given their renal metabolism, doses and intervals should be adjusted in renal impairment. Dosing for these drugs is summarized in Table 6.

Emicizumab

Emicizumab is a novel therapy for hemophilia A. It consists of a recombinant, humanized, bispecific monoclonal antibody (much like activated FVIII), which bridges activated FIX and FX and thus bypasses the need for activated FVIII. It is currently approved in several countries for routine prophylaxis of bleeding episodes in patients with hemophilia A with or without inhibitors. Given its subcutaneous administration every 1–4 weeks, it has revolutionized the prophylactic treatment of hemophilia A in recent years, significantly improving quality of life and enabling the start of prophylaxis from a very early age [38]. As mentioned above, APCC should not be used, or should be with significantly reduced doses, for bleeding complications in patients on emicizumab because of the risk of thrombosis with this combination (see Chapter 8).

Table 6. Antifibrinolytic agents

Product	Dose
Tranexamic acid[a]	
Intravenous	10–30 mg/kg per dose preprocedure and then 10 mg/kg per dose TID to QID after procedure until able to take orally (maximum 1,000 mg/dose) May also be given as a continuous IV infusion at 5–10 mg/kg/h following the loading dose
Oral	25 mg/kg per dose TID to QID beginning the evening preprocedure or with bleeding and for up to 5–7 days thereafter (maximum 1,500 mg/dose)
Mouthwash	Tranexamic acid 5% (7.65 g of tranexamic acid in 150 mL sterile water) mouthwash: every 6 h starting on the day of dental/oral surgery, beginning 5–10 min preprocedure and for 7 days after
Topical	Cotton gauze soaked with tranexamic acid 10% (e.g., 500 mg of tranexamic acid in 5 mL sterile water) applied topically, e.g., into a bleeding nostril
ε-Aminocaproic acid	
Oral, intravenous	Loading dose: 100–200 mg/kg (maximum loading dose: 10 g) Maintenance dose: 50–100 mg/kg per dose every 4–6 h for 5–7 days Maximum daily dose: 30 g

IV, intravenous; QID, four times a day; TID, three times a day. [a]Dose adjustment if renal impairment.

Acknowledgments

Our special thanks go to Mira F. Leibman, Ewurabena Simpson, Wendy Lau, and Heather A. Hume who were authors of this appendix in the previous editions of this Handbook, which provided a valuable background for this updated appendix.

Conflict of Interest Statement

Alexandra Zabeida and Alicia Koo have no conflicts of interest to declare. Nancy Robitaille is an employee of Héma-Québec. She is recipient of research grants from Agios and Forma-Therapeutics. Victor Blanchette reports receiving consultancy and speaker fees from Bayer HealthCare, Sanofi, Novo Nordisk, Pfizer, Roche, Takeda, and Spark Therapeutics. He is recipient of research grants from Sanofi, Bayer HealthCare, and Takeda and serves as a member of Data Safety Monitoring Boards for Octapharma and Takeda. He is Chair of a nonprofit organization, the International Prophylaxis Study Group (IPSG).

Author Contributions

Alexandra Zabeida and Nancy Robitaille drafted the appendix, critically revised it, and approved the final version. Alicia Koo and Victor Blanchette critically revised the chapter and approved the final version.

Abbreviations

APCC	Activated prothrombin complex concentrate
CMV	Cytomegalovirus
CSP	Cryosupernatant plasma
DDAVP	1-Deamino-8-D-arginine vasopressin (desmopressin)
DIC	Disseminated intravascular coagulation
FIX	Factor IX
FV	Factor V
FVII	Factor VII
FVIII	Factor VIII
FXI	Factor XI
FXIII	Factor XIII
FFP	Fresh frozen plasma
FP	Frozen plasma
HLA	Human leukocyte antigen
HMB	Heavy menstrual bleeding
HPA	Human platelet antigen
INR	International normalized ratio
ITP	Immune thrombocytopenia
IVIG	Intravenous immunoglobulin
PAS	Platelet additive solution

PCC	Prothrombin complex concentrate	SD	Solvent detergent
PPP	Plasma protein product	TDT	Transmissible disease testing
PRT	Pathogen reduction technologies	VKA	Vitamin K antagonist
rFVIIa	Recombinant activated factor VII	VWD	von Willebrand disease
RBC	Red blood cell	VWF	von Willebrand factor
RhIG	Rhesus (Rh) immune globulin	WHO	World Health Organization

References

1 Gupta A, Bigham M. Chapter 2 blood components. In: Clinical Guide to Transfusion. Canadian Blood Services; March 2023. Accessed August 20, 2023. https://professionaleducation.blood.ca/en/print/pdf/node/120

2 World Health Organization. Blood Safety and Availability, Key Facts. June 2023. Accessed August 20, 2023. https://www.who.int/news-room/fact-sheets/detail/blood-safety-and-availability

3 World Health Organization. Global Status Report on Blood Safety and Availability; 2021. Accessed August 20, 2023.https://apps.who.int/iris/bitstream/handle/10665/356165/9789240051683-eng.pdf

4 Callum JL, Pinkerton PH, Lin Y, Cope S, Karkouti K, Lieberman L, et al. Bloody Easy 5.1:Blood Transfusions, Blood Alternatives and Transfusion Reactions: a Guide to Transfusion Medicine. 5th ed. Ontario Regional Blood Coordinating Network; 2022:143 p. Accessed August 20, 2023. https://transfusionontario.org/en/bloody-easy-5-blood-transfusions-blood-alternatives-and-transfusion-reactions-a-guide-to-transfusion-medicine-fifth-edition-handbook/

5 Canadian Blood Services. Red Blood Cells, Leucocytes Reduced. Circular of Information for the Use of Human Blood Components, January 2021. Accessed August 20, 2023. https://www.blood.ca/sites/default/files/1000104991_2021-01-25.pdf

6 Kopko PM, ed. Transfusion Reactions. 5th ed. AABB Press; 2021:732 p.

7 Rebulla P, Prati D. Pathogen reduction for platelets-a review of recent implementation strategies. Pathogens. 2022;11(2):142.

8 Valentine SL, Bembea MM, Muszynski JA, Cholette JM, Doctor A, Spinella PC, et al: Consensus recommendations for RBC transfusion practice in critically ill children from the Paediatric Critical Care and Anemia Expertise Initiative. Pediatr Crit Care Med J. 2018;18:884–98.

9 Nellis ME, Karam O, Valentine SL, Bateman ST, Remy KE, Lacroix J, et al. Executive summary of recommendations and expert consensus for plasma and platelet transfusion practice in critically Ill children: from the Transfusion and Anemia EXpertise Initiative-Control/Avoidance of Bleeding (TAXI-CAB). Pediatr Crit Care Med. 2022;23(1):34–51.

10 World Health Organization. Educational modules on clinical use of blood, December 2021. Accessed August 20, 2023. https://www.who.int/publications/i/item/9789240033733

11 National Standard of Canada. CAN/CSA-Z902:20. Blood and Blood Components, 2020:162 p.

12 National Advisory Committee of Blood and Blood Products. Recommendations for use of irradiated blood components in Canada: a NC and CCNMT collaborative initiative, May 2018. Accessed August 20, 2023. https://nacblood.ca/sites/default/files/2021-08/Recommendations_Irradiated_Blood_Components.pdf

13 Foukaneli T, Kerr P, Bolton-Maggs PHB, Cardigan R, Coles A, Gennery A, et al. Guidelines on the use of irradiated blood components. Br J Haematol. 2020;91:704–24.

14 Wiersum-Osselton JC, Slomp J, Frederik Falkenburg JH, Geltink T, van Duijnhoven HLP, Netelenbos T, et al. Guideline development for prevention of transfusion-associated graft-versus-host disease: reduction of indications for irradiated blood components after prestorage leukodepletion of blood components. Br J Haematol. 2021;195:681–8.

15 Canadian Blood Services. Circular of information for the use of human blood and blood components. Plasma Components. March 2023. Accessed August 20, 2023. https://www.blood.ca/sites/default/files/IM-00004_Revision_2.pdf

16 Levy JH, Goodnough LT: How I use fibrinogen replacement therapy in acquired bleeding. Blood. 2015;125:1387–93.

17 van der Meer PF, de Korte D. Platelet additive solutions: a review of the latest developments and their clinical implications. Transfus Med Hemother. 2018; 45(2):98–102.

18 Canadian Blood Services. Circular of information for the use of human blood and blood components. Platelets. Ottawa; 2022. Accessed August 20, 2023. https://www.blood.ca/sites/default/files/IM-00003_Revision_1.pdf

19 Canadian Blood Services. Circular of information for the use of human blood and blood components. Pathogen Reduced Platelets Concentrates. Ottawa; 2022. Accessed August 20, 2023. https://www.blood.ca/sites/default/files/IM-00050_Revision_1.pdf

20 Nahirniak S, Slichter SJ, Tanael S, Rebulla P, Pavenski K, Vassallo R, et al. Guidance on platelet transfusion for patients with hypoproliferative thrombocytopenia. Transfus Med Rev. 2015; 29:3–13.

21 Burnouf T. An overview of plasma fractionation. Ann Blood. 2018;3:1–10.

22 Canadian Blood Services. Clinical Guide to Transfusion, Chapter 7. Fractionated blood products and associated pathogen safety; 2019. Accessed August 20, 2023. https://professionaleducation.blood.ca/en/transfusion/clinical-guide/fractionated-bloodproducts-and-associated-pathogen-safety

23 Horstman EE, Tormey CA. Plasma products for transfusion: an overview. Ann Blood. 2022;7:1–13.

24 Klamroth R, Groner A, Simon TL. Pathogen inactivation and removal methods for plasma-derived clotting factor concentrates. Transfusion. 2014; 54(5):1406–17.

III

25 Callum J, Farkouh ME, Scales DC, Heddle NM, Crowther M, Rao V, et al. Effect of fibrinogen concentrate vs cryoprecipitate on blood component transfusion after cardiac surgery. The FIBRES Randomized Clinical Trial. JAMA. 2019; 322:1966–76.

26 Rajpurkar M, Croteau SE, Boggio L, Cooper DL. Thrombotic events with recombinant activated factor VII (rFVII1) in approved indications are rare and associated with older age, cardiovascular disease, and concomitant use of activated complex concentrates (aPCC). J Blood Med. 2019;10:335–40.

27 Franchini M, Mannucci PM. Von Willbrand factor (Vonvendi®): the first recombinant product licensed for the treatment of von Willebrand disease. Expert Rev Hematol. 2016;9:825–30.

28 National Advisory Committee of Blood and Blood Products. Recommendations for the use of prothrombin complex concentrates in Canada. 2014. Accessed August 20, 2023. http://www.nacblood.ca/resources/guidelines/PCC-Recommendations-Final-2014-05-16.pdf

29 Liumbruno G, Bennardello F, Lattanzio A, Piccoli P, Rossetti G. Recommendations for the use of antithrombin concentrates and prothrombin complex concentrates. Blood Transfus. 2009; 7:325–34.

30 Rachid R, Bonilla FA: The role of anti-IgA antibodies in causing adverse reactions to gamma globulin infusion in immunodeficient patients: a comprehensive review of the literature. J Allergy Clin Immunol. 2012;129(3):628–34.

31 Pendergrast J, Armali C, Callum J, Cserti-Gazdewich C, Jiwajee A, Lieberman L, et al. A prospective observational study of the incidence, natural history, and risk factors for intravenous immunoglobulin-mediated hemolysis. Transfusion. 2021;61:1053–63.

32 Daw Z, Padmore R, Neurath D, Cober N, Tokessy M, Desjardins D, et al. Hemolytic transfusion reactions after administration of intravenous immune (gamma) globulin: a case series analysis. Transfusion. 2008;48:1598–601.

33 Kahwaji J, Barker E, Pepkowitz S, Klapper E, Villiacana R, Peng A, et al. Acute hemolysis after high-dose intravenous immunoglobulin therapy in highly HLA-sensitized patients. Clin J Am Soc Nephrol. 2009;4:1993–7.

34 Neunert C, Terrell DR, Arnold DM, Buchanan G, Cines DB, Cooper N, et al. American Society of Hematology 2019 guidelines for immune thrombocytopenia. Blood Adv. 2019;3:3829–66.

35 Huang L, Liu GJ, Kaye AD, Liu H. Advances in topical hemostatic agent therapies: a comprehensive update. Adv Ther. 2020;37:4132–48.

36 Gabay M, Boucher BA. An esssential primer for understanding the role of topical hemostats, surgical sealants, and adhesisves for maintaining hemostasis. Pharmacotherapy. 2013;33:935–55.

37 Relke N, Chornenki N, Sholzberg M. Tranexamic acid evidence and controversies: an illustrated review. Res Pract Thromb Haemost. 2021 Jul 14;5(5): e12546.

38 Young G. Management of children with hemophilia A: how emicizumab has changed the landscape. J Thromb Haemost. 2021;19:1629–37.

Published online: December 5, 2024

Blanchette VS, Brandão LR, Carcao MD, Kumar R, Rand ML, Revel-Vilk S (eds): SickKids Handbook of Pediatric Thrombosis and Hemostasis, ed 3, rev. and ext. Basel, Karger, 2024, pp 463–469 (DOI: 10.1159/000538204)

Connective Tissue Disorders Associated with Bleeding (Ehlers-Danlos Syndrome and Hereditary Hemorrhagic Telangiectasia)

Laura Banov[a] Kevon Dindial[b] Constance O'Connor[c]
Roberto Mendoza-Londono[d] Manuel D. Carcao[e]

[a]Hemostasis and Thrombosis Unit, Department of Pediatric Hematology/Oncology, Gaslini Children's Institute, Genova, Italy; [b]Eric Williams Medical Sciences Complex, San Juan, Trinidad and Tobago; [c]Ehlers-Danlos Syndrome and Connective Tissue Disorders Program, Department of Paediatrics, The Hospital for Sick Children, Toronto, ON, Canada; [d]Clinical and Metabolic Genetics, Department of Paediatrics, The Hospital for Sick Children, Toronto, ON, Canada; [e]Division of Haematology/Oncology, Department of Paediatrics, The Hospital for Sick Children, Toronto, ON, Canada

Although most bleeding disorders are disorders of platelets, coagulation factors (e.g., von Willebrand disease and hemophilia), or fibrinolysis, sometimes patients bleed when there is nothing wrong with any of these things. Instead, they bleed because of defects in the connective tissue surrounding and supporting blood vessels (connective tissue disorders) or in the blood vessels themselves, as in hereditary hemorrhagic telangiectasia (HHT). While connective tissue disorders include several very rare conditions such as Marfan syndrome, Loeys-Dietz syndrome, and homocystinuria, the most classic and common type of connective tissue disorders are hypermobility syndromes such as Ehlers-Danlos syndrome (EDS).

Ehlers-Danlos Syndrome

EDS are a group of rare inherited conditions that affect collagen and, as such, connective tissues (skin, bones, blood vessels, and other organs). According to clinical, pathological, and genetic features, the 2017 International Classification for EDS recognizes 13 subtypes of EDS (see Table 1) [1]. There does not appear to be any significant ethnic or racial predisposition to EDS.

For most of the EDS subtypes, the associated genes are known except for the most common form of EDS (hypermobile EDS [hEDS], which accounts for 80–85% of all EDS diagnoses) (Table 1). Most EDS is inherited in an autosomal dominant (AD) fashion, with some cases being inherited in an autosomal recessive (AR) fashion and many cases being sporadic.

Table 1. Subtypes of EDS and associated genes, inheritance pattern, and main clinical features (subtypes sorted according to prevalence)

Subtype (estimated prevalence)	Associated gene (inheritance pattern)	Most common hallmark features[a]
Hypermobile EDS (hEDS) (1/5,000–20,000)	Unknown (AD)	1. Generalized joint hypermobility with subluxations/dislocations, frank joint instability, and/or persistent joint pain 2. Skin hyperextensibility 3. Tissue fragility Note: Typically, not able to diagnose before puberty
Classical EDS (cEDS) (1/20,000–40,000)	*COL5A1*, *COL5A2*, *COL1A1* (all AD)	1. Skin hyperextensibility and atrophic scarring 2. Generalized joint hypermobility
Kyphoscoliotic EDS (kEDS) (1/100,000)	*PLOD1*, *FKBP14* (both AR)	1. Congenital early onset kyphoscoliosis 2. Congenital muscle hypotonia 3. Generalized joint hypermobility with subluxations/dislocations
Vascular EDS (vEDS) (1/200,000–250,000)	*COL3A1*, *COL1A1* (both AD)	1. Family history of arterial rupture/dissection in individuals <40 years 2. Thin, translucent skin 3. History of arterial rupture 4. History of spontaneous pneumothorax 5. Joint hypermobility (generalized or small joints) 6. Distinctive facial features
Classical-like EDS (clEDS) (very rare)	*TNXB* (AR)	1. Generalized joint hypermobility 2. Skin hyperextensibility Note: The absence of atrophic scars
Musculocontractual EDS (mcEDS) (very rare)	*CHST14*, *DSE* (both AR)	1. Generalized joint hypermobility 2. Contractures of small joints, including adducted thumbs 3. Clubfoot 4. Skin hyperextensibility and fragility 5. Severe bruising +/– large subcutaneous hematomas 6. Distinctive facial features
Arthrochalasia EDS (aEDS) (very rare)	COL1A1, COL1A2 (both AD)	1. Congenital bilateral hip dislocation 2. Generalized joint hypermobility with dislocations 3. Distinctive facial features
Spondylodysplastic EDS (spEDS) (very rare)	*B4GALT7*, *B3GALT6*, *SLC39A13* (all AR)	1. Short stature 2. Muscle hypotonia 3. Joint hypermobility (generalized or small joints) Note: features variable depending on affected gene, including: 4. Osteoporosis or osteopenia with fractures 5. Contractures of small joints 6. Kyphoscoliosis 7. Intellectual disability 8. Distinctive facial features
Periodontal EDS (pEDS) (very rare)	*C1R* (AD)	1. Early onset, extensive periodontal destruction 2. Pretibial plaques 3. Tissue fragility 4. Joint hypermobility (generalized or small joints)
Dermatosparaxis EDS (dEDS) (very rare)	*ADAMTS2* (AR)	1. Extreme skin fragility with redundant and lax skin 2. Severe bruising susceptibility 3. Absent/mild joint hypermobility at birth; more pronounced over time
Myopathic EDS (mEDS) (very rare)	*COL12A1* (AD or AR)	1. Muscle hypotonia present in infancy or childhood 2. Proximal large joint contractures 3. Distal joint hypermobility
Cardiac-valvular EDS (cvEDS) (very rare)	*COL1A2* (AR)	1. Severe cardiac-valvular disease 2. Skin hyperextensibility ± atrophic scars 3. Joint hypermobility (generalized or small joints)
Brittle cornea syndrome (BCS) (very rare)	*ZNF469*, *PRDM5* (both AR)	1. Thin, fragile cornea 2. Joint hypermobility (generalized or small joints) 3. Distinctive facial features

Adapted from Brady et al. [2] and Malfait et al. [1]. AD, autosomal dominant; AR, autosomal recessive; EDS, Ehlers-Danlos syndrome. [a]Easy bruising is a feature in most subtypes – where bleeding is more prominent, it is specifically mentioned.

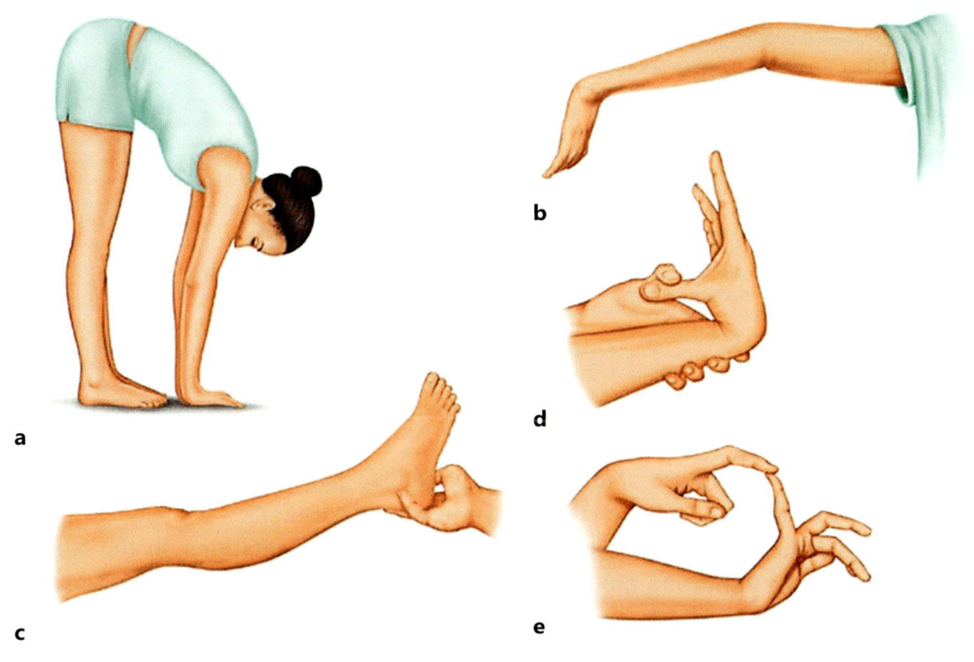

Fig. 1. The Beighton score [3] consists of the following five maneuvers, which patients are asked to perform. **a** Ability to hold the hand flat on the floor with the knees held in full extension. **b** Hyperextension of the elbow beyond 10° with the forearm supinated. **c** Hyperextension of the knee beyond 10°. **d** Apposition of the thumb to the volar aspect of the forearm (passive movement – as above). **e** Hyperextension of the fifth finger >90° (passive movement, i.e., examiner performs the movement). Reused with permission from Springer Nature (Rudin [4]).

Patients with EDS may experience excessive mucocutaneous bleeding, such as bruising and heavy menstrual bleeding. Additionally, some patients with certain subtypes of EDS may experience intracranial hemorrhage, gastrointestinal bleeding, and perioperative hemorrhage. One of the most feared subtypes of EDS is the vascular subtype (vascular EDS [vEDS]), which predisposes to arterial dissection and rupture (can affect any large- or medium-sized arteries) and, consequently, sudden death. The bleeding phenotype of patients with EDS varies from mild bruising in those with classical EDS (cEDS) and hEDS subtypes to severe and sometimes fatal bleeding in those with vEDS [5].

Patients with EDS have no abnormalities in primary or secondary hemostasis. Nevertheless, a comprehensive study of hemostasis is advisable, as abnormalities of hemostasis may further contribute to the risk of bleeding in patients with EDS [6].

The diagnosis of EDS is mainly clinical and is based on the presence of generally accepted diagnostic criteria [7]. Assessment of EDS relies primarily on a detailed clinical history and a careful physical examination [8] with evaluation of joint mobility using a widely used and verified score, the Beighton score (described by Beighton et al. in 1973 [9]) (Fig. 1).

Table 2. Beighton scoring system

Finding on clinical examination	Negative	Unilateral	Bilateral
Passive dorsiflexion of the 5th finger >90°	0	1	2
Passive flexion of the thumb to the forearm	0	1	2
Hyperextension of the elbows beyond 10°	0	1	2
Hyperextension of the knees beyond 10°	0	1	2
Forward flexion of the trunk with knees fully extended and palms resting on floor	NEG = 0	POS = 1	

Taken from Beighton score – Physiopedia (physio-pedia.com). NEG, negative; POS, positive. Maximum score = 9. A person is defined as having joint hypermobility if a score of ≥5/9 is achieved (in adolescents/adults) or ≥6/9 (in prepubertal children).

The Beighton score (Table 2) is a useful tool to investigate and detect joint hypermobility (JH) in children referred to rule out a bleeding disorder. JH defines the capability of a joint (or a group of joints) to move, passively and/or actively, beyond normal limits along physiological axes. Although validated for use in children 6 years and older, the Beighton score loses specificity in younger children who usually have quite mobile joints and may have difficulty performing certain tasks.

Some of the JH that might be present in the initial phase of the disease (hypermobility phase) may be lost later in life (adolescents and adults) because of chronic damage to joints associated with recurrent dislocations/subluxations and the development of chronic articular pain and progressive stiffness [10].

Therefore, applying this score may only be helpful in some situations. Specific populations, such as females and prepubertal individuals, are more flexible than others. Moreover, many joints and groups of joints are not considered in the clinical examination. Finally, JH decreases with age both in normal individuals as well as in subjects with hypermobility syndromes such as EDS. A further limitation is the Beighton score's lack of specificity, as approximately 10% of the general population will score as having a positive Beighton score. However, most of these cases will not be proven to have an underlying hypermobility syndrome such as EDS.

Despite these limitations, in the context of a bleeding disorders clinic, the Beighton score is a valuable screening tool to identify subjects with mucocutaneous symptoms in whom a careful family history looking for individuals with similar symptoms should be obtained, with consideration given to referral of individuals with a positive Beighton score to a genetics service for further investigation and counseling of the subject and parents/guardians as appropriate.

The management of EDS is multidisciplinary and based on specific symptoms and is beyond the scope of this appendix.

Hereditary Hemorrhagic Telangiectasia

The most well-known disorder of blood vessel development is HHT, also known as Osler-Weber-Rendu disease. HHT is characterized by the presence of multiple arteriovenous malformations (AVMs) that lack intervening capillaries and result in direct connections between arteries and veins. These manifest on skin and mucosal surfaces as telangiectasias, which can lead to epistaxis and gastrointestinal bleeding, leading to iron deficiency anemia. In addition, AVMs frequently

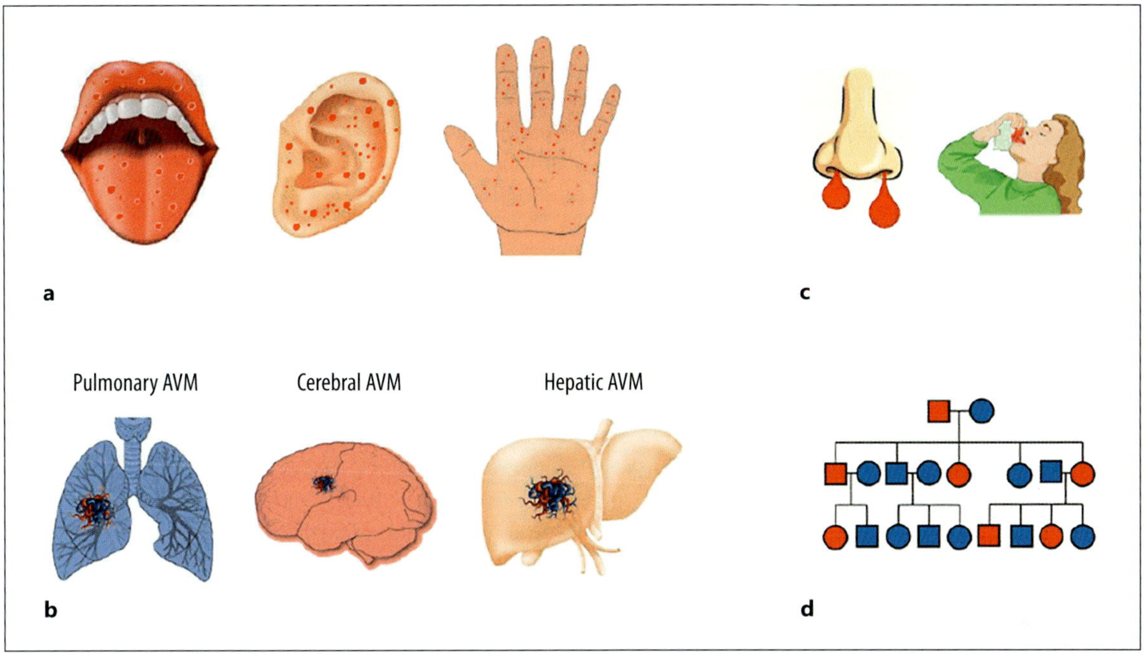

Fig. 2. Curaçao clinical criteria in HHT. **a** Multiple telangiectasias at characteristic sites, such as oral cavity, ears, and fingers. **b** Visceral lesions (AVMs) in the lungs, brain, liver or spinal cord, and gastrointestinal bleeding. **c** Epistaxis (spontaneous, recurrent nosebleeds). **d** An example of a family history of HHT; a genetic family tree with affected members in red and nonaffected members in blue is shown. Taken from Botella et al. [12].

affect the pulmonary, hepatic, and/or cerebral circulations, which may lead to sudden and catastrophic bleeding complications. Pulmonary AVMs can lead to cyanotic heart disease with subsequent secondary polycythemia and, ultimately, heart failure [11]. See Figure 2 for consensus clinical criteria, known as "Curaçao criteria" for HHT [12].

HHT is inherited as an AD trait with varying penetrance and expression (Table 3). Pathogenic variants in multiple genes can cause HHT. Two genes, *ACVRL* and *endoglin* (*ENG*), are responsible for most cases of HHT.

The diagnosis of HHT is established in a proband who has three or more of the following suggestive clinical features. Persons who only have two of these features are considered as having "possible or suspected" HHT:

- *Spontaneous and recurrent epistaxis.* Nighttime nosebleeds heighten the concern for HHT.
- *Multiple telangiectasias at characteristic sites.* Small blanchable red spots that are focal dilatations of postcapillary venules or delicate lacy red vessels composed of markedly dilated and convoluted venules; multiple, at characteristic sites, including lips, oral cavity, fingers, and nose. Transillumination of the digits is helpful for detecting vascular lesions not evident on the skin [13].
- *Visceral AVMs.* Typically, these are pulmonary, cerebral, hepatic, spinal, gastrointestinal, or pancreatic. AVMs outside these locations are uncommon and not suggestive of HHT.
- A *first-degree relative* in whom HHT has been diagnosed.

Table 3. Pathogenic genes associated with HHT (all are autosomal dominant)

HHT subtype	Gene	Protein	Proportion of HHT[a]
HHT1	*ACVRL1*	Serine/threonine-protein kinase receptor R3	52%
HHT2	*ENG*	Endoglin	44%
JPHT	*SMAD4*	Mothers against decapentaplegic homolog	1%
Other	Unknown[b]		~3%

HHT, hereditary hemorrhagic telangiectasia syndrome; JPHT, juvenile polyposis/hereditary hemorrhagic telangiectasia syndrome. [a]Note overall prevalence of HHT is 1/5,000–1/10,000. [b]Unknown includes variants in *GDF2*, *RASA1*, and *EPHB4*.

Patients with suspected HHT should be referred to a clinic specializing in HHT (usually, a genetics clinic) for further investigation and counseling of the subject and parents/guardians as appropriate. The management of HHT is multidisciplinary according to the presenting symptoms. From the standpoint of the hematologist, epistaxis (seen in 95% of patients with HHT) can be dealt with by humidification of the air, topical moisturizing therapies applied to the nasal mucosa, antifibrinolytic agents, such as tranexamic acid, as well as ENT procedures such as nasal cauterization. Anemia, found in 50% of patients with HHT, may require iron replacement and, in severe cases, red blood cell transfusions. The role of antiangiogenic agents, such as bevacizumab, for the above symptoms and others (pulmonary, hepatic, and intracranial AVMs) is being explored [14].

Conflict of Interest Statement

Laura Banov reports no conflict of interest. Kevon Dindial reports no conflict of interest. Constance O'Connor reports no conflict of interest. Roberto Mendoza-Londono reports having received research support from The Ehlers-Danlos Society and the SickKids Foundation and honoraria for speaking/participating in advisory boards from the Ehlers-Danlos Society. Manuel Carcao reports having received research support from Bayer, Bioverativ/Sanofi, Novartis, Novo Nordisk, Pfizer, Roche, and Shire/Takeda and honoraria for speaking/participating in advisory boards from Bayer, Bioverativ/Sanofi, CSL Behring, LFB, Novo Nordisk, Pfizer, Roche, and Shire/Takeda.

Funding Sources

No funding was received for this appendix.

Author Contributions

Laura Banov and Kevon Dindial wrote the first draft of the appendix, and then all the other authors (Constance O'Connor, Roberto Mendoza-Londono, and Manuel Carcao) revised the appendix and approved the final draft.

Abbreviations

AD	Autosomal dominant
AR	Autosomal recessive
AVM	Arteriovenous malformation
cEDS	Classical Ehlers-Danlos syndrome
EDS	Ehlers-Danlos syndrome
hEDS	Hypermobile Ehlers-Danlos syndrome
HHT	Hereditary hemorrhagic telangiectasia
JH	Joint hypermobility
vEDS	Vascular Ehlers-Danlos syndrome

References

1 Malfait F, Francomano C, Byers P, Belmont J, Berglund B, Black J, et al. The 2017 international classification of the Ehlers-Danlos syndromes. Am J Med Genet C Semin Med Genet. 2017;175(1): 8–26.

2 Brady AF, Demirdas S, Fournel-Gigleux S, Ghali N, Giunta C, Kapferer-Seebacher I, et al. The Ehlers-Danlos syndromes, rare types. Am J Med Genet C Semin Med Genet. 2017;175(1):70–115.

3 Clinch J, Deere K, Sayers A, Palmer S, Riddoch C, Tobias JH, et al. Epidemiology of generalized joint laxity (hypermobility) in fourteen-year-old children from the UK: a population-based evaluation. Arthritis Rheum. 2011;63(9): 2819–27.

4 Rudin NJ. The hypermobile patient. In: Abd-Elsayed A, editor. Guide to the Inpatient Pain Consult. Springer, Cham. 2020. p. 407–413. https://doi.org/10.1007/978-3-030-40449-9_27.

5 D'Hondt S, Van Damme T, Malfait F. Vascular phenotypes in nonvascular subtypes of the Ehlers-Danlos syndrome: a systematic review. Genet Med. 2018;20(6):562–73.

6 Artoni A, Bassotti A, Abbattista M, Marinelli B, Lecchi A, Gianniello F, et al. Hemostatic abnormalities in patients with Ehlers-Danlos syndrome. J Thromb Haemost. 2018;16(12):2425–31.

7 Beighton P, De Paepe A, Steinmann B, Tsipouras P, Wenstrup RJ. Ehlers-Danlos syndromes: revised nosology, Villefranche, 1997. Ehlers-Danlos National Foundation (USA) and Ehlers-Danlos Support Group (UK). Am J Med Genet. 1998;77(1):31–7.

8 Castori M. Ehlers-Danlos syndrome, hypermobility type: an underdiagnosed hereditary connective tissue disorder with mucocutaneous, articular, and systemic manifestations. ISRN Dermatol. 2012;2012:751768.

9 Beighton P, Solomon L, Soskolne CL. Articular mobility in an African population. Ann Rheum Dis. 1973;32(5):413–8.

10 Castori M, Camerota F, Celletti C, Danese C, Santilli V, Saraceni VM, et al. Natural history and manifestations of the hypermobility type Ehlers-Danlos syndrome: a pilot study on 21 patients. Am J Med Genet A. 2010;152A(3):556–64.

11 McDonald J, Stevenson DA. Hereditary hemorrhagic telangiectasia. 2000 Jun 26 [updated 2021 Nov 24]. In: Adam MP, Mirzaa GM, Pagon RA, Wallace SE, Bean LJH, Gripp KW, et al, eds. GeneReviews® [Internet]. University of Washington, Seattle; 1993–2023.

12 Botella LM, Albiñana V, Ojeda-Fernandez L, Recio-Poveda L, Bernabéu C. Research on potential biomarkers in hereditary hemorrhagic telangiectasia. Front Genet. 2015;6:115.

13 Mohler ER III, Doraiswamy V, Sibley A, Bernhardt BA, Pyeritz RE. Transillumination of the fingers for vascular anomalies: a novel method for evaluating hereditary hemorrhagic telangiectasia. Genet Med. 2009;11(5):356–8.

14 Ardelean DS, Letarte M. Anti-angiogenic therapeutic strategies in hereditary hemorrhagic telangiectasia. Front Genet. 2015;6:35.

Published online: December 5, 2024

Blanchette VS, Brandão LR, Carcao MD, Kumar R, Rand ML, Revel-Vilk S (eds): SickKids Handbook of Pediatric Thrombosis and Hemostasis, ed 3, rev. and ext. Basel, Karger, 2024, pp 470–479 (DOI: 10.1159/000538186)

Abbreviations

International Standards

PO	Per oral
SC	Subcutaneous
IM	Intramuscular
IV	Intravenous
U	Unit
IU	International unit
L	Liter
dL	Deciliter
mL	Milliliter
fL	Femtoliter
Da	Dalton
kg	Kilogram
g	Gram
mg	Milligram
µg	Microgram
µmol	Micromole
QID	Four times a day
TID	Three times a day
BID	Twice a day
OD	Once a day
h	Hour
min	Minute
s	Second

A

α2-AP	α2-Antiplasmin
AAV	Adeno-associated virus
ABI	Ankle-brachial index
ABR	Annualized bleeding rate

ACA	Anterior cerebral artery
ACLA	Anticardiolipin antibody
ACT	Activated clotting time
ACTION	Advanced Cardiac Therapies Improving Outcomes Network
ACTN1-RT	α-Actinin1-related thrombocytopenia
AD	Autosomal dominant
ADAMTS13	A disintegrin and metalloproteinase with a thrombospondin type 1 motif, member 13
ADC	Apparent diffusion coefficient
ADP	Adenosine 5′-diphosphate
aHUS	Atypical hemolytic uremic syndrome
AIS	Arterial ischemic stroke
ALL	Acute lymphoblastic leukemia
ALPS	Autoimmune lymphoproliferative disorder
aMBQ	Adolescent menstrual bleeding questionnaire
AML	Acute myelogenous leukemia
ANKRD26-RT	Ankyrin repeat domain 26-related thrombocytopenia
Anti-Xa	Anti-factor Xa
APC	Activated protein C
aPCC	Activated prothrombin complex concentrate
APLA	Antiphospholipid antibodies
APML	Acute promyelocytic leukemia
APS	Antiphospholipid syndrome
aPTR	Activated partial thromboplastin ratio
aPTT	Activated partial thromboplastin time
AR	Autosomal recessive
ARC	Arthrogryposis-renal dysfunction-cholestasis
ASA	Acetylsalicylic acid
ASH	American Society of Hematology
AT	Antithrombin
ATE	Arterial thromboembolism/thromboembolic event
ATP	Adenosine 5′-triphosphate
AUB	Abnormal uterine bleeding
AVM	Arteriovenous malformation
AVWS	Acquired von Willebrand syndrome

B

β_2-GPI	β_2-glycoprotein I
BAT	Bleeding assessment tool
BCS	Budd-Chiari syndrome
BHS	Bowhunter's syndrome
BiVAD	Biventricular assist device
BSS	Bernard-Soulier syndrome
BT	Blalock-Taussig
BU	Bethesda unit
BUN	Blood urea nitrogen
BV	Bioprosthetic valve
BW	Body weight

C

CA	Coronary artery
CalDAG-GEFI	Calcium and diacylglycerol-regulated guanine exchange factor I
cAMP	Cyclic adenosine monophosphate
CAMT	Congenital amegakaryocytic thrombocytopenia
CAT	Cutaneovisceral angiomatosis with thrombocytopenia
CBC	Complete blood count
CC	Cardiac catheterization
CD	Cluster of differentiation
cEDS	Classical Ehlers-Danlos syndrome
CFB	Complement factor B
CFC	Clotting factor concentrate
CFH	Complement factor H
CFI	Complement factor I
CH	Congenital hemangioma
CHD	Congenital heart disease
CHS	Chediak-Higashi syndrome
CLOVES	Congenital lipomatous overgrowth, vascular malformations, epidermal nevi, and spinal/skeletal abnormalities syndrome
CLVM	Capillary-lymphatic-venous malformation
CM	Capillary malformation
CMV	Cytomegalovirus
CNS	Central nervous system
COCs	Combined oral contraceptives
COX	Cyclooxygenase
CPB	Cardiopulmonary bypass
CSP	Cryosupernatant plasma
CSVT	Cerebral sinovenous thrombosis
CT	Computed tomography
CTA	Computed tomography angiography
CTEPH	Chronic thromboembolic pulmonary hypertension
CTPA	Computed tomography pulmonary angiography
CTV	Computed tomography venography
CVAD	Central venous access device
CVC	Central venous catheter
CVS	Chorionic villus sampling
CYP2C9	Cytochrome P450 2C9
CYP3A4	Cytochrome P450 3A4

D

DDAVP	1-Deamino-8-D-arginine vasopressin (desmopressin)
DIC	Disseminated intravascular coagulation
DMPA	Depot medroxyprogesterone acetate
DOAC	Direct oral anticoagulant
DTI	Direct thrombin inhibitor
dTT	Dilute thrombin time
DUS	Doppler ultrasound
DVT	Deep vein thrombosis
DWI	Diffusion weighted images

E

EACA	Epsilon-aminocaproic acid (Amicar)
EBMT	European Group for Blood & Marrow Transplantation
ECLS	Extracorporeal life support
ECLSO	Extracorporeal Life Support Organization
ECMO	Extracorporeal membrane oxygenation
ED	Exposure day
EDAS	Encephaloduroarteriosynangiosis
EDS	Ehlers-Danlos syndrome
EDTA	Ethylenediaminetetraacetic acid
EEG	Electroencephalography
EHL	Extended half-life
EIC	Extremity indwelling arterial catheter
ELISA	Enzyme-linked immunosorbent assay
EN-RBD	European Network of Rare Bleeding Disorders
ETV6-RT	ETV6-related thrombocytopenia

F

FCA	Focal cerebral arteriopathy
FDA	Food and Drug Administration
FDP	Fibrin degradation product
FEIBA	FVIII inhibitor bypass activity
FFP	Fresh frozen plasma
FII	Factor II (prothrombin)
FIX	Factor IX
FIXa	Activated factor IX
FLI1	Friend leukemia virus integration 1
FNAIT	Fetal and neonatal alloimmune thrombocytopenia
FP	Frozen plasma
FPD-AML	Familial platelet disorder with propensity to acute myelogenous leukemia
FV	Factor V
FVII	Factor VII
FVIII	Factor VIII
FVIII:C	Factor VIII coagulant
FVIIIa	Activated factor VIII
FVL	Factor V Leiden
FX	Factor X
FXI	Factor XI
FXII	Factor XII
FXIII	Factor XIII

G

GA	Gestational age
GGCX	γ-Glutamyl carboxylase
GI	Gastrointestinal
GnRHa	Gonadotropin-releasing hormone analogs
GP	Glycoprotein
GPS	Gray platelet syndrome
GT	Glanzmann thrombasthenia
GVHD	Graft versus host disease

H

HAT	Hepatic artery thrombosis
HA-VTE	Hospital-acquired venous thromboembolism
hEDS	Hypermobile Ehlers-Danlos syndrome
HEEADSSS	Home, education, eating, activities/employment, drugs, suicidality, sex, safety
HHT	Hereditary hemorrhagic telangiectasia
HIT	Heparin-induced thrombocytopenia
HIV	Human immunodeficiency virus
HLA	Human leukocyte antigen
HMB	Heavy menstrual bleeding
HMW	High-molecular-weight
HMWK	High-molecular-weight kininogen
HPA	Human platelet antigen
HPLC	High-performance liquid chromatography
HPS	Hermansky-Pudlak syndrome
HRQoL	Health-related quality of life
HSCT	Hematopoietic stem cell transplantation
HTC	Hemophilia treatment center
HTS	High-throughput sequencing
HUS	Hemolytic uremic syndrome

I

ICH	Intracranial hemorrhage
IE	Infective endocarditis
IgG	Immunoglobulin G
IgM	Immunoglobulin M
IH	Infantile hemangioma
IL-6	Interleukin-6
INR	International normalized ratio
IPD	Inherited platelet disorder
IPF	Immature platelet fraction
ISI	International Sensitivity Index
ISTH	International Society on Thrombosis and Haemostasis
IT	Inherited thrombocytopenia
ITGA2B/ITGB3-RT	ITGA2B/ITGB3-related thrombocytopenia
ITI	Immune tolerance induction
ITP	Immune thrombocytopenia
IVC	Inferior vena cava
IVIG	Intravenous immunoglobulin

J

JH	Joint hypermobility

K

KHE	Kaposiform hemangioendothelioma
KLA	Kaposiform lymphangiomatosis
KMP	Kasabach-Merritt phenomenon
KTS	Klippel-Trenaunay syndrome

L

LAC	Lupus anticoagulant
LADIII	Leukocyte adhesion deficiency syndrome type 3
LAHS	Lupus anticoagulant hypoprothrombinemia syndrome
LDH	Lactate dehydrogenase
LDL	Low-density lipid
LIC	Localized intravascular coagulopathy
LM	Lymphatic malformation
LMAN1	Lectin mannose-binding protein 1
LMWH	Low-molecular-weight heparin
LNG-IUS	Levonorgestrel-releasing intrauterine system
Lp(a)	Lipoprotein(a)
LTA	Light-transmission aggregometry
LUMBAR	Lower-body hemangioma, urogenital abnormalities/ulceration, myelopathy, bony deformities, anorectal malformations/arterial anomalies, and rectal anomalies
LVAD	Left ventricular assist device

M

MAHA	Microangiopathic hemolytic anemia
MAIPA	Monoclonal antibody-specific immobilization of platelet antigens
MBQ	Menstrual bleeding questionnaire
MCA	Middle cerebral artery
MCAP	Megalencephaly-capillary malformationpolymicrogyria
MCFD2	Multiple coagulation factor deficiency protein 2
MCS	Mechanical circulatory support
MCV	Mean corpuscular volume
MDS	Myelodysplastic syndrome
MECOM	MDS1 and EVI1 complex locus
MGUS	Monoclonal gammopathy of uncertain significance
MI	Myocardial infarction
MIS-C	Multisystem inflammatory disease in children
MIS-N	Multisystem inflammatory disease in neonates
MLT	Multifocal lymphangiomatosis with thrombocytopenia
MMCA	Malignant middle cerebral artery
MMF	Mycophenolate mofetil
MMR	Measles, mumps, rubella
MPN	Myeloproliferative neoplasm
MPV	Mean platelet volume
MRA	Magnetic resonance angiography
MRI	Magnetic resonance imaging
mRNA	Messenger RNA
MRPA	Magnetic resonance pulmonary angiography
MRV	Magnetic resonance venography
MTHFR	Methylenetetrahydrofolate reductase
MV	Mechanical valve
MVT	Mesenteric vascular thrombosis
MYH9	Myosin heavy chain 9
MYH9-RD	Myosin heavy chain 9-related disease

N

NEC	Necrotizing enterocolitis
NGS	Next-generation sequencing
NHF	National Hemophilia Foundation
NICH	Noninvoluting congenital hemangioma
NICU	Neonatal intensive care unit
NIPT	Noninvasive prenatal testing
NO	Nitric oxide
NSAIDs	Nonsteroidal anti-inflammatory drugs

O

OR	Odds ratio

P

PAI-1	Plasminogen activator inhibitor type 1
PAS	Platelet additive solution
PBAC	Pictorial Blood Loss Assessment Chart
PBQ	Pediatric Bleeding Questionnaire
PCC	Prothrombin complex concentrate
PCOS	Polycystic ovarian syndrome
PCR	Polymerase chain reaction
PDA	Patent ductus arteriosus
PE	Pulmonary embolism
Pedimacs	Pediatric Interagency Registry for Mechanical Circulatory Support
PedNIHSS	Pediatric National Institutes of Health Stroke Scale
PedsQL	Pediatric quality of life inventory
PEG	Polyethylene glycol
PF4	Platelet factor 4
PFA	Platelet function analyzer
PFA-100®/200®	Platelet function analyzer-100®/200®
PFD	Platelet function disorder
pfHb	Plasma-free hemoglobin
PGD	Preimplantation genetic diagnosis
P-gp	P-glycoprotein
PHACES	Posterior fossa anomalies, hemangioma, arterial anomalies, cardiac anomalies, and eye anomalies
PI3K	Phosphatidylinositol 3-kinase
PICC	Peripherally inserted central catheter
PICH	Partially involuting congenital hemangioma
PIOPED	Prospective investigation of pulmonary embolism – diagnosis
PISAPED	Prospective investigation study of acute pulmonary embolism – diagnosis
PIVKA	Protein induced by vitamin K absence
PJP	*Pneumocystis jirovecii*
PK	Pharmacokinetics
POCUS	Point of care ultrasound
PPP	Plasma protein product
PROS	PIK3CA-related overgrowth spectrum
PRP	Platelet-rich plasma
PRT	Pathogen reduction technologies

PT	Prothrombin time
PT/INR	Prothrombin time/international normalized ratio
PT-Fg	Prothrombin time-derived fibrinogen
PTS	Post-thrombotic syndrome
PTT	Partial thromboplastin time
PT-VWD	Platelet-type von Willebrand disease
PVT	Portal vein thrombosis

Q

QPD	Quebec platelet disorder

R

RAB27B	Ras associated binding protein 27B
RAM	Risk assessment model
RAT	Renal artery thrombosis
RBC	Red blood cell
RCT	Randomized controlled trial
rFIX	Recombinant factor IX
rFVIIa	Recombinant activated factor VII
rFVIII	Recombinant factor VIII
rFXIII	Recombinant factor XIII
RhD	Rhesus D
RhIG	Rhesus (Rh) immune globulin
RICH	Rapidly involuting congenital hemangioma
RIPA	Ristocetin-induced platelet agglutination
RNA	Ribonucleic acid
ROTEM	Rotational thromboelastometry
RPM	Revolutions per minute
r-tPA	Recombinant tissue plasminogen activator
RUSAT1	Amegakaryocytic thrombocytopenia with radio-ulnar synostosis
RVAD	Right ventricle assist device
RVO	Retinal vein occlusion
RVT	Renal vein thrombosis

S

SAH	Subarachnoid hemorrhage
SARS-CoV-2	Severe acute respiratory syndrome coronavirus-2
SCD	Sickle cell disease
SCPC	Superior cavopulmonary connection
SD	Solvent detergent
SGA	Small for gestational age
SHL	Standard half-life
siRNA	Small interfering RNA
SLE	Systemic lupus erythematosus
SOC	Standard of care
SOS	Sinusoidal obstruction syndrome
SpVT	Splenic vein thrombosis
SSC	Scientific and Standardization Committee
STEC	Shiga toxin *Escherichia coli*

SVAD	Single ventricle assist device
SVC	Superior vena cava

T

TA	Tufted angioma
TAFI	Thrombin-activatable fibrinolysis inhibitor
TAH	Total artificial heart
TAM	Transient abnormal myelopoiesis
TAR	Thrombocytopenia absent radius
TA-TMA	Transplant-associated thrombotic microangiopathic disorder
TBX1	T-box transcription factor 1
TCD	Transcranial Doppler
TDT	Transmissible disease testing
TE	Thromboembolism/thromboembolic event
TEG	Thromboelastography
TEM	Transmission electron microscopy
TF	Tissue factor
TFPI	Tissue factor pathway inhibitor
TIA	Transient ischemic attack
TMA	Thrombotic microangiopathic disorder
TORCH	Toxoplasmosis, rubella, cytomegalovirus, herpes simplex virus-2
TP	Thromboxane-prostanoid
tPA	Tissue plasminogen activator
TPO	Thrombopoietin
TPO-RA	Thrombopoietin receptor agonist
TPO-RT	TPO-related thrombocytopenia
TT	Thrombin time
TTP	Thrombotic thrombocytopenic purpura
TxA_2	Thromboxane A_2

U

UAC	Umbilical artery catheter
UFH	Unfractionated heparin
ULVWF	Ultra large von Willebrand factor
uPA	Urokinase plasminogen activator
UVC	Umbilical vein catheter

V

V/Q scan	Ventilation/perfusion scan
VA	Venoarterial
VAD	Ventricular assist device
vEDS	Vascular Ehlers-Danlos syndrome
VKA	Vitamin K antagonist
VKDB	Vitamin K deficiency bleeding
VKOR	Vitamin K epoxide reductase
VKORC1	Vitamin K epoxide reductase complex subunit 1
VM	Venous malformation
VSD	Ventricular septal defect
VTE	Venous thromboembolism/thromboembolic event

VUS	Variant(s) of unknown significance
VV	Venovenous
VWD	von Willebrand disease
VWF	von Willebrand factor
VWF:Act	VWF activity
VWF:Ag	VWF antigen
VWF:CB	VWF collagen binding assay
VWF:RCo	VWF activity (ristocetin cofactor assay)

W

WAS	Wiskott-Aldrich syndrome
WASp	Wiskott-Aldrich syndrome protein
WBA	Whole-blood aggregometry
WBC	White blood cell
WES	Whole exome sequencing
WFH	World Federation of Hemophilia
WGS	Whole genome sequencing
WHO	World Health Organization

X

XLT	X-linked thrombocytopenia

Subject Index